THE COMPLETE GUIDE TO

HEALTH & WELL-BEING

THE ONE-STOP REFERENCE TO YOUR HEALTH OPTIONS
FROM TRADITIONAL THERAPIES TO MODERN MEDICINE,
NATURAL TREATMENTS TO HOME REMEDIES

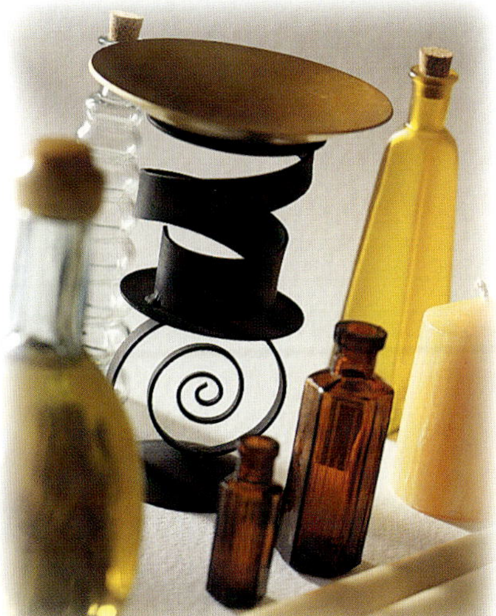

Compiled by TONI EATTS
Medical Consultant DR GISELLE COOKE

LANSDOWNE

CONTENTS

FOREWORD

I am honoured to have been asked to be the medical consultant for this book. I have a firm belief that we need to arm ourselves with as much information as possible about our minds, our bodies, and their diseases so that we can make well-considered decisions about how we would like to restore an ideal state of well-being. I believe this can only be achieved by a collaborative process between patient and carer, utilising the science of diagnosis alongside personal intuition about what our bodies need. This is how true healing takes place.

The world is currently facing a revolution in health care: self care. With greater availability of self-help information on illness and well-being and the aid of enlightened health care practitioners, individuals are reclaiming their right and ability to manage their own health.

The medical profession holds sacrosanct the teachings of Hippocrates and claims to uphold his philosophy yet much of Hippocrates' doctrine has a distinctly naturopathic direction. His overall belief was that to effect a cure we must assist nature. This is where I believe the path of modern medicine has diverged from that of natural healing and it is this essence of healing that modern, inquisitive patients are seeking. This is where I believe there is an essential role for a book such as this one to provide up-to-date, authoritative and balanced information on health conditions as a basis for early intervention for minor health complaints, or as an introduction to further research into the range of treatment options for more serious illness.

This guide has all the elements a first-time reader in natural health needs. There is an exhaustive survey of natural therapy techniques to explore and the list of health conditions is comprehensive and current. The inclusion of modern medicine in the recommended treatments in each ailment section provides more balanced information and makes this compendium different from most natural health manuals. I am particularly pleased with the level of emphasis given to the role of modern medicine for treating each condition: intervention advice is offered when appropriate without nervously deferring every minor problem to a doctor.

Often the place to start your health revival is with your mental well-being. The mind-body connection is, in my opinion, responsible for most chronic illnesses. This book addresses the subject up front. It also looks at protecting your immune system — an approach that holistic doctors now employ for cancer prevention and many natural therapists use when advising patients on how to manage recurrent infections and allergies. There's the importance of diet, exercise and posture, which forms the basis of my consultations for problems such as fatigue, chronic pain and digestive complaints. But my consultations are often built on relaxation and dealing with stress, and this book covers the subject from a number of angles. Stress is an inescapable factor which challenges our health today but if you master relaxation techniques a great deal of unnecessary illness may be avoided.

The power to heal ultimately resides within us, and this book provides the information to start that journey.

Dr Giselle Cooke, MB, BS, Dip Acup, DBM

INTRODUCTION

Medicine in the 20th century has made huge advances in testing for and treating illness and it continues to break new ground. Yet increasing numbers of health consumers are today returning to the ancient, well-ploughed fields of traditional therapies. Acupuncture, herbalism and massage, for example, trace their roots back across centuries and, at different times and in different cultures, have been the main approach to health maintenance.

These so-called "alternative" health practices tend to differ from modern medicine in one basic way: they take a holistic perspective. That is, they consider the whole body, not just the obvious symptoms of illness. And not just the physical body with all its interconnected systems and functions but also your mind, emotions and spirit, your lifestyle and the way you are affected by the world around you.

Holistic therapists work with the idea of homoeostasis, or a natural return to balance. In good health, your body is in balance. On the other hand, poor health or disease is really "dis-ease", a disturbance in this harmony. The aim of the holistic therapist is to encourage your body's inbuilt tendency to return to balance by creating the best conditions for this to happen.

These days more and more medical doctors are returning to this way of thinking and people are often seeking to combine the best of both worlds — technological and traditional. There is also a greater emphasis on prevention and taking responsibility for your own health. This is part of a growing realisation that one consultation, one course of tablets, one operation is not necessarily going to fix a health problem, and that one practitioner or one treatment approach may not have the complete answer to our health questions, particularly if the illness or reaction to standard treatment falls outside the "average" response.

Many conditions only respond to a well-executed plan of recovery. This may take a long time and require effort on our part: to change our diet, alter our habits, regularly practise the exercises that have been advised.

To return to health, the best route may be a multi-disciplinary approach, combining a number of different complementary therapies.

There is a variety of health options available and this can get confusing. Different ones suit different people. In making your choice, and in getting well, it is important that you get to know yourself so that you can establish what works for you.

This book is designed to inform you and help you with your choices. It includes an outline of some of the more commonly available therapies, then a look at how these may be applied to a range of health conditions. Sometimes it will suggest remedies or exercises you can try at home. However, taking an active role doesn't mean going it alone. Caring for your health is best done with the advice and care of qualified and experienced health professionals...of your choosing.

THE MIND BODY CONNECTION

If you are wondering about the impact thoughts have on your body, take a moment, and imagine you are biting into a big, juicy lemon. Did you feel your salivary glands instantly respond? Remember being angry and how that emotion flared through your body, making your heart beat faster — perhaps your face became red or you clenched your fists automatically, or held your shoulders rigid.

There is a theory that your body is like a map to your inner thoughts, your inner emotional make-up. For example, a person who has experienced considerable sadness will look permanently sad and someone who has cultivated a sense of inner calm will radiate that peacefulness.

This theory is based on the idea that each cell in your body responds to every thought you think, and these manifest in the lines on your face, your posture or certain behaviours, or in a particular illness.

Although emotions are important, if negative feelings are prevented from running their course or if they keep recurring, they can have a negative impact on your body. It is not unlikely, for example, if you are in a situation in which you are constantly arguing with your partner or at loggerheads with your boss, that you will become ill.

Traditional Chinese Medicine does not separate our emotions from our bodies. An important part of its health theory is the link between all emotions, the function of various organs and the manifestation of certain disease states.

In more recent years, other health practitioners have been paying an increasing amount of attention to this link and taking into account the personality and emotions of the individual in their treatment.

EMOTIONS, ENERGY AND THE BODY

Although somewhat hard to define and categorise in health terms, TRADITIONAL CHINESE MEDICINE recognises five emotions: anger, joy, contemplation, sorrow and fear.

Each is associated with particular organs. For example: anger with the liver/gall bladder, joy with the heart, and fear with the kidneys. Worry and anxiety are also recognised, but these do not relate to the organs in the way the other five emotions do.

These are all emotions we experience during the normal passage of our lives, but in excess they generate imbalance and disharmony in your body.

Many similar links are evident in Western culture, revealing themselves in a more subtle way through our language. Angry people were once described as "liverish". Passion is described as "heart-felt". It is common to speak of being so scared as to wet oneself — the link of fear to the kidney is evident.

HOW THERAPIES USE THE LINK

The notion of a link between your thoughts and your health is not a new one. It seems that healers in ancient cultures had people imagine certain images or scenes to kick-start the body's healing powers or try to unravel the complexity of a confused mind. Similarly, some Western doctors now encourage people with cancer to visualise such things as their healthy immune cells munching up their cancer cells (see AFFIRMATIONS AND VISUALISATIONS).

Meditation, too, is literally a thought-therapy that uses the disciplining of the mind to affect the overall functioning of the body. And achieving harmony between mind and body is the aim of both YOGA and Tai Chi (see page 186).

Therapies such as BACH FLOWER REMEDIES and HOMOEOPATHY are based on the observation that before a diseased state there is an imbalance in the emotions and thinking which predisposes a person to certain physical conditions.

Other therapies such as ACUPUNCTURE, SHIATSU and TRADITIONAL CHINESE MEDICINE go further; they link emotional imbalances to particular organs (see BOX above). For example, the liver is associated with anger. If you tend to be an angry person, this may have an impact on your liver or a disturbance in your liver may be what is making you feel angry.

In addition, many of the body-based therapists such as those who teach the ALEXANDER TECHNIQUE or the FELDENKRAIS METHOD believe that the way we think and feel can be seen in how we hold or carry our bodies. If you feel insecure or lack self-esteem, it is unlikely you will walk comfortably and with confidence. Therefore, it could be these feelings of inadequacy, not simply poor posture, that are the cause of the tension and pain in your neck and shoulders.

So whichever path you choose to travel in order to restore or maintain good health, it is likely to lead you to take stock of your emotions and deal with your negative mind-sets.

THE MIND BODY PROCESSES

Your body and its functions (including the important immune response, see page 31) are regulated through a complex series of chemical processes. This may be through hormones, for example, or through nerve pathways.

What we perceive as "a state of mind" can directly impact on these processes. Stress (which can be any kind of highly emotional state) can alter almost every chemical level in our body — stimulating the adrenal and thyroid hormones, for example — and, when chronic, can even change the structure and genetic make-up of cells such as lymphocytes (an important part of the immune system). It may also cause you to lose the nutrients needed for these chemical processes or for the rebuilding and maintainance of cells. See RELAXATION AND DEALING WITH STRESS.

Researchers are continually uncovering evidence of the mind-body link. In one study, the lymphocyte cells of recently bereaved people were found not to respond when the immune system was attacked.

HOW THE BRAIN WORKS

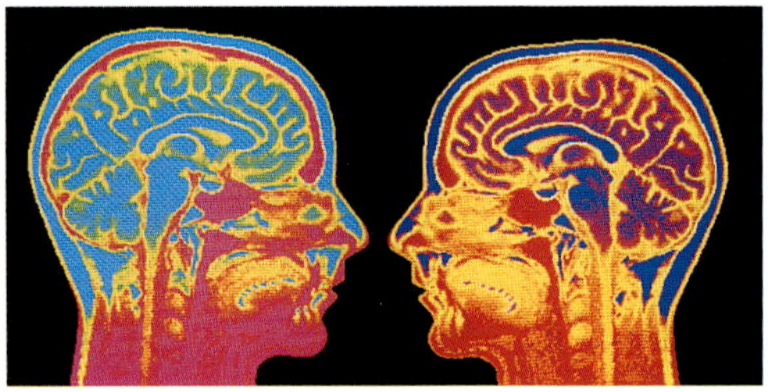

It is helpful to understand a few things about the workings of your mind and your brain.

The higher cortex of your brain is made up of a left and right hemisphere. The left hemisphere controls the right side of your body and the right hemisphere controls the left side. Research has also shown that the two hemispheres have an inbuilt capacity for different functions. The left brain appears to think in logical and sequential steps, has the ability to analyse, thinks in symbols and is responsible for language. The right brain thinks in pictures and tries to understand by seeing the overall pattern. It is the part of the brain involved in unconscious thoughts, dreaming and altered states of consciousness which occur during meditation. The left brain is dominant in most people.

The brain also operates within various brainwave frequency bands. Some researchers have linked these with four states of consciousness. The brainwave frequency bands are:

- Beta — this is the band you operate in when you are awake and conscious. It contains your critical faculties, your will and judgment. In this band your left brain is dominant.
- Alpha — your brainwave drops to this frequency when you are asleep, involved in a creative process, problem-solving and healing. This is also the area of dreams and rapid eye movement. It is the level reached during meditation. Here your right brain is dominant.
- Theta — this is the area in which you can experience super strength, stop pain and stop bleeding. You can access it during deep meditation.
- Delta — the slowest of the frequencies and little is understood about it.

Alpha, theta and delta are normally associated with sleep and are collectively known as the "unconscious". They are believed to be the area of memory and where you store your positive and negative thoughts, beliefs, habits and "programs"; they may also be where psychic awareness and altered states of consciousness are accessed.

THE IMPORTANCE OF DIET, EXERCISE AND POSTURE

The foundation of good health is a balanced diet and regular exercise. You have probably heard the terms "five main food groups", "the healthy diet pyramid" and of the need for "regular aerobic exercise". We are encouraged to eat more fibre, less salt and sugar, less fat, less cholesterol, and drink less alcohol. Our chances of heart disease, cancer, and a whole host of other diet-related illnesses will then, we are told, be minimised.

All of this makes perfect sense; however, many of us find it difficult to incorporate these demands into our busy lifestyles. But if you want to feel healthy, remain healthy or return to health, you have to monitor what you eat, you need to exercise regularly and — something you may not be aware of — you need to have good posture.

THE IMPORTANCE OF DIET

How you feel emotionally, how clear-headed you are, your energy levels and how your body functions all depend on what you eat. But these things are not what many people are thinking of when they eat. Pleasure, habit, filling an emotional need are common reasons why people eat and will often determine what they eat. Many of these people don't make the connection between the aches in their joints, their fatigue or their feelings of anxiety and the food they eat.

Your body won't run without fuel and it won't run efficiently unless it has the right kind of fuel — and that comes from a balanced diet.

Apart from physical activity, almost three-quarters of the energy you consume is used in keeping your organs functioning, your body temperature normal, and your cells renewed. This food energy is measured in kilojoules or calories and is essential to life. It is only if the amount of kilojoules you consume is more than your body needs that the excess is stored in your body as fat.

THE FOOD YOU EAT

The nutrient value of food can be summarised as six basic components:

- carbohydrates
- fibre
- vitamins
- minerals
- fats
- proteins.

About half your energy comes from complex and simple carbohydrates — starch and sugar — and the other half comes from protein and fat.

It is the simple carbohydrates that can cause you problems.

If you eat a slice of chocolate cake, you are mainly eating simple carbohydrates which your body can dump straight into your bloodstream.

All this sugar gives your body an energy high for a short while. This activates your pancreas to produce insulin which metabolises the sugar before it does any damage.

However, because your pancreas is efficient, it produces so much insulin that you are usually left with too little sugar in your blood.

This is the low you might feel which often follows the high after eating food such as chocolate cake. You might lack energy and feel depressed.

Coupled with this, the cake raises the fat level in your blood which can add to your weight by being stored as excess fat. Because the chocolate cake contains few nutrients your body has to call on its own vitamin and mineral store to metabolise it.

Complex carbohydrates, in contrast, are foods such as grains and vegetables. These take longer to digest. The sugar is released into your bloodstream at a rate that your pancreas can deal with, keeping your blood sugar level stable over a longer period.

Fruit contains the simple sugar, fructose, but also has high amounts of fibre which slows the release of this sugar into the bloodstream. Fruit juices, however, are devoid of fibre so the sugar is immediately absorbed.

Foods containing complex carbohydrates also contain many vitamins and minerals. So while your body is expending energy to digest the food, it is also receiving nutrients.

Vitamins and minerals are needed because they each have a role in maintaining the body's health (see tables on pages 12 to 15).

For example vitamin C strengthens connective tissue, vitamin E improves circulation and oxygenation and the B-complex vitamins help release energy from your cells.

Deficiencies in vitamins and minerals also cause specific diseases. For instance, a lack of vitamin C can lead to scurvy, a deficiency in vitamin D can cause rickets and an iron deficiency results in anaemia.

Protein is also essential because it is needed for the growth, maintenance and renewal of every cell in your body. Enzymes, antibodies, haemoglobin and other components of your blood are made from proteins or are proteins combined with minerals.

PROTEINS

Protein comes from animal and plant foods. Each protein molecule is made up of combinations of amino acids. These are the building blocks of your body. They are essential to the repair and replacement of bones, muscles, connective tissues and the walls of hollow organs. Some proteins are enzymes which are involved in the release of energy for cell activities such as the contraction of muscles.

Your best source of protein is lean meat and fish, eggs and dairy products. Proteins from these sources are complete proteins in that they contain the amino acids which your body cannot make itself.

Protein from plants falls into three groups: (1) nuts and seeds (2) beans and peas (lentils, soybeans etc) and (3) whole grains (wheat, rice, barley etc). These proteins are not complete and two of these groups must be eaten in combination to give you the complete protein you need. This is especially important if you follow a vegetarian diet.

FATS

It is vital to consume a small amount of fat to stay healthy, but most Western diets contain too much fat or the wrong type of fat.

When fat is digested, fatty acids, glycerol and triglycerides form. All three are used in cell growth and repair and as a source of energy. Any excess fat is stored under the skin causing weight gain.

There are three types of fat:

- saturated — found in animal and dairy products, these fats increase the amount of cholesterol and are linked with coronary heart disease.
- polyunsaturated — extracted from nuts, seeds and fish and eaten as oils or in margarines, they should only be eaten in moderation.
- monounsaturated — found in olives, peanuts and avocados, and in oils made from these foods or from canola. These fats have been linked with reducing the risk of heart disease but only if used in moderation.

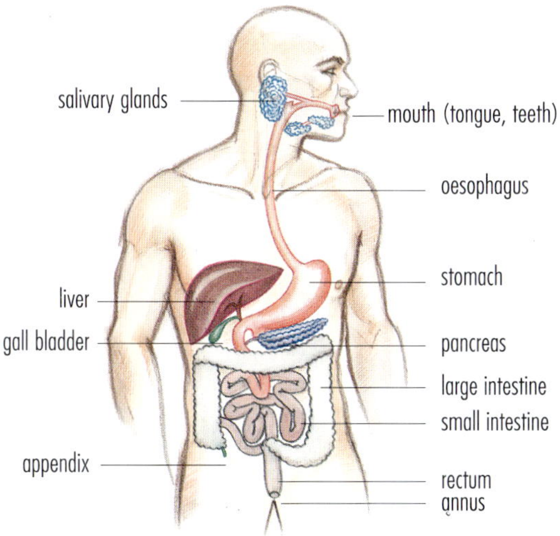

THE DIGESTIVE PROCESS

When you eat a meal, the first stage of digestion takes place in the mouth. Enzymes in saliva break down starch and the teeth grinds the food into smaller pieces before it moves down the oesophagus to the stomach.

In your stomach, your digestive process reduces this meal to a soft, moist mass. After about an hour this mass moves into your small intestine where your pancreas and gall bladder supply more digestive juices which convert complex carbohydrates into glucose, protein into amino acids and fats into fatty acid and glycerol. These then move into your bloodstream. The fibre or roughage that can't be broken down helps undigested food residue move through your small intestine to the large intestine and the bowel.

CHOLESTEROL

Most of the cholesterol in your blood has been made by your liver from foods rich in saturated fats. Your body uses cholesterol to produce hormones involved with growth and reproduction. It is also essential to the digestion of fats.

Cholesterol is transported in your bloodstream. The cholesterol that is not used by your cells remains in circulation and may soon build up to abnormally high levels. If there are not enough antioxidants (such as vitamins A, C and E), the cholesterol oxidises and then clings to the artery walls as fatty deposits, obstructing blood flow to organs such as the heart and brain.

Stress can affect cholesterol levels as more cholesterol is produced to make "stress hormones".

In addition, if the liver is not functioning well enough, it will not break down cholesterol efficiently.

You can counter this by encouraging healthy liver function (see page 329) and eating fibre, which will "drag" the cholesterol out of your body.

You can reduce your cholesterol levels by cutting fatty foods from your diet, particularly LDLs which are lipids from animal products (HDLs from vegetable oils and fish oils are seen as good lipids).

Foods that are naturally rich in cholesterol include eggs, liver, kidneys and some shellfish such as prawns and lobster. If you want to reduce cholesterol in your diet you also need to avoid food high in saturated fats such as cream, butter, hard cheese and fatty meats.

FIBRE

One of the problems with our modern diet of refined, processed foods is its lack of fibre. Previous generations did not have the luxury of white flour which we regularly use in bread and pastries. The cost of more refined white flour meant that it was only used by wealthy classes or for special treats. As a result the bread most people ate was made using wholemeal flour which is naturally high in fibre.

Fibre in our diets is found in unrefined grains such as brown rice, wholemeal pasta or cereals such as oat bran, the skin and flesh of fruit and vegetables, and other fibre-rich foods such as nuts, seeds and legumes (beans, peas etc).

MINERAL TABLE

MINERAL	FUNCTION	SOURCE	REC. DAILY AMOUNT
Calcium	Builds and maintains bones/teeth; important for muscle contraction (including heart) and relaxation (via the nervous system)	pilchards, sardines, clams, mussels, parsley, spinach, broccoli, haricot beans, sesame seeds, sunflower seeds, almonds, Brazil nuts, kelp, molasses, carob, bran, yogurt and other dairy foods, soya bean products	800 mg 1200 mg during growth periods, breast-feeding, pregnancy, and for the aged
Chlorine	Helps cell metabolism and red blood cell function; needed for production of stomach acid; activates many enzymes; helps nervous system with co-ordination	fish, meat, carrots, celery, lettuce, tomatoes, watercress, salt, milk	600 mg (but estimated daily intake is 3600–6000 mg as sodium choride — see sodium entry)
Chromium	Regulates blood-sugar levels; involved in stress response and immune function	shellfish, chicken, green vegetables, fruit, bran, whole wheat and whole rye bread, nuts, honey, brewer's yeast	10–30 mcg but requirements may be higher
Cobalt	Is part of vitamin B12 — see vitamin B12 entry	meat, green vegetables, wholegrain cereals, yeast, eggs, fruit	0.045–0.09 mcg
Copper	Helps enzymes and the formation of red blood cells; important in metabolism of iron and excretion of uric acid and cholesterol; necessary for utilisation of glucose	liver, shellfish, bran, wheatgerm, wholegrain cereals, soy lecithin, dry split peas, almonds, Brazil nuts, yeast, molasses, cocoa powder, bag tea, drinking water (from copper pipes)	2.5 mg
Fluorine	Strengthens bones; prevents tooth decay	seafood, fluorinated water	1 mg
Iodine	Used for thyroid hormone	seafood, spinach, lettuce, sea salt, kelp	50–300 mcg
Iron	Helps carry oxygen to cells and forms haemoglobin; necessary for functioning of many enzymes; acts against various microbes	liver, kidneys, meat, sardines, shellfish, molasses, parsley, spinach, watercress, sunflower seeds, nuts, spirulina, kelp, eggs, red wine	women 18 mg men 10 mg
Magnesium	Necessary for nerve and muscle function (including heart) and muscle relaxation; necessary for cell metabolism; agent in utilising other vitamins and minerals; helps prevent kidney stones; important in bone structure	seafood, meat, avocados, haricot beans, tofu, brown rice, muesli, wheatgerm, buckwheat, rye, almonds, Brazil nuts, cashews, kelp, spinach, molasses	300 mg 450 mg during pregnancy and breast-feeding

MINERAL TABLE

MINERAL	FUNCTION	SOURCE	REC. DAILY AMOUNT
Manganese	Helps balance blood-sugar levels; activates enzymes; helps reproductive processes; has anti-oxidant action; involved in breakdown of fats/cholesterol	kidneys, lentils, parsley, watercress, alfalfa, almonds, walnuts, pecans, Brazil nuts, bran, barley, rye, apricots	4–6 mg
Phosphorus	Helps growth and repair of cells (part of cell membrane); passes on genetic hereditary patterns; used in bones and teeth; essential for energy and transport of nutrients in the body	all dairy and all protein (including liver, fish, meat, wheatgerm, brewer's yeast, cheese, eggs, whole grains, legumes, nuts, seeds), soft drinks	600–800 mg
Potassium	Helps muscle control and water balance; important in many enzyme reactions and for energy metabolism; involved in production of insulin	dried beans, lentils, soya beans, potatoes, spinach, parsley, kelp, avocado, dried apricots, almonds, Brazil nuts, brewer's yeast, molasses, sunflower seeds	2–4 mg
Selenium	Antioxidant; interacts with vitamin E; involved in regulation of blood pressure; protects against mercury and cadmium toxicity; may prevent some cancer	kidneys, liver, nuts, seafood, wholegrain cereals, wheatgerm, butter, garlic, cider vinegar	100–300 mcg requirements increase with age
Sodium	Cellular metabolism; prevents excess fluid loss, balances acid-alkali levels; necessary for nerve impulses; involved in production of digestive juices	chicken, green vegetables, carrots, bran, salt, water, lentils, peas, pulses	1200 mg (although average diet gives 6000–15,000 mg)
Sulphur	Helps formation of body tissues; detoxifier; antioxidant; important for water balance	protein foods, onions, garlic, cabbage, molasses	800 mg
Zinc	Essential in many enzyme reactions; necessary for protein digestion; involved in energy production, calcium metabolism, detoxification of alcohol, lactose breakdown; involved in vision; needed for repair of wounds; major role in immune system; impacts on sperm and foetus.	liver, seafood, sunflower seeds, nuts, legumes, eggs, bran, wholemeal flour, buckwheat	10–15 mg requirements can increase due to stress, pollution, pregnancy etc (the term elemental zinc refers to the amount of zinc in a compound such as zinc sulphate)

VITAMIN TABLE

VITAMIN	FUNCTION	SOURCE	REC. DAILY AMOUNT
A	Essential for night vision; necessary for proper bone development and strength of mucous membranes; reduces susceptibility to infection; role in reproductive system	liver, kidneys, beans, cod liver oil, parsley, any green/yellow/orange vegetable	5000 IU
B1 Thiamine	Functioning of nervous system, heart and liver; important part of energy production	liver, beef, lamb, port, asparagus, brown rice, brewer's yeast, wholemeal bread, bran, pine nuts, Brazil nuts, peanuts, sunflower seeds	1.5 mg
B2 Riboflavin	Good vision and clear eyes; essential for normal growth and reproduction; protects against birth defects	liver, kidneys, meat and yeast extract, beans, avocados, mushrooms, peas, spinach, almonds, wheatgerm, yogurt	2 mg
B3 Niacin	Breaks down fats, protein and carbohydrates; reduces blood cholesterol levels; stabilises blood sugar levels; vital for energy production; improves circulation; important for mental health	liver, kidneys, meat, chicken, tuna, sardines, salmon, mackerel, spinach, eggs, peanuts, wheatgerm, wholemeal bread	15 mg
B5 Pantothenic	For functioning of adrenal gland; essential for all energy metabolism; important in manufacture of haemoglobin for red blood cells and production of antibodies; important for functioning of digestive system; prevents premature aging/wrinkles	liver, kidneys, mushrooms, peanuts, bran, wheatgerm, brewer's yeast	5–10 mg
B6 Pyridoxine	Aids metabolism (including metabolising energy and yeast, vitamins B3, B5 and B12); forms antibodies and red blood cells; role in nervous system function	liver, chicken, mackerel, bananas, brewer's yeast, wholemeal bread, wheatgerm, brown rice, Brazil nuts, walnuts	2 mg
B9 Folic Acid	Aids proper functioning of B12, formation of red blood cells and use of proteins, fats and carbohydrates; vital for normal pregnancy reproduction of cells; prevents miscarriage, birth and premature birth; role in prevention of cervical cancer	liver, kidney, meat, green vegetables, fresh fruit, brewer's yeast, yeast extract, wheatgerm, pulses	0.2 mg 0.4 mg during pregnancy

VITAMIN TABLE

VITAMIN	FUNCTION	SOURCE	REC. DAILY AMOUNT
B12	Proper functioning of B9 folic acid; red blood cell formation; healthy nervous system, synthesis of neucleic acids and proteins; metabolism of fats, proteins, carbohydrates; prevention of cell degeneration	liver, meat, kidney, fish, egg yolk, dairy products — especially cheese, fortified cereals, brewer's yeast, spirulina	3 mcg 8 mcg during pregnancy and breastfeeding
Biotin	Metabolism of fats and cholesterol; synthesis of glucose when diet is low in carbohydrates; metabolism of amino acids; involved in activation of some B vitamins; important for hair production	brewer's yeast, liver, soya beans, egg yolks, brown rice. Up to 90% supplied by intestinal flora.	0.1 to 0.2 mg
C	Maintains the essential protein collagen; helps healing of tissue; antioxidant; prevents viral and bacterial infection; involved in energy metabolism, adrenal function and stress response; reduces cholesterol levels; detoxifier; antihistamine; important for calcium and iron absorption	capsicum, parsley, liver, asparagus, broccoli, cabbage, grapefruit, guavas, oranges, lemons, blackcurrants, bananas, melons, watercress, leeks, lettuce, red chilli	50 mg
D	Essential for absorption of calcium; helps bone building; involved in production of digestive juices and synthesis of thyroid hormone; role in eyesight	sardines, herring, mackerel, cod liver oil, halibut liver oil, apples, carrots, cabbage, parsley, leeks, tomatoes, sunshine on the skin	400 IU
E	Helps circulation system; increases stamina; used to increase fertility; antioxidant; retards aging; important for normal cell growth; protective action on heart muscle; can lower blood pressure; essential for thyroid hormone production	tuna fish, cod's roe, cod liver oil, olive oil, apples, avocado, mango, kiwi fruit, carrots, cabbage, parsley, leeks, tomatoes	20 IU, although recent research shows that more than 150 IU has a protective effect on the heart
K	Prevents haemorrhaging	broccoli, brussels sprouts, cabbage, lettuce, cauliflower, spinach, potatoes, wheatgerm, alfalfa, strawberries. Eating acidophillus yogurt will encourage healthy intestinal bacteria which synthesise this vitamin.	150 mcg

The fibre does not contribute energy to your body but adds roughage to your diet. Because it can't be broken down during digestion, it is not absorbed by the body and instead passes through the stomach and intestine thus preventing constipation. It has been linked with the slight lowering of blood cholesterol levels by reducing the absorption of digested fats. A high-fibre, low-fat diet has also been found to reduce the incidence of bowel and breast cancers.

It is recommended that you eat around 30 grams of fibre each day. As a quick guide, an apple contains around 3 grams of fibre, a bowl of whole grain about 6 grams and a slice of wholemeal bread about 2 grams.

FOOD ADDITIVES

During the processing and manufacture of many foods, substances are added to improve flavour, colour and texture and to help the food stay fresh longer. While these additives have passed testing and safe levels are set, some people react badly to these acceptable levels.

The most commonly recognised link affecting health is between food colouring additives and hyperactivity in children. If you suffer from allergies, your health practitioner will probably recommend allergy testing and warn you about the dangers of food additives.

If you are concerned about food additives, make a habit of reading the labels on packaged food items. Preservatives, artificial flavourings, colours and sweeteners, emulsifiers, thickeners and antioxidants are additives that may cause you harm. These additives are coded by numbers and there are books available which give you detailed information on the codes and what they mean.

A QUICK GUIDE TO HEALTHY DIET CHANGES

• **Reduce fats** — eat only moderate amounts of lean red meat and poultry without the skin. Avoid butter, margarine and oil. Use monounsaturated oils such as canola or olive oils, if necessary, for cooking. Avoid take-away food. (Remember, however, that fatty acids are an essential vitamin and can be sourced in your diet from fats from deep-water fish and vegetable sources e.g. nuts, seeds and cold pressed vegetable oil.)

• **Reduce sugar** — buy only foods with no added sugar. Cut out sweets, desserts, cakes, jam and soft drinks.

• **Reduce salt** — cut down on processed foods as these are usually high in salt. Choose low-salt options where possible. Avoid using salt in cooking or adding it to your meals. (Note: salt does play a function in maintaining a healthy body. Some conditions benefit from higher salt intakes: see sodium entry, page 13, and consult your health practitioner for advice.)

• **Reduce alcohol** — limit your intake to one to two standard drinks per day for women and no more than four for men. Don't drink if you are pregnant.

• **Increase fibre** — eat a minimum of four servings per day of wholemeal bread, cereal, whole grains, fruit and vegetables together with nuts, seeds and legumes.

• **Drink water** — keep up your fluid intake by drinking eight glasses of water per day. Where possible, avoid tap water and invest in a water purification system or drink bottled water. Choose bottled water that carries an analysis of its contents because some disreputable companies sell water taken from the city water supply.

DIET RECOMMENDATIONS

While there are some general rules about nutrition your body has its own particular set of needs.

Eating red meat suits some body types, being a vegan is great for others. You might crave cheese and yet your system reacts as if it were poison.

You are going to have to discover which style of eating best suits you. You should also remember that your needs will change throughout your life so, in a way, it is best to think of food as an ongoing study.

This is especially important if you are facing a health challenge. For a time you may have to adopt a strict approach to your diet. Then as you return to health your body's needs will change and you will have to reassess your diet.

Just as there may be many ways of treating any one health problem, there are dozens of approaches to diet to suit any number of people.

There is debate over cooked food versus raw food and the role of supplements. Many people swear by organically grown food, and some feel it is okay to eat veal, lamb, free-range chicken and fish but no pork or beef.

Many naturopaths recommend you cut salt and

THE FOOD PYRAMID

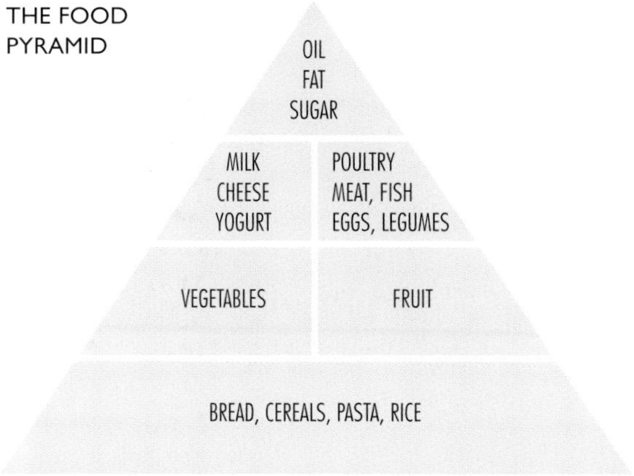

sugar from your diet totally, others recommend sea salt and honey. Some say no dairy products, others believe goats milk is superior to cows milk, while another group advocate soya bean products as a dairy substitute.

Protein foods such as meat, fish, chicken, milk, eggs and dairy products have been considered by many diet specialists to be the most important part of a balanced diet.

THE FOOD PYRAMID

"The healthy diet pyramid" is a diet philosophy supported by a great number of nutritionists. It gives prime importance to complex carbohydrate foods such as cereals, grains, pasta, fruits, vegetables and pulses such as beans and lentils.

Starting at the bottom of the pyramid, it is recommended that you make complex carbohydrates the basis of your meals.

You should eat moderately from the next level — protein foods such as poultry, fish, lean meat, eggs, nuts, milk, cheese, yogurt and pulses. It is recommended you eat 40–50 grams of protein a day. This can be a little difficult to estimate, but as a rough guide, this amount of protein is contained in an average sized piece of steak and a wedge of cheese.

On top of the pyramid are the foods you should eat least — butter, margarine, oil, sugar and salt.

Nutritionists also encourage a diet based on a wide variety of food and a mix of raw and cooked foods as well as fresh and processed foods.

VEGETARIAN DIET

People choose a vegetarian diet for a variety of reasons. It can be for health or it could be because they oppose the killing of animals.

There are three types of vegetarian diet:

- lacto-ovo-vegetarian — includes dairy and eggs
- ovo-vegetarian — includes eggs
- vegan — includes no dairy or eggs.

In contrast to the food pyramid, naturopaths in favour of a lacto-vegetarian diet place emphasis on three basic food groups, in this order of priority:

1. seeds, grains and nuts
2. vegetables
3. fruits.

They would supplement these foods with milk and milk products such as yogurt, and with cold-pressed vegetable oils, honey, brewer's yeast and other vitamin and mineral supplements.

The term vegeterian is often used by people who eat a diet mostly of fruit and vegetables, grains, seeds and nuts, but who may add fish if they eat out.

MACROBIOTIC

This form of eating was introduced to the West by Michio Kushi and Georges Ohsawa. It is based on the philosophy of yin and yang and foods are defined as yin or yang (see page 182). For example, "extreme yang foods" include eggs, meat, poultry and fish such as salmon and tuna and "extreme yin foods" include dairy products, sugar, processed food and tropical fruits and vegetables.

The aim is to balance your body energies (Qi, Ch'i or Ki) by eating a diet balanced in yin and yang foods. For this reason the extreme yin and yang foods are not recommended. A diet based on salads, for example, would not provide you with enough yang energy. The moderate yin and yang foods are favoured and these include whole grains, seeds and nuts, vegetables and fruits.

Macrobiotics requires some study but built into it is a health philosophy. You can treat illnesses and rectify imbalances by altering the yin/yang ratio of the food you eat.

Often SHIATSU therapists have an interest in macrobiotics and will be able to offer assistance.

RAW FOOD DIETS

The people who advocate raw foods believe that cooking causes a loss of nutrients and enzymes. They are advocates of uncooked fruit and vegetables and fresh juices consumed immediately.

FOOD COMBINING

This way of eating is based on the idea that different foods need different enzymes to digest them properly. For example proteins need an acid environment while starches need an alkaline environment. So the theory is that if you eat them at the same time you are not able to digest either fully. In addition fruit should only be eaten by itself or with food with which it is compatible. Therefore, if you combine foods correctly you will eat sweet fruits with starches and acid fruits with proteins (animal or vegetable) and never proteins and starch together. Neither is it recommended that you drink with meals.

ELIMINATION DIETS

These are often prescribed to overcome certain health problems. For example, if you are allergic to dairy products or are lactose intolerant you could be placed on a diet which replaces these foods with dairy substitutes such as tofu or soya bean products.

There are also diets aimed at eliminating toxins from your body.

These are usually tailored to your specific needs to deal with a health problem you are facing.

THE DIET EXPERTS

There are a number of health philosophies in which diet plays an essential part, including NATUROPATHY, SHIATSU and TRADITIONAL CHINESE MEDICINE.

Western medicine is increasing its interest in the role of diet in a person's health. Specialists in this field are dieticians or nutritionists, university or college-trained professionals who can be consulted directly or through a doctor's referral. Dieticians can assist in the medical treatment of conditions such as heart disease, diabetes, constipation and irritable bowel syndrome and give advice on diet for those with food allergies or weight problems, or those with special needs such as babies or pregnant women.

FASTING

Another form of diet is fasting. This is usually recommended for therapeutic purposes and can be a juice fast, water fast or herbal tea fast. See PROTECTING YOUR IMMUNE SYSTEM for an inner-cleansing fast you can do at home.

THE IMPORTANCE OF EXERCISE

It is important to find an exercise program that suits you. The most commonly recommended form of exercise is aerobic exercise — power walking, swimming, running, jumping, bicycling, or running up stairs — for 20 minutes, three times a week, at a sufficiently energetic level to cause your heart to beat a good deal faster than normal.

Exercise not only burns up kilojoules to help you lose weight or maintain your ideal weight, it also:

- tones muscles
- improves your body shape
- delivers more oxygen to your cells
- improves your energy levels
- reduces your stress levels
- helps to condition your heart.

The positive effects exercise has on your heart are important. Your heart is a pump which, if it is healthy, will work as often and as hard as you demand.

If you exercise in a controlled way and build up your levels of exercise, your heart will learn to respond. It becomes stronger in much the same way as your biceps will if you lift weights. However, you do need to gradually increase your level of activity, otherwise you can damage your heart.

If you have a history of heart problems, pulmonary or kidney disease, have a full physical check-up with your doctor before beginning any aerobic or exercise progam. You should also discuss your intended exercise program with your doctor or seek professional advice.

HOW TO START

When you decide to improve your fitness, the best thing to do is start moving. This doesn't have to be walking or jogging distances. It can be as simple as walking an extra bus stop in the morning before you catch the bus, or climbing a couple of flights of stairs at work before taking the lift.

Fitness trainers say that once you begin moving, you realise how much your body enjoys it. If you exercise correctly it will become a natural, health-enhancing addiction.

There are dozens of ways you can improve your fitness — dance classes, tennis, football, going to the gym, walking the dog, roller-blading, swimming — to name a few.

Whatever you decide on, try to incorporate these five elements into your physical fitness program:

1. **Flexibility** — this involves lengthening muscles and increasing the suppleness of your body. Yoga, Tai Chi, dance and aerobic classes and stretching exercises increase flexibility.
2. **Strength** — to become stronger you need to incorporate into your exercise program either weight training or using your own body weight to provide necessary resistance. Increase the resistance not the repetitions when you exercise. Yoga, Tai Chi, martial arts, weight training, aerobics, dance and specifically designed exercises will increase your strength.
3. **Muscle endurance** — this can be achieved by increasing the number of repetitions when you are exercising a group of muscles, either with weights or using your own body weight. Yoga, martial arts, weight training, aerobics, dance and specifically designed exercises will increase your muscle endurance.
4. **Stamina** — you can build up your staying power by increasing the intensity of your exercise until your heart rate is between 60 percent and 85 percent of its maximum. Your maximum heart rate per minute is worked out by subtracting your age from 220. Aerobic exercise, swimming, jogging, cycling and dancing are all exercises that will increase your stamina.
5. **Motor fitness** — this relates to your co-ordination, balance and reaction time and involves the connection between your brain and your muscle actions. Ball sports, team games, martial arts and Tai Chi will help develop your motor fitness.

SENSIBLE ADVICE ABOUT EXERCISING

Before you exercise make sure you warm up your body first. This allows your muscles, heart and lungs to prepare. Always take your joints gently through a range of movements (see examples on page 20). These will help the joints secrete lubricating fluid.

After you have finished your exercise session end it with some stretching. This is especially important to ease out contracted muscles if you have been working hard aerobically or using your muscle strength.

Be careful never to overwork or over stretch your body. Pain, faintness, nausea or headache are signals from your body indicating that it has had enough. Many therapists advise against the "no pain, no gain" philosophy and pushing your body too hard. They are critical of joggers who insist on running even when they are ill or nursing an injury. These experts believe that stressing your body does more harm than good. It draws energy away from your body's natural healing processes, compromising your immune system. This could make you susceptible to flu or other infections, and the wear and tear on joints could cause long-term problems such as arthritis.

Other points to consider:

- keep your movements smooth — jerky movements may cause injuries.
- allow at least 90 minutes after a meal before exercising so you have fully completed the digestive process.
- make sure you wear the correct protective clothing, such as knee pads or a helmet.
- wear footwear that supports your feet and ankles and suits the activity you are undertaking.
- avoid clothing that will make you hot; drink water so you do not become dehydrated, and keep warm after exercising.
- if you haven't exercised for a while, take it easy. Begin slowly and increase your level of activity as your fitness increases.
- become aware of your body and feel the muscles you are working. Your body is able to tell you a good deal in this way. For example, you will soon be able to tell how tense you are by the tightness you find in certain areas of your body.
- incorporate some discipline into your program. Exercise at the same time each day if you can.

EXERCISE CAN BE FUN

What is most important is that you have fun. Exercise with friends if you can, enjoy the environment if you are exercising outside, play music to lift your spirits — choose activities that you enjoy, and vary the exercise so you don't become bored.

People who look forward to exercising the most are the people who incorporate it into their social lives. They go bike riding in the park at weekends with friends, they head for the country or a walk through a national park, they go out on a Saturday night and they dance. Exercising doesn't always have to be at a class or on a bench pressing weights. Incorporate exercise into your life and make it as pleasurable as sharing a meal or seeing a movie. If you are able, involve the whole family. That way you will all be fitter and much more healthy.

WARM-UPS AND STRETCHES

WARM-UPS

Wrists: Rotate the wrists clockwise in large, slow circles; then rotate anticlockwise.

Ankles: Stand on one leg and extend the other in front of you, raised a little from the ground *(see Figure 1)*. Flex the raised foot towards you, then point it away from you. Rotate the foot in both directions. Repeat to other side.

Neck: Gently roll your head to one shoulder, centre, then roll to the other shoulder. Bring your head to the centre again and then allow it to roll forward, chin to chest, then roll backward.

Shoulders: Place your hands on your shoulders, then rotate, drawing large circles with the elbows in one direction then the other.

Hips and legs: "Cycling" is an excellent way to lubricate the joints of the lower limbs. Lie flat on the floor on your back. Raise the legs and make large, cycling movements in the air. Keep the motion flowing as you cycle forwards, then backwards. *(See Figure 2.)*

Whole body: Finish with a gentle twisting movement which loosens all the joints of the body. Stand with legs about a metre (3–4 feet) apart, knees bent and arms held straight at shoulder level *(see Figure 3)*. Let all your joints hang loose as you twist the upper body and head to the right, allowing your hands to slap the body wherever they naturally fall *(see Figure 4)*. Twist right around to the left side in one smooth movement. Keep the knees very loose and springy as you continue to twist from side to side. Develop a gentle, rhythmic motion and feel your whole body relax.

After these, you should prepare your cardiovascular system by raising your pulse a little. Try running on the spot or star jumps. A few rounds of Salute to the Sun (see p 190) will also help to get the blood flowing.

STRETCHING EXERCISES

Before doing any strenuous exercise, stretch your muscles gently so they become warm and more pliable. This prevents injury.

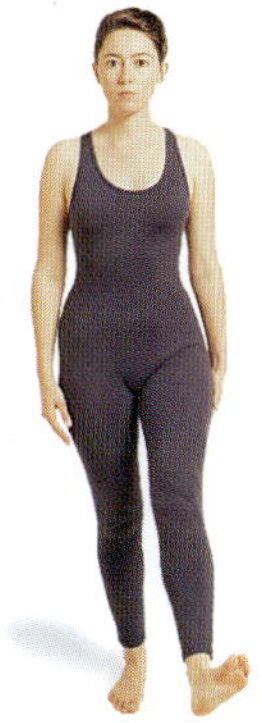

FIGURE 1

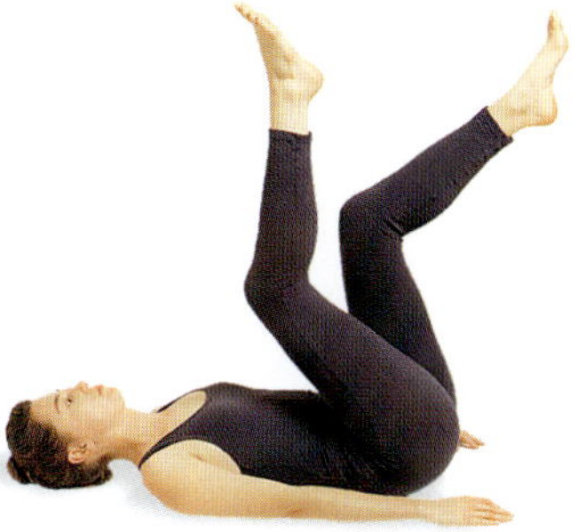

FIGURE 2

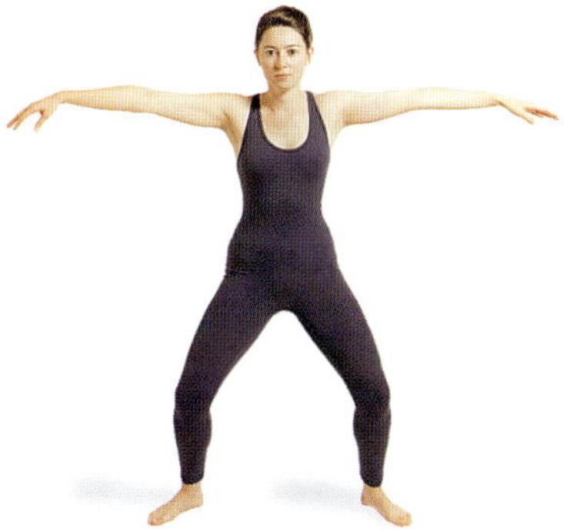

FIGURE 3

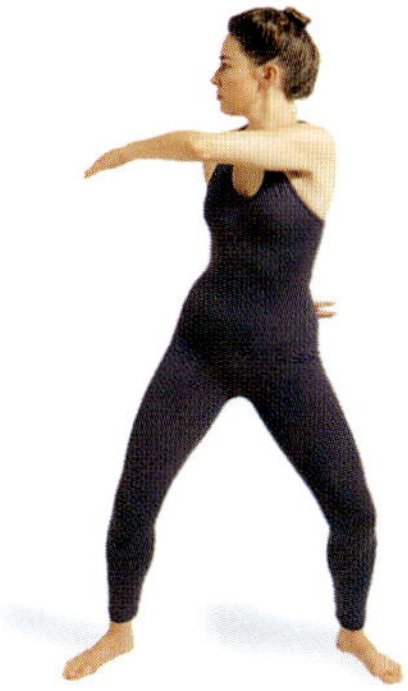

FIGURE 4

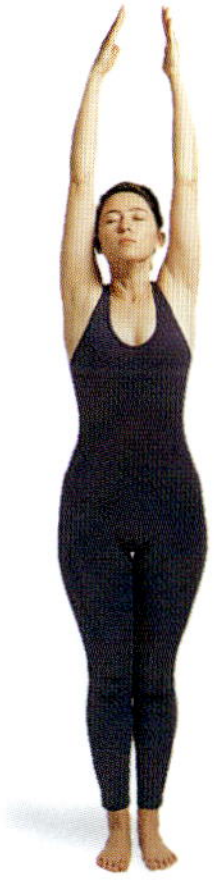

FIGURE 5

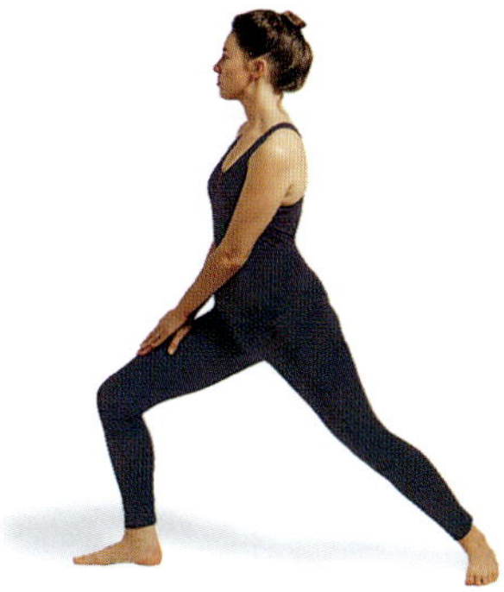

FIGURE 6

STANDING STRETCHES

Whole body: Begin by raising the arms above the head, palms facing each other, and stretch the whole body upwards from the toes to the fingertips *(see Figure 5)*. Repeat several times.

Lower limbs: Side lunges stretch the thigh and calf muscles, and open the pelvic area. Stand with the legs a metre (3–4 feet) apart, feet parallel with toes pointing forward. Swivel your hips to the right so that the right foot is pointing sideways, while the left remains in the original position. Keep the hips aligned and the upper torso straight (do not bend forward). Bend the right knee keeping the left leg straight, and feel the stretch in both legs. *(See Figure 6.)* Repeat to other side.

Upper torso: Try side stretches to warm the muscles of the arms and waist area. Standing with feet about a metre (3–4 feet) apart, raise the right arm in the air and let the other arm rest on the left thigh. Keeping the body straight (not falling forwards or backwards), bend the upper torso and right arm to the left and let your left arm move further down the leg *(see Figure 7)*. Do not strain or hold for longer than comfortable. Bend the knees if you feel discomfort. Gently bring your body to the upright position, and repeat to the other side.

SITTING STRETCHES

Forward stretches from a sitting position help prepare the hamstrings, calves, back muscles and open the whole pelvic region.

Lower limbs and back: Sit on the floor and place a rolled towel beneath your buttocks, legs stretched straight in front of you. Open your legs as wide as possible and stretch your arms above your head, lengthening the spine *(see Figure 8)*. Bending from the hip joints, stretch as far down the right leg as possible, as if trying to lower your upper torso onto the leg *(see Figure 9)*. Hold for as long as comfortable, stretching further and lower with each exhalation. Return to centre, arms stretched above the head; then repeat other side.

Calves and hamstrings: Sit on the floor with your left leg stretched out in front of you, toes pointing to the ceiling, and bend the right leg so the heel is close to your buttocks *(see Figure 10)*. Keeping the back straight, glide your hands down the extended leg, bending from the lowest part of your back *(see Figure 11)*. Do not hump your upper back and do not strain. Return to centre position, and repeat other side.

Inner legs, pelvis and hips: To stretch and loosen lie on the left side, supporting the body with the elbow. Raise the right leg and hold *(see Figure 12)*. Raise a little higher, hold. Lower leg slowly, then repeat other side.

Shoulder region: Sit with your legs bent beneath you and your buttocks resting on your toes. Bend and raise the right arm so the elbow is touching the head and the hand is reaching down the spine. Simultaneously, bend the left arm so the elbow is close to the waist and the hand is reaching up the spine. If possible, clasp the hands together *(see Figure 13)*. Hold for several seconds, release and repeat other side.

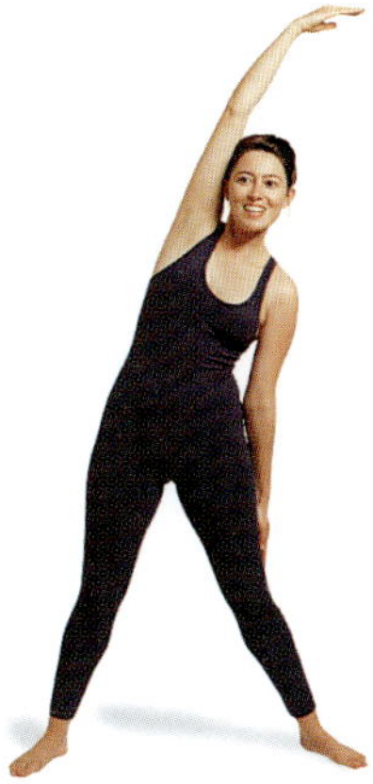

FIGURE 7

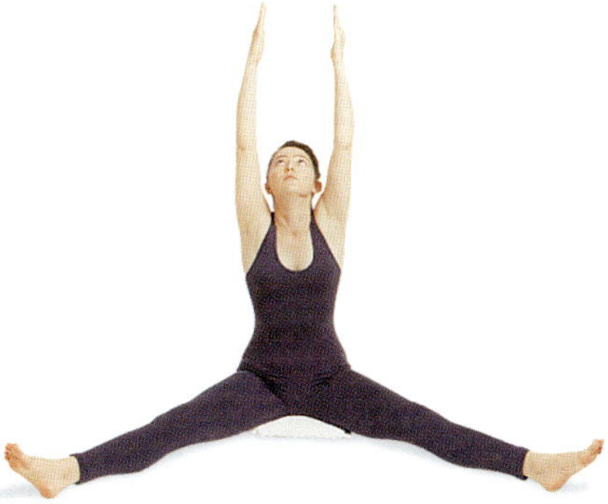

FIGURE 8

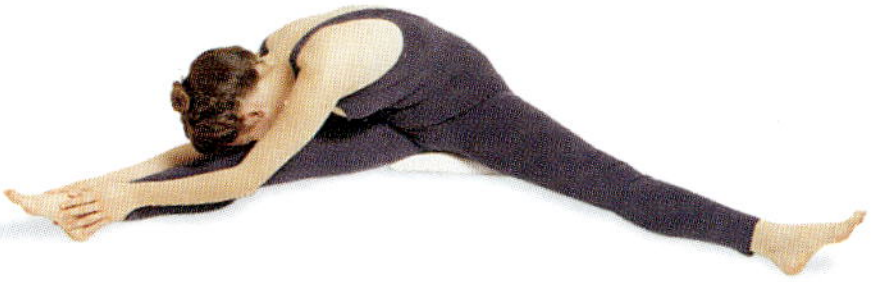

FIGURE 9

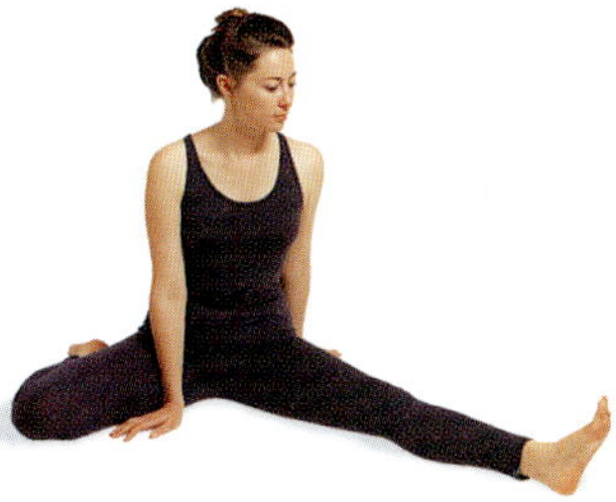

FIGURE 10

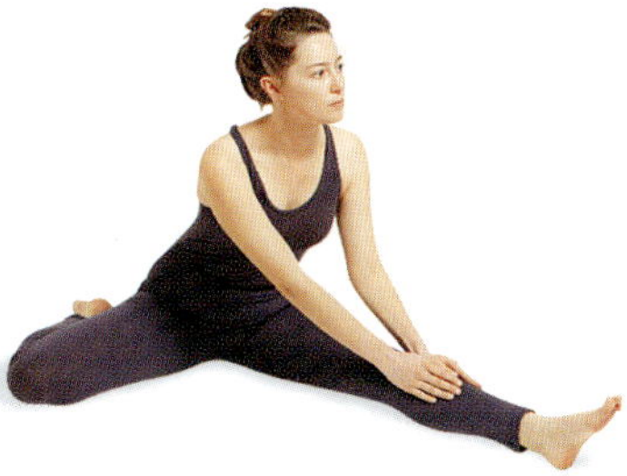

FIGURE 11

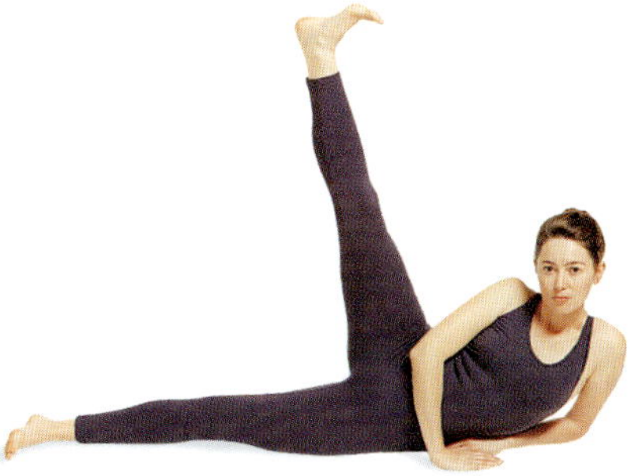

FIGURE 12

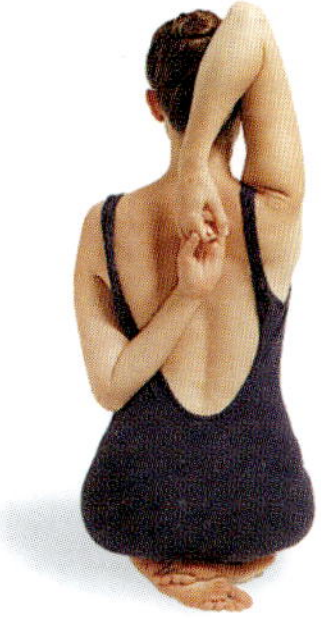

FIGURE 13

THE IMPORTANCE OF POSTURE

If you have aches and pains, suffer from headaches or migraines or have some joint soreness, it would be worthwhile to examine your posture.

Posture means the way you hold, carry and move your body during all the activities you undertake — sitting at your desk, moving up from a table, walking, running, bending, lifting, even brushing your teeth.

Our body movements are usually learnt movements imitated from our parents. That's why you can see similarity in the habits of family members. The problem is that many of these learnt behaviours are not the best movements for your body. Despite the fact that they come to feel natural and correct, often they are not correct nor are they efficient ways of moving. In time your body will protest against the strain caused by bad posture.

Signs of incorrect posture can include such problems as:

- Repetitive Strain Injury
- Asthma
- Digestive Problems
- Arthritis
- Headache and Migraine, Neck Pain
- Back Pain
- stiff and sore shoulders
- Foot Soreness, Bunions and Corns
- knee problems
- hip problems.

Changing habits of a lifetime is not as difficult as it might first seem. There are therapists such as those who teach the Alexander Technique and the Feldenkrais Method who can help you retrain your body through a series of lessons.

These teachers believe that your body has an inbuilt memory of what it feels like to move freely, easily, gracefully and without pain. Once it is reminded and you increase your awareness of correct movement you will soon move back into balance.

SOME REASONS FOR POOR POSTURE

- birth defect
- weight problems
- muscle imbalance
- tiredness
- sleeping on a poor mattress
- straining from poor eyesight
- stress, both physical and mental.

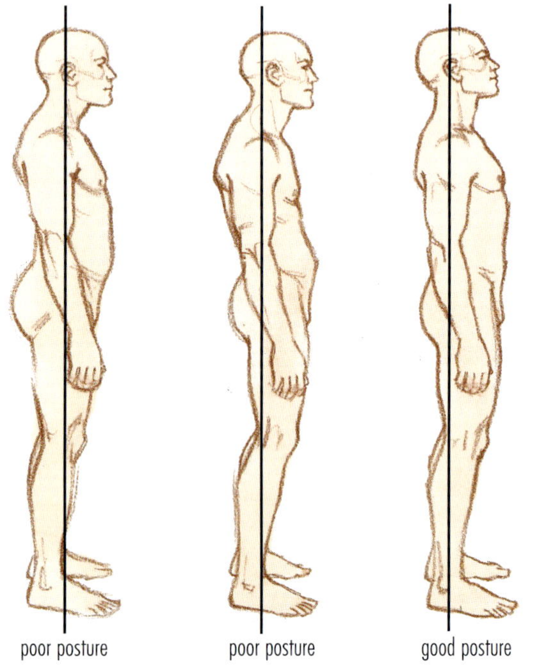

Good posture is not about being rigid, or sticking out your chest or pulling in your buttocks. It is about balance. The lift comes first from the crown of the head and your feet should be evenly grounded. Think about how you stand, sit and move. Are you slumping now? Look at the heels of your shoes: are they worn down more on one side?

THE IMPORTANCE OF BREATH

Although breathing is an automatic response in your body, the way you breathe greatly affects your general health. This is because all the cells of your body need a constant supply of oxygen to perform the process of metabolism which provides your body with energy. Blood pumped by the heart picks up the oxygen in the lungs and carries it to the cells then returns to the lungs with carbon dioxide which is breathed out of the body.

During exercise your rate of breathing increases as your heart pumps faster to bring more oxygen to your muscles. You are probably aware of these changes. However, your rate of breathing also changes according to your emotions. If you are calm your breathing is gentle and rhythmic. If you become angry or frightened your breathing will speed up. If you have long-term stress, you can develop a hyperventilation pattern of breathing, where the balance between oxygen and carbon dioxide becomes disturbed (your body actually needs a proper amount of carbon dioxide to make use of oxygen).

In Eastern terms your breath is your connection to the "life force" — the Ch'i, Qi, Ki or Prana. If you breathe poorly you will have poor energy levels and feel more tension. That's why physical disciplines such as YOGA and Tai Chi (see page 186) pay so much attention to your breath and how you can enhance it.

Most of us, however, are not very effective at breathing. We breathe well enough to live but not well enough to really flourish.

If you are not breathing properly you are starving your cells, muscles and organs of the thing that makes them work. Little wonder that so many of us suffer from stress, fatigue and depression — all of which can be helped by improving the quality of breath.

Lack of exercise, over-exercise and stress are the major factors that disturb breathing.

BREATH AND POSTURE

It is important to remember that good breathing and good posture go hand in hand. You cannot breathe properly if you are slumped in a chair or tied in a knot on the couch. The lungs cannot expand to their full capacity when the body is contracted or contorted. To breathe properly the body should be relaxed with the spine straight, the neck centred, the shoulders held gently backwards to expand the chest and the abdomen loose. See The Importance of Diet, Exercise and Posture.

BREATHING WITH AWARENESS

To improve the quality of your breath you should practise breathing with awareness. This means being conscious of the breath as it enters and leaves the body. Mostly we are not conscious of the fact that we breathe at all. Being able to observe the breath is the first step towards being able to breathe at the optimum level and releasing abnormal breathing patterns in your muscles. Most people find their breathing slows down when they breathe with awareness.

Exercise: Lie on your back and allow your body to be relaxed and heavy. Listen to the sounds around you. There may be traffic noises, voices, clocks ticking. See how many different sounds you can hear. Now, let these sounds fade away and begin to concentrate only on your own breath. Let the breath be natural — do not hold your breath or alter your normal breathing pattern.

Follow the air as it enters your nostrils and travels down the airways to reach your lungs. Sense your whole body expand without force or muscular effort. As the air leaves your lungs feel your body relax.

As you breathe in, imagine your body being filled with fresh life and as you breathe out imagine peace coming over your body.

Allow your whole awareness to become nothing more than the rhythm of the breath in and out, expansion then release.

Practise this exercise from time to time and you will become more aware of your own breath and how intrinsic it is to your existence. Also, the breath intimately connects you with the world around you, as air enters and leaves your body. Of course, it is not necessary to breathe with full awareness all the time — just take a moment every now and then to stop, observe and appreciate your breath.

WAYS TO BREATHE

If the first step to improving the quality of the breath is being aware that you breathe, the second step is being aware of *how* you breathe.

The way you breathe depends a lot on the activity in which you are engaged and your emotional state. For example, you will breathe differently when you are running to catch a bus than when you are relaxing in a warm bath. Generally, however, there are two ways in which we breathe: (1) *chest breathing* (2) *diaphragmatic breathing.*

CHEST BREATHING

This is the term used to describe how our respiratory system automatically functions during exercise and times of stress, anxiety or fear. The ribs contract and the air is drawn into the upper chest area.

BREATHING FOR RELAXATION

Try this exercise that involves breathing, body awareness, mental focus and relaxation:

Begin by making sure your spine is straight. At first you may find it easier to either sit or lie on your back with your knees bent.

Breathe in gently.

As you breathe out, focus your mind on the feeling of relaxation that comes with exhalation. Use no force or muscular effort with the exhalation...just follow the exhalation to its end point by allowing the muscles to let go.

When your exhalation has reached its end point, WAIT until you feel the urge to breathe coming from your diaphragm. Feel the peace and stillness that exist at this point of the breath. You can repeat the word "peace" if you wish. Put your mental focus into waiting for the sensation that is the desire to inhale coming from your diaphragm area.

Breathe in again — gently. Keep repeating this sequence.

As you relax while you do this exercise, the period at the end of each exhalation will get longer. It will take a few complete breaths before you get into a steady rhythm. Then, your breathing will slow and your respiratory muscles will relax. (When you are tense, your breathing speeds up or you hold the in-breath, and there is less of a break after the out-breath.)

Practise this exercise regularly until it becomes an unconscious signal for your mind and body to relax. This breathing will create chemical changes in your body that will make you relax automatically. You can do it when you are walking, taking a work break or any time when you need release. It can also be used to bring relief in a stressful situation.

Chest breathing occurs when your breathing becomes rapid. It may be useful in certain situations; however it can become a habit and is very unhealthy if maintained as a regular breathing pattern.

Generally, chest breathing will overstress and tire rather than relax the body. People with chronic chest breathing patterns will often have a tense and tight abdomen. Chest breathing is the type of breathing used in hyperventilation. When we hyperventilate we actually utilise less oxygen. Those people with severe hyperventilation problems often gasp, sigh, yawn and feel breathless.

The tendency to predominantly chest breathe is very common in our society. This is because we have "unlearnt" our natural breathing pattern of babyhood. This has a lot to do with the encouraged body image of "chest out and tummy in", which forces us to breathe in a shallow manner. Daily stress and anxiety is also a contributing factor.

Exercise: Place your hands on your upper chest area. As you inhale force your chest upwards and outwards so the air moves into the upper portion of your lungs only. Feel the expansion of your chest beneath your fingers. This is chest breathing — the abdomen remains still and only the chest expands. Repeat the breath five or six times only. Observe how this style of breath makes you feel.

There is nothing wrong with using the upper portion of your lungs, as you do in chest breathing. The problem arises when you use *only* the upper portion. It is better to utilise the whole of your lung cavity, as is the case with diaphragmatic breathing.

DIAPHRAGMATIC BREATHING

This is the best way to breathe for your overall health. It is the normal, natural way we are all designed to breathe but many of us lose the habit during childhood and as a result breathe poorly.

When you breathe in this manner, the air is taken down into the abdominal region filling your lower lungs first, and then the middle and upper regions. Your breathing quietens and slows. More oxygen is released into the body tissues and less muscular effort is used in breathing (thus less energy is wasted). With the proper balance of gases, your metabolism improves and less lactic acid is produced.

You can use the exercise opposite to improve diaphragmatic breathing.

BREATH AS A TOOL

Once you understand the nature of the breath and how it can be manipulated, you can begin to use it as a tool in everyday life.

You can use it to calm the emotions and alleviate stress. Notice how your breathing increases and how you tense your abdomen and hold your breath when you are under pressure or feeling angry, anxious or afraid. Try three or four long diaphragmatic breaths (see opposite) and you will be able to deal much better with any situation.

The breath can also be used to combat tiredness. Often we become tired because the body is not receiving enough oxygen to function at optimum level. Learning to breathe well will help greatly with fatigue.

In turn, an increase in relaxation and energy levels will stimulate the working of the immune system, improving overall health.

The value of breath work has been recognised for thousands of years by Eastern culture. Today the breath is an intrinsic part of many physical therapies such as THE FELDENKRAIS METHOD, THE ALEXANDER TECHNIQUE, SHIATSU and YOGA. If you are interested in learning more about the power of the breath, try attending classes or visiting practitioners within these disciplines. There is also extensive information available on self-help breathing techniques in books and on tape, and several yoga breathing exercises are included in this book; see page 187.

IMPORTANT

It is a general rule that if you are prone to respiratory problems you should only do breathing exercises under the supervision of a breathing specialist. Unsupervised breathing exercises can cause hyperventilation, headaches and even asthma attacks.

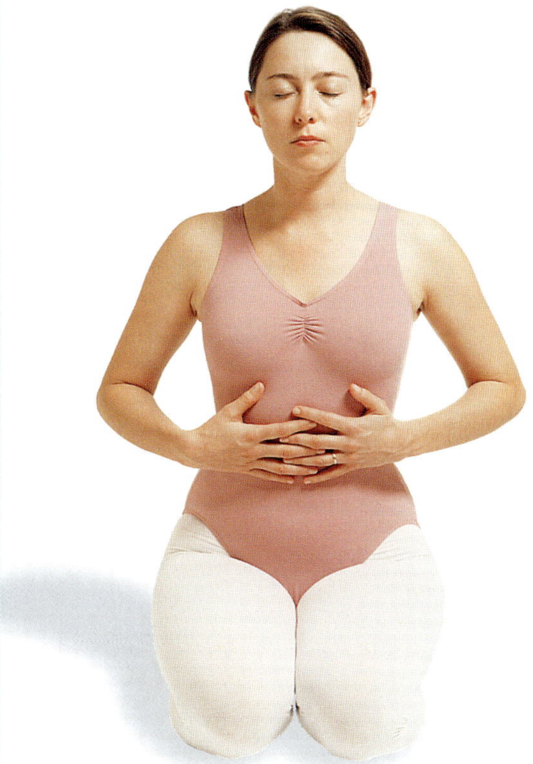

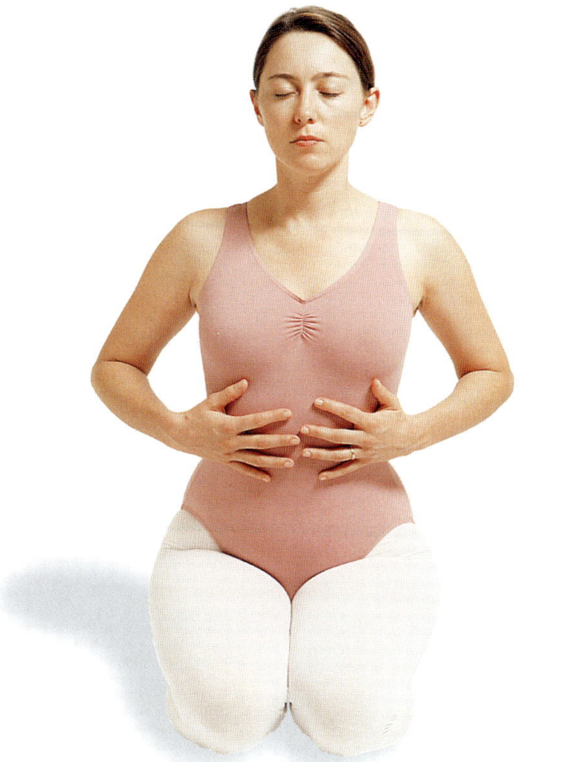

DIAPHRAGMATIC BREATHING EXERCISE:

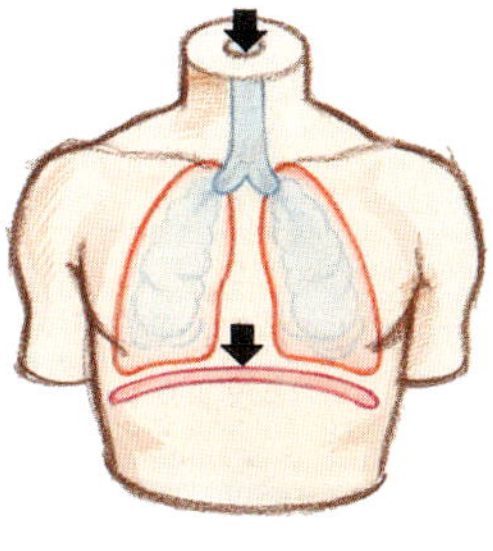

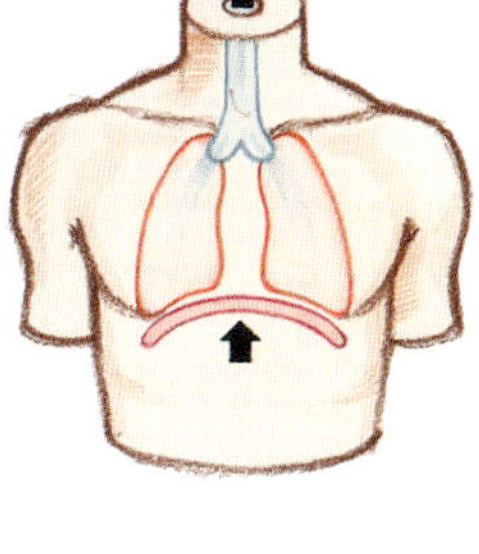

Place your hands above your waist with your fingers interlaced on the stomach. As you breathe in, allow the air to travel down into the abdominal area. Feel the stomach area filling and rising. Let the tummy be loose and relaxed. If you are breathing in the proper diaphragmatic way, you will notice your fingers moving outwards on each side and a space forming between the fingertips of each hand.

As you practise the diaphragmatic breath, notice how calm and relaxed this style of breathing makes you feel. Compare it with the effect of chest breathing. From time to time, practise breathing with the diaphragm and before long this method of breathing will seem completely natural once again.

In essence, the breath comes naturally with the rhythmic contraction and relaxation of the diaphragm. You can feel your diaphragm as the dome-shaped muscle between your ribs and abdominal cavity. When you use your diaphragm to inhale, it contracts, flattens and moves downwards, increasing space in your chest so that air is sucked into the lower lungs. As the diaphragm relaxes and moves up into your chest, air is forced out of the lungs.

THE BUTEYKO BREATHING TECHNIQUE

The quality of breath has become paramount in the discovery of ways to control debilitating conditions like asthma, emphysema and breathing disorders such as sleep apnoea (where breathing pauses during sleep), and for those who rely on breathing in their work or anyone involved in physical labour.

The effectiveness of breathing techniques is particularly attractive given the side effects of bronchodilator medication and other asthma drugs, but care should be taken in reducing any steroid medication and only in consultation with a doctor and a breathing specialist.

One very effective method of breath control is the Buteyko Breathing Technique.

The technique has been gaining international recognition since its development in Russia in the 1960s by Dr Konstantin Pavlovich Buteyko. It achieved a greater than 90 percent success rate in trials held at the Hospital for Children in Moscow with children suffering from asthma. An Australian study showed asthmatics were able to reduce the use of bronchodilators by 90 percent after six weeks and steroids by 50 percent after three months.

The technique uses breath-control to alter your breathing pattern. The average asthmatic is known to hyperventilate or "over-breathe" three to five times the recommended amount. It is simply the hyperventilation that can and often does trigger an asthma attack.

Hyperventilation triggers an asthma attack because it causes a loss of carbon dioxide (CO_2) from the body. This is a problem because when the level of CO_2 is too low the lungs spasm, thus the body uses CO_2 as a marker for correct breathing.

The correct level of CO_2 in the lungs is 6.5 percent. If it gets down to 2.5 percent the body systems begin to shut down. When the body gets used to a low CO_2 level chronic problems like asthma can develop from the body's automatic defence mechanism.

The theory that the body has an automatic defence mechanism when it thinks the CO_2 level is too low, was formulated by Buteyko. The defence mechanism is as follows:

- the bronchi and blood vessels spasm
- the mucus and phlegm production is increased
- the production of cholesterol in the liver is increased which makes the cell membranes in the lungs and blood vessels thicken which means that less blood will reach areas of the body
- the blood vessels spasm to try to slow CO_2 release from the body, affecting blood pressure.

Carbon dioxide is also needed for oxygen to be properly released into the tissues. If you hyperventilate and there is too little CO_2, the blood cells become sticky which makes it harder for the oxygen to travel around the body.

The Buteyko method's object is to achieve the optimum CO_2 level — by altering a person's breathing pattern to increase the "control pause".

If you breathe in then out then hold your breath the "control pause" is the number of seconds before your first level of discomfort before you take the next breath in. It's the "space" between each breath.

The control pause is a Buteyko method of measuring the percentage of CO_2 in the lungs and the severity of asthma or abnormality of breath. A sixty second control pause is the ideal and ten seconds or less is not very good.

Buteyko should also help your nervous system to get back to a better state because hyperventilation or "overbreathing" makes your nervous system become hyperactive. Asthmatics can be taught to use the Buteyko technique to control an attack by enlisting the natural properties of CO_2 that dilate the bronchi. They can also be taught to alter their breathing pattern between attacks to improve their general condition and prevent attacks.

The technique is not hard to learn but it needs to be supervised and monitored by a trained Buteyko practitioner while your breathing pattern is altering, particularly if your condition is severe. Initially, you will need to attend workshops and classes. Children as young as four can start learning the technique.

PROTECTING YOUR IMMUNE SYSTEM

AN IMMUNE SYSTEM QUIZ

As a quick check on the state of your immune system answer the following questions:

- Are you easily susceptible to colds, influenza and viruses?
- Do you feel tired even after a good night's sleep?
- Do you take longer to heal cuts and scratches than you used to?
- Are you developing more allergic reactions than you used to?
- Are you less able to cope with stress?

If you have answered yes to any of the above, you're in need of an immune system tune up.

THREE TYPES OF IMMUNITY

We are all born with a general type of immunity which is then reinforced via our mother's milk. This initial immunity can be weaker in some people than others or contain a genetic predisposition for certain weaknesses or strengths. It is called passive immunity.

Physical barriers (such as the skin or hairs in the nostrils) and chemical barriers (such as enzymes in the saliva) provide what is called mediated immunity.

The third and most powerful form is called humoral immunity. It is known as acquired immunity because it depends on how your body responds when it comes into contact with each new bacterium or virus.

Your immune system has the astounding ability to recall harmful bodies it has done battle with, recognise them and then switch on the necessary response. This is the theory behind immunisation. You are deliberately exposed to a small amount of dead or weakened bacteria or virus. Your body reacts to it and then in later life the defence system has the antibodies it needs to immediately deal with those substances if it encounters them again.

WHAT IS THE IMMUNE SYSTEM?

Your body's very complex defence system against infection and damage from micro-organisms is known as the immune system. It is perceived as the system which battles with foreign bodies which threaten the delicate ecology of your body.

One major component in this defence is the lymph system. Lymph vessels throughout your body link up in a similar manner as your blood vessels. They start off microscopic and become larger and larger until they drain back into your veins.

Every cell in your body is surrounded by an extracellular fluid and it is the job of your lymph system to purify this fluid to ensure that your cells live in a healthy environment. All the nutrients that feed your cells pass from your blood across the extracellular fluid. The waste products from your cells also cross back to your blood. However, some waste products cannot pass into your blood and they accumulate in the extracellular fluid.

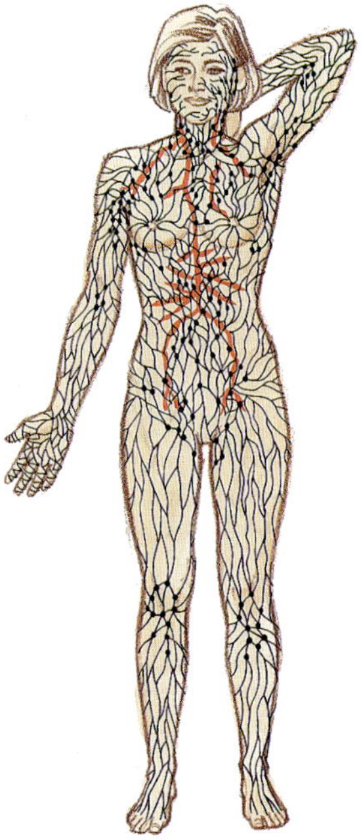

The system of lymph vessels spreads throughout the body, although the nodes are located in your armpits, neck, groin and behind your knees and elbows.

Unlike your blood circulation system, the lymph system is not pumped by your heart. Its movement depends on muscular contraction assisted by valves in the lymph vessels. This is why regular exercise or lymphatic drainage massage are of great assistance to your immune system. Lymphatic drainage can be poor, creating a polluted environment for your cells.

Meanwhile, the polluted fluid circulates along the lymph vessels and through lymph nodes. These nodes are found in your armpits, neck, groin and behind your knees and elbows. The nodes are a type of filter, filtering out infections so they won't spread around the body. This is why your nodes can become swollen and painful when you are fighting an infection.

In addition, the nodes — along with organs such as the thymus gland — manufacture lymphocytes, a type of white blood cell which fights infection. Certain types of lymphocytes also produce antibodies which are important in the "search and destroy missions" to rid the body of invaders such as bacteria or microbes. These antibodies circulate in the blood.

Your bone marrow forms another part of your immune system, producing another type of white blood cell. Your spleen is actually the largest mass of lymphatic tissue, cleansing the blood of foreign organisms, and your liver works to clear the debris such as dead cells and toxins from your blood.

THREATS TO THE IMMUNE SYSTEM

The most common forms of microbe to invade your body are bacteria, protozoa, fungi and viruses.

BACTERIA

Bacteria are micro-organisms consisting of a single cell without a nucleus. They are everywhere and most cause no harm. In fact, many kinds of bacteria are essential for good health, for example, those that are found in your bowel. However, there are bacteria that can trigger disease. They are able to penetrate healthy tissue and multiply in huge numbers. These bacteria can cause inflammation, invade or destroy cells and tissues, or produce toxins which can enter the bloodstream and cause poisoning.

Pneumonia, conjunctivitis and an infected wound are examples of conditions which can be caused by bacteria. Often your doctor will be able to tell what type of bacterial infection is causing a problem. The diagnosis can be confirmed by a pathology report.

PROTOZOA

Protozoa are single-celled animals similar to bacteria except they are larger. They are found in the soil, wet grass and almost all bodies of water, even the sea. Most are harmless but some can cause serious health problems. Toxoplasmosis is a relatively common form of disease triggered by protozoa and transmitted by cats and raw meat. It can be difficult to recover from and can cause severe damage, even death, to the unborn child. Other varieties of protozoa cause vaginitis in women and urethritis in men, and amoebic dysentery.

FUNGI

Mushrooms, toadstools, moulds, mildew and yeasts are all familiar forms of fungus. Fungi reproduce by spore and are found everywhere in the soil and in the air. Most cause no ill-effects to human health. However, there are fungi that do cause problems such as thrush and ringworm (which is not a worm at all).

Fungal infections are most common on the skin. While fungal growths on the body surface (such as tinea/athlete's foot) are preventable, they often recur because the active fungus may be killed but the spores remain in the skin's pores.

Like bacteria, useful fungi also live normally in the digestive tract but these may cause problems if their numbers grow too large or they move to other areas of the body.

It seems virtually impossible to avoid internal fungal diseases caused by inhaling the fungi in the air, but serious fungal infection of the internal organs, such as the lung, brain and sinuses, is relatively rare.

VIRUSES

Viruses are difficult to detect. They are so small that they can only be seen using powerful microscopes. Made up of molecules of protein and nucleic acid, they are not "alive" as such but they do have the ability to multiply inside a living cell. They are little damaged by temperature or by disinfectants.

Viruses affect your body by invading your cells, preventing the cells from functioning normally and making them instead serve the needs of the virus.

Viruses have been linked with countless disease conditions including the common cold, cold sores, measles, hepatitis, chickenpox and glandular fever through to cancer and smallpox.

Millions of viruses continually enter your body via your nose or mouth and are quickly destroyed by your immune system. Sometimes, however, your immune system is overwhelmed and you may feel below par for a day or two. If this condition develops into a cold, for example, then viral infection symptoms will appear. Your throat could become sore and swollen and phlegm and mucus are produced. As your body destroys the viruses, poisons are created which circulate around your bloodstream to cause fever or muscle pain. Your body will keep producing the number of antibodies necessary to destroy the virus. When this is completed, the symptoms of the disease will disappear.

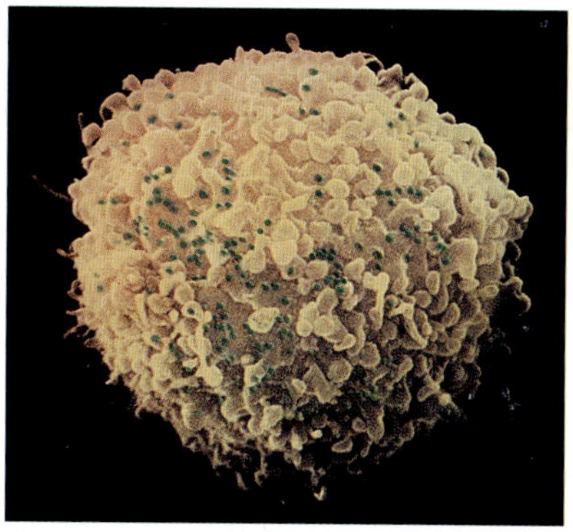

Lymphocytes are a type of white blood cell that fights infection. This one has been infected with the HIV virus.

INDIVIDUAL IMMUNITY

Often your immune system is called your body's first line of defence. This may be an oversimplification because your immune system does not operate in isolation from the rest of your body systems or your emotional or mental situation. It is inextricably linked with your whole being.

This connection with your whole being (along with a genetic predisposition and acquired immunity) is one of the reasons why some people will come down with a virus while other people who are exposed to the virus do not appear to be affected. It is not the bacteria, virus or toxin which is the real problem but how your body deals with it.

BUILDING YOUR IMMUNE SYSTEM

One of the best things you can do to remain healthy is to protect your immune system. This is particularly true for viral infections, as viruses are little affected by elements outside your own body's system; they are often unfazed by extremes of temperature or disinfectants. Prevention, therefore, is extremely important. Virus infections are best avoided by eating a well-balanced diet, exercising regularly, reducing stress, keeping your body at a constant warm temperature and reducing intimate contact with anyone who is already infected.

To give your immune system the optimum conditions it needs to restore and repair your body follow these guidelines:

NUTRITION

- Eat nutritious, whole foods. Fresh fruits and vegetables that are in season should make up the bulk of your daily food intake. These help to detoxify and regenerate cells. You can also try making your own fruit and vegetable juices as it is easy for your body to absorb vitamins and minerals in this form.
- Avoid toxins and artificial colourings, flavourings, sweeteners, emulsifiers and preservatives.
- Wash food well before eating to remove as much insecticide, pesticide and herbicide as possible.
- Avoid foods to which you have allergies. A naturopath can help you establish if you have any food intolerances.
- Avoid refined sugar, salt, alcohol, cola, coffee, tea, chocolate, and nicotine.
- Take mineral and vitamin supplements if necessary to ensure adequate intake of antioxidants such as vitamins C, A, E, amino acids, L-lysine, selenium and zinc — substances vital to your immune system. See pages 12 to 15.
- Drink bottled or filtered water — eight glasses a day.
- Avoid overeating as your body requires energy to digest food.

INNER CLEANSING

When your nutrition has improved to the extent that a cleansing diet will not add stress to your body, undertake an internal spring clean. It is best to do this under the supervision of a naturopath or other health professional. Many natural health centres offer cleansing diets as part of their service and this can be a supportive environment if you have no experience of fasting.

Inner cleansing is great for your immune system. When you are eating lightly or not at all, your body burns up fat cells — the same place it also stores toxins. Toxins are substances such as drugs and chemical poisons in the air, water or foods — pesticides, herbicides, heavy metals and the like — which accumulate in your body tissues. If this load becomes too heavy it can trigger allergic responses and even mood swings and depression. (See BOX on page 36.)

EXERCISE

Regular exercise is also essential for a healthy immune system. This is because your body needs sound circulation, lymphatic drainage and efficient breathing for the immune system to function properly. Exercise improves all these plus it can help reduce your stress levels, help you maintain your proper weight and increase the oxygen supply to all your organs.

Choose an exercise you enjoy, do it at least three times a week and make sure it increases the delivery of oxygen throughout your body, tones your muscles and increases flexibility.

MEDITATION

If you are unable to increase the hours you sleep then consider learning how to meditate. Meditation has numerous health benefits, expecially for busy people. See page 152.

REDUCE STRESS

Stress is known to reduce immunity. For example, you are probably aware of people who become ill around the time of examinations, stressful work situations or after the death of a loved one. It is often easier to recognise this in others than yourself. See page 40.

A POSITIVE ATTITUDE

Your immune system is unlikely to be in top condition if you persistently think negative thoughts about yourself and your life. See the chapter on THE MIND BODY CONNECTION. Try cultivating a positive attitude. This doesn't mean falling into "denial" by sugarcoating your life. Rather, adopt a life philosophy like the one expressed in the Serenity Prayer of Alcoholics Anonymous: "God grant me the serenity to accept the things I cannot change, to change the things I can, and the wisdom to know the difference". Even if you can't immediately change much around you, you can change your attitude and with time your circumstances and your well-being will also change for the better.

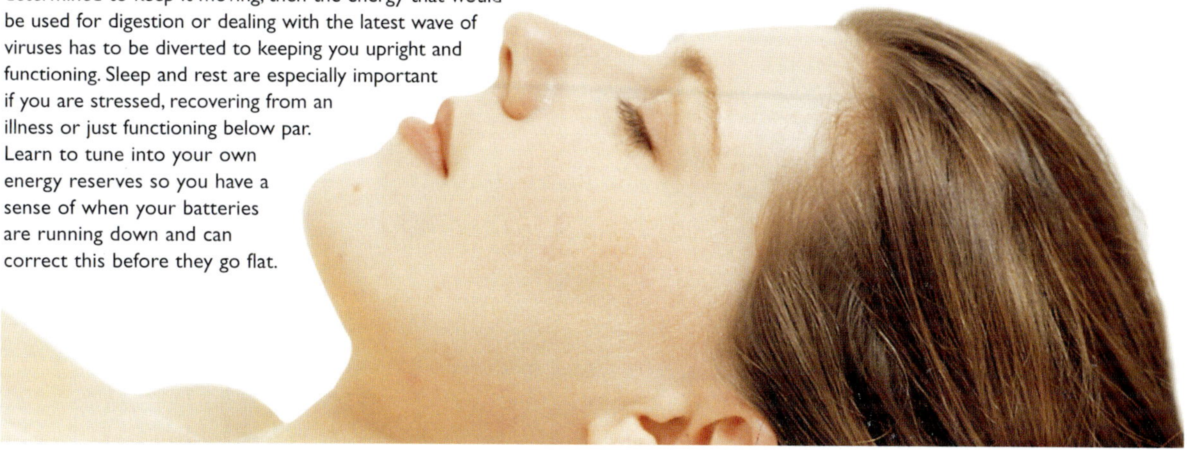

Never underestimate the importance of sleep. In our culture sleep is often seen as an indulgent waste of time but think of it this way: if your body is physically tired yet your mind is determined to keep it moving, then the energy that would be used for digestion or dealing with the latest wave of viruses has to be diverted to keeping you upright and functioning. Sleep and rest are especially important if you are stressed, recovering from an illness or just functioning below par. Learn to tune into your own energy reserves so you have a sense of when your batteries are running down and can correct this before they go flat.

DEALING WITH YOUR FEELINGS

A feeling of inner peace is as important as any change in diet or improved exercise plan in keeping your immune system strong. Unresolved emotional issues from the past and in your present will undermine your immune system. Counselling may help you find resolution.

HOW VARIOUS THERAPIES CAN HELP

A weakened immune system can lead to major health problems such as chronic fatigue syndrome, chronic allergies, chronic anxiety, depression, asthma attacks and cancer.

For a number of reasons, the immune system is not dealing with the challenges presented to the body. Often these challenges can be a combination of external pressures such as carcinogens, allergens and stress and inadequate internal conditions such as poor nutrition, poor detoxification, liver/kidney/bowel dysfunction and negative thoughts and feelings.

Various health therapies can assist your immune system and help your body to return to a state of balance or to protect it and build it to optimum level.

INNER CLEANSING FAST AT HOME

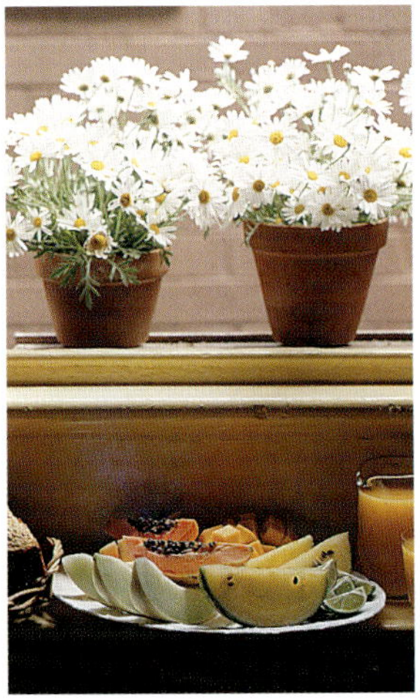

If you are in good health you can undertake a short cleansing fast at home.

Choose a time when you are not going to encounter much stress — over a long weekend is good if you work. You will not be eating so your energy levels will be low and it is best to remain inactive.

A few days before the fast, reduce the amount of meat, fats, tea, coffee and sugar in your diet and stop smoking. Eat mainly fresh fruits and vegetables, especially for the final two days.

Then for three to four days take only filtered or bottled water, plus freshly squeezed fruit or vegetable juices mixed 50-50 with water at meal times. Drink at least eight glasses of liquid a day, more if you are thirsty.

During this time rest. Make this your aim. Realise that your body needs all the energy it has to clean itself so sleep, read, listen to music and relax. Take short walks if you wish but don't push yourself in any physical exertion.

You may find you suffer from headaches, a bad taste in your mouth, indigestion, aches and pains, discharges or other flu-like symptoms. These are part of the detoxifying process and usually disappear within 48 hours. They are an indication that the cleansing process is taking place.

To end your fast, gradually add small quantities of fresh fruit and steamed vegetables. Remember not to overload your digestive system which has been enjoying the rest. It is also a good idea to add yogurt that contains acidophilus cultures as this will aid digestion.

Then move onto whole grains and finally protein foods such as fish, meat and dairy products. Do this over a few days. By this time you should be feeling refreshed and energised and your eyes, skin and hair will look shiny and clear.

A WARNING: Consult your doctor before undergoing any cleansing diet, particularly if you have a serious health condition, such as diabetes or cancer, which will require supervision.

ACUPRESSURE

As an addition to other therapies, acupressure can help to improve your immune system if used regularly. Although it can be used at home, it is best to seek the advice of an acupressure therapist to locate the points you will need to stimulate. Pressure points are considered in relation to each individual condition to support the defence system and weaken the antagonist in the body.

As a general boost to the immune system that you can try at home, activate the points Colon 4, Liver 3 and Spleen 6 (see page 87).

ACUPUNCTURE

Acupuncture can help stimulate your immune system and improve overall function. You will probably require a series of treatments and for serious immune system problems you could be advised to have acupuncture in conjunction with taking Chinese herbal remedies or other treatments, depending on the methods preferred by the practitioner you consult.

AROMATHERAPY

Aromatherapy essential oils strengthen the immune system by maintaining the vitality and health of the organs in the body. They also stimulate the body to protect itself from invading organisms and help it to eliminate the overload of toxins that can make you prone to infection. A lot of essential oils have antibacterial and antiseptic qualities (see page 99).

BACH FLOWER REMEDIES

The removal of emotional blocks that affect your immune system can be encouraged by the use of Bach flower remedies (see page 106). As a general rule, rescue remedy may help if there is stress involved.

CHINESE HERBS

There are many Chinese herbs that are known to stimulate the immune system: Ren Shen (ginseng), Huang Qi (astragalus) and Dang Gui (angelica sinensis) are among the best known. However, not all people simply need immune boosting — the aim in Chinese medicine is to make fine adjustments to the immune system that suits the individual. It is unwise to self-prescribe herbal tonics, particularly in the early stages of an acute infectious disease, as they have sophisticated effects that can suppress certain actions of the immune system while enhancing others. By self-prescribing, you may prolong the course of the illness rather than repel it. Consult a trained practitioner to find the herbal combination that best suits your own constitution.

CHIROPRACTIC

Chiropractic adjustment can help your body to heal itself and in effect strengthen your immune system. The adjusting of the bones in your body ensures nothing disrupts the function of your tissues and organs, which are connected through your nervous system. When your general spinal function improves, your nervous system function will improve too as well as your general health and immunity to illness.

HERBALISM

The herbs that are good for protecting the immune system include echinacea, poke root, St John's wort, thyme, golden seal and marshmallow. Rosemary, calendula, ginger and sage are immunity stimulating.

Apart from these herbs there are many herbal combinations and formulas available from health food shops that greatly help to improve your immune system. Five mushroom extract is a popular one.

HOMOEOPATHY

Various homoeopathic remedies are available over the counter that can relieve the symptoms of an infection, but for general immune-boosting a homoeopath will prescribe a consititutional remedy. Each client is assessed individually for a unique treatment scheme.

MASSAGE

Massage can help in your overall health plan to strengthen your immune system by giving relief from stress. There is also a form of massage known as lymphatic drainage that can be used by a qualified practitioner to stimulate your lymphatic system.

MODERN MEDICINE

Antibiotics can be extremely effective, even life-saving, in treating infection. They work by killing bacteria and fungi, but the appropriate antibiotic must be prescribed to deal with the particular problem-causing micro-organism. This identification may be made by a doctor, but making an accurate diagnosis may be difficult from just the observation of outward signs — a pathology test may be needed for confirmation. Broad-spectrum antibiotics are available which are effective against several types of bacteria. A full course of antibiotics must be taken, even though symptoms may have disappeared.

However, antibiotics (especially broad-spectrum ones) can harm the beneficial bacteria in your body (those needed for digestion, for example). As a result, common side effects of antibiotics include diarrhoea or thrush. The side effects of some antibiotics may lead to photosensitivity, stained teeth, nutritional deficiency or even liver damage.

Some people are also allergic to particular antibiotics with reactions ranging from rashes and nausea to potentially fatal.

Overprescription of antibiotics can lead to the breeding of drug-resistant strains of bacteria. Too-low dosages can have the same effect, and may also lead to bacteria actually producing more toxins.

It is worthwhile exploring all these issues and limitations, as well as the potential benefits of antibiotics, with your doctor.

Because viruses are not really "alive", they cannot be "killed" and modern medicine has no real cure for them. Antibiotics have no effect on viruses and can only be used to treat a secondary (bacterial) infection that may flare up due to a viral infection lowering your body's immunity.

Other medication can be used to relieve the symptoms of viral infection such as general pain or a runny nose.

Some anti-viral drugs have also been developed and while these cannot stop the virus invading the body, they do appear to slow down or prevent the virus from spreading through your cells.

There have been some vaccines developed for bacterial and viral infections (see page 159).

Usually lotions and creams are used to treat fungal infections but sometimes the fungus can occur in various organs such as the lungs or the gut. These conditions are more difficult to treat and may require the use of anti-fungal drugs.

Immune-stimulating medication that synthesises the body's own substances is being developed with limited success.

You should be aware that some medication such as cortisone, cytotoxics and chemotherapy suppresses the proper function of the immune system.

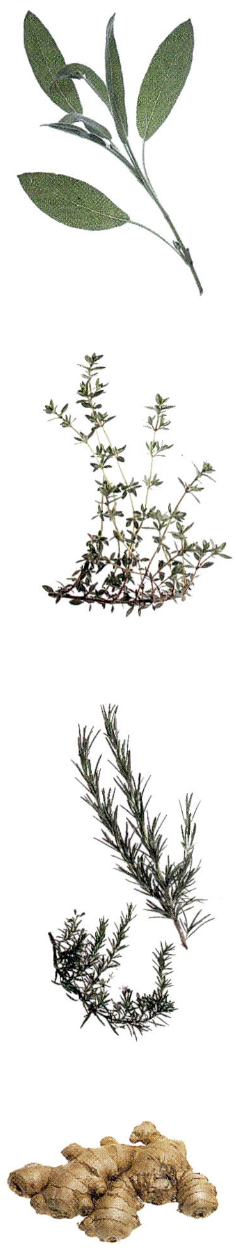

Sage, thyme, rosemary and ginger are among the herbs that have a beneficial effect on the immune system.

NATUROPATHY

Vitamins A, C, E, zinc, magnesium phosphate, and many of the B group vitamins are important for the immune system. A naturopath can recommend specific dosages and may suggest you avoid all sugars and test for potential allergens such as dairy foods which can greatly affect the immune system.

You can also try including immune-stimulating foods in your diet such as garlic, lemons, cabbage, cloves, parsley, carrots, honey, mustard, leeks, onions and watercress.

It is important too that you are consuming a full compliment of amino acids (complete protein) to manufacture antibodies and enzymes and to make and repair cells.

It is recommended that you avoid smoky atmospheres and reduce your own smoking as smoke can hinder the function of your immune cells. Coffee (even decaffinated) should also be avoided.

OSTEOPATHY

If the structure of your body is in order, it will help to support all your body systems. Your immune system depends on a harmonious balance with the nervous and endocrine systems. Osteopathy, by treating the neuro-musculo-skeletal system, can minimise or alleviate the mechanical stresses that upset the efficient working relationship between the different systems. Many osteopathic techniques are specifically designed to enhance the nervous, circulatory and lymphatic systems as well as ensuring that your automatic nervous system is correctly balanced. This helps control processes such as breathing, digestion and the release of secretions to fight the body's invaders. As well as gentle manual treatment, an osteopath can advise you on lifestyle, diet and exercise that can enhance your immune defence.

REFLEXOLOGY

If your immune system is low a reflexologist can work on points on your feet and hands to establish what parts of your body need help. They will then activate these points to help your body to function better. A reflexologist can show you which points you can use at home. To begin, try working the spleen, thymus and lymph; see page 172.

SHIATSU

A weak immune system in shiatsu terms is a weakness of defensive Ki energy in the body. A shiatsu therapist will "tonify" the kidney, lung, spleen and large intestine to strengthen this Ki. Total shiatsu treatments are a good way to maintain health and enhance your immune system.

YOGA

There is an ancient Indian exercise to strengthen resistance against illness which yoga teachers use today. It involved swinging a thick branch back and forth. Tension in the shoulders was known to increase susceptibility to illness, and this exercise loosens the shoulders and promotes circulation and therefore good health. The yoga mudra posture is based on these principles.

YOGA MUDRA

1. Sit on your heels with the knees held together. Rest the toes of one foot on the other, with the heels apart.
2. Lower your head and place it on the floor in front of your knees. Clasp your hands together behind your back.
3. Inhale and begin to gradually lift your arms towards your head as far as possible. Do not jerk. If possible, your arms should form a straight line to the ceiling.
4. Exhale then breathe normally in this position for a few moments.
5. Inhale and gently stretch your arms further.
6. Exhale and lower your arms to the floor.

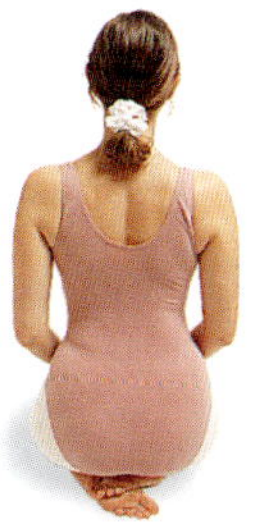

STEP 1

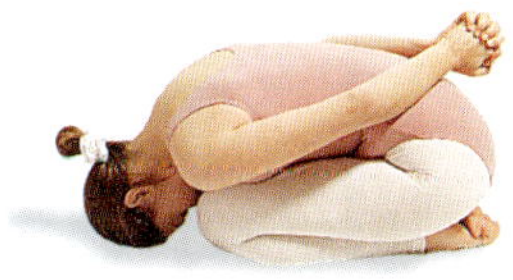

STEP 2

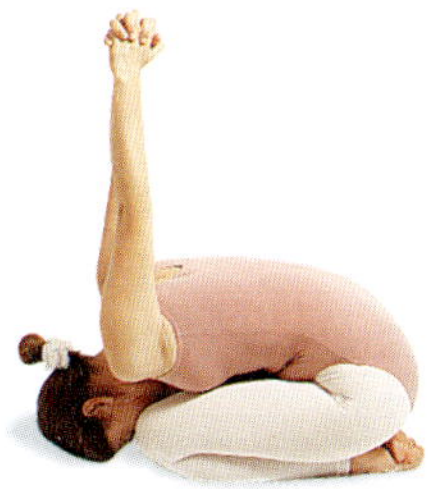

STEP 3

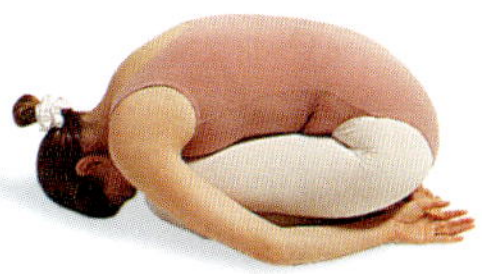

STEP 6

RELAXATION AND DEALING WITH STRESS

There are few people who do not encounter some form of stress during their daily lives. Stress is a normal part of life and it should be remembered that not all stress is bad. What might be termed "good stress" or "reactive tension" is what motivates you to come up with positive solutions to a dilemma. The stress you experience when you play sport or are excited by a new prospect, perhaps a date, job or social outing adds an enjoyable edge to life.

Everyone should be able to deal with occasional negative stress. The problem with stress arises when it is excessive or prolonged. Then it is as though your body has the stress switch permanently turned on. When this happens you can even become addicted to the stress. The term "adrenalin junkie" is often used to describe people who have come to rely on the cut and thrust of the stock exchange or a weekend dose of parachuting in order to feel alive.

For the rest of us, our stress levels rise gradually. Usually we are sailing along and then a few events occur and suddenly we discover we are no longer coping as well as we used to.

No doubt you can easily identify someone else who is stressed; you may even be able to identify the early signs of stress in others. But it may not be until you become ill or someone close to you suggests that you might be under a lot of pressure, that you realise just how stressed you are.

Your body reacts to stress. The "fight or flight" response is activated, which results in altered hormone levels (such as an increase in adrenalin), a change in breathing, higher heart rate and blood pressure, and tensed muscles. This response is helpful if you are fleeing from a tiger, but if you are upset because a friend can't make it to dinner, it is not only a waste of valuable energy, it can be very damaging to your health.

Stress impacts directly on the nervous, endocrine and immune systems, and because all the body systems are interconnected, the effects can be wide-ranging. The bodily reactions that are triggered by stress can cause physical discomfort such as an aching head, neck or shoulders and also affect our mental and emotional states.

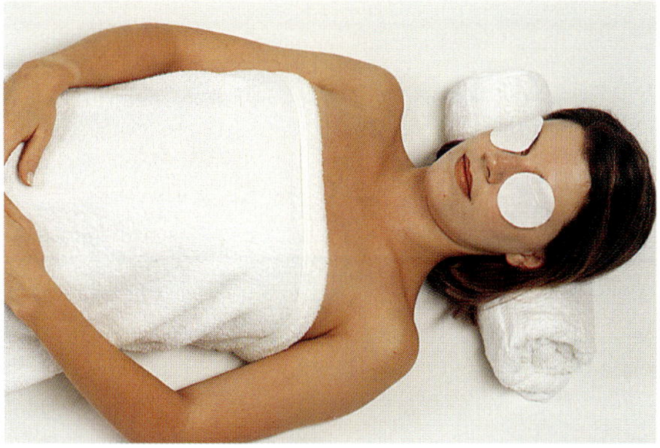

Stress is a contributing factor to almost every illness. If you leave yourself stressed all the time your immune system weakens, leaving you open to infection.

If you are under stress you need to find a way to deal with it. This can involve changing the circumstances or changing yourself. Often it is easier to start with yourself by learning to relax.

When you are relaxed, your heart rate slows down, your blood pressure is reduced, muscle tension decreases and the blood flow to your skin and organs improves. Because your energy levels are not being unnecessarily drained, you have plenty of physical and emotional strength to deal with day to day events.

HOW TO START RELAXING

Relaxation is something you can achieve by simply looking at a sunset or taking a walk. To relax can mean doing anything that helps you unwind.

But being relaxed is more than just not doing anything. You can sit in silence and still feel tense and anxious. Unless you were lucky enough to be raised in an environment that cultivated relaxation, you'll need to practise relaxing. After you have learnt relaxation techniques and have a physical sense of what relaxation feels like, you will be able to obtain this state in less formal circumstances.

To experience relaxation, try the following exercise. You may find it helpful to read the instructions — slowly — onto an audio cassette to play back while you do the exercise. Other alternatives for experiencing the process of conscious relaxation are pre-recorded audio cassette or video tapes, or you might like to join a yoga class which usually ends with a relaxation exercise.

ARE YOU STRESSED?

You could be feeling stressed if more than one or two significant events have taken place in your life during the past 18 months such as:

- the birth of a child
- the start of a new relationship or marriage
- the end of a major relationship
- the death of someone you love
- a move to another job
- a change in where you live
- you or someone close to you suffering a serious illness
- the death of a pet
- a new supervisor at work
- being overlooked for a promotion or a pay rise
- your child or children being ill.

SYMPTOMS OF STRESS

If you are stressed you may be experiencing some of the following symptoms of stress:

- an increase in headaches or migraines
- broken sleep, nightmares or insomnia
- feeling tired
- tight neck and shoulder muscles
- chest pain
- nausea or actually vomiting
- feeling out of breath, particularly when you are in a stressful situation
- high blood pressure
- skin problems
- diarrhoea or constipation
- allergies
- menstrual problems
- other health problems
- a change in eating habits, for example: a desire for sugary or junk foods or a loss of appetite
- feeling more like drinking alcohol, smoking cigarettes or using other forms of drugs
- feeling dizzy and "on edge" as if you could crack at any moment
- feeling tearful, moody or depressed
- feeling irritable with a tendency to get angry more quickly than before.

1. Ask anyone who make demands on your time to give you 20 minutes to yourself. Take the phone off the hook. Find a quiet, comfortable place to sit or lie down. If you wish, play relaxing music — ambient music, a relatively new form of music especially suitable for relaxation, is recommended because even classical music can tug at your emotions. What you are trying to create is a total sense of peace and calm.
2. Now you are comfortable, focus your attention on your feet. Experience how they feel. If they are tense or sore, mentally say "relax". Feel the tension in your feet go and let them become heavy.
3. Move your attention to your ankles and do the same. Then to your calves and shinbones. Experience how they feel and mentally say "relax". If you find an area of tension, breathe in slowly and deeply and imagine your breath flowing to that area. You might see it as blue healing energy. Visualise the blue energy ease out the tension and let that tension flow out of your body with your exhalation, perhaps visualising it as a dark, muddy colour.
4. Work up your body in this manner:

knees	chest	fingers
thighs	upper back	throat
buttocks	shoulders	neck
pelvis	upper arms	jaw and tongue
stomach	lower arms	scalp
lower back	wrists	mouth and eyes
middle back	hands	forehead.

5. Feel your whole body relax. Let all the tension go.
6. Allow yourself to drift for a moment. Observe your thoughts flit through your mind like sparrows. Notice how busy your mind is.

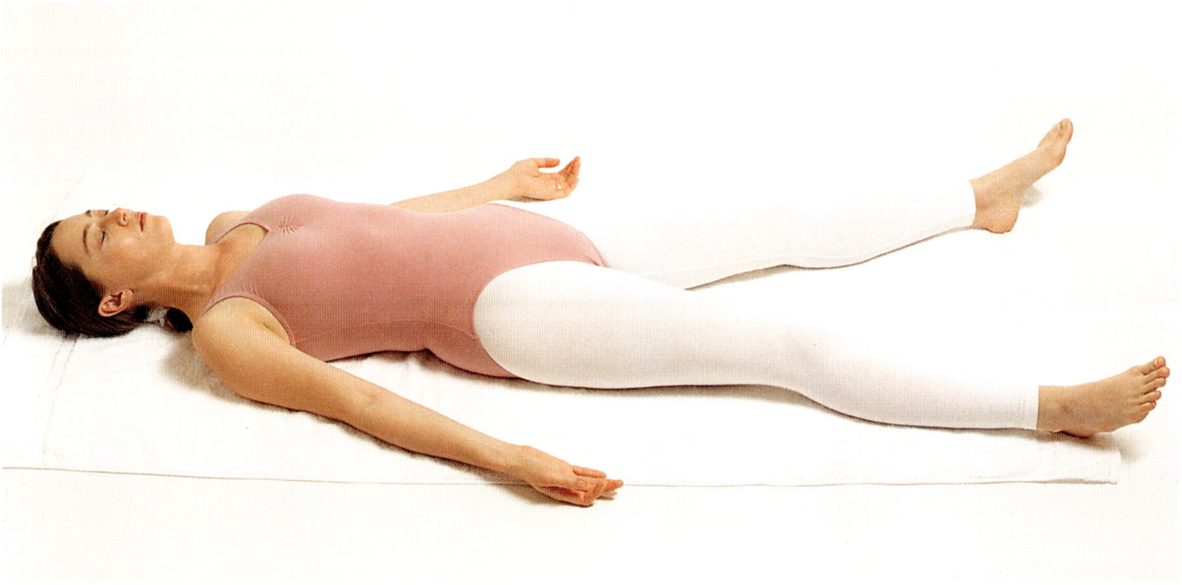

7. Now imagine you are walking down seven steps, count your way down from seven to one. See yourself in a beautiful place. It could be a garden, a park, a forest, a beach or any other place you associate with peace and happiness. If the images don't come clearly, don't worry.
8. Imagine this special place any way you want it. See the trees or the water, feel the air on your skin, smell the fragrance of the flowers and find a safe, comfortable place where you can lie down.
9. Now you are lying down in your special place, take your attention back to your feet and run through the relaxation process again.
10. Feel any tension in your feet and breathe it away. Then move up through your body, noticing any tension as you did before. You may discover that you can relax even further.
11. When you have completed relaxing all parts of your body, return your attention to your whole body. Notice how different it feels. Enjoy this feeling of relaxation and luxuriate in it for as long as you can permit yourself. Just let your mind drift. If you need a focus, use your imagination to take you for a walk in your beautiful place and discover what you can see.

You can do this exercise whenever you wish. Once you have mastered it, and can identify when you are holding stress in your body, you can do this exercise in a less formal way — for example, during your lunch break or on buses, trains or planes.

If you've had a tense day and haven't had a chance to unwind, give yourself a mini-relaxation exercise just before you fall asleep. As you lie in your bed focus your attention on each part of the body, beginning with your feet, and feel the tension drain away.

LEARNING HOW TO RELAX

- If you find yourself feeling tense, imagine your special place in your mind's eye and while imagining the tension leaving your body, say "relaaaaax" slowly to yourself and in time with a few, deep breaths.
- If you are feeling angry when you are stressed, shake a rug or go for a quick walk. Activity will dispel your excess negative energy and calm you down so that you can use your energy more effectively.
- Try to incorporate a relaxing leisure activity into your routine — at least once a week. You will be healthier and happier for it.
- Exercise regularly. It has been proven that exercise produces endorphins that create a sense of well-being in the body. Fit people suffer less from depression than unfit people and depression creates stress. Exercise also provides a healthy outlet for excessive nervous energy. Exercise frees you from mental restraints and gives your body a purpose. It takes you away from everyday drudge and can be socially rewarding.
- Be aware of your breathing. Your breath is perhaps the single most important stress-relieving tool you have. When stressed, your breathing is likely to be shallow. Make it deeper and fuller without force and you will soon have a greater sense of well-being. For more information see THE IMPORTANCE OF BREATH.

Sometimes if you have a restless night or disturbing dream you can wake feeling physically and emotionally stressed. Before getting out of bed, take a minute to two to relax each part of your body and imagine all the tension draining away. Then take three or four deep, even breaths. Now you are ready to begin the day.

NATURAL THERAPIES FOR STRESS

Many natural therapies can help you deal with excessive stress and better manage stressful events in your life. See also entries under symptoms such as ANXIETY, DIGESTIVE PROBLEMS, HEADACHES, INSOMNIA and NECK PAIN.

ACUPRESSURE AND ACUPUNCTURE

These ancient Chinese healing arts can relieve stress by clearing the energy channels in your body to allow the energy to flow. While acupressure works by using finger pressure on the relevant points, an acupuncturist will insert needles into the same points. For more information see pages 87 and 92.

THE ALEXANDER TECHNIQUE

This technique relieves the amount of muscular strain and tension on your body which in turn reduces stress. An Alexander teacher can do this by helping you to discover new ways of holding yourself and moving that are more efficient and less detrimental to your system. For more information see page 96.

AROMATHERAPY

Aromatherapy offers some effective ways of reducing stress in your body. Essential oils may be used in your bath or as part of a massage routine. They can even be used as a preventive stress measure: for example, you can carry a tissue or handkerchief sprinkled with oil on a potentially stressful day and sniff it whenever you need calming. Alternatively, have an oil burner in your office or home ready to light when you feel the need.

The oils you can use for reducing stress are numerous. Any of the sedative and antidepressant oils are good for relaxing the mind and body. The main oils in this category are: chamomile, bergamot, clary sage, jasmine, lavender, marjoram, neroli and rose. Your own senses will tell you which oils work best for you.

If you are feeling really stressed and need immediate help, see a professional

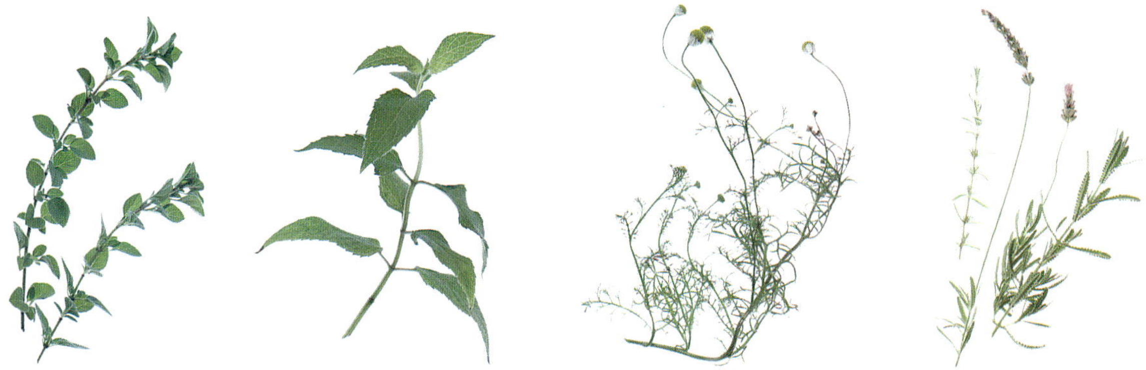

Among the essential oils recommended for stress are (left to right) marjoram, bergamot, chamomile and lavender.

aromatherapist. They will advise you on what oils are best for your condition and give you a massage to relax tight muscles.

For more information see page 99.

BACH FLOWER REMEDIES

Bach flower remedies can be very effective, although it is important to choose the right remedy for your condition. There are many causes of stress, each of which might require a different Bach remedy. For instance, mimulus is suitable for anxiety of a known cause, such as a problem at work or in your personal life or the worry you might have over the health of a loved one. If your stress is the result of shadowy causes — ones you can't quite put your finger on — then aspen may suit you. Rescue remedy is very suitable for emergencies and treating shock. Try it if you are about to sit an exam or attend an important interview, or if your stress is caused by the death or serious illness of a loved one. White chestnut relieves persistant unwanted thoughts, walnut is good if you are feeling vulnerable and elm if you are feeling overwhelmed. For more information see page 106.

CHIROPRACTIC

Chiropractic adjustment can be very beneficial as it reduces any blockages that may be irritating your nervous system. When these are released your body feels freed up and less stressed.

One common symptom of stress is stiff, tired muscles in the neck and shoulder areas. Chiropractic care can release the tension from these areas and give you a feeling of looseness in your body which will in turn provide you with greater strength to deal with problems.

For more information see page 110.

COUNSELLING

A counsellor can help reduce excessive stress levels by giving advice on how to avoid or cope with stressful situations. When you are in a state of stress, relatively minor situations can take on major significance. Simply talking about the problems in your life can often help put things back into perspective. Counsellors find that many people who suffer stress demand too much of themselves. For more information see page 113.

THE FELDENKRAIS METHOD

Once you understand how stress is held in your body and learn movement and breathing strategies to combat it your stress can be greatly reduced. The Feldenkrais Method teaches such a technique and has helped many people reduce their stress. For more information see page 116.

HEALING MEDITATION AND VISUALISATION

This relaxation technique is especially beneficial in the relief of stress. It involves learning to see energies as light in your mind's eye and making them work for you. For a detailed explanation see page 120.

HERBALISM

The herbs that are most often prescribed for stress include valerian, skullcap, chamomile, lime blossom, passion flower and hops. Your stress could be due to a variety of factors and the mix of herbs prescribed will depend on the other factors in your life (for instance, are you also overtired? Do you have muscular aches?).

You can try drinking a herbal infusion that contains the herb valerian whenever you feel a stressful feeling coming on, but for significant long-term results see a herbalist for a full assessment.

HOMOEOPATHY

There are many homoeopathic remedies for reducing stress that homoeopaths can prescribe along with suggestions for changes in your diet and lifestyle. Treatments are worked out on an individual basis. For more information see page 131.

MASSAGE

Massage is a wonderful way of relieving stress. Swedish and aromatherapy massage particularly will give effective relief, and can even be practised at home. For more information see page 135.

MODERN MEDICINE

Doctors may recommend that patients see a counsellor or psychologist to work on the cause of stress and may suggest an exercise program and other lifestyle changes to help you deal with stress effectively. Medication, particularly sedatives, antidepressants and benzodiazepines, is sometimes prescribed but it is not a cure and should be used with caution as it is potentially addictive.

NATUROPATHY

Naturopathy generally involves a combination of natural therapies. A naturopath can give you a complete assessment if you are feeling stressed and will identify factors like diet and environment that might be contributing to your condition.

Vitamin C (2000 mg per day) and high potency B complex (take as directed on the label) are the most important vitamins to take when under stress. Vitamin B helps nourish the nervous system and vitamin C is for the adrenal glands.

Naturopaths also recommend that you give up smoking and reduce alcohol consumption. These substances put an extra load on the nervous system by constantly stimulating it and this can increase stressful feelings and raise blood pressure.

OSTEOPATHY

All body systems are inter-related so by treating your physical body osteopathy can inflence your ability to deal with stress. An osteopath will use gentle, hands-on techniques to relax muscle tension, improve connective tissue health and correct the mobility of joints, including your spine. This will encourage good circulation and balanced functioning of your nervous system. An osteopath may also give you exercises and advice on lifestyle. In these ways, osteopathy can better equip your body to deal with stress. For more information see page 168.

REFLEXOLOGY

Reflexology is a very relaxing and non-stressful activity (especially for those who like their feet massaged). When a reflexologist discovers what parts of your feet and hands are tender, they will know which of your internal organs are not coping with the stress you are putting on them and can work to restore optimum functioning. For more information see page 172.

SHIATSU

Shiatsu practitioners are expert at relieving stress. The system of touch that they use is caring and gentle, and sometimes this alone can be enough to reduce stress. They will also ensure that Ki energy flows unimpeded through your body. For more information see page 178.

YOGA

Exercise is recommended to reduce stress and yoga is perhaps one of the best forms because of its gentleness and its calming effect. For more information see page 187.

HEALING MEDITATION AND VISUALISATION

This relaxation technique is especially beneficial in the relief of stress. Follow the self healing technique described in the HEALING ENERGIES chapter. Bring your attention to your breath and visualise the blue healing energy coming into your crown chakra with each inhalation. Then see the stress and tension leave your body on each exhalation. This may be through your mouth and nose or it could flow out of your fingers and toes. You may also wish to visualise this stress as a colour, perhaps brown or grey.

When you have done this a few times, run your attention around your body and notice any places which feel tight or tense. Focus your breath on these areas and visualise the tension effortlessly flow away from you.

When your body is relaxed focus your attention on how you feel emotionally. You may find that you can feel certain emotional sensations in parts of your body. For example, around your heart area there could be the tight feeling of grief, or in your fists you could feel anger.

Move around your body and sense each of the feelings separately. While you do this keep breathing in the blue healing energy into your emotions as you did with your tense body parts. Visualise the emotional tension draining away as effortlessly as did the physical tension.

Then focus your attention on any mental tension you may have. This might be a fear such as: "I'll never make that deadline" or "I won't be able to cope when my parents come to stay."Again hold your attention on the thought and feel how it affects you. Bring your attention away from your future fear and back to the present moment. Breathe blue light into that thought. Then visualise the thought dissolving. As the thought dissipates from your mind replace it with a positive affirmation such as "I am relaxed and capable at all times. I cope effortlessly with all challenges. I am at peace."

When you have completed your healing meditation, see the blue light leave your body. Feel how relaxed you are and take your relaxed feelings into your daily life.

Do this healing meditation once a day if you are under stress or whenever you feel the need.

AFFIRMATIONS AND VISUALISATIONS

One of the most powerful changes you can make in your life is to become conscious of your thoughts. There is a view that what you believe about yourself creates your experiences. And it is certainly true that your thoughts have an impact on your emotional and physical well-being.

This claim is easily tested. Try the following exercise:

Think of a person or a situation which makes you angry. As you bring this to mind, notice what happens to your body — you might feel an internal tightening or a quickening of your pulse; perhaps you feel a surge of adrenalin or find you are gritting your teeth. Whatever sensations you feel be aware of how they change you physically and realise that these emotions also alter your body chemistry, however subtly.

Now think of a time recently when you felt happy, loved and contented. Perhaps it was during your last holiday or at a family gathering for your birthday. Whatever the situation, let the images come to mind and feel the changes that take place in your body.

Perhaps you feel yourself relax, your muscles softening, your heart rate slowing a little; and you might find yourself smiling, the result of a feeling of joy. These positive thoughts also affect your body. Compare them with the sensations that accompanied the anger-provoking thoughts.

The above exercise can help you recognise two important points:

1. Your thoughts affect you physically, mentally and emotionally.
2. Thoughts can easily be changed; as easily as it was for you to swap from angry thoughts to positive thoughts.

NEGATIVE BELIEFS

We all have beliefs that we have unconsciously accepted. Usually they are established in childhood, and many of them can be negative. Examples include:

- Boys don't cry.
- Good girls never get angry.
- I never do anything right.

Some we accepted because they were linked to our survival. For example, if you were told that you would become ill unless you ate everything on your dinner plate, you might have believed this and still be overeating. Other unconscious conditioning may have come from the opinions of others, especially adults you respected. You may have heard statements such as:

- You'll never amount to anything.
- You'll be the death of your mother.
- You were a "mistake".

Often we are not conscious of these beliefs because they are the building blocks of our personalities, but they can be particularly relevant to a health issue.

As adults we tend to treat ourselves in the same way as we were treated as children. If you grew up in a household in which you were criticised rather than praised, or abused rather than loved, then you are likely to be unconsciously

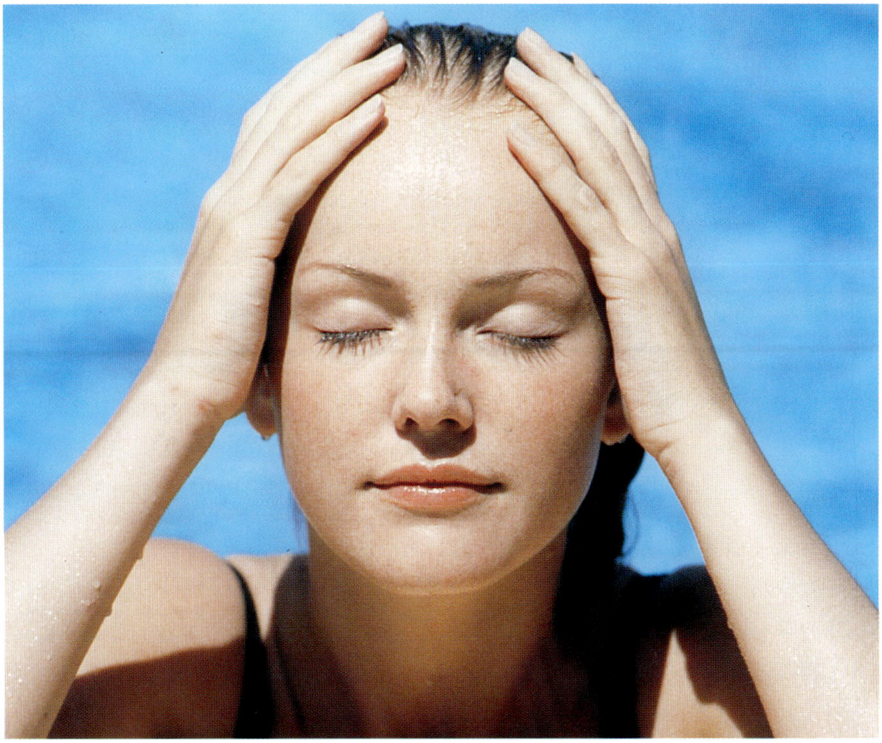

Affirmations and visualisations may be used in many different circumstances but they can be particularly effective when combined with relaxation techniques such as meditation.

continuing this behaviour on yourself. If you've been programmed with a lot of negative thoughts, it makes sense that your body might be feeling their ill-effects.

The power of your mind is such that you can change this conditioning, your "program" of thoughts, beliefs and habits. All programs can be remade, but it does require vigilance. One of the easiest, most effective ways of doing this is with affirmations and visualisations.

AFFIRMATIONS

Affirmations are positive statements repeated to yourself over and over again, either out loud or in silence, until their message is accepted by your subconscious mind and they are manifesting in your life. They help to "make firm" your new ideas and beliefs. The transforming effect of a specific affirmation can be used for health as well as in other aspects of your life.

Cultivate the habit of watching your thoughts. When you hear yourself say or think something negative, say the word "stop" or "cancel" and replace the old thought with a new positive thought. See the BOX for some examples.

You can also use an affirmation like a mantra, a statement repeated for the purpose of meditation. But you don't need to meditate to use your affirmation. Say your affirmations out loud or over and over again in your head. You can set time aside for this or you can repeat your affirmation as you go about your everyday routine, while driving your car, for instance, or doing housework.

To enhance the effect, you may like to write out your affirmations, sing them, or record them onto an audio-tape and play them while you are going to sleep. You may also like to incorporate them into a visualisation (see page 51) or MEDITATION.

Choose or make up affirmations to suit your own particular condition. To design an affirmation to assist the healing of a health or emotional problem take a careful look at the influences in your life.

If you have a throat condition, it may indicate that you have difficulty "voicing" your thoughts or feelings. On the other hand, it may have more to do with a food intolerance. You will need to observe yourself closely while being very honest.

EXAMPLES OF AFFIRMATIONS

OLD BELIEF	AFFIRMATIONS
• Everyone is out to get me.	• I am safe and secure at all times.
• I am a failure.	• I have skills and I now welcome success.
• Life is frightening.	• My life is filled with joy.
• I am worthless.	• I am beautiful and lovable just the way I am.
• I can't cope.	• I feel great. I feel happy. I attract all the help I need.

A good starting point is to focus on the 48 hours or so before you exhibited any symptoms of the illness. It may have been an emotional flashpoint or stressful circumstance that contributed to your ill-health. Once you have identified the source, you can create an affirmation to counter the negative influence, and use it throughout the day.

Root problems often involve basic feelings that destroy your self-esteem such as fear, anger, frustration, guilt, disappointment — anything which contributes to a negative frame of mind.

To create affirmations to suit your particular condition, you will have to define the basic problem — that is, learn to identify your true feeling by asking yourself what brought on the feeling. Once you have done this, you can create a positive statement which directly replaces the negative.

For example, if you find you are constantly thinking "I feel tired", replace it with "I have all the energy I need".

When you are repeating your affirmations, try to inject some feeling and enthusiasm into them, even if you feel otherwise. Act as if these changes are already happening in your life.

It is important that you make efforts to deal with the cause of your problem and use affirmations as a support, not as a substitute for action. If you have low energy, for instance, you will still need to closely examine your general health and either improve your diet and exercise routines or get adequate rest.

AUTOSUGGESTION

"Every day, in every way, I am getting better and better" was a phrase made popular by French chemist and psychotherapist Emile Coué (1857–1926). It formed part of his technique known as autosuggestion or Couéism, which was a simple form of hypnotism. Coué proposed that the repetition of a positive phrase (without concentrating on its meaning or thinking of it as a command) would empty the mind and induce relaxation. That phrase would then become implanted in the subconscious where it could positively affect the body and the mind.

Coué believed that the imagination was more powerful than the will, and that as long as the will did not intervene, autosuggestion could influence the imagination to heal all types of physical and emotional problems.

VISUALISATIONS

Another way to reshape your life along the same principles is to combine MEDITATION with visualisations, using the power of your alpha and theta brain wave patterns to by-pass your conscious mind and reshape your unconscious mind (see THE MIND BODY CONNECTION).

You can create a visualisation to suit the changes you want to make in your life. Read the example on page 52 for a guide on how to structure a visualisation. Experiment with different techniques and images to find what feels comfortable for you. Imagining your scenarios on a movie screen is one method you may like to try, especially if you do not find it easy to build mental images.

Visualisations can also be simple and yet effective. If you have a headache, you could choose to visualise the pain localised in your head as the colour red, bold and vivid. You may then see and feel it slowly losing colour intensity transforming to a pink then a mauve then to a cool peaceful blue.

It is important to involve all your senses whenever you visualise a new situation for yourself — see your new behaviour and beliefs, and taste, smell, touch and hear them.

The first time you do a new visualisation do it in two parts. In the first part see the situation as it is right now. For example, if you have chronic fatigue, see how you wake up feeling so tired that you are unable to get out of bed. If you are projecting this onto a movie screen in your head, you may also like to shout "stop" or "cancel" or see the screen go black or the image disappear in a puff of smoke — whatever feels best for you.

In the second part of the visualisation, forget about the first scenario and see only the best possible outcome of the situation — see and feel yourself waking up full of energy, being excited about the new day. Feel the fresh morning air on your cheeks filling you with energy and joy. See yourself leaping out of bed with such enthusiasm that you can feel it in every cell of your body. Taste your breakfast filling you with health and vitality; hear your family members and friends telling you how wonderful you look. See yourself giving one of them a hug and smiling and laughing because you feel so fabulous. Then see yourself moving with vigour and joy throughout your day. As you are watching yourself in your mind, relax and become involved with the scene. You are the director and the writer of your script. Create it as you want it to be.

When you next repeat this particular visualisation see only the best possible outcome — do not repeat the first part, your current situation.

When you finish a visualisation, go about your daily business and try to bring the feelings from the visualisation with you. Every now and again think of your visualisation and how you felt and recreate those feelings.

THE KEY TO AFFIRMATIONS

To be effective, the phrases you use as an affirmation should be:

- specific — contemplate what it is you want
- in the present tense — use "is", not "was" or "will be"
- in the first person — use "I"
- positive — state what you want, not what you don't want
- repeated — either in your mind, audibly or by writing it down.

If you are working on a specific problem, do your visualisation at least once a day.

You can also incorporate affirmations into your visualisations. If you are dealing with improving your immune system your affirmation might be: "Every cell in my body is full of health and vitality". You can then repeat this affirmation as you visualise energy pouring into your body.

AN EXAMPLE OF A VISUALISATION

Sit or lie in a comfortable position and relax your body. Begin at your feet and, as you take your attention to each part of your body, say the word "relaaaax" — feet, ankles, calves, knees, thighs, buttocks, abdomen etc until you reach your head and finally your scalp.

Now that you are totally relaxed, use your imagination to see yourself walking along a winding path through the bush or forest. As you walk feel the ground beneath your feet, the sun on your face and take in the beauty of the nature which surrounds you.

Walk around a bend in the path. You come upon seven magical rainbow steps descending into a beautiful garden which beckons you.

Walk down the steps, and notice how each colour lights up as you step — red .... orange .... yellow ....green .... blue .... purple .... and clear white.

The garden feels fresh and slightly damp, but you are intrigued so you walk through it until you come to a clearing.

There, in a brilliant patch of golden sunlight, is the house of your dreams.

Take time to visualise this house. See the detail on the windows and doors, look at the roofing. Notice what surrounds it and how it sits in its environment. Create whatever pleases you.

Now you have your dream house in your mind's eye, walk to the door. There is a key in the lock.

The door opens easily. You take the key and you walk through. Look at the key and notice its shape and colour. Know that you can come back to this house whenever you want and that only you have the key. You are safe in your house and only people you want to invite in can pass through the front door.

Inside the house you discover a beautiful room furnished in a way which delights you.

Take time to look at all the furniture and decorative features, adding touches such as fresh flowers, music, carpets and the view outside the window.

When you have done this notice that the far corner is set up like a cinema for one. There is a comfortable chair in front of a huge white movie screen.

Walk over and sit in the chair. On the screen you see ....

This is where you need to create a visualisation to suit the changes you want to make in your life. Whatever it is you want to change, you should now see the situation as it is in the present, then as you want it to be. (For advice on how to do this, see page 51.)

When you have completed that aspect of the visualisation, leave your house, walk back through the garden and up the seven rainbow steps counting ...7...6...5...4...3...2...1.

Feel yourself back in the room you are sitting or lying in, then close the visualisation. You may wish to do this ritualistically, by giving thanks.

NATURAL APPROACHES TO CLEAR SIGHT

Eyesight problems and their causes are many and varied. In some cases they are due to the natural process of old age; sometimes deterioration of the eye is the result of disease or physical malformation. In other cases, blurry eyesight can be caused by bad habits of vision such as straining. There may be double vision, problems with seeing at night or with depth perception. You may have a "lazy" eye or "crossed" eyes. Your eyes may become irritated or tired easily. See also CONJUNCTIVITIS and FIRST AID: EYE INJURIES.

Some of the most common eyesight problems include:

- **myopia** (short-sightedness) — when objects cannot be seen far away due to light focusing short of the retina. This usually occurs from a young age but may develop at any time.
- **hypermetropia** (long-sightedness) — when objects cannot be seen close-up due to the light focusing behind the retina.
- **presbyopia** — when reading or close-up vision problems develop due to a difficulty in the process of "accommodation" i.e. the lens's ability to change shape and focus on near objects. This commonly happens in middle age, as the lens becomes stiffer.
- **astigmatism** — caused by uneven curvature of the cornea.

The shape of the eyeball is affected by various muscles that surround it and are responsible for its movement. In many conditions, it is the tensions and foreshortening of these muscles that can cause problems in focusing.

Vision problems, therefore, can be assisted by relaxing and strengthening these muscles and other associated muscle systems. Living with defective sight or glasses is not your only option, whether young or old.

WHAT YOU CAN DO

Your deterioration of vision may not be caused by physical factors but can be related to emotional and psychological factors such as trauma, excessive anxiety, and fear. In some cases, this can be linked to a particular event. Such stresses can lead to muscle tension which in turn has a negative effect on the muscles of the eye that control vision.

Eyesight problems are more likely to be reversed if eye exercises are accompanied by an understanding of the non-physical factors that may be linked to eyesight. In addition, environmental and lifestyle factors have to be considered and, most importantly, the desire to see.

There are many therapists working in natural vision improvement who can be contacted through natural health clinics.

A lot of contemporary treatment builds on the work of Dr William Bates (1860–1931), an ophthalmologist who in the early 20th century developed a revolutionary method of visual re-education based on his theory of straining and the emotional and psychological factors he proposed as a basis of defective vision.

There has been considerable success in treating a range of eyesight problems, although the therapy is not intended as a cure for pathological and physiological problems such as cataracts, glaucoma or colour blindness.

RELAX, BLINK AND BREATHE

This is the essential principle of natural vision improvement, based on avoiding staring and letting go of the tension in your eyes. The technique involves:

- relaxing your shoulders, neck and jaw
- blinking your eyes a few times
- breathing easily and rhythmically.

You should use this technique when you catch yourself staring and when taking breaks while doing close work. Regular breaks are essential when doing any work that requires visual concentration, especially if you are working on a computer. A computer screen has an almost hypnotic effect on your eyes, inducing you to stare at it.

Other forms of relaxation include:

- closing your eyes for a minute or so whenever possible (e.g. while talking on the phone, travelling on a bus)
- **swinging** — let your body sway from side to side in a rhythmic, easy movement and allow your eyes to move along too
- **palming** — warm your hands by gently rubbing them together then place them firmly over your eyes, gaze into this dark space and let your eyes relax until the tension melts away
- **massage** — use stroking and light friction to your whole face, scalp, jaw, neck and shoulders (see page 58). You can also incorporate the acupressure points on page 57.

SHOULD YOU GET GLASSES?

If you have problems with your sight, a doctor will usually refer you to an ophthalmologist (a medical doctor specialising in visual defects and diseases) who may advise glasses, contact lenses or medication, depending on the problem. Many conditions that involved having to wear glasses in the past can now be corrected with surgery. Also those people who could not wear contact lenses may now have access to new kinds of lenses as the result of technical developments.

A medical examination is recommended for all eye problems to rule out other causes of poor vision such as diabetes or high blood pressure (see pages 268 and 234). An optometrist can examine your eyes for visual problems and prescribe optical aids but cannot provide any form of medical treatment.

You will need to get specific advice from a natural vision improvement practitioner to find out whether you should use glasses when you are practising natural vision techniques. This will very much depend on how bad your eyesight is. The point to note is that glasses will prevent your eyes from improving as any change in your vision (for better or worse) will result in distortion when looking through your prescription lenses. However, you may need to use them or other types of glasses (such as pin hole glasses) as a transitional aid. Prescriptions can usually be substantially reduced, even at the outset, giving the eyes a better chance to improve.

DAILY EXERCISES

There are several easy-to-learn and simply executed activities which will help improve your eyesight that can be done at odd moments during the day. They need to be practised regularly if they are to make a difference. Be careful, however, not to overwork your eyes — the idea is to relax them, not strain them further. Do not wear glasses or contact lenses while practising these exercises.

(1) accommodation — move your gaze from near to far and back again.

(2) fusion — focus on a near point, such as your finger or a pencil, and then beyond it at a further point, such as the opposite wall — your finger will become a double image. Then bring your focus back to the finger which will become a single image again.

(3) visualisation — while palming your eyes, imagine a symbol or image in great detail, as if you were really seeing it. This form of exercise can reactivate your visual brain and reprogram it with a positive expectation which will improve your capacity to receive clear images.

(4) the magic paintbrush — imagine that you have a paintbrush at the end of your nose that directs your eyes to one small point at a time. Using your paintbrush, draw an infinity symbol or number eight on the wall opposite you, moving upwards along the diagonals and downwards at the sides to activate both the right and left hemispheres of your brain.

WAYS OF SEEING

When looking an arm's length away, the eye can only clearly see an area equivalent in size to your thumbnail. This is because of the way the majority of light receptor cells are clustered in one spot on the retina. If you try to focus on large chunks of visual information, you will not see as clearly and the eye will start to strain.

To solve this problem, apply the "magic paintbrush" technique described above. Following the paintbrush will keep your head moving and make your eyes more relaxed and mobile. By moving your head to point your nose towards small areas of information, "centralisation" and "scanning" is encouraged. You will avoid staring at large visual fields and trying to see too much at one time.

Centralisation is the ability to focus on a small area of visual information at one time. *Scanning* is the ability to shift that focus from one small spot to the next, keeping the vision mobile and relaxed. The visual brain constantly needs new information if it is not to suffer visual stress. If the image you are looking at doesn't change in size, colour or luminance, and remains constant and stationary relative to the retina, your visual brain will cease to function within one to three seconds.

Staring is the opposite of scanning. Trying to see large chunks of information is usually accompanied by tension in the neck, shoulders, face and jaw, and a pause in blinking and breathing. The habit of staring underlies most visual problems and can be broken by blinking, breathing, relaxing, yawning, stretching, and using the magic paintbrush and "infinity swing".

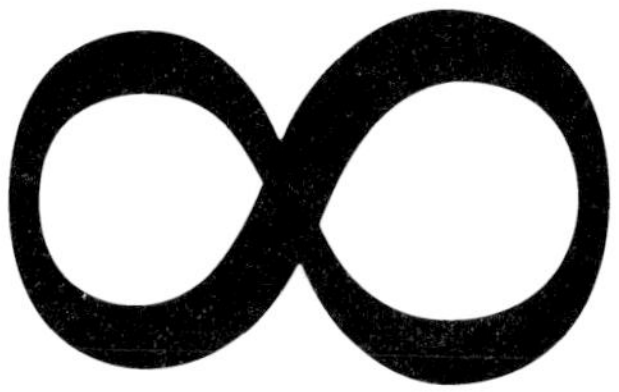

The magic paintbrush technique involves drawing an infinity sign or figure eight in your mind's eye.

POSTURE

There is actually a typical short-sighted and a long-sighted posture. You can imagine what these are as you either strain forwards to see or back off from seeing what is in front of you.

Good posture for close work is really a matter of common sense. The main things to remember are:

- sit up straight (use a chair with adequate lower back support)
- sit facing straight on to your task, not at an angle
- make sure your desk and chair are compatible (room for your knees and no hunching)
- keep a good distance (the distance between your middle knuckle and elbow point for reading material and 2–3 metres (6–8 ft) from the TV).

In addition, if you are working at a computer, you should be aware of the following:

- place all your reference material near the screen to avoid large head movements
- place the screen and hard copy equidistant from your eyes to avoid frequent changes of focus
- make sure your screen is 20 degrees down from your eye level
- avoid lifting your arms and rotating your wrists inward to reach the keyboard
- make sure the screen is at least 50 cm (20 inches) away from you. You can tell how far away you need it by observing your posture — are you leaning your head forward or back?
- fix any problem glare with a glare-proof screen
- yawn occasionally to release tension in your jaw
- "scan" your material using the magic paintbrush technique so that you do not stare at the whole screen at once
- look away from the screen every few minutes
- remember the golden rule: "Relax, Blink and Breathe".

THE FELDENKRAIS METHOD and the ALEXANDER TECHNIQUE can also assist you to learn impoved posture.

Poor physical habits (as well as injury) can lead to cranial and neck problems and interfere with the upper nervous system which will, in turn, affect your vision. These problems can be assisted by CHIROPRACTIC and OSTEOPATHY.

You will also find YOGA exercises to help your posture as well as ones that will work specifically to strengthen your eyes.

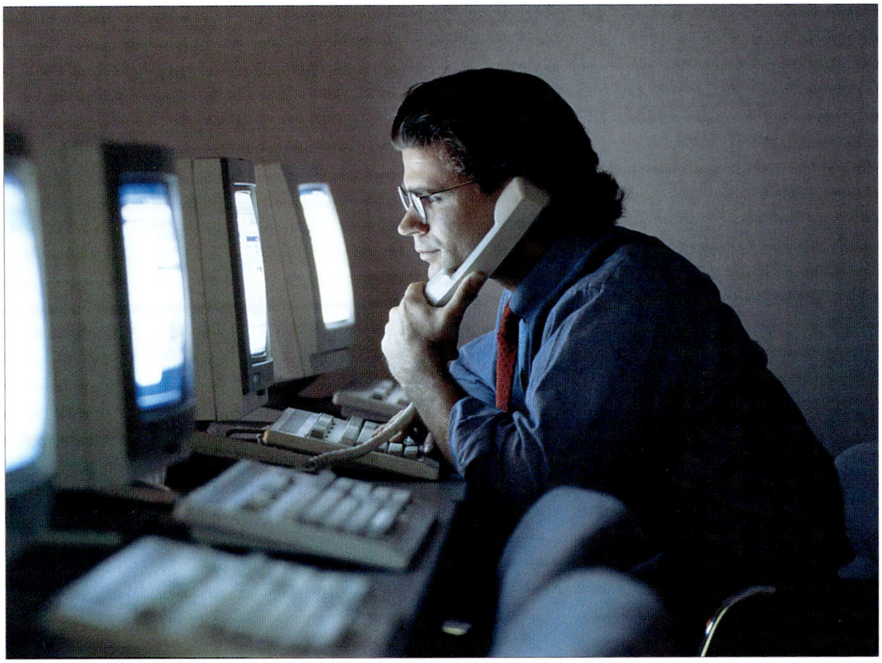

Poor posture at the computer can be the cause of eye strain as well as other health problems.

SORE, TIRED EYES?

• Gently bathe tired eyes in a weak herbal solution containing eyebright and golden seal eye drops in warm water or saline. The bottles should tell you the correct dilution rate which will depend on the brand. You could also try cool compresses soaked in a herbal tea, or slices of cucumber placed on closed eyes.

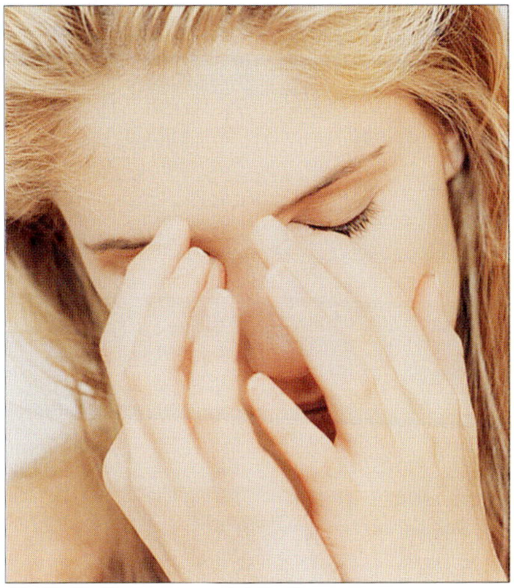

• Eye problems can be alleviated by stimulating stagnant energy in your body through shiatsu massage or acupuncture. For tired eyes with an ache behind them, you can try the following acupressure points at home: Bladder 1, Liver 3 and 4, and Taiyang (see page 91). (They may also prevent a migraine which is often associated with this kind of pain.)

• For all problems with the eyes, try activating the reflexology points for the eyes and kidneys plus all the fingers or toes as these correspond to the head area. Do this on both feet or hands for a total of 15 minutes twice weekly. See page 172.

CORRECT LIGHTING

Natural light is the best but if this is not possible use incandescent (not fluorescent) light bulbs of 150 to 200 watts. Fit these into overhead or table lamps; the wattage is too strong for reading lamps. For a reading lamp whose bulb is contained within a small shade area which could cause overheating, you should use a special reflector bulb with a wattage of about 60, but make sure the light is directed on your work.

NUTRITION

Vitamins A, C and B complex can help your eyes. These can be taken in tablet form or through your diet. Calcium, magnesium and silica can also be of benefit. See the table on pages 12 to 15. For further information on how certain foods can improve your vision, a naturopath may be consulted.

ATTITUDE

Most physical tensions have an emotional factor, and attitude to your eyesight is a crucial factor in vision improvement. Trying too hard to see will only increase tension; relax with your vision to allow it to improve. If you believe your eyesight will deteriorate no matter what you do, then that is likely to happen. There have also been cases where the eyesight of a person has been dramatically improved when some aspect of their life has been properly examined and dealt with.

RELAXING SELF-MASSAGE

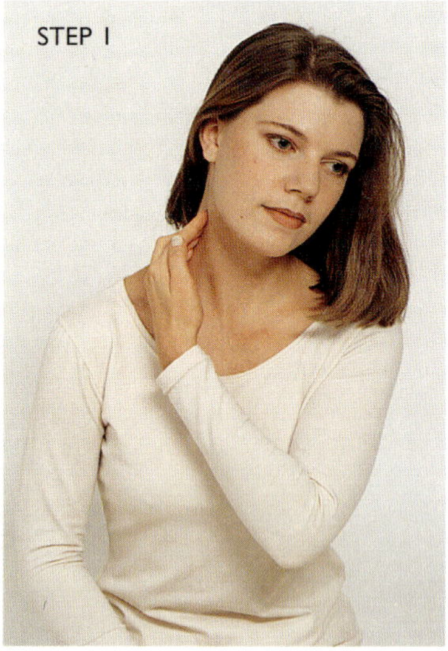

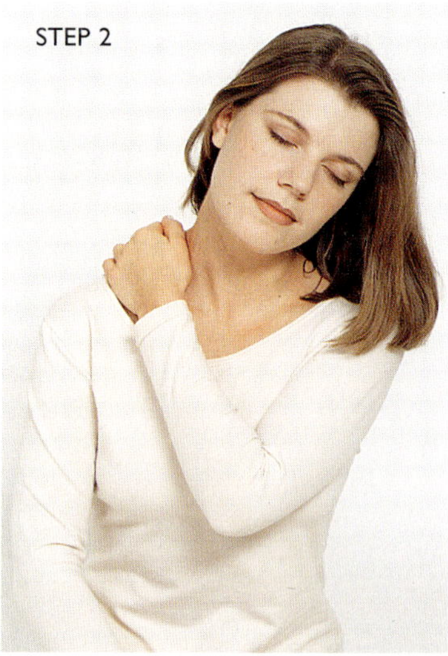

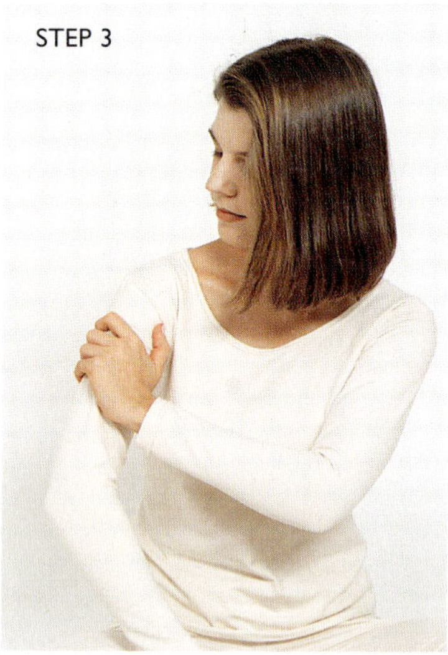

NECK AND SHOULDERS

1. With palm and fingers, stroke from the base of your scalp to the collarbone. This will gently relax the neck muscles. Work both sides.

2. Bringing one hand across your body to your other shoulder, knead the area by squeezing and releasing.

3. Continue this movement all the way down the arm to the wrist, and then back up again.

4. Work your shoulder area more deeply, with finger tip frictions.

5. Repeat steps 2 to 4 to other side of your body, using the other hand.

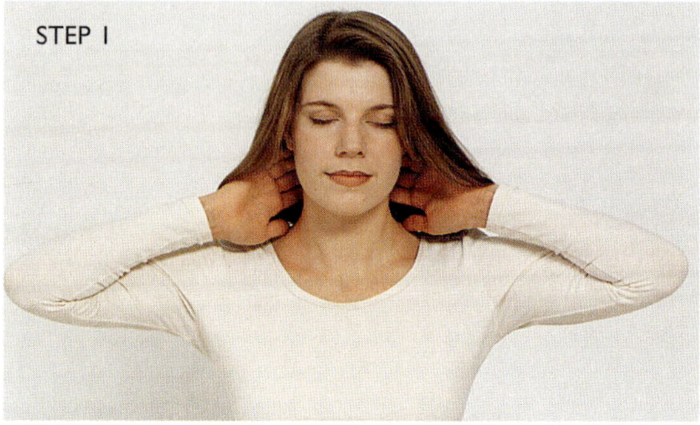

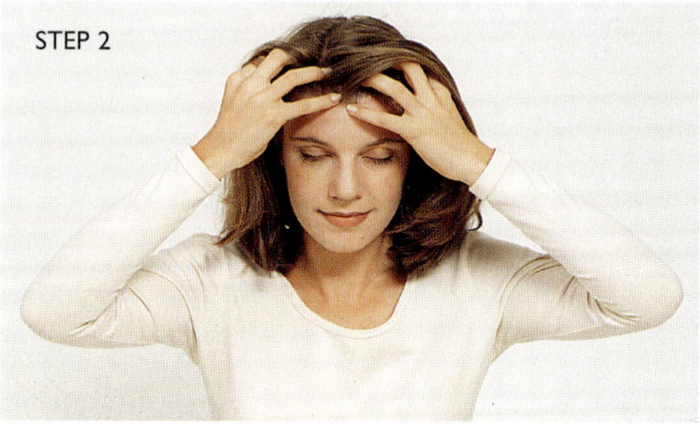

SCALP

1. Moving to the base of your skull, start just behind the ears and work around the ridge to the middle of your neck, using small deep finger frictions. You are likely to find many tender spots in this area. If you find one, work gradually to soothe away the tension.

2. Follow this movement with a relaxing massage to the whole scalp, using all your fingers in small circular movements. Feel the skin move under your fingertips.

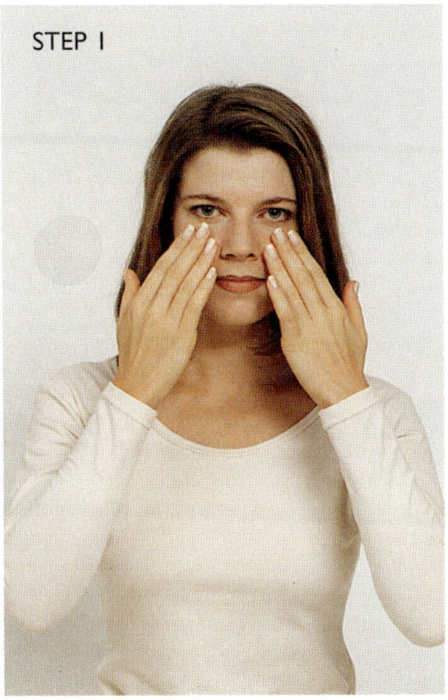

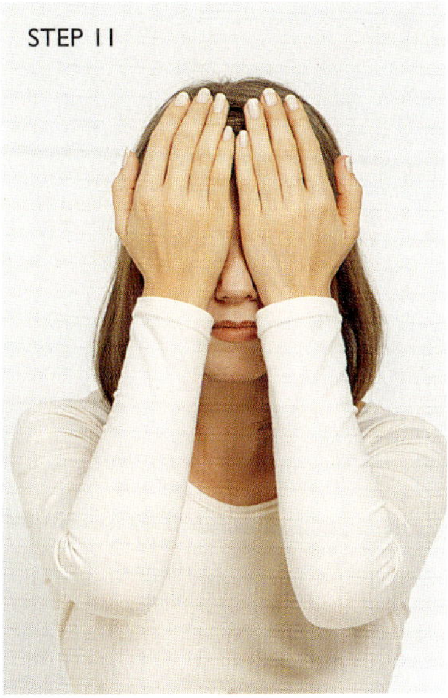

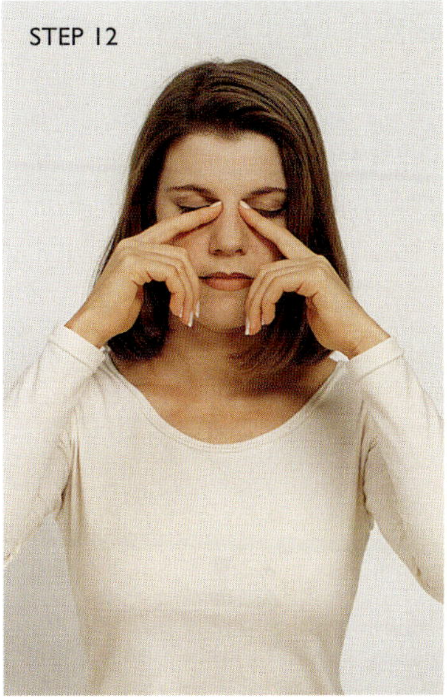

FACE

1. Stroke over the cheek area with your fingertips.

2. Smooth the nose area and over your lips with your fingertips.

3. Stroke along your jaw line from chin to your ears.

4. Knead the chin area by gently squeezing and releasing along the jaw line. Use your thumbs and fingers and work from the chin to the ears.

5. Squeeze along the edge of your ears.

6. Very gently "slap" your face, your cheeks, and neck.

7. With small circular movements, massage the mouth and cheek area.

8. Use the same movements to massage along the sides of your nose.

9. Very carefully massage around the eyes with the pads of fingers, not forgetting to stroke your eyelids.

10. Stroke over your eyebrows with your fingers.

11. Rub your hands together until they are warm, and then place palms or fingers over your eyes, applying a gentle pressure. Stay like this for a minute or so. Feel the penetrating warmth. It is surprising how comforting and relaxing this simple movement is. You can use it during the day to relieve tired eyes.

12. Using your index or middle fingers, press each side of the eye socket at the top of your nose, as illustrated. Be careful of long fingernails. Hold for several seconds.

13. Now massage the whole of your forehead and temple area using the pads of fingers in small circular movements.

14. Finish by gently stroking your entire face, and running fingers softly down your throat.

15. Your self-massage is now complete. Allow yourself some time to relax before slowly rising.

NATURAL THERAPIES FOR PREGNANT WOMEN

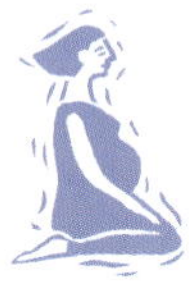

Pregnancy is a major life experience which you can enhance by combining the best modern medicine has to offer with the age-old wisdom of many other health therapies. Refer to the A–Z of Health Conditions (page 211 to 385) for advice about problems such as Sciatica, Fatigue, Insomnia, Constipation, Digestive Problems, Blood Pressure Problems, Haemorrhoids and Fluid Retention.

Take heed, however, of warnings below about specific natural therapies which are not suitable when you are pregnant. It is always best to consult a qualified practitioner and to tell them that you are pregnant.

CONSCIOUS CONCEPTION

Conscious conception is where you make a deliberate decision to have a baby and then prepare physically, emotionally, mentally and spiritually. Ideally this preparation should begin about 12 months before conception as it's important that both partners are fit and healthy. In addition to the woman's egg, the quality of the man's sperm has an impact on all sorts of things, not the least of which is fertility. It's a good idea to consult with a range of health practitioners who can assist you with this process.

This could involve undertaking a detoxification program, increasing your levels of aerobic fitness, adjusting your diet or optimising health and minimising stress through activities such as meditation or yoga.

A VISUALISATION FOR MOTHER AND UNBORN CHILD

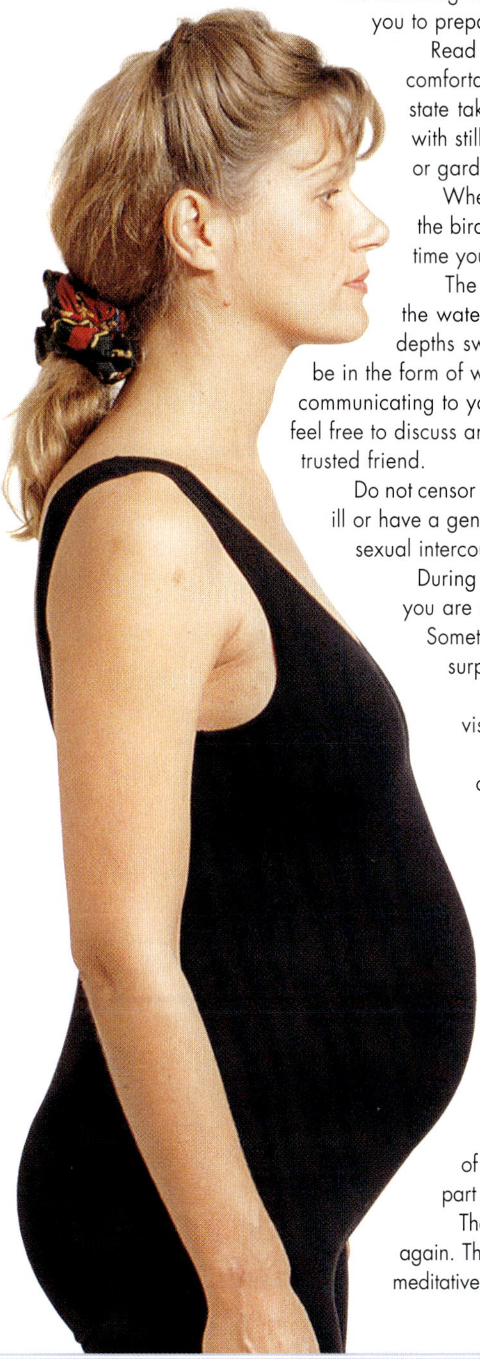

The following visualisation may reduce your fears during your pregnancy and help you to prepare for the birth.

Read AFFIRMATIONS AND VISUALISATIONS and prepare yourself by settling in a comfortable position and relaxing your body. When you are in a meditative state take your mind to a special place of your choice. Choose somewhere with still water — a windless beach, rainforest rock pool, crystal clear lake, or garden with a beautiful fish pond.

When you have chosen your spot, see the details of it (the trees, the grass, the birds); take in the smells and the sounds. Return to this special place each time you do this visualisation and make it your own.

The water at this special place is so still that it is like a mirror. You sit by the water and see your reflection in it. As you gaze into the water, from its depths swims up the face of your baby. Your baby speaks to you. This could be in the form of words, thoughts or feelings. You clearly understand what your child is communicating to you, knowing that the two of you are equals. Understanding this, you feel free to discuss any fear you may have with your child as you would with a close and trusted friend.

Do not censor your fears, discuss them all: your fear that the baby may be deformed, ill or have a genetic disease; your fear that you and the baby may die; your fear that sexual intercourse may harm the baby.

During these discussions do not censor your child's replies. Even if you think you are making up or directing the responses simply let the process happen. Sometimes you will not hear anything of value. At other times you will be surprised at what you learn.

If the conversation is long, you might like to save the next part of this visualisation for another session.

After you have finished speaking, the water ripples over with a silver colour. Then you, with the spirit of your child watching on, visualise the type of labour and delivery you want. Make this as perfect as you can imagine it.

See yourself in your ideal situation; see yourself surrounded by loving support as you capably deal with the contractions; see your cervix dilating without difficulty and your baby voyaging down the birth canal easily and effortlessly to be delivered into a calm and loving atmosphere; see you and your support people welcoming the child; see all of you happy and contented and wrapped in a cocoon of love; see the baby bond with you; see the afterbirth being delivered effortlessly; see everyone congratulating you on a job well done and see your baby take to your breast with gusto.

Add your own perfect outcome to this visualisation and relish each of the details until you feel it in your body, as a part of you and a natural part of your future.

Then when you have finished this visualisation, the water ripples with silver again. Thank your child for visiting. When you are ready slowly come out of the meditative state by wriggling your fingers and toes.

The best preparation you can do for birth is looking after yourself, physically and mentally. Other chapters in this book contain advice on how you can optimise your health; see RELAXATION AND DEALING WITH STRESS, for example.

ACUPRESSURE AND ACUPUNCTURE

As pregnancy is an energy-gathering process, some experts recommend that you avoid acupuncture and acupressure during pregnancy. The incorrect stimulation of energy flow in the body can result in abortion or premature labour. However, correctly applied these techniques can be very useful in preventing miscarriage, relieving morning sickness and managing other symptoms after an extensive consultation. Be sure to seek advice from both your doctor and a qualified practitioner before you embark on any treatment. Obviously, acupressure is not suitable for use at home during this time, except under the guidance of a practitioner.

THE ALEXANDER TECHNIQUE

This technique can be helpful during pregnancy because it can teach you easier ways of sitting, bending and walking as your weight and shape changes. It can also reduce the amount of muscular tension that is put on the body through movement. See an Alexander teacher for lessons.

AROMATHERAPY

A professional aromatherapist will be able to advise you on what aromatherapy practices are safe during your pregnancy. As a general rule, it's best to avoid all essential oils for the first three months of pregnancy, or for the whole term if you have a history of miscarriage. **There are some oils that all women should avoid during the entire pregnancy** because they can induce menstruation and deplete fluid in the foetal sac. These oils include: aniseed, angelica, arnica, basil, birch, camphor, cedarwood, clary sage, cypress, fennel, hyssop, jasmine, juniper berry, lovage, marjoram, myrrh, origanum, pennyroyal, peppermint, rosemary, sage, savoury, sweet fennel, thyme, true melissa, and wintergreen (this oil is actually on the toxic list). However, it is best to seek the advice of a professional aromatherapist before using any oils at home during this time.

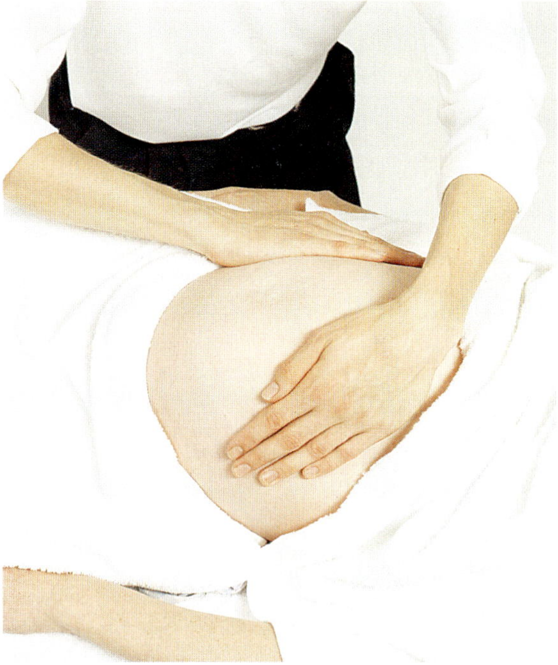

A gentle abdominal massage with suitable essential oils can be beneficial in late pregnancy.

Essential oil baths can be great for relaxation and relieving back pain during pregnancy, as can gentle massage in the later months. It's also claimed that regular aromatherapy massage can create a calm baby.

Massage from a professional aromatherapist during some stages of labour is an option — it can help relieve pain and calm you. Alternatively, the aromatherapist can advise you on oils to use during labour such as lavender compresses to soothe or clary sage in an oil burner to strengthen contractions.

After the birth, allow yourself time (at least 15 minutes each week) for regular baths with uplifting oils, particularly if you are suffering postnatal depression. Try sprinkling 3 drops of any of the following oils into your bath, making sure it is well dispersed: camphor, chamomile, jasmine, thyme, basil, bergamot and clary sage.

You can also use 1 drop each of lavender and tea tree in a warm bath to promote healing of your perineum.

BACH FLOWER REMEDIES

As these therapeutic tools work on an emotional, physical and energy level they can help support and nurture you and your partner.

Rescue remedy is great for reducing shock — both emotional and physical — at the time of delivery, especially if it is combined with homoeopathic Arnica which helps reduce bruising and trauma to your body. Take 4 drops of each a week before the baby is due and a week after the birth. You can take 4 drops of each more frequently (every 10 minutes) during the birth.

There are also many Bach flower remedies you can take to help reduce postnatal depression. These include walnut to help you with the change in your life, cherry blossom for loss of control, mustard for depression and sadness, and elm for feelings of being overwhelmed.

CHINESE HERBS

There are many wonderful Chinese herbs that can help prepare you for conception and assist you during pregnancy. They can also balance your hormone levels after delivery. However, because many of the herbs have such a powerful effect, they should only be used under the guidance of a qualified practitioner.

CHIROPRACTIC

If you are thinking of becoming pregnant it can be helpful to get a chiropractic adjustment before you do so to get your pelvis, lower back and spine in the healthiest condition to support your baby and assist with the delivery. Chiropractic care before and during pregnancy can increase your chances of a normal delivery.

Gentle chiropractic adjustment is safe even in the first trimester as long as your chiropractor has full knowledge of your pregnancy. They will not have X-rays taken in your first trimester and will only use gentle specific techniques when they adjust you.

After delivery, chiropractic adjustment can help restore balance to your frame, normalise your nervous system and increase circulation around your body which, in turn, will lift your mood and help to balance your hormones.

COUNSELLING

This is a time of change in your life and it's important to consider the emotional aspects of deciding to conceive. These can include anxiety about the change the pregnancy will have on your relationship, financial concerns regarding a loss of income, the need for more space in your home, and fears about the pain of labour or whether you will cope with the demands of parenthood.

With this in mind you might seek counselling from a midwife who is familiar with the emotional aspects of pregnancy or your health practitioner if they also happen to do counselling. You could turn to a trusted person who has experienced parenthood or consult a professional counsellor. Don't be afraid to ask for advice or assistance when you need it.

A counsellor may be able to help you understand what you are feeling and communicate your needs to others. They might also suggest practical ways to help.

For example, counselling can offer much to a mother with postnatal depression, depending on the cause. If it is fatigue, they may encourage you to accept assistance from others or help you to establish your priorities.

If your depression is because you feel alone, counsellors can support you in finding friendships

TAKING CARE OF YOUR BACK

If you haven't done body awareness work before your pregnancy, this is a good time to start. Lessons in areas such as the Alexander Technique or the Feldenkrais Method can help you avoid some of the back and postural problems associated with pregnancy. Even a course in belly dancing (after your first trimester) will increase your connection with your body and reduce the likelihood of you accidentally injuring yourself.

As your pregnancy progresses you will find that you can no longer sit, stand, walk or lift without some strain unless you learn how to do these common movements with some degree of consciousness.

It is best to learn from a teacher as they can help you adjust your habitual movements into the correct ones. On page 64 are some tips to begin. See also BACK PAIN.

SITTING

Push your lower back into the chair as far as it will go and keep your spine straight, your shoulders naturally lowered. Make sure your thighs are well supported by the chair, your legs slightly apart and your feet flat on the floor. Don't cross your legs as this can aggravate back pain as well as limit circulation to your legs.

Many modern chairs are shaped in a way that encourages you to slump. Where possible avoid these and seats without back support.

Don't sit for long periods. Rise every 30 to 60 minutes — take a break, walk, stretch. Remember to use the arms of the chair for support when you rise.

Give your feet a rest and ease swelling by elevating your legs.

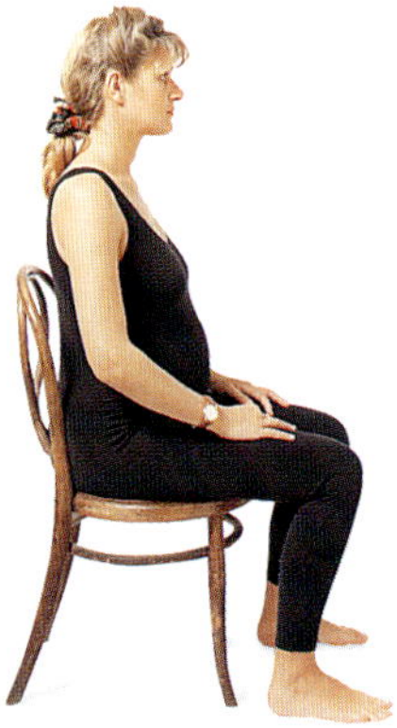

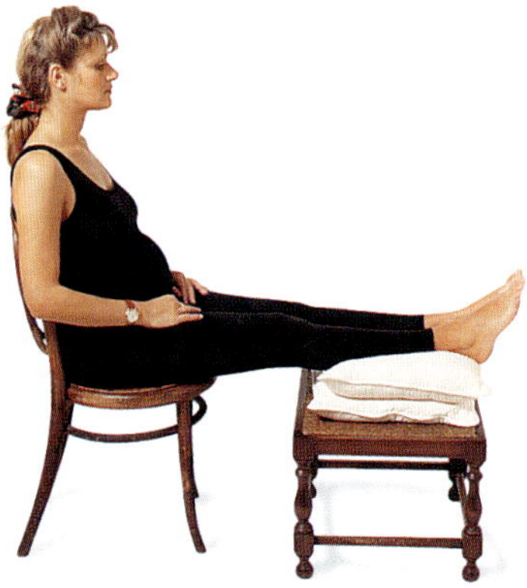

STANDING

Stand on both feet with your weight spread evenly between them. Keep your spine stretched, your head and neck free and your shoulders naturally relaxed. It helps to relax your knees and tuck your bottom under a little.

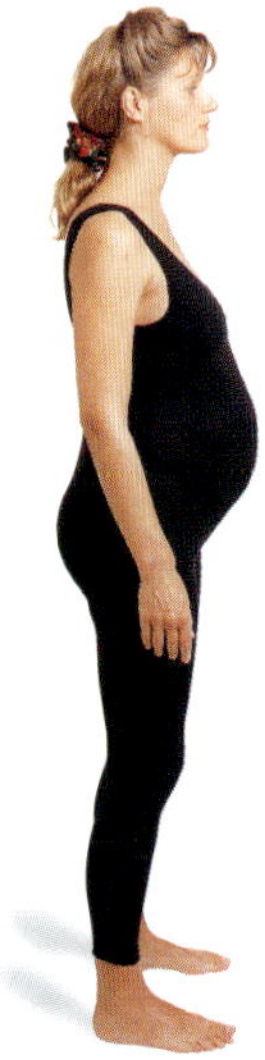

RESTING

To minimise back pain, try sitting on the floor with your knees wide apart then lean forward on your elbows. You can read a book in this position or listen to music. Take care that your lower back doesn't curve inward. If you keep your back straight, it will be supported by your abdominal muscles, taking pressure off your spine.

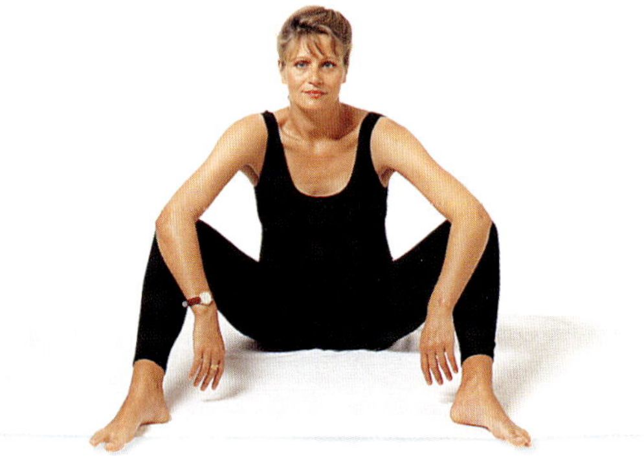

LIFTING

Squat down, bending your knees and keeping your back straight. Rest the object against your body and keep your elbows bent. Then use the muscles in your legs to straighten up. Do this slowly and as smoothly as possible.

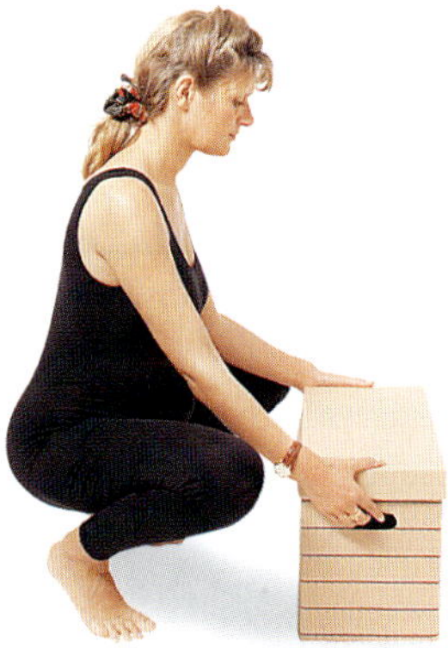

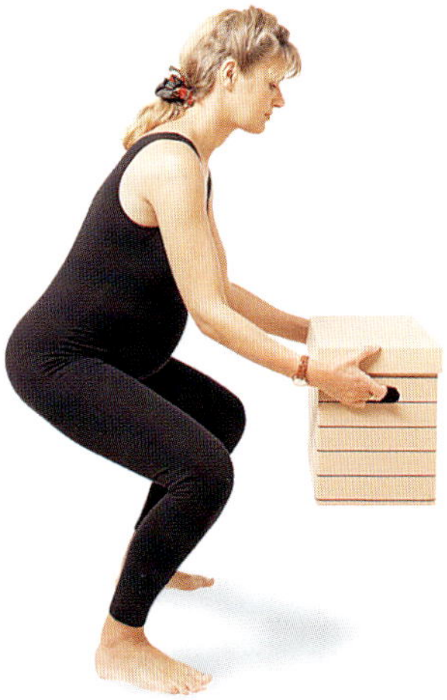

with other new mothers. While isolation is not generally a good idea if you are depressed, they may encourage you to satisfy a need for solitude if you need time to re-establish yourself before returning to normal social interaction.

THE FELDENKRAIS METHOD

The Feldenkrais Method may be beneficial during pregnancy. It can help you adjust to the different movements you need to make due to your changing shape. Improving movement in your spine, pelvic area and hip joints will enable you to have an easier birth. The method can also show you how to move more efficiently with less strain as you look after your baby.

HERBALISM

In the first trimester of pregnancy you should not take herbal medicine of any kind except if prescribed by a qualified herbalist for a serious condition, such as the prevention of miscarriage. Once you are into your second trimester you can safely take herbal remedies to treat a wider range of conditions, such as morning sickness, but only on the advice of a qualified herbalist. If correctly prescribed, these are very effective yet without side effects for you or your baby.

Some herbs should be avoided during pregnancy as they are oestrogenic or can cause contractions of the uterus and lead to miscarriage. They include: barberry, black cohosh, calendula, feverfew, golden seal, hawthorn, juniper, liquorice, mugwort, nutmeg, pennyroyal, poke root, rue, sage, tansy, thuja, wormwood and yarrow. Large doses of laxative herbs, such as aloe, cascara sagrada and senna pods, should also be avoided.

A herbalist can advise you on herbs that are useful during childbirth. For example, raspberry leaf tea is known to be helpful to women during labour and as preparation after the first trimester. A herbal remedy for ineffective, weak contractions is to drink extracts of golden seal root or blue cohosh. For short sharp contractions, you can drink herbal infusions of any of the following herbs individually or combined: cramp bark, wild yam and squaw vine. In the early stages of labour, a sponge bath using rosewater, lavender water or an infusion of rosemary is very soothing.

After the birth, you can try an infusion of leaves and seeds of borage, dill seeds, aniseed and fennel seeds, taken three times a day, to stimulate milk flow.

Different herbs work on different people so a herbalist will design a postnatal prescription especially for you. To balance hormones they may recommend blue cohosh, false unicorn root or St John's wort. If you have a progesterone deficiency that is causing postnatal depression, they may suggest wild yam, fenugreek or chaste tree.

An ointment containing St John's wort and comfrey can speed healing of your perineum. Comfrey and calendula, in a cream or ointment, applied three times a day to your skin can help reduce stretch marks, and a weak infusion of golden seal root used as a wash will soothe the itchy skin that is often an associated problem. Calendula cream is soothing and anti-inflammatory and can be used on the nipples after every feed to prevent cracking.

HOMOEOPATHY

Many homoeopathic remedies are useful during and after pregnancy, but you should only take them under the supervision of a homoeopath who will direct you on remedies and dosages. Some of these remedies are Sepia for morning sickness and *Arnica montana* which is often used during labour.

MASSAGE

If you are pregnant and would like to be massaged, check with your doctor or midwife before proceeding. Professional massage can be of great benefit but you can also use simple massage techniques at home (see page 135). It can provide a wonderful way of

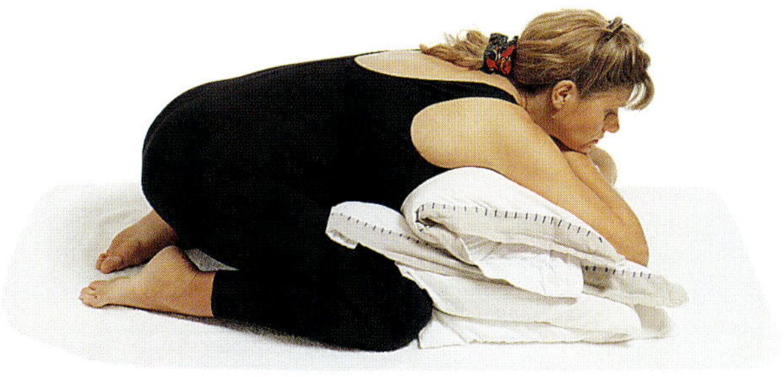

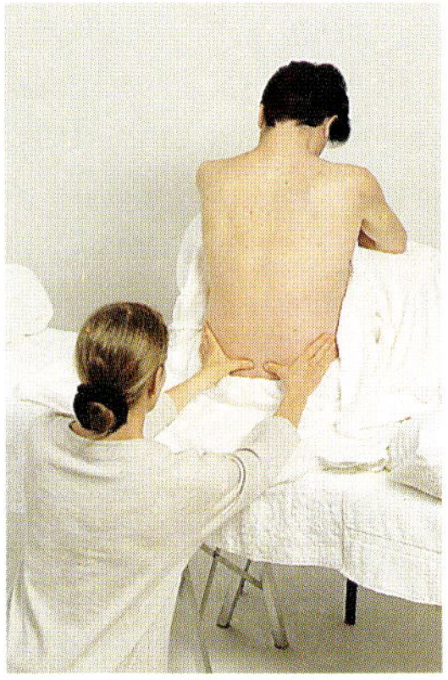

Sitting on the side of a bed provides a comfortable position for back massage. Support the legs on a chair if the bed is high.

bonding with your partner, and abdominal massage can be experienced by the baby in the womb (which can have a calming effect on an overactive child).

When massaging a pregnant woman, avoid deep pressure and keep the movements smooth. Sweet almond oil is recommended as it will also help with dry skin and stretch mark prevention.

Try a seated massage (see page 151) to release a stiff neck and shoulders, or a leg massage for tired feet.

A seated position is also good for back massage: either on the side of the bed, or curved forward over a pillow or bean bag (see page 65).

Abdominal massage may be performed with the woman lying on her back and slightly tilted to the left side by placing a cushion under the back. In later pregnancy, however, it is unwise for a woman to lie on her back for prolonged periods so the massage can be done sitting up with the back well supported. Ensure you massage lightly in a clockwise direction, using the palms and fingers.

Before childbirth, perineal massage can prepare the area and reduce the risk of it tearing. Start at least six weeks before delivery and massage for at least 5 to 10 minutes each day. You can use a base carrier oil such as sweet almond oil and a mirror to check your positioning. Ensure your hands are clean, your nails are short and your bladder empty.

For perineal massage: place your thumb inside your vagina and gently press towards your anus. Gently but firmly and with a steady pressure, massage the lower wall of the vagina in a "U" shape for about 30 to 60 seconds until you feel a burning or tingling sensation. Release and repeat.

Massage during childbirth can be of immeasurable value: it can relax, relieve backache, and help create a feeling of comfort and reassurance while promoting pain relief through the release of endorphins which in turn increase energy and reduce stress. If the feet and legs are massaged during labour, enlist the support of another person as both legs should be massaged simultaneously.

New mothers will benefit from the emotional and physical balancing provided by massage, as well as the personal attention and time. This relaxation process will help you feel more able to cope and thus able to give to your child. Ask your doctor or midwife how soon after the birth you can start having massages.

You can massage your own breasts when they feel sore or after each feeding session. Use a base carrier oil — add a small amount of an essential oil as recommended by an aromatherapist, if you desire. Massage from the outer edge of your breast inwards but avoid the nipple. Don't forget your underarm area and remove all traces of oil before the next feed.

Your baby too can experience the direct benefits of massage. It can help soothe the child, encourage the parent-child bond and may relieve conditions such as colic. Keep the strokes light and gentle and move down the body and limbs away from the heart. Connect your movements so that they flow smoothly.

MODERN MEDICINE

There is a lot of information available on how doctors and obstetricians deal with pregnancy and postnatal care. The general trend these days is to move away from intervention and closer to achieving the most "natural" environment for mother and child. However, there are still obstetricians who prescribe drugs during childbirth when they are not always needed, so it is important that you seek a medical practitioner you can trust, who will support you in your choice of options.

NATUROPATHY

Naturopaths can give you great assistance with advice on a variety of natural treatments from natural fertility methods to simple home remedies for new mothers. For example, placing a soft fresh cabbage leaf between the breast and bra cup will help nursing mothers with breast soreness.

Naturopaths will help you work out your diet, which is more important than ever during this time of your life. Sound nutrition can help you avoid problems such as morning sickness, constipation and indigestion and give your child the best possible start.

A naturopath can also advise on dosages and brands of vitamins and minerals. Taking a good multi-vitamin supplement as well as an iron and calcium supplement can help you maintain excellent health throughout your pregnancy.

When planning your pregnancy, folic acid (0.8-1.2 mg per day) may be recommended. Research studies have shown that folic acid, taken about the time of conception, reduces the risk of neural tube defects such as spina bifida. However, since the baby's need for all nutrients is strong very early in pregnancy, you may wish to consider taking a balanced supplement for several months before conception.

After pregnancy, high potency vitamin B supplements (taken as directed), calcium (800 mg per day), magnesium (400 mg per day) and zinc (25 mg elemental per day) are effective in balancing the body and calming the nervous system. And vitamin E (500 iu per day), zinc (25 mg elemental per day) and silica (taken as directed on the label) will help your skin to heal and your body to return to shape.

OSTEOPATHY

Osteopathic treatment prior to conception can be of benefit as it can assist the position and mobility of the pelvis, enhancing the blood supply and nerve control of the ovaries and uterus, and perhaps assisting conception and pregnancy.

Osteopathy is used in pregnancy to optimise your health, labour and delivery through manipulation of your body structure. The osteopath does not enforce "symmetry" but rather helps your body achieve its best functional position for both you and your baby.

You may choose to consult an osteopath for lower back pain caused by your increasing weight and postural changes. Osteopathy can assist your muscles and skeleton to accommodate the growing baby by adjusting your pelvis and lumbar spine to a more comfortable position. This will increase your mobility, enhance circulation and prepare your pelvis for the birthing process.

Women who experience lower back pain after the birth of their child can also be helped by osteopathy.

Others find that they become more round-shouldered, with discomfort in their upper back and neck due to breast enlargement. An osteopath can help with the movement of your upper thorax so there is a better blood supply around your breasts to help lymphatic drainage, which also aids breathing and digestion. Gentle osteopathic treatment is often accompanied by advice on breastfeeding positions to minimise neck problems.

REFLEXOLOGY

It is not advisable to have reflexology if you have a history of unstable pregnancies or if you are in the first trimester of your pregnancy. Apart from these rules reflexology can be useful in pregnancy as it can relieve pain, nausea etc, but should only be administered by a trained reflexologist.

After delivery, you can use reflexology at home to help bring your hormones back into balance. Regularly work the following points on both feet or hands for a total of 15 minutes: ovaries, uterus, pituitary and, specifically for postnatal depression, all the fingers or toes as they correspond to the head and neck areas.

SHIATSU

It is important that your Ki flows freely around your body when you are pregnant to provide nourishing energy for both you and your baby. Gentle shiatsu treatment will keep that energy flowing without blockage, lessen the strain on your body and increase your general vitality.

It is advisable to avoid self-treatment with shiatsu but rather see a trained shiatsu practitioner. Treatment is usually given while you are on your side or in a sitting position in order to make you and your baby as comfortable as possible. The lower body (leg area) is generally avoided because disturbance of these areas may affect the balance of your reproductive system.

If your pregnancy is going well, it is advisable to avoid shiatsu treatments that include deep pressure on specific points.

However, if you are experiencing pain from the disturbance of your centre of gravity and other postural changes you could see a shiatsu practitioner. Particularly good is the shiatsu technique that involves stretching of the neck — this reduces the pressure in your lower back.

Shiatsu from a practitioner during labour can speed up your contractions and reduce the pain. It can also be administered by a support person who has done a short course in shiatsu and provide a caring bond between the two of you. To be effective the pressure on various points needs to be as strong as the pain that is experienced. Shiatsu on your neck, shoulders and lower back is good for relieving the pain of contractions.

After delivery, shiatsu treatments can work to restore the balance of Ki in your body.

YOGA

Because yoga is such a gentle form of exercise it is perfect for pregnant women who can use it to keep fit without putting strain on their bodies, to achieve a calmer state of mind and to create a peaceful environment for their babies. Specific yoga exercises during your pregnancy can increase the strength in your pelvic area which will assist your baby during the journey through the birth canal. The breathing techniques can also be very useful when you give birth. Yoga practice will help you to cope better with the demands of motherhood (e.g. disturbed sleep), through relaxation techniques and exercises that tone stretched muscles.

Whether you are starting yoga for the first time or practise regularly, it's important that you take it at your own pace. If you feel tired, don't rush the exercises. They will benefit you more if you take them slowly.

A word of caution. When you are pregnant you will be producing increased amounts of oestrogen which alters collagen and other substances to allow body tissue to soften and stretch in preparation for childbirth. This can sometimes allow you to hyper-extend your body when you shouldn't, so take things easily and only go as far as you feel comfortable.

Some yoga exercises are not safe to do during pregnancy. These include all exercises done for extended periods on your back and inverted postures.

A yoga teacher can give you specific exercises suitable for your stage of pregnancy and fitness level but here are a couple of daily exercises you can try to get you started.

Specific instructions are given about the position of your body. In the first months, you can lie on your back with your knees bent and feet about hip width apart. Support your head and shoulders with a cushion. As your pregnancy progresses beyond the fourth month, however, do these exercises standing, sitting or squatting (as suggested).

THE BUTTERFLY

1. Sit up straight on the floor. You may like to sit on some folded blankets to make it more comfortable for you.
2. Bring the soles of your feet together, pulling them into your body with your hands. Gently push your knees towards the floor. *(See Figure 1.)*

FIGURE 1

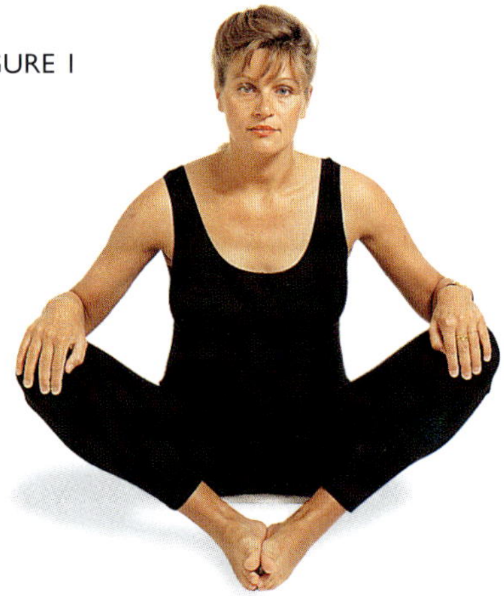

Be conscious of the gentle stretch of your inner thigh muscles while you breathe deeply and slowly, but don't force your knees any further than they can comfortably go.

This position is good for preparing your pelvic area for childbirth.

THE FROG

1. Kneel down on the floor and sit on your heels (you may like to kneel on some folded blankets if this is more comfortable). Make sure your big toes are touching and your knees are apart.
2. Put your hands on the floor in front of you and breathe in as you sit up straight *(see Figure 2)*.
3. Breathe out as you stretch out in front of you, lowering your body. Relax into this position *(see Figure 3)*. You can widen your legs also so that your baby fits neatly between your thighs but be careful not to put too much pressure on this area and squash the baby. When you feel totally relaxed, breathe in and sit up straight again.

This exercise is good for relaxing your body as well as stretching your lower pelvic area. Squatting is an excellent way to prepare yourself for birth in your last trimester so do this exercise once a day during this period of your pregnancy.

FIGURE 2

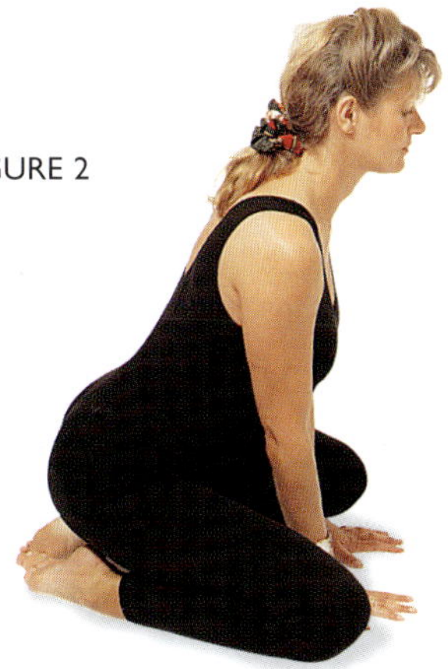

FIGURE 3

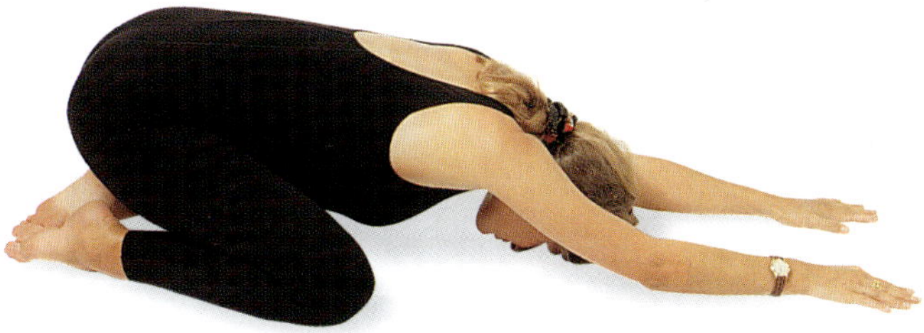

KEGEL EXERCISE

1. Tightly squeeze the muscles around your vagina, anus and pelvic area. Hold for as long as you can — aim for 10 seconds.
2. Slowly release the muscles. Focus on control here and count to five on an outward breath. Then relax.

Do these at least 30 times a day. Three sets of ten are good if you can manage it.

PELVIC TILT

Up to the fourth month do this exercise in the lying position but after that do it standing with your back against a wall. Try to increase your awareness of your pelvic area so you have a sense of being able to isolate the movement there.

1. Exhale as you press the small of your back against the floor or wall.
2. Inhale and relax your back. Repeat this several times.

DROMEDARY DROOP

1. Get down on your hands and knees with your knees directly under your hips. Hold your spine straight but keep it relaxed and hold your head in line with your spine. *(See Figure 4.)*
2. Breathe in and arch your back upwards into a hump *(see Figure 5)*. Begin at your tail bone and imagine each vertebrae moving into the arch so that the last to move is your neck, as your head drops down. At the same time tighten your abdomen and buttocks.
3. Breathe out, relaxing your spine — again move from your tail bone first. Finish with your head in its original position.

Do this exercise several times a day. It is particularly effective at relieving the pressure placed on your spine as your uterus enlarges.

FIGURE 4

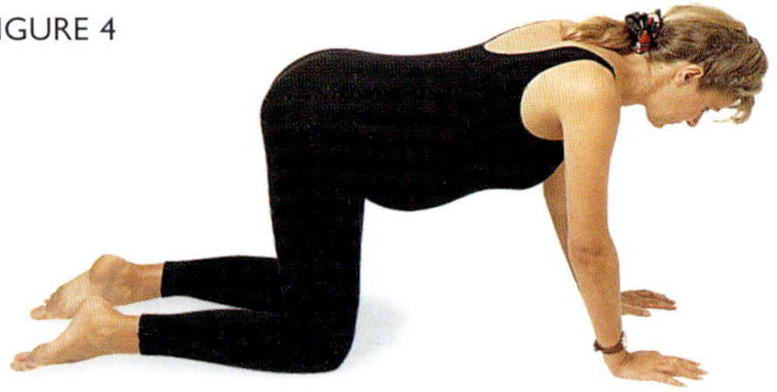

FIGURE 5

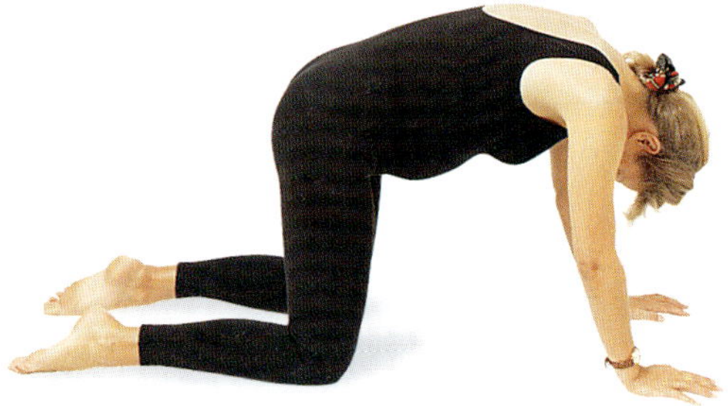

STRETCHING AND OPENING

1. Stand and hold onto the back of a chair for support. Place your feet hip-width apart. (*See Figure 6.*)
2. Unlock your knees. Taking care to keep your back straight, lower your body as far as you can comfortably go *(see Figure 7)*. You should feel the stretch along your inner thighs.

Do this a few times a day and gradually build up strength in your thighs, so you can go more deeply into the squat.

Take the opportunity during this exercise for a visualisation. See your body stretching and opening like a beautiful, great bloom. See all your pelvic area relaxing and expanding so that you become accustomed to the idea of opening to deliver your baby.

FIGURE 6

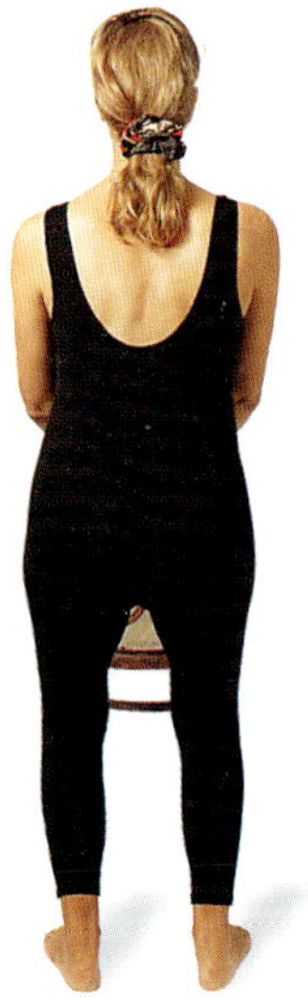

FIGURE 7

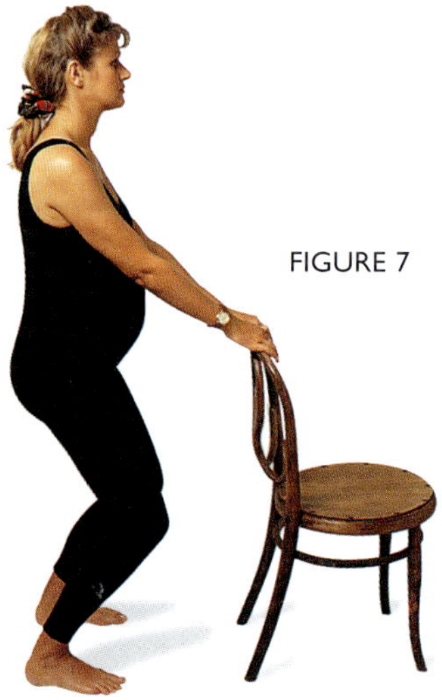

NATURAL HEALTH FOR CHILDREN

It can be distressing for everyone when a child is ill. If the child is too young, or too ill to express their feelings, it is difficult to know what the child is experiencing. Yet it befalls you, as the adult, to make judgments to ease your child's suffering. When should you give temporary relief aids like aspirin? At what point should you seek professional help? How do you know if you are being overly protective?

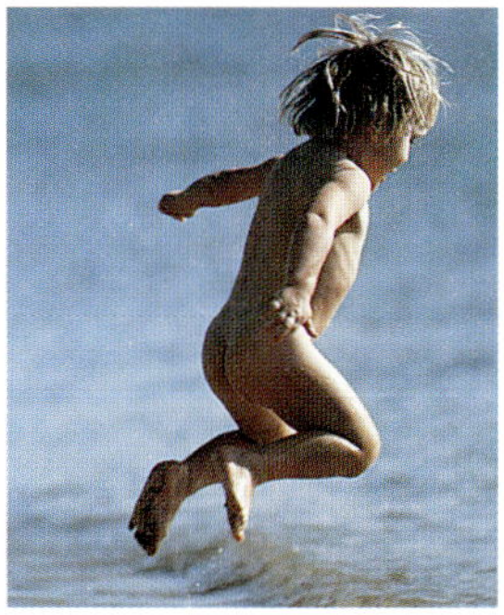

Fortunately most children are fairly resilient to the usual childhood illnesses; others, however, have to deal with chronic conditions such as asthma or allergies.

If you are concerned about any aspect of your child's health it is always best to seek medical guidance from your doctor, even if you are unsure about the need for it. This will, at the very least, offer reassurance, especially if your child becomes agitated by your distress.

However, there is a place for home remedies and natural therapies to enhance health, providing commonsense is used.

HOW NATURAL THERAPIES CAN HELP

Many natural therapies are particularly suitable for children — their gentle action is effective on young immune systems.

Many "normal" illnesses that children experience, from coughs and colds through to mumps, can be viewed as nature's way of strengthening your child's immune system. There are therapies that aim to support and encourage your child's immune response rather than suppress it.

You may like to consult a general practitioner sympathetic to other therapies. Usually they will be pleased to discuss treatments such as antibiotics with you and will be supportive of other natural therapies you may use to improve your child's health.

ACUPUNCTURE

Although it can be effective, acupuncture is not often recommended for children because they tend to be frightened by the needles. It is best to try other natural therapy methods such as acupressure that are less intrusive.

ACUPRESSURE

Acupressure is an effective natural crisis treatment for children, especially those who are prone to allergic reactions to food or who experience discomfort from climatic changes, particularly the cold.

Children may feel some discomfort with acupressure as it does hurt slightly when the pressure point is first pressed by the thumb. But after a few moments the discomfort will pass. If your child reacts against the firm pressure, a light massage will be sufficient until they get used to the idea.

You can use acupressure at home on a child over seven but consult a professional if you are unsure about what acupressure point to activate.

The only rule is that acupressure should not be used as a home remedy on children under the age of seven, although a professional practitioner — especially those who have specialised knowledge of children — can be consulted.

AROMATHERAPY

Aromatherapy is a gentle natural therapy children respond to well. The fragrances are pleasurable and the oils can help them, unobtrusively, feel calmer when they are distressed. As well, the oils boost their immune system to prevent or tackle minor ailments.

Chamomile, lavender and mandarin are the most common oils used to treat children because of their gentleness. See page 102 for information on specific oils and their uses — but it is best to check with an aromatherapist about which oils are most suitable for your children. They can pinpoint those which are not only most effective but also safe. Some essential oils should not be used on babies and young children.

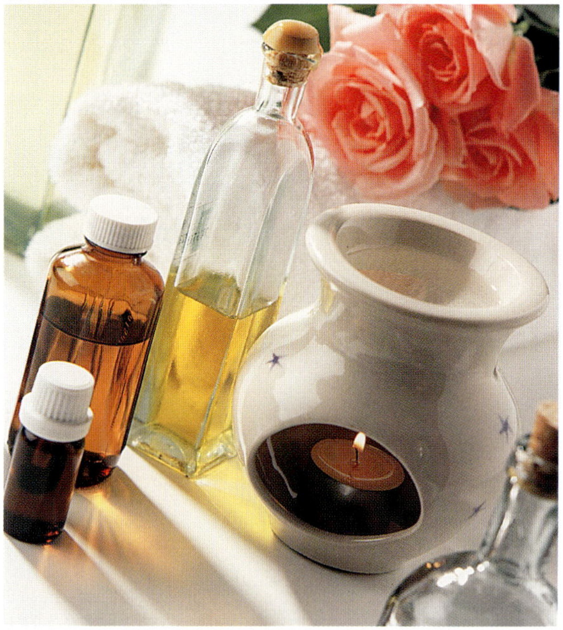

Aromatherapy is a gentle natural therapy. Children respond well to the pleasant scents and unobtrusive application.

The simplicity of use also makes aromatherapy an attractive option. The oils can be diluted in children's baths or in oil burners around the home. After-bath massages with mild essential oils can prevent conditions such as nappy rash and assist parent-child bonding.

Aromatherapy is an effective preventative treatment for children. If your children feel a little off-colour, overexcited or are not sleeping, a warm bath with two drops of pre-diluted chamomile or lavender oil can often bring them into balance.

Despite their versatility there are some cautions you should take when using essential oils with children:

- Use less oil than you would on an adult — for a child over three years old, use half the recommended adult dosage; for three years and under, use a quarter of the adult dosage; for babies under 18 months, add only one drop of oil to their bath.
- Make sure that children don't apply the oils or lotions themselves but are properly supervised.

- Keep all your essential oils and glass bottles out of your child's reach.
- Keep oil burners out of children's reach.
- If you are giving a child a steam inhalation, never leave them alone with the bowl of hot water and don't make the water so hot they can burn themselves. When they inhale the steam, make sure it is only for about 15 seconds at a time, as children have a shorter tolerance of inhalations than adults. Avoid using a towel "tent" for young children; hold the baby and sit the bowl close-by.

BACH FLOWER REMEDIES

Children's health problems can come hand-in-hand with emotional states such as overexcitement or fear, and this is the level at which Bach flowers work effectively. Children can take the same dosage of Bach flower remedies as adults on their tongue — check the bottle to determine the amount as the remedy may be concentrated or already diluted. For babies, just wet their lips with the remedy and let them absorb it.

CHINESE HERBS

When prescribed by a herbalist, Chinese herbs are safe for children to take and can assist a great many childhood ailments. It may be difficult for a child to drink the large quantity of herbal tea required and they may find the taste unpalatable, but the practitioner can prescribe the herbs in other forms such as pills, syrups and powders.

CHIROPRACTIC

Chiropractic adjustment can work very well on children as their nervous systems are generally healthy and they have not yet developed the chronic spinal problems that come with bad posture, stress and injury in adulthood.

Most chiropractors will use a different adjustment technique on children to that used on adults, involving a small instrument called an activator. This device exerts a small impact when triggered by a release switch. It is gentle, not fast or frightening, and there is no "cracking" involved. It is also useful for getting into the smaller joints of a child's body.

A caring chiropractor will generally talk to the child before an adjustment to let them know exactly what is happening so they are calm and relaxed about the procedure.

Chiropractors treat children most commonly during their growing spurts when their spine and joints may be having trouble adapting to their new shape. Children's nervous systems may also need help in avoiding bouts of "growing pains" and associated problems.

Chiropractors can safely treat babies and chiropractic care is one of the most effective ways to treat those with colic or croup. The adjustments that qualified chiropractors use for these ailments are very, very gentle.

THE FELDENKRAIS METHOD

Lessons in the Feldenkrais Method can improve function in children with movement difficulties. Children with altered muscle tone can learn to move with reduced effort and those with poorly coordinated movement can learn to stabilise and organise their movement.

HERBALISM

There is no minimum age for taking herbal remedies but it is recommended that if a child is younger than six months a compress of herbs should be applied over the affected area rather than taking the herbs internally.

The mothers of children under six months should take the herbs if they are breastfeeding as the baby will absorb the herbs through their breast milk.

For older children, herbs can be given in warm teas or infusions (strained if the herb is loose). Let the tea sit for at least 10 minutes so that your child doesn't get burnt — it really doesn't matter if they drink the tea hot or cold as it will still have the same effect. You can add honey to sweeten, if desired.

You can also add the herbal tea to your child's bath — the solution should be 20 times stronger than the recommended internal dose. The herb will pass through the skin and into the body without distressing a child who is afraid of taking "medicine".

If the herb comes in powder form you can mix it with a banana and honey for a dessert.

Tinctures of herbs contain a small amount of alcohol and children generally quite like the warming effect this has on their tastebuds. If your child is two years or under, tinctures should only be taken with the advice of a herbalist.

Herbs also come in tablet form, but as children do not generally like taking tablets it may be better to administer herbs in some of the other ways described.

Herbal remedies are available over the counter, but for severe or chronic health problems or if you wish to use herbs regularly as part of your child's health maintenance, it is best to consult a herbalist. Though herbs have very few side effects, some children have allergic reactions (see page 214) to specific herbs. If this is the case, stop the herbal treatment immediately and consult a health practitioner.

HOMOEOPATHY

Children's young immune systems respond well to homoeopathic remedies, and the low dosage means side effects are extremely unlikely. The dosages recommended in The A–Z of Health Conditions (pages 211 to 384) need no further dilution for children.

You can administer the remedies to children in tablet form which they can suck until the tablet dissolves on their tongue or which can be dissolved in a teaspoon of water. Babies should take the remedy in the dissolved form.

Children usually like the taste as the tablets are often mixed with lactose or maize starch to make them more appetising. Some children may prefer the liquid form of the remedy, taken directly by the spoonful or diluted in fruit juice.

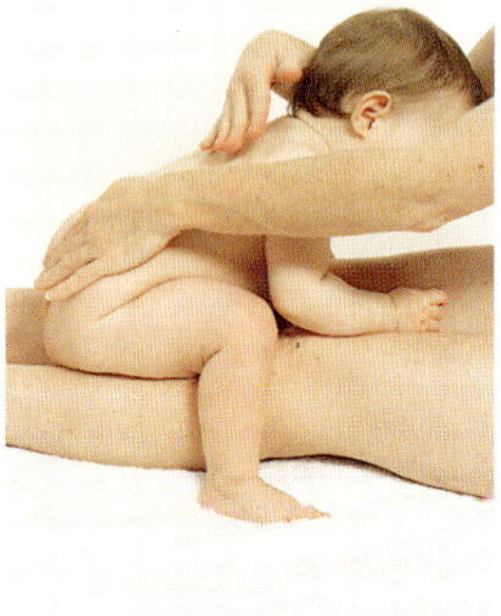

Baby massage provides a good opportunity for parent-child bonding.

NATUROPATHY

The value of a wholesome, balanced diet cannot be underestimated when it comes to health. The dietary advice a naturopath can give will provide children with a great start in life and help them avoid health problems later on.

Many children's health problems are actually associated with food allergies. A naturopath can help you pinpoint what foods are detrimental to your child's health and work out substitutes.

Vitamins and minerals are an important part of naturopathic treatment. Children are more likely to take the supplements in powder or liquid form (mixed into drinks) than in tablet form. There are also chewable vitamins and minerals with natural flavours that your children will think are "treats".

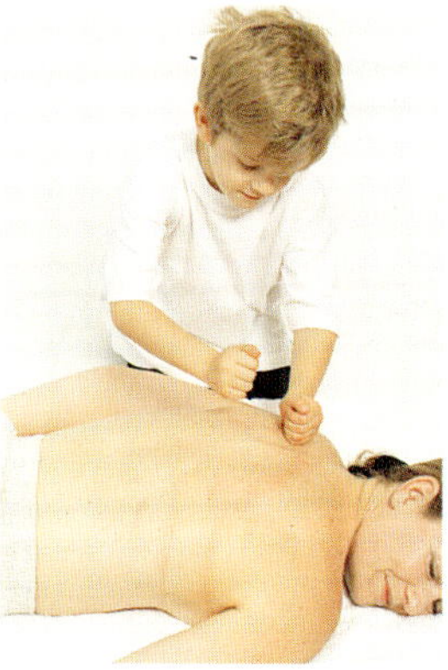

Older children may enjoy giving massages as well as receiving them.

MASSAGE

When you are bathing, changing or feeding your children it is easy to extend this contact into a gentle massage. They will enjoy the feeling of your touch, and as a parent it will help you bond with them.

Older children can also enjoy massage and you may incorporate it into a playing session. There is no need to undress as light clothes will not hinder the massage, nor are oils necessary.

Experiment with different techniques (see page 135) to discover those the child likes best, whatever the age. Many children are restless so keep the session short.

OSTEOPATHY

The calming and soothing approach of osteopathy is well suited to children and newborns. Osteopathy can be helpful in the prevention and treatment of structural problems stemming from a variety of causes including difficulties during pregnancy or birth, childhood accidents and falls, infections or inflammatory conditions and genetic disorders.

REFLEXOLOGY

Most children enjoy the feel of reflexology treatment on their feet. All the reflexology points used on adults can be used on children. However, you should use less pressure with your thumbs when working reflexology points on a child than with an adult.

It may be difficult to get your child to sit still during a reflexology treatment. Try doing it while they are involved in something stationary like watching television or when you are telling them a story.

After reading the section on reflexology, you could explain to your child how their feet and hands are like miniature bodies with all the parts. This usually fascinates older children; they can use their imagination to guess what parts of their feet and hands refer to what part of their body.

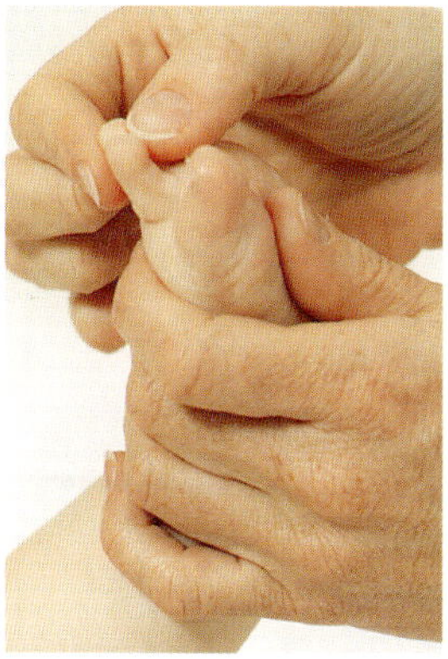

Most children will enjoy a reflexology treatment but they are liable to be ticklish. It is important to handle their feet gently but firmly.

SHIATSU

Shiatsu can be safely given to children of all ages and they usually respond well to it. Shiatsu practitioners generally find that the Ki energy in children's bodies flows well so they will use dispersing techniques rather than toning techniques. The most common technique used on babies is a light stroking shiatsu along their meridians. Children aged two to four years are also dealt with gently in shiatsu and are rocked and rubbed. For children over four, shiatsu practitioners will use normal shiatsu treatment although the session may be shorter because of a child's limited attention span. Shiatsu is especially useful for hyperactive children who become calmer and happier after a treatment.

Most children like shiatsu and find it comforting and energising. Parents in Japan practise shiatsu on their children from birth. You can undertake a shiatsu course so you can treat your own children at home. A greater bond may be achieved between parents and children if shiatsu is part of their general health program. Also parents are more likely to notice any changes in their children's health immediately so they are able to pre-empt illness and seek professional advice.

YOGA

Yoga seems like a game to children, not exercise. They can pretend to be animals when they do poses like the cat, the cobra and the dog (see page 76). These exercises are good for the back, kidneys, arms, legs, and general spinal fitness. In particular, the cobra is effective in activating the lymph glands.

It is best to start children on simple exercises under the guidance of a yoga teacher but your child can try these examples at home, finishing with the yoga resting position (*see Figure 1 on next page*).

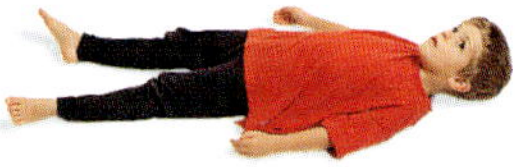
FIGURE 1

Children have short attention spans, so the poses are not held for long, and a number of poses are included for variety.

Any kind of exercise is worth encouraging. If children start yoga, particularly at a young age, it is likely they will keep their suppleness in later life. They will also learn some important techniques such as posture, breathing, relaxation, concentration and discipline, and their internal body system will be well-toned.

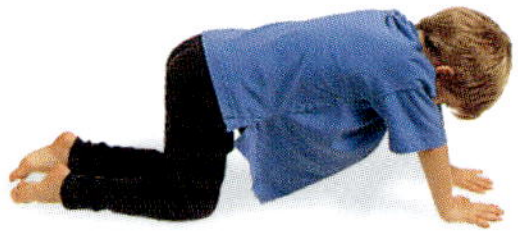
FIGURE 2

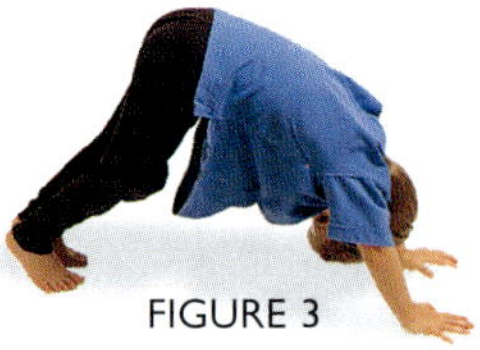
FIGURE 3

THE DOG

1. Get on the floor on your hands and knees *(see Figure 2)*. Breathe evenly so that the air flows in and out.
2. Lift your knees from the floor, tuck your toes under and straighten your legs while bringing your weight onto your arms.
3. Push your weight backwards onto your legs as if you are trying to get your heels on the floor and your bottom to the sky. This is how a dog stretches when it gets up from a nap. Hold this posture for a few breaths *(see Figure 3)*.
4. Relax your knees and lie on the floor on your stomach, your head turned to one side. Your arms should be relaxed beside your body.

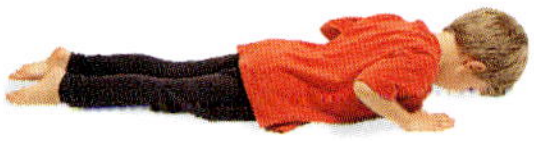
FIGURE 4

THE COBRA

1. Lie on your stomach with your forehead and forearms on the floor and your hands beneath your shoulders, palms down *(see Figure 4)*. Breathe gently in and out while you are doing the exercise.
2. Stretch your upper body towards the ceiling with your head up *(see Figure 5)*. Keep your shoulders down and back (it is not necessary to straighten the elbows).
3. Now relax and lower yourself to the floor, letting out a "hissing" noise like a snake.
4. Relax on the floor with your head to one side and your arms by your side. Repeat this exercise twice with rests in between.

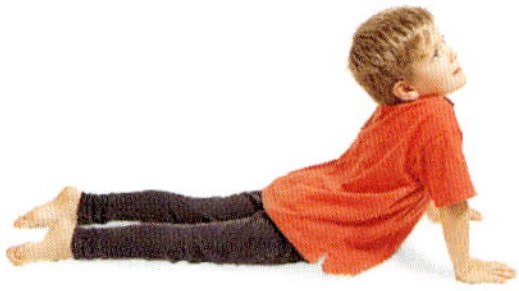
FIGURE 5

THE CAT

1. Kneel on the ground and rest your forehead on the floor with your arms beside you *(see Figure 6)*. Breathe evenly and deeply but do not force your breath.
2. Get up on all fours and arch your back upwards with your head pointing down *(see Figure 7)*.
3. Then push your back down the other way and your head back *(see Figure 8)*.

   Repeat three times then rest lying on your back on the floor with your palms facing upwards in the yoga resting position *(see Figure 1)*.

   Encourage children to do this exercise slowly, pointing out that a cat takes its time when stretching. They can use cat noises if they like to add imagination to the exercise.

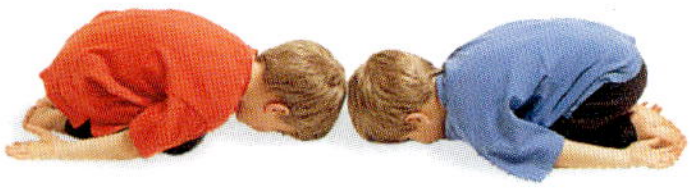
FIGURE 6

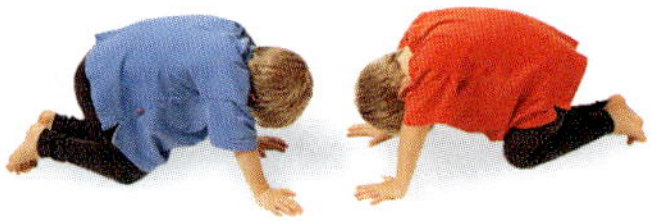
FIGURE 7

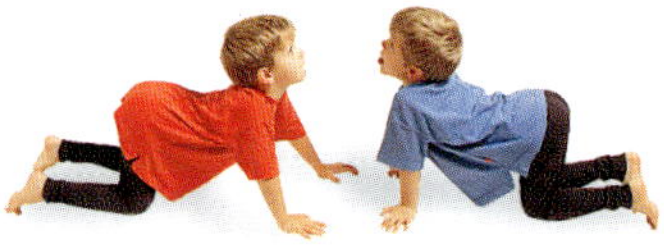
FIGURE 8

USING THE MIND BODY CONNECTION TO IMPROVE YOUR CHILD'S HEALTH

Children are very open to the positive benefits of affirmations, visualisations, healing energy and meditation. Their young minds readily absorb new information and their imaginations are not as constrained as those of adults.

Read the chapters on AFFIRMATION AND VISUALISATIONS and HEALING ENERGIES. If you are exploring any psychological factors in your child's ill-health, be careful not to make strong generalisations. Be honest too — as a parent, you may be involved in the underlying issues and the problems may be difficult for you to see.

AFFIRMATIONS

You can design affirmations on behalf of your child as you would for yourself. Incorporate the affirmations into play — ask your child to sing them to you as a game. With very young children and babies you can try repeating affirmations to them "mantra-like" while they are asleep.

VISUALISATIONS

Choose a quiet time when the child is comfortable and relaxed and you have their attention. Make up a visualisation/story in which your child is the central character and there is a positive final outcome. For example, if your child is troubled by earaches:

Ask the child to imagine they can see a tiny spaceship come down and land on the pillow next to them. Out climbs a favourite character with magical powers who offers to take your child on a magical journey inside the child's ear (use your imagination to describe the details). When the sore part of the ear is reached, ask your child what it looks like. Then get your child and the character to do something to reduce the pain (perhaps zapping it with icy water). Ask your child what the ear looks like after this "magic" has occurred. Then suggest that all pain is gone.

The same idea can be used to disperse an emotional crisis. The important point is for your child to imagine themselves as they would wish to be — happy, strong, peaceful, capable.

HEALING MEDITATION

Parent-child bonds are often so strong that channelling healing energy can happen naturally and unconsciously. You can also consciously practise techniques such as those outlined in the HEALING ENERGIES chapter, both when your child is ill and as a preventative measure.

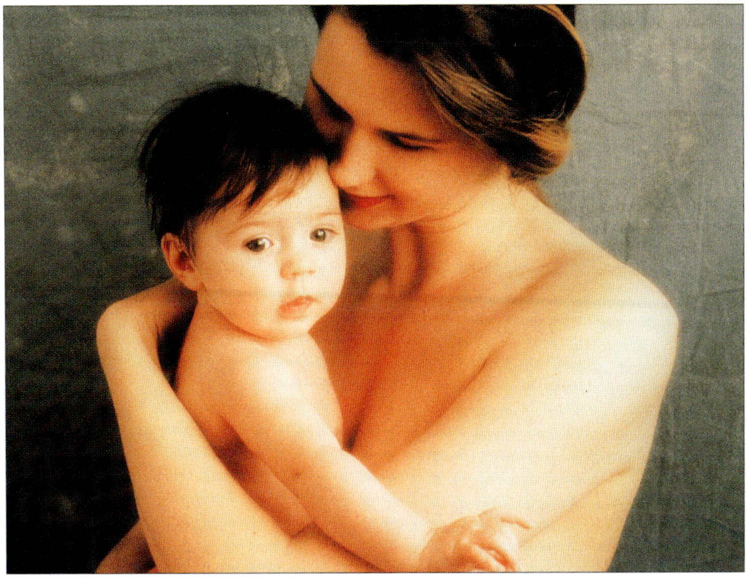

AN A TO Z OF CHILDREN'S HEALTH CONDITIONS

CAUTION

Seek medical advice if your child:

- has a fever above 40°C (104°F)
- has pain in the chest
- wheezes or has difficulty breathing
- becomes increasingly disinterested and tired.

See also WHEN TO CALL THE DOCTOR, page 386.

CHICKENPOX

Chickenpox can take two to three weeks to appear after a person is exposed to the herpes zoster virus that is its cause. Symptoms usually begin with fever, loss of appetite, lethargy and HEADACHE followed by the characteristic rash that starts as small red spots and progresses to blisters and then scabs. The blisters are very itchy and can scar if scratched too vigorously. The condition is extremely contagious from the beginning of the symptoms until the scabs have disappeared.

Usually chickenpox only lasts a week, leaving the person immune to another attack, but the virus does remain in the body and can cause shingles later in life. In rare cases, complications may arise. Adults who don't have immunity can get chickenpox. Adult-onset chickenpox is often more severe and longer lasting than the childhood condition.

IMPORTANT: *Medical advice should be sought if the fever is high or persists, if there is vomiting, or if the neck is painful when stretched.*

WHAT YOU CAN DO

- It is most important that children are isolated so they do not pass on this infection.
- Do not give aspirin as it has been linked to complications. You can choose a child's dose of paracetamol if desired.
- It is difficult to resist scratching. Cut nails to stop damage to the skin and keep them clean to avoid infection. Cover hands in gloves or mittens, if necessary.
- The itching can be relieved by the application of calamine lotion or bathing in a cool bath to which 1/2 cup baking soda has been added. Cool compresses can also help.
- Clean cotton clothing or pyjamas will cause the least irritation and help keep the skin temperature soothingly cool.
- During the fever, keep the child quiet and give plenty of fluids. The rest of the time the child may not feel sick and need not be kept in bed.

AROMATHERAPY

Aromatherapy from a professional can be used for a child over the age of four to reduce the length of the illness and its discomfort.

CHINESE HERBS

In Chinese medical terms, chickenpox symptoms are due to dampness, heat and toxins which need to be eliminated from the body. A Chinese herbalist can help your child gain a speedy recovery from chickenpox.

HERBALISM

Herbs that are useful when your child has chickenpox include echinacea, St John's wort, golden seal, cleavers, calendula and poke root. Only administer these herbs with a herbalist's advice.

However, there are herbal creams you can use at home which are very good for healing the skin. To heal the pox marks try chickweed and/or calendula — they sometimes come in the one cream. Apply to the skin three times a day when the pox marks have formed scabs. Use comfrey cream when the scabs begin to heal to speed recovery and prevent scarring.

Aloe, either as a pure extract or straight from the fleshy leaves of the plant, can be soothing when applied to the skin. Chamomile tea may be applied externally as a wash or taken internally for its soothing effect.

HOMOEOPATHY

Homoeopathic remedies are effective in reducing the length of illness. Try one of the following remedies that best fit your child's symptoms but see a homoeopath if in any doubt.

If your child's spots are very itchy and your child is restless, give them one 12C potency of *Rhus toxicondendrona* three times a day. If your child is emotional and has a fever but won't drink much fluid, give them one 12C potency tablet of *Pulsatilla nigricans* three times a day.

MODERN MEDICINE

Local creams may be recommended to stop the itch. Antihistamines may be prescribed to reduce irritation.

If the sores become infected, antibiotics may be prescribed.

NATUROPATHY

To aid the healing of sores, give your child vitamins C, A and E plus zinc in doses prescribed by a naturopath to suit the age. Vitamin E can be used in cream form to heal the pox marks after itching has stopped.

REFLEXOLOGY

To help your child recover faster, gently work all the points corresponding to the glands as well as the diaphragm for relaxation and the toes/fingers as they correspond to the head area. Try this for a total of 15 minutes daily on both feet or hands until the condition clears.

COLIC

Colic refers to severe cramping pain in the abdomen, due to muscular spasm in the walls of an organ. Colic may strike adults but is very common in babies during their first three months.

The symptoms in babies include prolonged crying at night and sometimes screaming — they often draw up their legs and go red in the face when they cry — and wanting to suck something constantly. The belly may be distended and there may be a tense expression on the face.

The cause of colic in babies may include a sensitive nervous system, an immature digestive system, food ALLERGIES, inappropriate food or feeding problems, as well as physical problems such as a HERNIA.

WHAT YOU CAN DO

- What works for your child is personal — experiment with different approaches.
- Babies will often be calmed by sucking on a dummy (pacifier) or by rocking, carrying, feeding or burping them.
- Some babies need stimulation or company at this time, others are over-stimulated and need to be left to lie passively (in your arms or on their own) with no eye contact.
- Overly-sensitive babies seem to respond well to structure and organisation, including a regimented feeding time.
- Hold babies upright, not horizontal, when feeding to prevent swallowing too much air. Burp them well.
- If breastfeeding, mothers should avoid foods that may cause irritation to babies such as onions, garlic, coffee, cabbage, cauliflower, broccoli, legumes, chickpeas. Raw bananas, cucumber, lettuce, yogurt and apples can also cause problems and may need to be avoided by some young children or nursing mothers. This is also true for food that may cause an allergic reaction such as dairy, wheat, gluten or eggs.
- Similarly, helpful substances can be passed on — use basil, dill, fennel, cumin and caraway in cooking.
- Make sure you get some time away from the colicky child; do something that will revive your energy and positive feelings about yourself and your baby.

AROMATHERAPY

Chamomile is an essential oil that helps relieve colic by releasing the gas from a baby's stomach. When your baby has colic, make up a mixture of 2 drops of chamomile in 10 tsp (60 ml/2 fl oz) base carrier oil or lotion and use a little for an abdominal massage (see picture next page).

CHINESE HERBS

There are many Chinese herbal remedies and tonics that may be effective in relieving colic, depending on a herbalist's diagnosis of the child's specific symptoms.

CHIROPRACTIC

Professional chiropractic adjustment is a safe and effective way of treating your baby for colic. Chiropractors have found that children who have had a forceps delivery or a delivery involving problems with their mother's pelvis are more prone to bouts of colic.

COUNSELLING

Parents and carers can really benefit from support when dealing with a colicky child. It can be difficult to maintain positive feelings about yourself and your child when your baby seems to do nothing but scream. As well as trained counsellors, observers and instructors who can offer advice, there are support groups formed by parents in similar situations.

HERBALISM

The herbs that are most effective in reducing the occurrence of colic in babies include peppermint, dill, fennel seed and chamomile. If you are breastfeeding a baby with colic, you could drink 4 strong cups of these herbs in infusions per day. Allow the tea to brew for 15 minutes and only use one tea bag or heaped teaspoon of the herb per cup.

As a herbal remedy for colic in older babies, you can place 1/4 teaspoon of dill seeds in 1/4 cup of boiling water and let it stand for 30 minutes. Give 1/2 teaspoon of this to your baby and repeat every 15 minutes until their condition improves.

HOMOEOPATHY

If your baby's fists are clenched and you hear a gurgling in the stomach, give one 6C potency of *Cuprum metallicum* crushed up in milk as often as needed, or if you are breastfeeding take the remedy yourself.

If your baby quietens down by being carried around but is inconsolable most of the time, give one 6C potency of *Chamomilla vulgaris* crushed up in milk as often as the symptoms dictate, or take it yourself if you are breastfeeding. If in any doubt see a homoeopath.

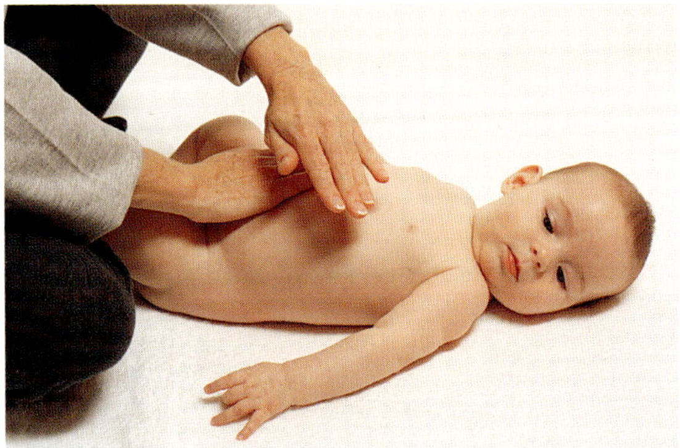

A gentle abdominal massage in a clockwise direction (thereby following the path of the intestine) may bring some relief to a colicky baby.

MODERN MEDICINE

Antispasmodic and analgesic medications may be prescribed.

NATUROPATHY

As well as the impact of various foods, there may be a deficiency in the breast milk that is contributing to the problem. A naturopath may recommend zinc, magnesium and calcium supplements.

REFLEXOLOGY

Gently work on the following points on your child: diaphragm, large intestine, small intestine and stomach. Try these points for a total of 15 minutes on both hands or feet.

SHIATSU

A shiatsu practitioner may give your child light shiatsu to their stomach and lower back to help relieve the colic. Sometimes just simply holding this area can make a difference. The knees may be stretched gently towards the stomach to expel wind and the legs may be moved in a gentle cycling motion. You could try stroking your child's index finger from where it meets the thumb to the tip — this can help the large intestine meridian.

EARACHE

Earache can be caused by a middle ear infection due to a viral or bacterial infection. The outer ear may also become infected. This may be the result of bacteria thriving in moist conditions (when there is an excessive amount of wax, for example) or due to an irritation. This can in turn spread to the middle ear.

As the middle ear is connected to the nose and throat by small tubes, an infection in these areas can spread and an earache may accompany a head cold or sore throat. In young children, the tubes tend to get swollen and blocked with phlegm when an irritation is present, causing painful pressure and the condition known as glue ear. Impacted ear wax and water can also cause blockages. A middle ear infection often follows. Earaches are thus common in the young but the tendency decreases with age.

Earaches usually start with a pain in the ear, then fever and a loss of balance — our sense of balance is maintained by fluid levels in the inner ear.

IMPORTANT: *Earaches should always be investigated by a doctor — there is always the possibility the earache is indicative of a more serious problem, particularly if the ache is persistent. Recurrent infections may also lead to permanent damage. After a diagnosis, if the condition is not serious, you could seek help from a number of therapies. Glue ear requires long-term treatment.*

WHAT YOU CAN DO

- Rest the ear on a hot water bottle (wrapped in a towel) or a heating pad. The neck or throat should also be kept warm.
- If giving eardrops, avoid trapping air in the ear canal. Have the person lie on the side with the ear up and apply the drops slowly so they run down the side of the canal.
- Treat COLDS AND INFLUENZA, TONSILLITIS, SINUSITIS and other infections quickly.
- Allergies can irritate the mucous membrane. Do not smoke around children. If a child has chronic ear infections it may be worth checking for an allergy to dairy foods, animal hair or dust.
- Breastfeeding your baby seems to decrease the chance of ear infections. When nursing a child (by bottle or at the breast), keep them in an upright position to avoid regurgitated milk flowing into the tubes to the ears.
- Prevent "swimmer's ear" by maintaining the cleanliness of your own pool and using ear plugs (even petroleum jelly coated cotton wool) in public pools and spa baths.

AROMATHERAPY

Warm compresses can be very effective in relieving the pain of earaches for children and will help them to sleep. Make up a warm compress (see page 127) with 1 drop each of lavender and chamomile essential oils and hold on the ear for 10 minutes. Do this every morning and night.

CHINESE HERBS

Chinese medicine is very effective in quickly relieving the symptoms and cause of earache. A Chinese herbalist can give your child a herbal prescription.

CHIROPRACTIC

Subluxations in the upper neck of your child can contribute to earache. These can be treated by a chiropractor.

HERBALISM

Earache can often be helped with ear drops made from the herb mullein. Other herbs known to strengthen your child's immune system against infection include echinacea, fenugreek, golden seal and poke root.

These herbal remedies should be used under the supervision of a herbalist — more damage can be caused by incorrect use at home.

HOMOEOPATHY

The following homoeopathic remedies should clear an earache that has no complications, but if your child's illness continues see a homoeopath for a full assessment.

If the pain in your child's ear is throbbing, is worse in the right ear and is worse if they move, give them one 30C potency of *Atropa belladonna* every half an hour for one day then reduce the dosage to three times a day for the next two days.

If your child's ear is too sore to touch and they feel the cold, give them one 30C potency of *Chamomilla vulgaris* every half an hour for one day and then reduce the dosage as above.

MASSAGE

Lymphatic drainage from a qualified practitioner may be of assistance, depending on the cause of the earache. If the ear is badly inflamed or there is an abscess present, do not massage.

MODERN MEDICINE

Analgesics are often prescribed by doctors to reduce the pain and a full course of antibiotics are given for middle ear infection. Antibiotic or antifungal drops or ointment may also be prescribed. Excess wax may be removed using ear drops or a water wash with a syringe.

In cases of glue ear, medications may be prescribed to liquefy the mucus in the ear and antihistamines to reduce swelling and dry up the phlegm. In some cases, a doctor may insert a ventilation tube into the ear to drain the fluid in the middle ear.

NATUROPATHY

Vitamins A and C can help stem an ear infection — ask a naturopath for the correct dosage for your child.

If the problem is glue ear, potassium chloride will be prescribed to help fight the infection. Your child should also avoid products containing sugar, wheat and dairy foods, and dilute all fruit juices as they increase the production of mucus in the body. It is advisable to take these steps in any case of earache.

REFLEXOLOGY

Gently work the points for the ear, throat and neck as well as all toes or fingers as they correspond to the head. Try this for a total of 15 minutes daily on both feet or hands until the condition clears. The reflexology treatment will also help divert the child's attention from the painful ear.

SHIATSU

The blockage of Ki energy in the gall bladder is often the cause of earaches in both children and adults. A shiatsu practitioner would treat the side and back of your child's head with shiatsu to disperse the Ki energy and bring them back into balance.

MEASLES

Measles is a viral infection that may start with a fever, cough, sore eyes, runny nose and tiny white spots in the mouth on the inside of the cheeks. A pink rash then spreads over the face and body; it is not itchy. The condition is extremely contagious — from five days before the rash appears until it disappears.

Complications can include middle ear infections (see pages 80 to 81), SINUSITIS or pneumonia. Immediately after a bout of measles, the immune system is often susceptible to other infections.

Usually measles only lasts about ten days from fever to end of rash, leaving the person immune to another attack.

WHAT YOU CAN DO

- Isolate the child from those who are not immune.
- Make sure they drink lots of fluids, eat lightly and get plenty of rest — don't let them resume normal activity in a hurry.
- A lukewarm sponge bath can relieve the discomfort of fever.
- Protect sensitive eyes from light. Flushing the eyes with saline solution may be soothing.

RUBELLA

Also known as German measles, rubella is a totally different virus to common measles. Contracting one does not give you immunity to the other. Rubella also produces a fine rash over the body, but this is often mild and is not accompanied by the cold-like symptoms of measles. The glands at the back of the neck may be enlarged.

The main concern is that rubella can cause severe birth defects if contracted during the sixth to 12th week of pregnancy. Immunisation is available.

AROMATHERAPY

The antiviral, antibacterial and anti-infectious qualities of eucalyptus and tea tree essential oils can help guard against secondary infections and/or alleviate many of the symptoms. Eucalyptus is also an expectorant and will help make breathing easier. Use a few drops of each oil in an oil burner or atomiser.

To reduce fever, sponge the child's body with tepid (not cold) water to which chamomile, bergamot and/or lavender have been added. Use 2 or 3 drops of these essential oils in a medium bowl of water and mix to disperse the oils.

CHINESE HERBS

The Chinese divide the measles into three stages of illness: first stage — fever and chills; second stage — skin pustules and rash appear; third stage — rash starts to disappear, convalescence. There are different Chinese herbal remedies which should be taken at different stages of this illness. The particular remedies depend on the specific symptoms your child is displaying.

HERBALISM

Garlic and onion (fresh or in tablet form) and echinacea are useful home remedies when fighting the measles infection. When fever is present the herbs boneset, yarrow and peppermint can be of assistance. There are also expectorant herbs such as marshmallow for treating the cough. Chamomile tea may be applied externally or taken internally for its soothing effect. A herbalist can advise you as to which of these herbs your child should take for their specific condition.

HOMOEOPATHY

It is best to see a homoeopath for the most effective remedy to reduce your child's period of illness. Homoeopathic remedies most commonly used to treat measles include *Pulsatilla nigricans, Gelsemium sempervirens, Apis mellifica* and *Atropa belladonna*.

MODERN MEDICINE

As a viral infection, there is no actual cure but there is immunisation available which as a parent you will have to consider for your child (see page 159) — make sure you discuss any allergies or other conditions with the doctor.

For those with measles, paracetamol is suggested for relief of pain and fever. Doctors also watch measles closely for further complications and may prescribe antibiotics in such cases.

NATUROPATHY

Give your child plenty of fresh fruit juices as this may help. Doses of vitamin A and C and zinc appropriate to the child's age will help the immune system recover faster.

REFLEXOLOGY

Gently work the following points: chest and lung for the cough, eyes to reduce soreness, diaphragm for relaxation, all glands and the lymph to boost the immune system, and all the fingers or toes as they correspond to the head area. Try this for a total of 15 minutes daily on both hands or feet until the condition clears.

MUMPS

Mumps is a viral infection that makes the salivary glands in the head and neck painful and swollen. Other symptoms include fever, difficulty swallowing and Headache. Occasional complications, especially if the infection occurs after puberty, include inflammation of the testes or ovaries. This can cause sterility in men.

Mumps usually passes in about a week. It is highly contagious from the onset until the end of symptoms and so your child must be isolated from people who have not had the mumps, and cutlery, towels etc. should be kept for their exclusive use. There is a remote chance of catching mumps twice.

IMPORTANT: *Mumps should be diagnosed by a doctor as other conditions can cause swelling of the glands. Seek medical attention if the condition is accompanied by vomiting, abdominal pain, swelling or pain in the testes, a high fever, stiff neck or severe headache.*

WHAT YOU CAN DO

- Make sure the child gets ample rest even if they do not appear particularly sick — adults with the mumps will require immediate bed rest.
- Avoid strongly flavoured, sour or acidic foods (including fruit juices) as they can aggravate the pain in the salivary glands.
- Chewing can be painful and saliva may not be being produced efficiently, so moist or soft foods such as soups are a good choice.
- Warm compresses on the swollen area may bring some relief. In other cases, ice packs may help by reducing swelling.

CHINESE HERBS

The two stages of mumps, firstly the headache and fever and then the swollen glands, are treated in Chinese herbalism with different remedies. These can be obtained after assessment from a Chinese herbalist.

HERBALISM

Give your child 1/2 cup of chamomile or dandelion root tea three times a day, making sure it is not too hot for them to drink. Echinacea in a tea form is also excellent for fighting infection. Mullein, calendula and red clover may be recommended by a herbalist.

HOMOEOPATHY

The same principle applies for mumps as it does for measles. Homoeopathic remedies most commonly used to treat these conditions are *Apis mellifica, Atropa belladonna, Pulsatilla nigricans, Rhus toxicondendrona* and *Aconitum napellus*. This viral infection should be referred to a homoeopath for the best results.

MODERN MEDICINE

There is no specific treatment or cure. Analgesics may help ease the pain.

REFLEXOLOGY

Gently work the points for the head and neck/throat, the ear, all glands, lymph and kidneys, as well as all the toes or fingers as they correspond to the head area. Try this for a total of 15 minutes daily on both hands or feet until the condition clears.

NAPPY RASH

Nappy rash is a rash which occurs around the area of a baby's bottom due to constant contact with ammonia in urine and dampness, providing an ideal atmosphere for bacterial growth. It is often also complicated by yeast infection (see page 374).

Seek medical attention if the nappy rash persists or is severe.

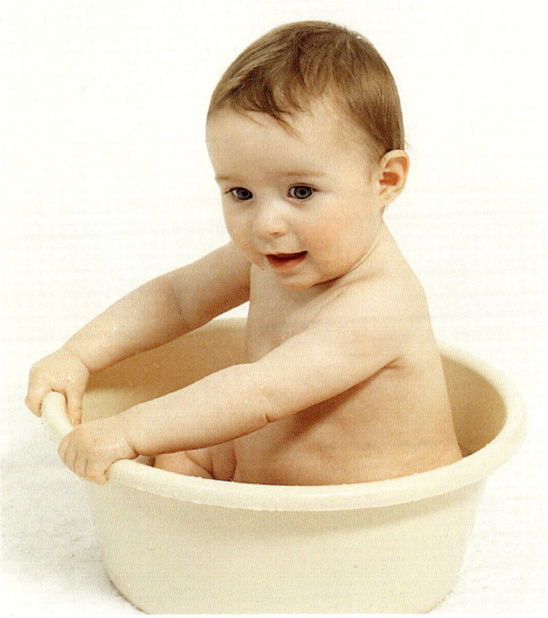

Bathing will help relieve nappy rash but dry your child well.

WHAT YOU CAN DO

- Try a sitz bath in a few inches of warm water for 5 minutes a few times a day.
- Keep your child as dry and clean as possible.
- Clean your baby with plain water as some soaps or alcohol may irritate skin. Avoid skin products with chemical additives including commercial wipes with alcohol, perfume and soap. If you do use soap, make sure it is mild and natural. Similarly, avoid strong detergent when washing nappies; try natural soap flakes or a low-allergy washing powder plus a final rinse in diluted vinegar.
- Don't scrimp on clean nappies; change them as soon as they are wet or soiled.
- Avoid plastic pants as they keep the moisture in and can further irritate some children. You may like to try cloth nappies.
- Changing the nappy during the night can help.
- Let your child be without nappies or pants as often as possible to let air get to the area.
- Snugly fitting nappies can be a problem as they prevent air flow. It is best if there is space around the waist and legs.
- Make sure your child drinks plenty of fluids so that the urine is not overly concentrated.

AROMATHERAPY

Before washing, soak your baby's nappies in a bucket full of water sprinkled with 8 drops of tea tree essential oil. This is preferable to chemical disinfectant because it will not irritate the skin. Lavender oil can also be effective in promoting cell renewal. Add 2 drops to the washing machine on the final rinse cycle. A mild tea tree antiseptic cream may be applied directly to the rash.

HERBALISM

There are a variety of herbal creams and ointments that help reduce nappy rash. These contain either paw paw or calendula and/or chickweed — their suitability varies from baby to baby. Apply after each change.

MODERN MEDICINE

Local creams and barrier creams are recommended by doctors for nappy rash. Hydrocortisone creams are available over the counter but, although effective, they can cause severe side effects. Also avoid boric acid and mercury preparations. Methylbenzethomium chloride in ointment or powder form may be a preventative.

NATUROPATHY
It helps if you bathe your child with non-alkaline soap or an oatmeal bath. Make an oatmeal bath by putting 2 cups of rolled oats in an old stocking and run the bath water through this.

You can also apply dry cornflour, arrowroot powder or bicarbonate of soda (baking soda) directly to the area. Castor oil cream may help some cases.

Dietary changes can cause nappy rash. If it appears after you have introduced a new food to the diet, try eliminating that food for two weeks to see whether it has an effect.

Highly acidic urine, which can cause irritation, comes from a diet too high in sugar — both the baby's diet and that of the breastfeeding mother can be responsible. Under the guidance of a naturopath, dairy products, wheat and meat may be cut from the diet and replaced with plenty of fruit, vegetables and brown rice. Goat's milk yogurt is an excellent protein and calcium source to replace dairy foods, as are soya bean products (such as soy milk). Nuts and seeds are good sources of protein.

TEETHING PROBLEMS

The majority of children experience problems when their teeth come through. These problems include sore gums, excessive dribbling, INSOMNIA, moodiness and crying.

WHAT YOU CAN DO

- Rub the gums with your finger or with a small clean gauze pad or with an ice cube wrapped in cloth. You could also try rubbing lemon juice into the gums to reduce sensitivity.
- Teething babies love to chew. A clean washcloth soaked in cold water or chamomile tea, or kept in the refrigerator is ideal to chew on and will bring some pain relief. A chilled fluid-filled teething ring will work in the same way. Foods that are suitable for chewing (while the baby is sitting upright) include raw carrot and celery sticks, cucumber, apple slices, hard crusts and rusks.
- Wipe away drool and change drool-drenched clothes as the moisture can cause a rash. If excessive, apply a barrier cream such as petroleum jelly around the mouth for protection.

BACH FLOWER REMEDIES
Rescue remedy soothes the child's emotional state and can also ease pain to some extent.

HERBALISM
The herbs lobelia and marshmallow are known for their healing effect on the gums. Give your child a stick of marshmallow root that has been peeled and washed. Chewing on it can relieve the pain. Older children can sip cooled chamomile tea (with honey, if desired) and babies can be given 1 or 2 teaspoons every 2 hours.

HOMOEOPATHY
The best remedy for teething is *Chamomilla vulgaris* because it works well with many children. If your child expresses their pain through anger and impatience, give them one 30C potency three times a day for three days.

If your child has diarrhoea with a sour odour when they are teething give them one 12C potency of *Rheum officinale* three times a day for three days.

MODERN MEDICINE
Soothing oral creams or gels are recommended by doctors (these are also available over the counter) as well as mild analgesics, suitable for babies, for pain reduction.

REFLEXOLOGY
Gently work the point for the diaphragm and solar plexus to induce relaxation, and all the toes or fingers as they correspond to the head area. Try this twice daily for a total of 10 to 15 minutes on both feet or hands.

SHIATSU
With your child lying on the back, apply gentle pressure to Governing Vessel 26 located half-way between the upper lip and nose. Then apply pressure around the gum line in a circular motion. Massaging Stomach 6 in the hinge of the jaw on both sides can relieve pain and inflammation.

TREATMENTS & THERAPIES

PAGE 86

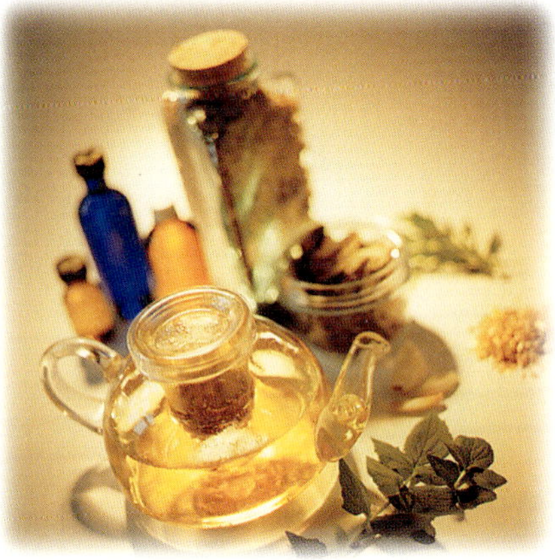

ACUPRESSURE

ACUPRESSURE IS PART OF THE SYSTEM OF TRADITIONAL CHINESE MEDICINE AND ITS TRADITIONAL MASSAGE TECHNIQUES. IT HAS AS ITS BASIS THE CONCEPT OF ENERGY FLOWING ALONG PATHWAYS IN THE BODY KNOWN AS MERIDIANS (SEE PAGE 182 FOR FURTHER INFORMATION).

Put simply, acupressure is when pressure is applied to acupuncture points with a fingertip, the knuckle of the index finger, a thumb — even the elbows and feet — instead of needles to stimulate points towards activity or inactivity (see page 92). The process may begin as pressure-then-release, pressure-then-release and develop to a deep and constant pressure. In other cases only one kind of pressure may be used. The finger may be rotated slightly in a very tight circle. The pressure must be in close proximity to the point for the treatment to be of benefit. Depths of pressure and the length of time it is applied are important aspects of the treatment.

PREVENTING ILLNESS

Though part of the treatment is concerned with resolving the presented symptoms, the major object of acupressure is to strengthen your overall health. Regular sessions of acupressure, in conjunction with other lifestyle changes, are potentially beneficial for health maintenance. You'll need to have a series of treatments before you feel the long-term benefits. It is probably best to have one treatment a week or one a month, depending on what your acupressure therapist advises.

If you are interested in acupressure as a way to sound health, you need to locate a properly trained practitioner. Your local acupuncturist or natural health centre may be able to refer you to one in your area.

A PROFESSIONAL CONSULTATION

An acupressure therapist is concerned with all aspects of your health — mental, emotional and physical. A good practitioner will explain the process to you and will need to gain an overview of your medical history, your job, diet and lifestyle activities. They will question you on the nature of your symptoms and even on your lack of specific symptoms. A diagnosis will be based on the 12 pulses (three places in each wrist, and two depths in each place), on the condition of the spine and abdomen, and on your facial expression. Based on their experience, practitioners also try to determine how you are "presenting" your energy — anger, nervousness, degree of relaxation are all great indicators of problem areas.

Acupressure can be performed when you are sitting or lying. It can help during a treatment to become conscious of your breath. Breathing a little more slowly and deeply will aid the energy flows in your body. Also be aware of how your muscles, particularly the one being worked on, begin to relax.

How long the treatment lasts depends on how your body reacts to the massage and the condition being treated. A point may be stimulated for 30 seconds, a few minutes, or for an extended time.

Acupressure massage can be incorporated within the framework of general relaxation as well as being condition-orientated. A whole body massage may take up to 1 hour but a more specific session is dependent on the responses of the client. Acupressure can be performed through clothing.

In general, no products are used but some practitioners may utilise liniments, egg white, ginger juice, garlic juice, water, heating pads or ice packs, all of which are applied externally.

IS ACUPRESSURE PAINFUL?

Responses to acupressure in regards to soreness or pain is relative to each individual's pain tolerance, the nature of the injury or ailment and the practitioner's skill in application. The same may be said about individual sensations during, immediately afterwards, and some 48 hours after treatment.

A SELF-HELP TECHNIQUE

Acupressure can be used as a self-help technique. It is important you locate the appropriate point, but once you know the general area a reliable indication of the exact location is the amount of tenderness triggered by your finger pressure. With a

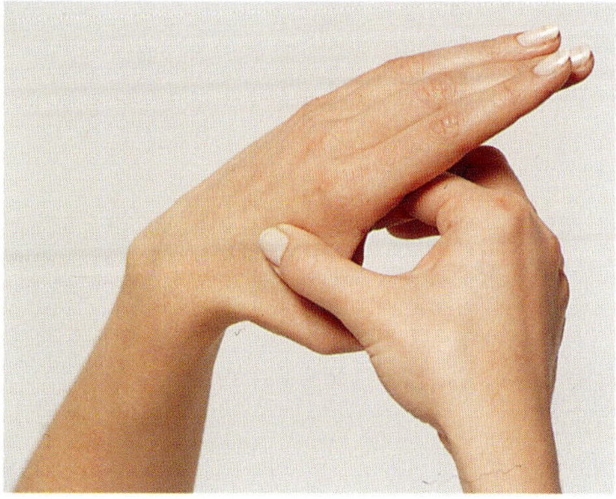

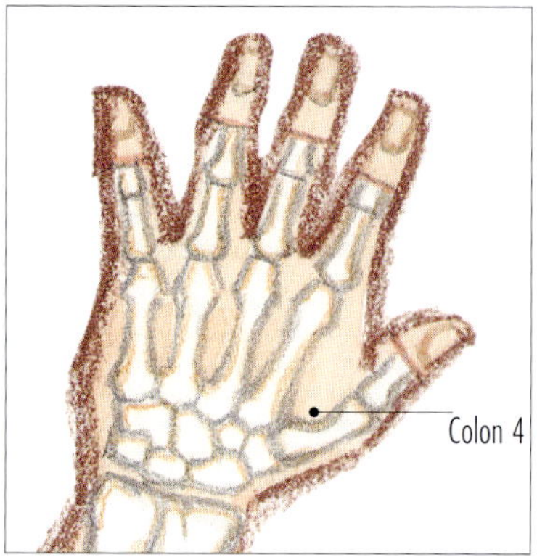

Finding the exact location of the point is important; that's why skeletal diagrams have been included. This point is Colon 4 which is very effective for the relief of nausea.

little experimentation you will become familiar with the particular sensation that accompanies an acupressure point.

Probably the best place to test this sensation is the point between your thumb and index finger on the back of your hand. This point is known as Colon 4 (Ho-Ku). Simply hold your hand out in front of you and follow the bone structure down to its natural V. With the thumb of your other hand, gently press into the base of the V until you find the tender spot. The pressure on this spot should feel strong and a little sore, but not acutely painful.

Press this point, varying the pressure until you feel the tenderness. Then move your thumb to another area on your hand, press and notice the difference. Do this a few times to "tune" yourself into the particular sensation of tenderness that indicates the correct acupressure point.

You can also look at the diagrams on pages 90 to 91 and experiment with other points on your body. Try the acupressure points listed in the A–Z OF HEALTH CONDITIONS, and notice how your body reacts to this therapy. With a little practice, you will soon be able to feel around until you locate the sensation that indicates you are right on the point.

Using acupressure at home is an effective way of treating simple complaints such as a minor headache, but seek the assistance of a professional for acute or chronic conditions. It is also important to see an acupressure therapist before you begin any lengthy home treatments to ensure you are activating the correct pressure points. If you self-administer acupressure and show no sign of improvement, consider seeking professional advice.

JIN SHIN DO — A MODERN VERSION

There are modern versions of acupressure blossoming as Westerners draw from the wisdom of the ancient Chinese healers, couple it with modern theories and adopt the whole to suit today's needs. One of these is Jin Shin Do.

This new form of acupressure has been developed in recent decades by an American woman, Iona Marsaa Teegurden. Aimed at releasing muscle tension, the therapy is a combination of Teegurden's research into acupressure, acupuncture, breathing techniques and modern psychology.

Jin Shin Do differs from acupressure in that it concentrates on releasing chronic stress in muscles, called "armouring". This is tension that has developed over many years, often initially as a result of a particularly stressful experience, and which has been gradually added to by other similar events that remind the person of the original trauma.

Because a Jin Shin Do therapist is working with underlying emotional conditions, they are inclined to apply a more gentle finger pressure than is used in traditional acupressure. They will begin with light pressure, increasing it gradually as the person relaxes and "invites" the deeper work.

While this pressure is concentrated on the point that contains the most tension, the therapist's other hand will work on several other points which are complementary to the release of tension. This combination helps the body return to balance.

WHEN TO AVOID ACUPRESSURE

- People with serious medical conditions should seek advice from a professional therapist or doctor before treatment.
- Areas of your body that have recent scar tissue, or are infected or bruised, should be avoided.
- Pregnant women, infants and young people are not suitable candidates
- The general rule: if in doubt, don't.

ACUPRESSURE DIAGRAMS

Throughout the A–Z OF HEALTH CONDITIONS section of this book, you will find references to acupressure points you can try at home. These diagrams show where the points can be found. However, it is best to consult with a professional acupressure practitioner who can provide a thorough diagnosis and treatment as well as advice on using acupressure for the greatest effect at home.

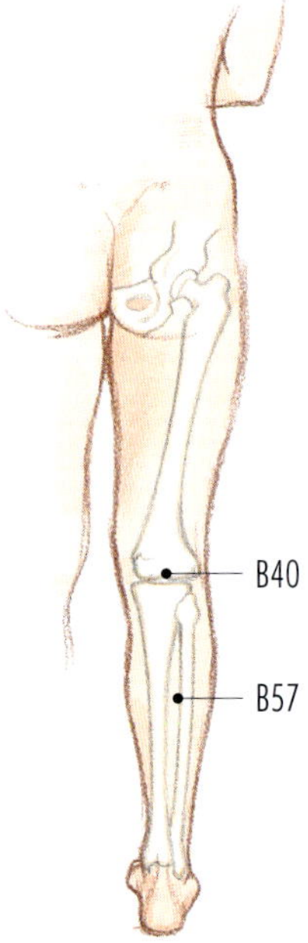

BACK

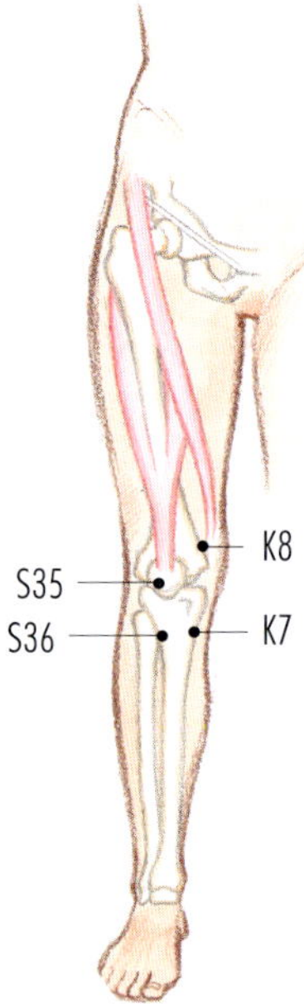

FRONT

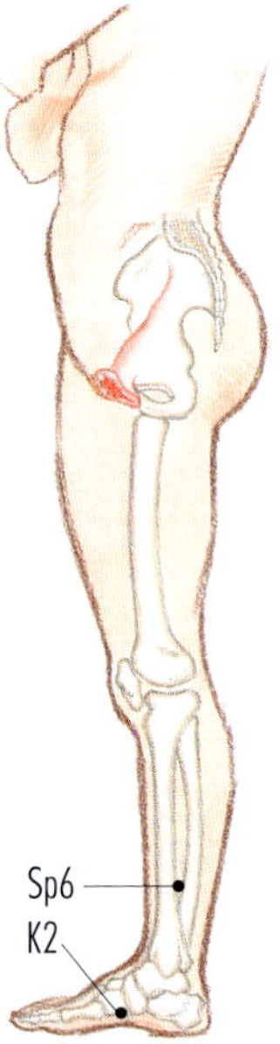

INSIDE

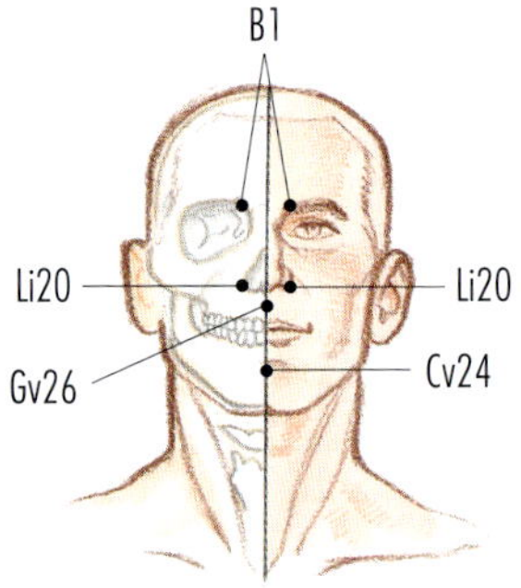

FRONT

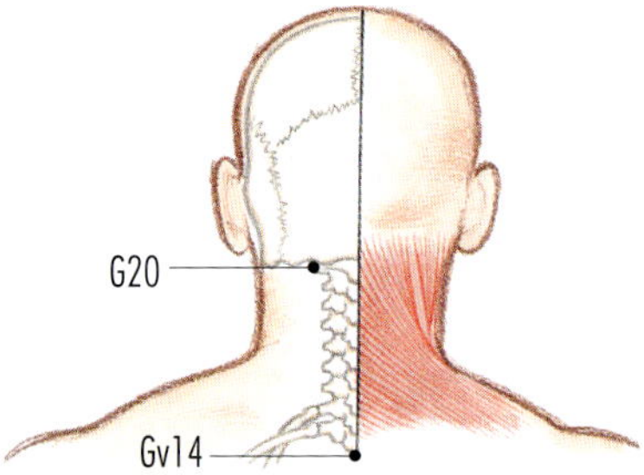

BACK

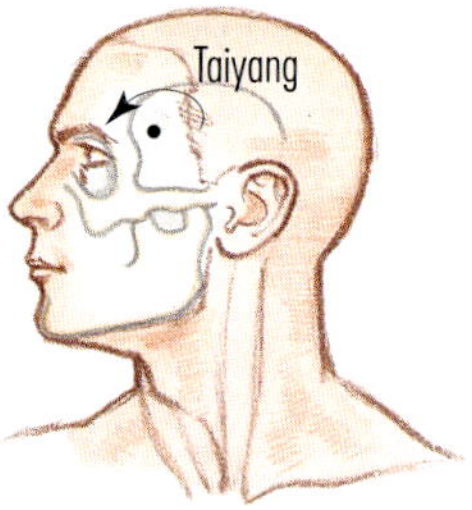

LEFT SIDE

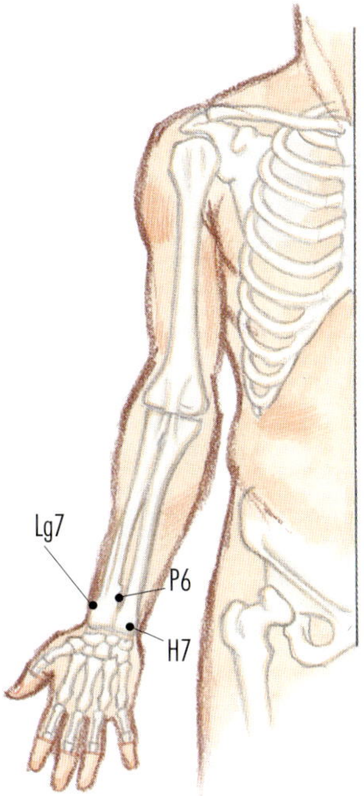

FRONT

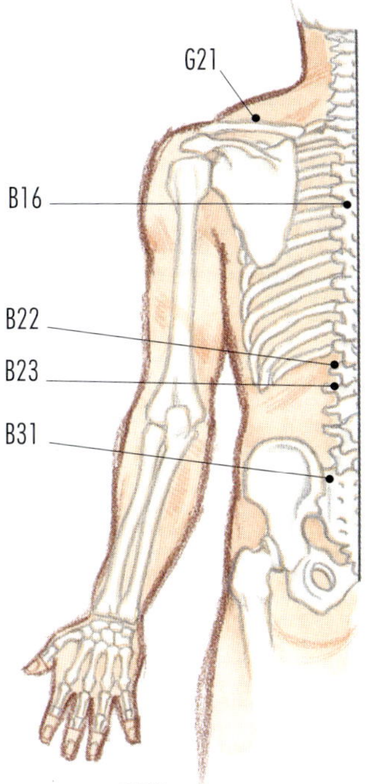

BACK

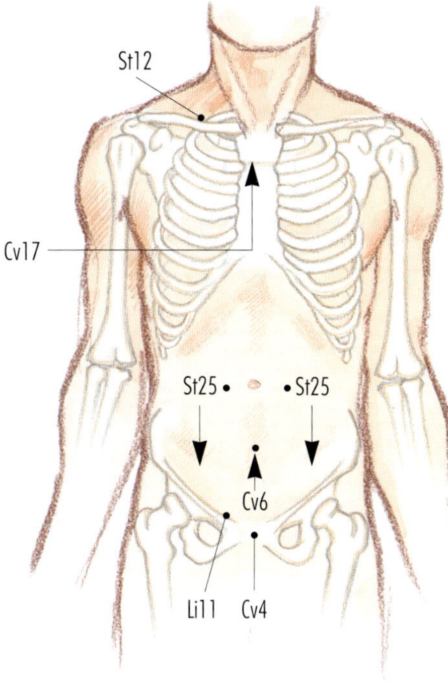

FRONT WHOLE

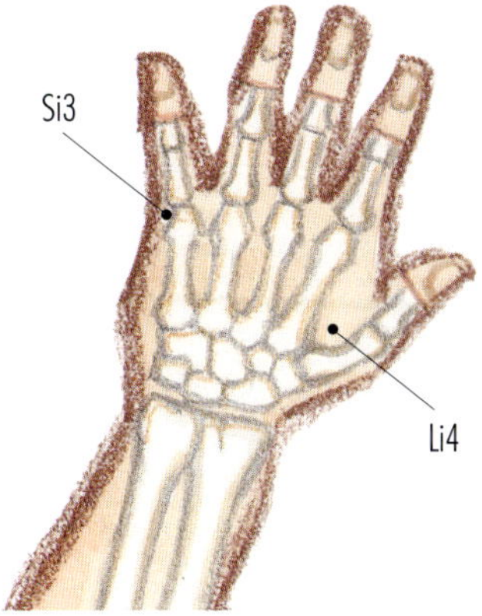

BACK

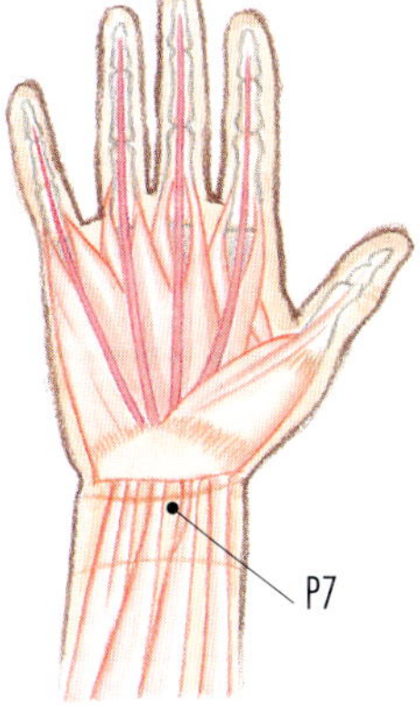

PALM

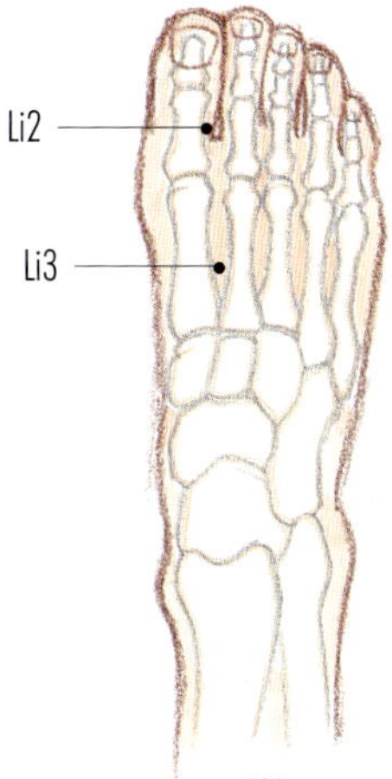

TOP

TABLE

ABBREVIATIONS FOR THE MERIDIANS

B = Bladder
Cv = Conception Vessel
G = Gall Bladder
Gv = Governing Vessel
H = Heart
K = Kidney
Lg = Lung
Li = Liver
P = Pericardium
Si = Small Intestine
Sp = Spleen
St = Stomach

ACUPUNCTURE

LEGEND HAS IT THAT ACUPUNCTURE BEGAN WHEN A MAN WAS LIFTING HEAVY ROCKS. HE HAD A HEADACHE SO SEVERE THAT HE ACCIDENTALLY DROPPED A ROCK ON HIS FOOT. SUDDENLY HIS HEADACHE STOPPED. THE ROCK HAD DROPPED ON THE POINT NEAR THE BIG TOE KNOWN AS LIVER 3. THIS POINT IS STILL USED TODAY TO RELIEVE HEADACHES, WITH NEEDLES REPLACING THE ROCK.

Acupuncture in its present form is believed to have originated from a text written during the first and second century BC. It is called the Huang di Nei Jing (translated as The Yellow Emperor's Manual of Corporal Medicine). The text discusses yin and yang, the five phases (fire, earth, metal, water and wood) and various acupuncture points. By the time of the Tang Dynasty (618–907 AD), the Imperial Medical College had a professor of acupuncture, an assistant professor and ten instructors.

In recent years, acupuncture has found increasing acceptance in Western medical practice, particularly in relieving pain.

HOW IT WORKS

Acupuncture is just one treatment in the broader system known as TRADITIONAL CHINESE MEDICINE which is based on the concept of an energy flow through the body called Ch'i or Qi. This energy circulates through the body along pathways known as meridians (see page 182 for further information).

It is believed that if the flow of energy is blocked, imbalances occur which in turn lead to health problems. This flow can be unblocked with the use of needles at specific points along the meridians. These points correspond to the various organs in the body. When needles are applied to the points, the organ function is stimulated.

Acupuncture and acupressure treatments are aimed at unblocking the meridians, easing muscle tension, and stimulating the energy and blood flow so the nutritive and defence energies within the body are adjusted, striking a balance between yin and yang, the active and passive aspects of your body.

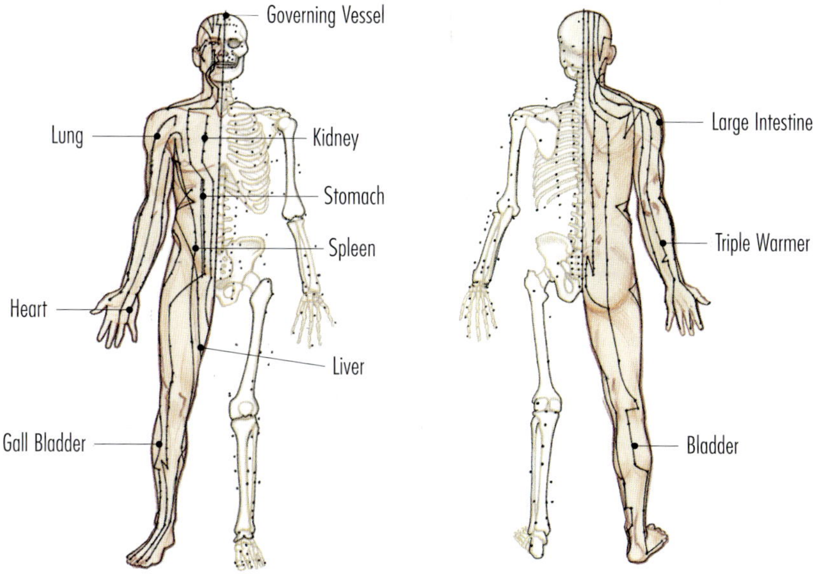

Acupuncture is based on the concept that there is an energy flow through the body. This energy circulates on specific pathways known as meridians. Each of the different meridians cover different parts of the body and are linked to particular organs.

WHO WILL BENEFIT

Acupuncture can be a valuable preventative tool. Rather than waiting until your body is in a state of imbalance and displaying physical symptoms, a one-off or regular acupuncture treatment can help maintain good health.

It is, of course, extremely effective in the management of acute and chronic conditions as well.

Some of the common conditions that can be successfully treated by acupuncture include:

- Headache and Migraine, dizziness
- nervous tension, Anxiety, Depression
- addictions such as Smoking
- Insomnia
- high or low blood pressure, poor circulation, Fluid Retention, angina
- Digestive Problems such as indigestion, Flatulence, Ulcers, Colitis, Diarrhoea, Constipation, Haemorrhoids
- Liver and Gall Bladder Problems
- Kidney and Bladder Problems
- hormone imbalances, Menstrual Problems including Pre-menstrual Tension and difficulties with Menopause and fertility
- Asthma, Bronchitis, Tonsilitis, Sinusitus and other respiratory problems, including Colds and Flu
- skin conditions such as Acne, Dandruff, Eczema
- muscle pain including Cramps, strains
- Arthritis, Sciatica
- toothache, Gingivitis and mouth Ulcers
- irritated eyes, Conjunctivitis and eye disorders including short-sightedness in children and some forms of cataracts.

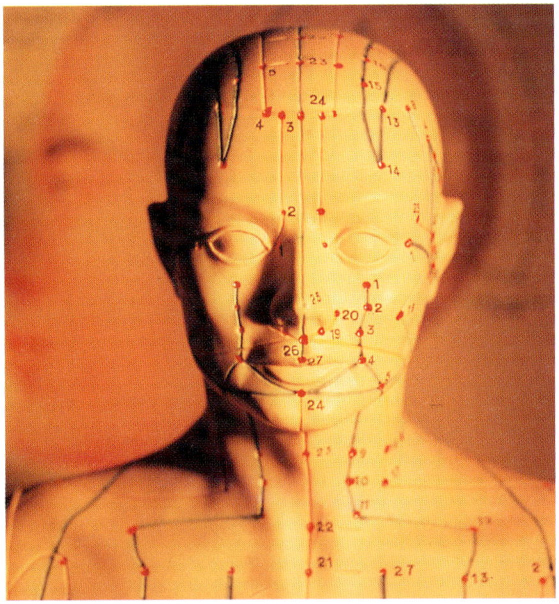

The placement of needles on points is very particular.

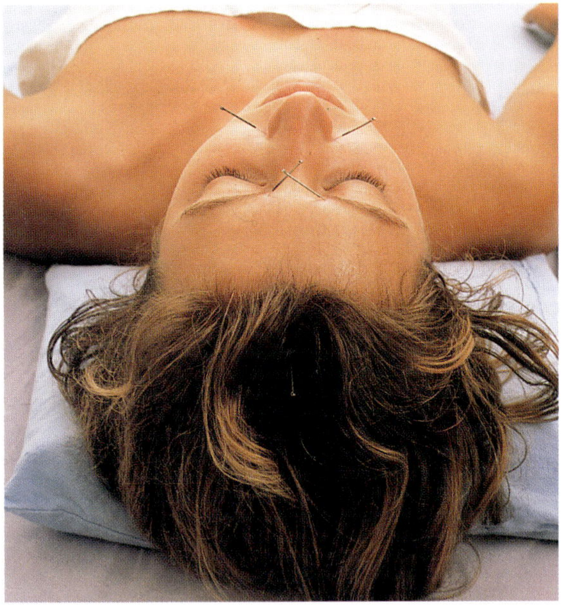

Many people feel relaxed, even sleepy, during treatment.

CONSULTING AN ACUPUNCTURIST

Acupuncture should only be performed by a qualified practitioncr — one with at least three to four years of full-time training and represented by a professional association.

A consultation with an acupuncturist will begin with a complete diagnosis (see page 184). The points for acupuncture will be selected based on this overview.

With traditional acupuncture, very fine "filiform" needles are used — these should be single-use needles, disposable and pre-sterilised. The insertion is quick, usually bloodless and basically painless. How far the needle goes in will vary according to the patient and the point being treated; it may only just break the surface of the skin (on the finger, for example) or it may go in several centimetres in fleshy areas such as the buttocks. You may feel a slight prick when a needle is inserted. Some people have a dull, heavy distended feeling around the needle site, others experience a tingling sensation along the channel or a warm spreading feeling. During treatment, many people become very relaxed and may feel sleepy.

The needle is usually left in place for 20 minutes in adults and 10 minutes in children. In some cases the needles may be manipulated once they are inserted; they may be strongly stimulated or just gently rotated once or twice. Some techniques use insertion-manipulation-withdrawal — the needle being in place for less than a minute with several points treated in quick succession. There are also thread-imbedding techniques and special needles, like tiny thumb tacks, that may be inserted and left for up to a week. They are covered with surgical tape to prevent them from falling out and to keep them clean.

The number of needles used in a treatment can vary considerably depending on the condition and the technique used.

You should feel an improvement immediately after a session. Some people feel very light, even euphoric, relaxed yet energetic. This is thought to be due to the release of endorphins stimulated by acupuncture. Other people may feel very tired and want to sleep more than usual. This is due to the relief from bodily tension and the lowering of stress levels. After treatment for muscular disorders, there may be some dull, residual pain but this soon wears off.

TYPES OF ACUPUNCTURE

Other than using the filiform needle alone, other treatment techniques include moxibustion, cupping, electro-acupuncture and laser acupuncture.

CUPPING is a technique often used for muscular-skeletal problems and chest congestion. A cup, usually made of glass, is flamed — the air inside is heated quickly with a lighted taper. This is then placed on the affected region (often on the back or over a large muscle area). As the air inside the cup cools, the skin and flesh covered by the mouth of the cup is subjected to a steady suction that relaxes the underlying muscle.

ELECTRO-ACUPUNCTURE involves attaching voltmeters to the inserted needles. Fewer needles need to be used with this form of acupuncture and practitioners of this method say the stimulation of the acupuncture points is stronger.

LASER ACUPUNCTURE has been used in Europe for more than 20 years but other countries have been slower to catch on. Laser light is transmitted from a hand-held wand to stimulate the acupuncture points.

MOXIBUSTION is a traditional type of acupuncture using moxa, the dried leaves of the herb mugwort, either alone or mixed with other herbs. In one form, a spongy substance known as moxa wool or loose moxa is moulded around the handle of a needle and burned. The moxa wool can also be moulded into a ball the size of a grain of rice. This is placed either directly on the skin to burn and create a tiny blister, or on top of ginger, salt or garlic, depending on the result desired. Special moxibustion cups may be used with this technique. Alternatively, a moxa roll (which looks a bit like a large cigar) can be lit and held over an acupuncture point to warm it.

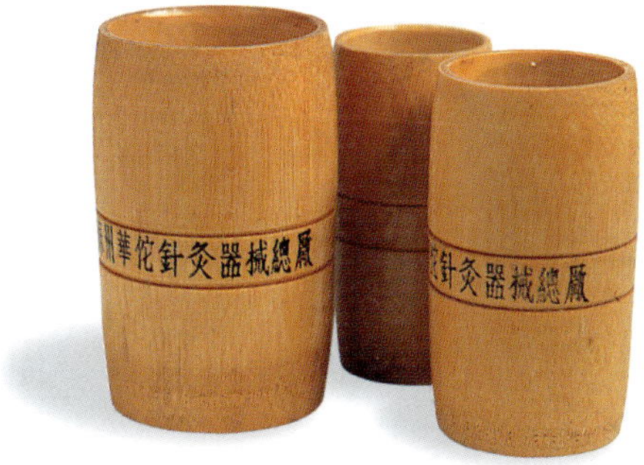

Moxibustion cups

THE ALEXANDER TECHNIQUE

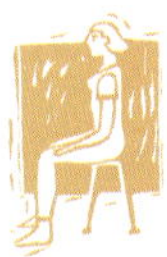

THE ALEXANDER TECHNIQUE IS ONE OF THE EXERCISE AND MOVEMENT TECHNIQUES THAT RELY ON RESTRUCTURING RATHER THAN MANIPULATION. IT IS BASED ON THE BELIEF THAT PEOPLE LEARN TO MISUSE THEIR BODIES IN WAYS THAT FEEL NATURAL BUT ARE, IN THE LONG TERM, DETRIMENTAL. JUST BECAUSE THE WAY YOU HABITUALLY MOVE FEELS RIGHT, DOESN'T MEAN IT IS RIGHT!

Body aches and pains or health problems can be an indication your body is not being moved as it was designed to be moved. The focus of the Alexander Technique concentrates on relearning the correct way to stand, sit, walk, lift objects and breathe. An Alexander teacher will help you "experience" this, but discipline is needed to practise the technique and discard old habits of posture and movement.

THE PERSON BEHIND THE TECHNIQUE

Tasmanian-born Fredrick Matthias Alexander (1869–1955) developed the Alexander Technique. For a period in his life he worked as an actor reciting Shakespeare and poetry. During this time, Alexander lost his voice regularly. He tried all that the modern medicine of his time had to offer, but nothing seemed to work.

Observing himself in a mirror as he recited, Alexander noticed how he would pull his head back and tighten the area around his larynx. He experimented and discovered that if he lifted his head vertically and freed his neck, his vocal quality improved. This new way of standing felt uncomfortable, but he persevered with it, retrained his body, and began to notice an additional pay-off: he felt healthier and more self-confident, and his voice trouble completely disappeared. The experience inspired Alexander to make a nine-year study of his own posture and how to improve it. This became the foundation of the Alexander Technique.

Alexander believed that the human body is designed to move with maximum balance and co-ordination using minimal effort.

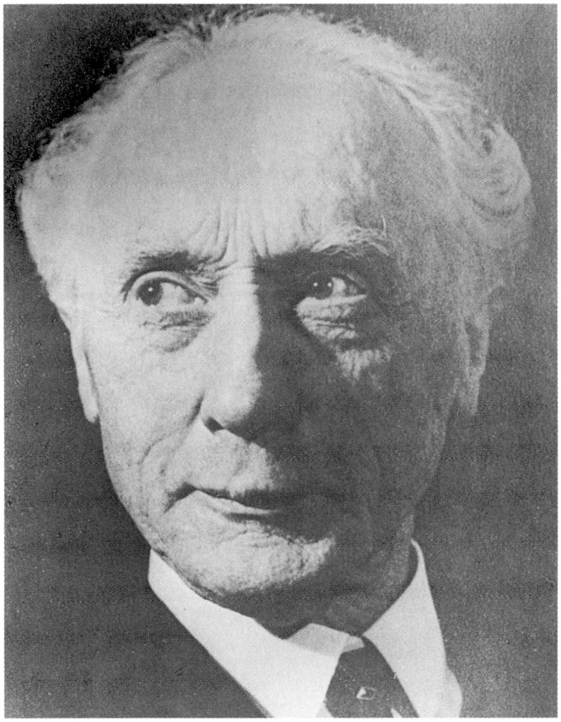

Fredrick Alexander developed an exercise and movement technique to help combat his recurring voice problems.

He noticed that most people have learned unnatural postures (chins held too high, shoulders rounded, heads pushed back) which stress the body. Alexander's answer to this was simple: "Let the neck be free to let the head be forward and up, and the back widen and lengthen". If you can achieve this natural posture, your body will be relaxed, and your breathing and blood circulation will improve, creating greater feelings of balance and well-being.

In the early 1900s, Alexander moved to London where he began teaching his technique. He also wrote books about it, the most popular being *The Use of the Self*. During the 1930s the Alexander Technique gained acceptance and recognition. Clients included the writers Aldous Huxley and George Bernard Shaw.

Over the years, the technique has also gained a good deal of acceptance from the medical profession, and in recent decades, other students of the technique have improved on Alexander's original teachings.

LEARNING THE TECHNIQUE

When you attend your first Alexander lesson, your teacher will observe how you stand, sit, walk, move and breathe. When they have assessed what you are doing incorrectly, they will attempt to give you a sense — an experience — of what it will mean to make these movements in a different, more natural way.

Often they will use visualisation techniques. You may be asked to think of your head as a balloon floating free above your body with the string as your neck and spine. You will be encouraged to release the unnecessary tension you are holding, to deepen your breathing, let your shoulders relax, and allow your back to lengthen and expand.

The teacher will usually guide you by touch. If the teacher is in natural balance, their guiding your body into its correct balance will reawaken your body's own memory. This gives you a physical sense of what is possible, and the task of discarding bad old habits for what is natural and correct is made much easier.

Often students report leaving an Alexander Technique lesson feeling taller and lighter, walking with more freedom in their movements.

It takes a series of lessons for students to properly integrate these new ways of being. It also takes practice and self-discipline to remain conscious of your body throughout the day and avoid falling back into the old habits.

One of the benefits of attending Alexander Technique classes is that the information you gain will stay with you for the rest of your life.

Alexander Technique students report that even decades after their lessons they can use what they learnt in times of stress (for example, before giving a public speech or attending an important interview). Once they become aware they are physically tense, they will consciously adjust their bodies and let their necks go free, they feel their heads float up vertically and their backs lengthen and widen.

The technique is useful for relaxation and tension release. It is also helpful to anyone suffering from a repetitive strain injury. It can assist sports people, athletes, dancers, actors and musicians to improve their breathing, and the use of their bodies to prevent soreness and injuries. And because the Alexander Technique demands that you increase your body awareness, your sense of self is also increased. Your body can tell you a great deal about yourself and how you relate to the world — the Alexander Technique is one way to understand those messages.

WHO IT CAN HELP

Some of the conditions that the technique may assist include:

- ASTHMA and respiratory disorders
- FATIGUE
- DEPRESSION
- ULCERS
- HEADACHES
- high blood pressure
- rheumatoid ARTHRITIS and osteoarthritis
- BACK PAIN
- SCIATICA.

It is likely to have an effect on your overall well-being, from improved sleep and mental alertness to greater emotional balance.

STANDING UP AND WALKING ALEXANDER STYLE

In essence, the Alexander Technique is about the appropriate relationship between the neck, head and back. When the body is in its natural state of balance, all movements only require a minimal amount of effort.

For example, to rise from a seated position to a standing position, it is easiest if you lean forward with a straight back so that your weight shifts to your feet, allowing an easy transfer. This is the correct way to rise.

The way most people rise from a chair, by pushing the body upright, requires an overall tightening of the body.

To walk with ease, the head moves upward and away from the body, and the body follows, head and shoulders relaxed, arms and legs moving in an easy rhythm.

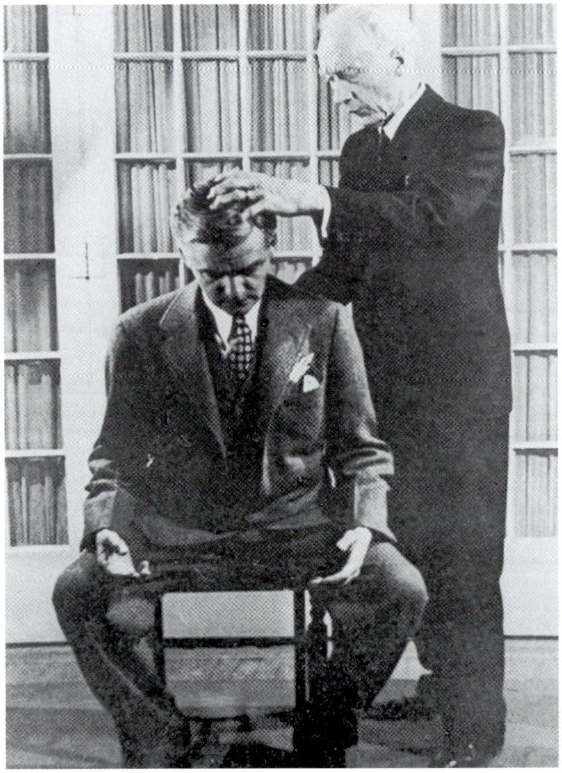

An Alexander teacher will observe how you stand, sit, walk, move and breathe. When they have worked out where the problems lie, they will teach you how to move in a more natural way. This is done by guiding you through touch so that you actually *feel* the different way of moving.

AROMATHERAPY

LEGEND HAS IT THAT CLEOPATRA HAD HER CLOTHES, CURTAINS, AND EVEN THE SAILS OF HER BARGE, PERFUMED WITH THE ESSENTIAL OILS OF ROSE AND JASMINE. IT SHOULD COME AS NO SURPRISE THAT AROMATHERAPISTS BELIEVE THAT ROSE IS AN APHRODISIAC AND USE JASMINE AS A RELAXANT. JULIUS CAESAR AND MARK ANTONY DIDN'T STAND A CHANCE!

While we will never know exactly how much power Cleopatra's oils exerted in the arena of romance, the ancient Egyptians are renowned for their knowledge of aromatic substances. It is acknowledged that Egyptian priests used them to embalm their pharaohs, but it is also believed the Egyptians understood the healing properties of oils and incorporated them in the treatment of nerve problems and depression.

Hippocrates apparently accepted the connection between the oils and their therapeutic use. He prescribed aromatic baths and scented massages, and recommended certain oils because they offered protection against contagious diseases. Centuries later, scientists have confirmed that some oils have antiviral, antibacterial, and antifungal properties — for example, the oil from Australia's tea tree.

The modern-day interest in oils began in the 1920s when a French chemist, Rene Maurice Gattefosse, was making fragrances. While working in his laboratory he burnt his arm, and with no cold water nearby, he plunged the arm into a jug of lavender oil. To his amazement the pain was less than he expected, the blistering was greatly reduced and the healing process sped up. Gattefosse was so impressed he spent the rest of his life researching the healing properties of oils; it was he who coined the term "aromatherapy".

WHAT ARE ESSENTIAL OILS?

Aromatherapists work with what are called "essential oils". Essential oils differ from perfume, or aromatic oils. While essential oils may smell as beautiful as perfume oils, they are distilled from plants and used for their healing properties rather than their scent.

Aromatherapists can choose from about 300 essential oils, and oils are now traded around the world. The oils are produced from all types, and parts, of plants — flowers, leaves, stalks, gums, seeds, and even roots. To ensure the best-quality oil product, the plant

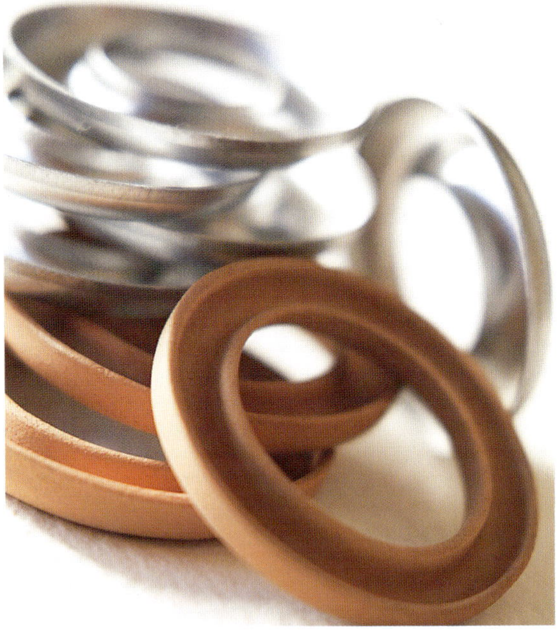

Light bulb rings are one way to distribute essential oils around a room.

must be picked at the optimum time. In the case of sandalwood, that means waiting 30 years until the tree has matured.

This explains the variations between the prices of different oils. Lavender is relatively inexpensive because it is easy to harvest and extract. Rose, on the other hand, is the queen of the oils and very expensive. It takes tens of thousands of rose petals to produce just one small bottle of oil. Sage oil is still extracted from the plant's leaves using traditional methods that have changed little over the centuries — the leaves are spread out on racks to dry naturally in the sun before they are distilled. Accordingly, sage oil is often slightly more expensive than most other essential oils.

HOW DO OILS WORK?

The essential properties of the oils can also be absorbed through the skin or mucous membranes. They are then transported around the body and affect various organs and body systems.

The oils can be used to aid the treatment of emotional and physical problems, relieve symptoms, or just add an enriching sensual quality to your life.

Aromatherapists use the oils singly or in combinations. They talk about "synergy", when the combination of the oils creates a chemical compound which is more powerful than the individual oils. For this reason, oil blend recipes should be followed because the aromatherapist will have experimented to find the best synergistic effect. This is particularly important if you are using oils as an adjunct to other treatments for serious health problems.

When consulting an aromatherapist, they will usually ask questions about your health and well-being to establish which oils will most benefit you. Often the aromatherapist will encourage you to select oils by your sense of smell. There is a belief you will be drawn to the fragrance that holds the properties which will help bring your body and emotions into balance.

This principle is useful to understand if you experiment with aromatherapy at home. Allow your intuition to guide you to the appropriate oils. Sometimes you will find yourself attracted to one oil — for example, sandalwood — for a few weeks then suddenly that scent will no longer appeal to you and you will be drawn to another oil.

SOME HELPFUL ADVICE

- Store oils and oil blends in dark glass bottles in a cool dark place.
- If blending oils, only make up enough for your immediate use — about a week's worth for oil blends, a day for water. You can keep water blends in the refrigerator.
- Do not confuse essential oils with fragrant oils which may smell good and are cheaper but do not contain the essential active ingredients. Read the labels carefully.

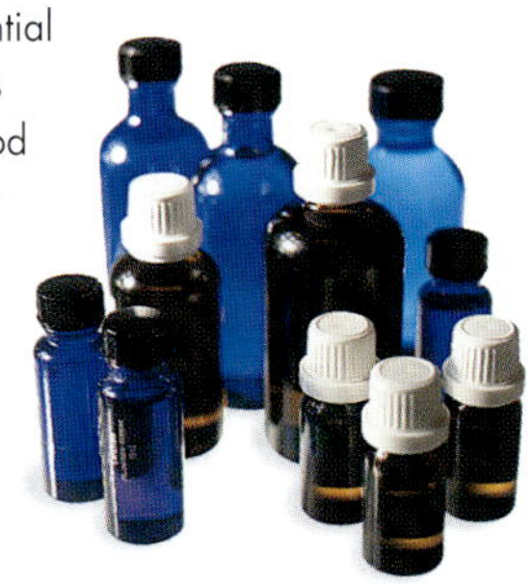

COMMON WAYS TO USE THE OILS

DIRECT APPLICATION Not usually recommended, but lavender and tea tree oils are exceptions. Apply to an affected area with a dampened cotton swab.

OIL BURNERS Also called fragrancers, vaporisers, aroma lamps and diffusers, these containers have a bowl at the top and an opening for a candle at the bottom. Fill the bowl with hot water and add 5 to 15 drops of essential oil. The candle keeps the water heated, releasing the fragrance and essential properties into the air. Take care not to let the water evaporate completely as the oils will leave a sticky residue.

AROMABATH Add 6 to 12 drops of essential oil to a bath, or use an oil blend, but wait until the bath is almost full of water because the oils evaporate quickly. Ensure they are well dispersed so they do not irritate your skin. Breathe deeply, and try to soak your entire body for 10 to 20 minutes. You can also have foot baths, hand baths, and sitz baths or hip baths.

SHOWERS You can add 2 to 3 drops of oil to a damp cloth or body brush and rub over your body as you stand under the shower. Remember to inhale deeply.

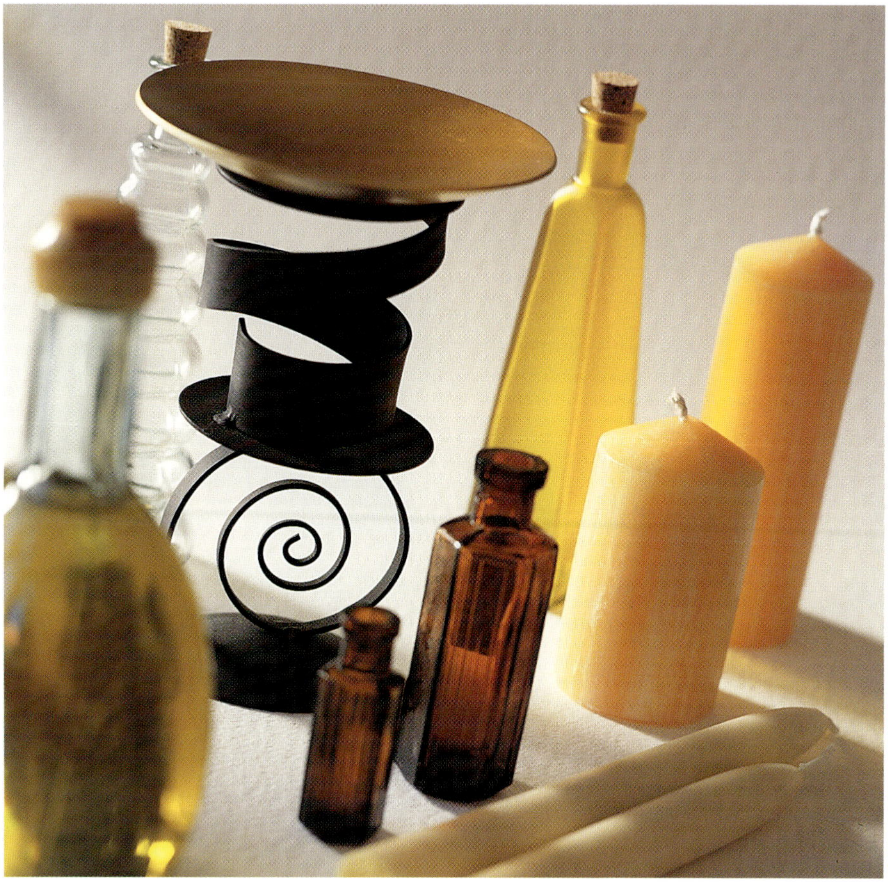

Essential oils can be used in oil burners or incorporated into cosmetics and massage oils, even candles.

THE ESSENTIAL OILS

NAME	PROPERTIES	CAUTION
Basil *Ocimum basilicum*	Digestive • respiratory • soothing • calming • relaxing to muscles • head-clearing • uplifting • clarifying • aphrodisiac • mentally stimulating • refreshing • aid to concentration • useful for soothing skin abrasions	Avoid use during pregnancy
Bergamot *Citrus bergamia*	Respiratory • uplifting • clarifying • antiseptic • digestive • treatment for skin, hair and scalp • refreshing • deodorising (personal) • antidepressant	Phototoxic — do not use on the skin in sunlight
Chamomile *Matricaria chamomilla (German), Anthemis nobilis (Roman)*	Soothing • mildly antiseptic • analgesic • calming • relaxing to muscles • digestive • balancing for the female system • refreshing • anti-inflammatory • treatment for skin, hair and scalp • treatment for insomnia • mild anaesthetic	Should not be used in the early months of pregnancy
Cedarwood *Juniper virginiana*	Antiseptic • digestive • astringent • skin toning • calming • aphrodisiac • harmonising • strengthening • sedative • soothing • diuretic	Avoid use during pregnancy
Cinnamon *Cinnamomum zeylanicum*	Antiseptic • digestive • respiratory • toning for skin • aphrodisiac • haemostatic • astringent • warming and soothing to skin • uplifting	Avoid use during pregnancy
Clary sage *Salvia sclarea*	Soothing • anti-inflammatory • calming • astringent • tonifying • warming • relaxing • uplifting • euphoria-producing • balancing female system • antidepressant	Avoid use during pregnancy, if you have high blood pressure or after alcohol
Clove *Carophyllus aromaticus*	Antiseptic • antispasmodic • slightly aphrodisiac • analgesic • carminative • digestive • nervine • respiratory • warming	Avoid use during pregnancy
Cypress *Cupressus sempervirens*	Balancing to the female system • stimulating • circulatory • respiratory • decongestive • head-clearing • antispasmodic • gently diuretic • refreshing • relaxing • astringent • treatment for skin • deodorising	Avoid use if you have high blood pressure and during pregnancy
Eucalytpus *Eucalyptus globulus*	Head-clearing • refreshing • stimulating • uplifting • invigorating • respiratory • decongestive • antiseptic • cooling • cleansing • anti-inflammatory • antispasmodic • analgesic	Avoid use if you have high blood pressure or are an epileptic
Frankincense *Boswellia thurifera*	Nervine • respiratory • restorative • beneficial to the female system • rejuvenating • comforting • relaxing • soothing • fear-dispelling	
Geranium *Pelargonium graveolens*	Antiseptic • antidepressant • anti-inflammatory • diuretic • balancing • tonifying • warming • refreshing • relaxing • harmonising • treatment for skin	

THE ESSENTIAL OILS

NAME	PROPERTIES	CAUTION
Jasmine *Jasminum grandiflorum*	Relaxing • uplifting • beneficial to the female system • aphrodisiac • strong sensual stimulant • soothing • confidence-building • antidepressant • fear-dispelling • skin-softening	Avoid use during pregnancy
Juniper *Juniperus communis*	Nervine • diuretic • analgesic • relaxing to muscles • cleansing • toning • balancing • relaxing • digestive • appetite-stimulating • circulatory • carminative • refreshing • invigorating • antiseptic	Avoid use during pregnancy
Lavender *Lavandula officinalis*	Head-clearing • respiratory • skin-healing • nervine • relaxing to muscles • digestive • sedative • calming • balancing to emotions • analgesic • antiseptic • antibacterial • decongestive • antidepressant • refreshing • relaxing • soothing	
Lemon *Citrus limomum*	Antiseptic • physically stimulating • skin tonic • antibacterial • astringent • diuretic • circulatory • refreshing • cooling • uplifting • stimulating • motivating • deodorising	Phototoxic — do not use on the skin in sunlight
Marjoram *Origanum majorana*	Antispasmodic • carminative • respiratory • nervine • calming • relaxing to muscles • digestive • sedative • warming • fortifying	Avoid use during pregnancy
Myrrh *Commiphora myrrha*	Healing • digestive • anti-inflammatory • respiratory • tonic • stimulating • antifungal • astringent • antiseptic • toning • strengthening • rejuvenating • expectorant	Avoid use during pregnancy
Neroli *Citrus aurantium*	Antibacterial • calming • healing to the skin • circulatory • nervine • digestive • sedative • antidepressant • aphrodisiac • relaxing • fear-dispelling	
Orange *Citrus aurantium*	Relaxing • astringent • refreshing • uplifting • antidepressant	
Patchouli *Pogostemon patchouli*	Nervine • anti-inflammatory • aphrodisiac • sedative • relaxing • insect repellant • antiseptic	
Peppermint *Mentha piperita*	Digestive • carminative • respiratory • anti-inflammatory • balancing to the female system • cooling (and warming) • clearing • relaxing to muscles • refreshing	Avoid use during pregnancy
Pine *Pinus sylvestris*	Respiratory • antiseptic • nervine • deodorising • stimulating • refreshing • invigorating	Pine oil should not be used by people with sensitive skin, as it may cause skin irritation

THE ESSENTIAL OILS

NAME	PROPERTIES	CAUTION
Rose *Rosa damascena (rose otto), Rosa centifolia (rose absolute)*	Antibacterial • balancing • astringent • antiseptic • antidepressant • anti-inflammatory • aphrodisiac • digestive • relaxing • soothing • sensual • confidence-building • beneficial to female system	
Rosemary *Rosemarinus officinalis*	Invigorating • digestive • nervine • respiratory • circulatory • muscular • uplifting • stimulating • refreshing • clarifying • treatment for skin, hair and scalp • memory-enhancing	Avoid use if you have high blood pressure, during pregnancy or if you are an epileptic.
Sage *Salvia officinalis*	Diuretic • analgesic • antiseptic • nervine • relaxing • decongestant • refreshing • appetite stimulant • healing to skin • • deodorant and antiperspirant • astringent • stimulating	Avoid use during pregnancy
Sandalwood *Santalum album*	Digestive • calming • relaxing • soothing • softening and healing to skin • antispasmodic • antidepressant • sedative • warming • confidence-building • grounding	
Tea tree *Melaleuca alternifolia*	Antiseptic • antifungal • digestive • healing to skin • antibacterial • respiratory • decongestive • strengthening to the immune system • insect repellent	
Thyme *Thymus vulgaris*	Antiseptic • disinfectant • circulatory • stimulating • respiratory • nervine • cleansing and toning to skin, hair and scalp • relaxing to muscles • refreshing • strengthens the immune system • fortifying	Avoid use during pregnancy
Ylang ylang *Cananga odorata*	Antiseptic • aphrodisiac • sedative • nervine • relaxing • soothing • euphoric • antidepressant • toning • balancing	

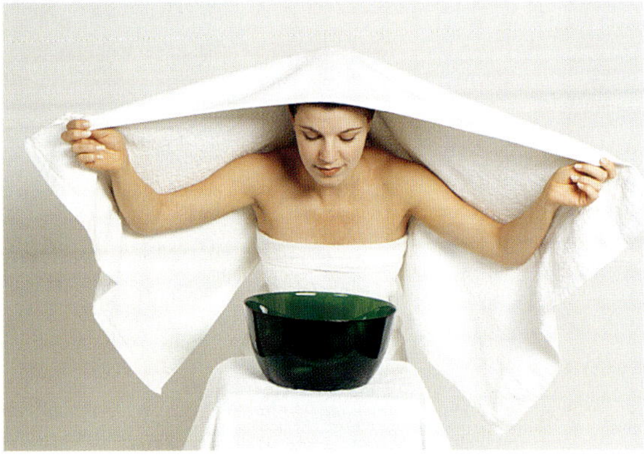

Steam inhalations can be enhanced with essential oils.

INHALATION These help to hydrate, cleanse and stimulate the skin and nasal passages, and are recommended for some skin and respiratory problems. Fill a bowl with near-boiling water and add 4 to 10 drops of essential oil. Drape a towel over your head, covering the bowl as well, and breath deeply for several minutes.

Another method of inhalation is to sprinkle the oil directly onto a handkerchief or tissue — the health-giving scent can be inhaled throughout the day.

AROMATHERAPY MASSAGE One of the best ways to experience aromatherapy. Dilute essential oil in a neutral base carrier oil, such as olive, jojoba,

IMPORTANT

Aromatherapy is generally safe enough for home use, if you follow the basic guidelines in this chapter and remember:

- do not ingest essential oils except with the guidance of a professional
- do not use the same oils for weeks and weeks without a break. Constant use may cause irritation and toxic constituents can build up in your body which can be dangerous.
- before using any oil, patch test a diluted quantity on a small part of your skin, in case you have an allergic reaction.

Essential oils can have powerful properties, and while a certain oil may assist some people, it may have a negative reaction on others — you will have to monitor this personally.

Some oils can be phototoxic, meaning they can react on your skin if exposed to sunlight — you can avoid this by applying the oil at night. Others can trigger menstruation, and should therefore be avoided by pregant women. See page 62. You should also be careful if you have high or low blood pressure, epilepsy, highly sensitive skin, or allergies.

Be aware that some oils can be strong enough to negate the effects of flower remedies and homoeopathic treatments. If you are undergoing chemotherapy, you should not use aromatherapy.

The chart on pages 102 to 104 gives some details but see a professional aromatherapist for further advice, especially if you have a serious health problem.

grapeseed, or peach or apricot kernel oil. Adding stabilised wheatgerm oil or vitamin E will stop the mixture oxidising and turning rancid. Usually the best blend for a body oil is around 5 drops of the essential oil to 2 teaspoons (10 ml/1⁄3 fl oz) of the carrier oil. Note: Massage with essential oils can be greatly beneficial but massage of all kinds should be avoided if you have a fever.

ATOMISERS These are also called sprays or spritzers. The container should be made of glass, not plastic. Fill with distilled, purified, spring, mineral, or cooled boiled water. Add 3 to 6 drops of essential oils to each 30 ml (1 fl oz) of water. Use to fragrance a room, freshen your face, or to apply the oils gently to your skin.

COSMETICS Make special cosmetic blends by diluting suitable essential oils in neutral, unperfumed moisturisers, balms, soaps, cleansers and shampoos.

HUMIDIFIERS You can add essential oils to the water.

COMPRESSES You can make hot or cold cloth compresses using essential oils diluted in warm or cool water. Soak cotton cloth in the water, squeeze out excess liquid and apply the cloth to the affected area.

LIGHT BULB RINGS Pour essential oils into these hollow clay, porcelain or metal rings and slip them over a light bulb. The heat from the light will release the essence into the room.

AN AROMATHERAPY HEALTH KIT

If you have the following selection of essential oils on hand, you should be prepared for most common ailments and injuries, especially when travelling.

Chamomile diarrhoea, exhaustion, insomnia

Eucalyptus colds, cramps, cuts, fever, heat exhaustion

Geranium blisters, dehydrated skin, exhaustion, heat cramps

Lavender burns, cuts, dehydrated skin, diarrhoea, fever, headaches, heat exhaustion, insects, insomnia, skin infections, sprains

Peppermint diarrhoea, exhaustion, fever, headaches, indigestion, insects, nausea, toothache

Tea tree colds, skin infections, thrush

BACH FLOWERS

IN THE NINETEEN-THIRTIES, THE BRITISH DOCTOR EDWARD BACH FORMULATED HIS BACH FLOWER REMEDIES, HERBAL MEDICATIONS TO ASSIST IN HEALING THE CONFLICT BETWEEN SPIRIT AND EGO WHICH HE SAW AS FUNDAMENTAL TO ILL HEALTH.

Bach flower remedies are chosen in line with psychological states. However, they can also be used to treat physical ailments — often linked to emotions — as they are designed to treat the whole person and their internal imbalance, not just an illness.

THE PATH TO DISCOVERY

Early in his distinguished, orthodox medical career, Bach decided that the best method of medical education was the observation of patients' reactions to disease, and that the main fault of modern medical science was to treat effects or symptoms rather than causes.

In the course of practising at University College Hospital, London, and at his private consultation rooms in Harley Street, Bach became dissatisfied with the success rate of orthodox medicine, noting that patients who enjoyed permanent recovery were rare while others made only scant improvement or suffered relapses.

He began to search for more effective treatment, a quest which led him to explore many fields of medical research. He won acclaim for his work on vaccines as Assistant Bacteriologist at the University College Hospital and during the First World War when his responsibilities included a huge war casualty ward.

In July 1917, Bach was given three months to live and he determined to complete his current research before his death. He noticed that far from declining quickly under this stress, his health improved. His experience led him to conclude that a sense of purpose in life was fundamental to good health.

Following his recovery, Bach continued to practise orthodox medicine, gaining further professional distinction during the influenza epidemic of 1918 when his vaccines saved the lives of thousands.

Soon after, he read *The Organon of the Healing Art* by Samuel Hahnemann, the founder of HOMOEOPATHY. Hahnemann's philosophy was to treat the sufferer, not the illness, and he obtained most of his remedies from animal, vegetable and mineral matter.

Inspired, Bach joined the London Homoeopathic Hospital while continuing to manage his increasingly popular private practice. He defined what he called the Seven Nosodes, oral vaccines that worked on organisms present in the intestines. He also advocated a diet of uncooked fruits, vegetables, cereals and nuts to reduce toxins in the intestines.

THE PHILOSOPHY

In 1928, Bach suggested that people could be categorised as personality types and that, although individuals may encounter a variety of illnesses, the people within each grouping would react in the same way. These similarities presented a useful frame of reference for diagnosis and treatment.

Bach also supposed that if distress could affect one's appearance it might also adversely affect internal bodily organs.

These theories and his study of Hahnemann encouraged Bach to abandon his London-based work and search for remedies that would work on an emotional level to change a person's temperament and increase their inner peace and vitality. He set out to investigate the effects of simple, herbal medicines on human thoughts and feelings, and believed that the sources of these remedies would be found in nature.

FINDING THE FLOWER REMEDIES

From 1930 until his death in 1936, Bach walked the countryside of England and Wales, observing nature and developing the Bach flower remedies. During this time, he discovered that his sensitivity to plants increased so that he could hold a flower and feel the effects of the bloom's properties in his body. Sometimes a flower would leave him feeling uplifted, at other times nauseous or faint.

Bach focused on flowers because he believed the essence of a plant was concentrated in its flower before seeding. He extracted the essence by placing picked flowerheads in a bowl of water left in the sun for several hours to receive solar energisation before being stabilised with brandy.

Bach listed 38 plants with healing properties, including the 12 plants he wrote about in *The Twelve Healers and Other Remedies*. His remedies can be used singly or in combination, and Bach urged their use in conjunction with other forms of treatment. Recent decades have witnessed renewed interest in Dr Bach's healing philosophy and his flower remedies which seem to be devoid of side effects.

WORDS OF WISDOM

In his book *Heal Thyself*, Bach wrote of the "medical school of the future" which he believed would move beyond the physical symptoms of the disease and beyond the administration of drugs and chemicals to "concentrate its efforts upon bringing about that harmony between body, mind and soul which results in the relief and cure of disease ... For those who are sick, peace of mind and harmony of the Soul is the greatest aid to recovery".

He also wrote: "Our conquest of disease will mainly depend on the following: Firstly, the realisation of the Divinity within our nature and our consequent power to overcome all that is wrong; secondly, the knowledge that the basic cause of disease is due to disharmony between personality and the Soul; thirdly, our willingness and ability to discover the fault which is causing the conflict; and fourthly, the removal of any such fault by developing the opposite virtue".

USING THE REMEDIES

Bach flower remedies can be prescribed by a health professional or can be administered at home. They are available for sale in health food stores and through therapists such as herbalists and naturopaths. Follow these guidelines if using the remedies at home:

- You probably can't be as objective as a professional in analysing your situation so it is always advantageous to consult a therapist but if self-prescribing be as honest as possible in examining yourself before selecting a remedy. Some remedies may be chosen to address your general personality type and taken long term; others may be taken for a specific, short-term problem.
- Do not use too many remedies simultanteously. One at a time is best, and not more than five remedies at once.

- The concentrated stock remedies that you purchase may need to be further diluted before taking. Add 2 drops of each to a small (about 30 ml/1 fl oz) dropper bottle filled with distilled or spring water. You can then keep this solution for about three weeks in the refrigerator or a cool dark place. For longer storage life, add a dash of brandy. Discard if there is any change in appearance or smell.
- Take 4 drops of the diluted remedy up to four times a day (including immediately after waking and before bed), or when needed. You can take the drops in a glass of water or drop directly onto or under the tongue.

RESCUE REMEDY

Rescue remedy is a composite remedy made up of:

- star of bethlehem for shock
- rock rose for terror and panic
- impatiens for mental stress and tension
- cherry plum for desperation
- clematis for the removed feeling which often precedes fainting or loss of consciousness.

It is to be used during emergencies and for trauma or sudden shock of any kind. It can also be used when you are feeling stressed — for example, before an exam or important interview. Rescue remedy is very effective on children and animals.

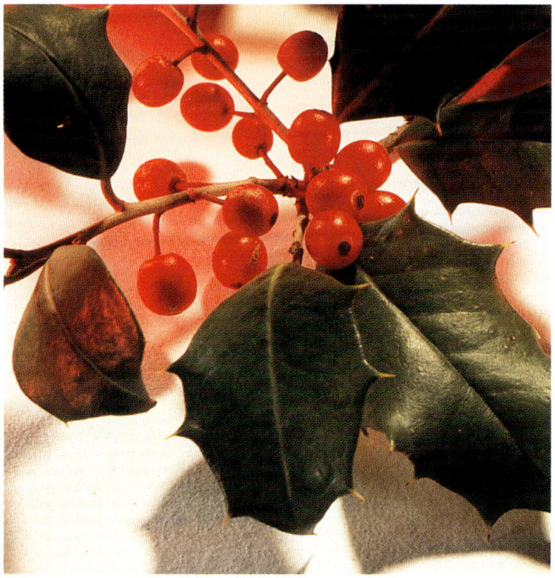

CHOOSING A REMEDY

There are many more moods and personality types and remedies for balancing them. The following is a list of some of the most common emotional states and the remedies that can help counter them. If you are in doubt as to which remedy to take, see an expert for a proper consultation.

- mostly unhappy — holly
- panicky — rock rose
- fear of losing control — cherry plum
- absorbed by memories — honeysuckle
- absorbed by self — heather
- desire to be alone — water violet
- dislike of being alone — chicory, heather
- lack of ambition — clematis, gorse, wild rose
- anxiousness — agrimony
- sulky — willow
- strict with others — beech, vine
- vexatious — holly, pine
- talkative — honeysuckle, vervain
- apathetic — clematis, wild rose
- worries over other people's troubles — red chestnut
- drains others' vitality — vervain, cerato, vine
- not clear about ambitions — oat
- feeling suicidal — aspen, cherry plumb, mimulus
- a struggler — oat
- tearful — scleranthus
- self-pity — heather, willow
- gives in to setbacks — gorse
- sensitive to noise — clematis, mimulus

BACH FLOWERS TABLE

The 38 remedies and the states that they treat:

AGRIMONY mental torture; worry that is concealed from others

ASPEN vague fears of unknown origin; anxiety; apprehension

BEECH intolerance; criticism; passing judgements

CENTAURY weak willed; too easily influenced

CERATO distrust of self; doubt of one's ability; foolishness

CHERRY PLUM desperation; fear of losing control of the mind; dread of doing some frightful thing

CHESTNUT BUD failure to learn by experience and lack of observation in the lessons of life — hence the need for repetition

CHICORY possessiveness; self-love; self-pity

CLEMATIS indifference; dreaminess; inattention; unconsciousness

CRAB APPLE the cleansing remedy; despondency; despair

ELM occasional feelings of inadequacy; despondency; exhaustion from over-striving for perfection

GENTIAN doubt; discouragement; depression

GORSE hopelessness: despair

HEATHER self-centredness; self-concern

HOLLY hatred; envy; jealousy; suspicion

HONEYSUCKLE dwelling upon thoughts of the past; nostalgia; homesickness

HORNBEAM tiredness; weariness; mental and physical exhaustion

IMPATIENS impatience; irritability; extreme mental tension

LARCH lack of confidence; anticipation of failure; despondency

MIMULUS fear or anxiety of a known origin

OAK despondency; despair; but never-ceasing effort

OLIVE complete exhaustion; mental fatigue

PINE self-reproach; guilt feelings; despondency

RED CHESTNUT excessive fear; anxiety for others

ROCK ROSE terror; panic; extreme fright

ROCK WATER self-repression; self-denial; self-martyrdom

SCLERANTHUS uncertainty; indecision; hesitancy; unbalance

STAR OF BETHLEHEM after effect of shock (mental or physical)

SWEET CHESTNUT extreme mental anguish; despair; hopelessness

VERVAIN strain; stress; tension; over-enthusiasm

VINE dominating; inflexible; ambitious

WALNUT oversensitive to ideas and influences; the line-breaker

WATER VIOLET pride; aloofness

WHITE CHESTNUT persistent unwanted thoughts; mental arguments and conversations

WILD OAT uncertainty; despondency; dissatisfaction

WILD ROSE resignation; apathy

WILLOW resentment; bitterness

CHIROPRACTIC

CHIROPRACTIC WAS PIONEERED BY AN AMERICAN HEALER, DANIEL DAVID PALMER (1845–1913), BASING IT ON THE CONCEPT OF A VITAL NERVE FORCE WITHIN THE BODY. PALMER DEVELOPED HIS APPROACH BY COMBINING TIME-HONOURED MANIPULATION TECHNIQUES AND MODERN ANATOMICAL KNOWLEDGE. HE HAD USED MESMERISM AND MAGNETIC HEALING (THE FORERUNNERS OF HYPNOSIS AND THERAPEUTIC TOUCH) AND HAD STUDIED OSTEOPATHY.

Chiropractic and OSTEOPATHY are often confused. While they have a lot in common, there are also significant differences. The emphasis in chiropractic is on the connection between the spine, the nervous system and disease while osteopathy is concerned with the soft tissues and a healthy blood supply as well as the skeletal framework and nervous system. The aim is to ensure the optimal functioning of all the body systems.

HOW IT ALL BEGAN

In 1895, Harvey Lillard visited Palmer after becoming suddenly deaf. He had strained his back some 17 years earlier and on examining the man, Palmer found a lump on the spine, which appeared to be a displaced vertebra. He adjusted the vertebra and the man's hearing improved. After follow-up adjustments, the vertebra was corrected and the client's hearing returned to normal.

Palmer concluded that the spinal column was connected to the nervous system, and so developed a set of techniques to lever misaligned vertebrae into place. He called his therapy chiropractic, combining the Greek words cheiro and praktikos which mean "done by hands".

Nerves branch from the entire length of the spinal column into the head, arms, torso and legs. Building on the osteopathic premise that structural problems can lead to health imbalances, Palmer deduced that problems with the spinal column upset the nervous system, and in turn the reduced neural signals lowered the body's natural healing ability.

THE PHILOSOPHY OF CHIROPRACTIC

Chiropractic care is primarily concerned with the location and adjustment of variations in the alignment of the spine. It is aimed at enhancing the environment of the body thus inducing a better and increased immune response and resistance to disease.

IMPORTANT

Treatment should only be given by a professional and experienced chiropractor. It is safe and hugely beneficial if performed by a fully trained expert. However, if the person is not qualified, such activity may cause bruising, and even serious injury such as fracture, or rupture to arteries.

If you are seeking a chiropractor, ask for recommendations, or contact the chiropractic association in your area.

Although there has been some conflict with orthodox medical practitioners in the past, chiropractic is now widely accepted by the general medical community and it is quite likely your doctor can refer you to a chiropractor.

The brain governs the body and is connected via the nervous system to the body's every cell. Chiropractors believe it is vital the nervous system's pathways to the brain are free of interference. Chiropractors use the term "subluxation" or "vertebral subluxation" to refer to the location of interference or blockage in the nervous system, or unnatural pressure upon it. The longer these subluxations exist, the greater the likelihood the body has compensated for the dysfunction. This compensation will, in turn, create extra stress within the body.

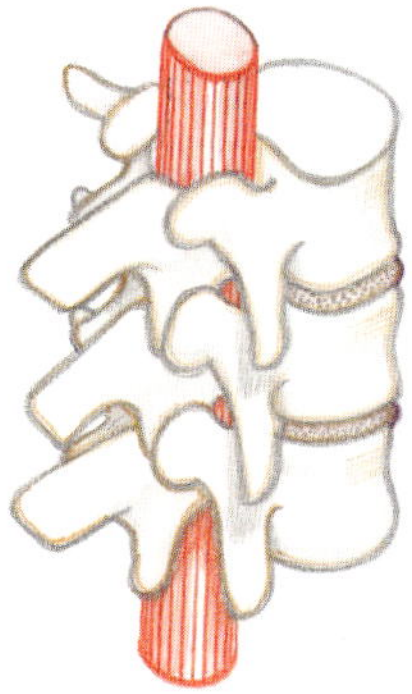

Chiropractors aim to locate and remove the blockages. They believe that people function better when all nerve channels are open and the brain can govern the function, repair and regeneration of the body tissues at all times.

Blockages in the nervous system can be the result of disease or dysfunction such as accident, stress, even poor posture. In either case, the chiropractic approach will be similar, though the extent of the problem will affect the techniques used (see below).

Chiropractic accepts the body has an in-built ability to heal itself and that the body's healing ability is determined by the amount of external and internal stress placed on it.

These stresses can be divided into three areas: physical, chemical and emotional.

Chiropractic care relieves the mechanical and structural stresses on the nervous system by keeping the spinal column balanced. Part of the strength of chiropractic is the pain relief it can give.

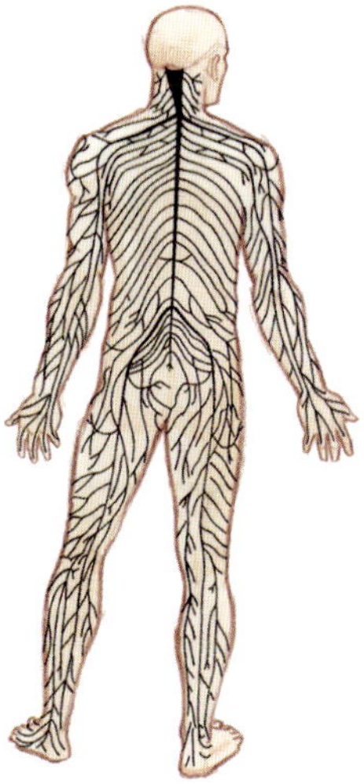

The spine and the nervous system are closely related. By working on the spine, chiropractic treatment can affect the entire body.

CHIROPRACTIC TREATMENT

Chiropractic adjustment involves changing the position of the vertebrae by specific direct force in a way that causes that vertebra to move normally with both the vertebra above and below. This allows the nerves between the vertebrae to also move more freely, restoring normal nerve function. Rotation, stretching and pressure may be used to relax muscles from spasm and restore normal position and movement.

Each chiropractor will have their own preferred method of adjustment. Some chiropractors follow a conservative approach and will incorporate various mechanical devices into their treatment. Others will have a softer approach and prefer to recommend subtle treatments such as postural and nutritional advice or breathing exercises along with their adjustments. Chiropractic does not use surgery or drugs to relieve muscle/skeletal problems.

A chiropractor will take you systematically through a range of tests to evaluate the present level of spinal health. For the first adjustment, it is usually necessary for the patient to undress to their underwear and then put on a robe. The chiropractor will want to know your complete health history, and some may request you have X-rays — in such cases, treatment may commence on the second visit or at a time when the X-rays have been thoroughly read and examined. Adjustments may not be performed until the practitioner is completely satisfied that they know how the spine is functioning or where the dysfunction exists.

Standard consultation time is 30 to 45 minutes for an initial consultation and 10 to 15 minutes on consecutive visits. Chiropractors may also recommend a series of adjustments over a number of visits, particularly if the primary problem has been present for some years.

A single treatment can reduce pain to the extent that you feel fully recovered. Your body, however, may take some time to "settle" after an adjustment so it is wise to take it easy. Try to schedule your visits so they are not followed by sitting for a prolonged period. You will benefit much more from the treatment if you combine it with a relaxing activity afterwards such as a gentle walk or a long, warm bath. Discuss what will best aid your recovery for your particular condition with your chiropractor.

Some people experience aching and stiffness following an adjustment, or even the next day.

CONDITIONS THAT CHIROPRACTIC CAN HELP

As well as being used to maintain a healthy body, chiropractic can assist in the treatment of many ailments, including:

- musculo-skeletal damage of all kinds including those caused by accidents
- sports injuries
- sprain, strains and damaged ligaments
- stress-related pain in the muscles or joints
- lower back pain
- back pain caused by pregnancy and childbirth
- arthritic or rheumatic conditions
- slipped discs
- lumbago
- sciatica
- neuralgia
- organ-related illnesses
- bladder problems
- some asthma
- some migraines or headaches, particularly those involving muscle tension.

COUNSELLING

IT IS OFTEN SAID THAT ALL OUR EMOTIONS CAN BE REDUCED TO COMBINATIONS OF THREE BASIC FEELINGS – SORROW, HAPPINESS AND ANGER, OFTEN SIMPLIFIED AS SAD, GLAD OR MAD. IMBALANCE IN THESE EMOTIONS OR A BLOCKAGE IN THEIR EXPRESSION CAN CAUSE PHYSICAL AND MENTAL PROBLEMS.

In Western culture it is often not acceptable to appear weak, feel wretched or be sorry for yourself. Many people also feel reluctant to ask for help or openly express and discuss feelings. And while there may be some "blame" attached to relationship or work difficulties, there is seldom any attached to illness.

These attitudes can establish patterns of behaviour. A child's anger, sadness or other "negative" emotion is often discounted by adults, who may cajole the child or simply tell them to cheer up. Yet, if the child is hurt or ill, these feelings are more accepted by an adult and attract real attention. Once grown, a person may fall back on this knowledge and become ill during a time of stress in an unconscious attempt to attract attention and support.

It is also common for people to be critical of their bodies, to obsess about their appearance and feel unhappy if they don't measure up to the fashionable body image. This can, in turn, lead to unhealthy or abusive patterns of behaviour, such as excessive dieting.

In addition, we all face challenges in our lives — the death of loved ones, the loss of a job, drug and alcohol abuse, family problems or the breakdown of an important relationship. With experiences like these, the emotional pain involved can be so overwhelming that you need help to find your way through it, hopefully before it seriously impacts on your mental and physical health. While these experiences can be painful, they do provide opportunities for you to learn about yourself and your emotional make-up, and this can be one of the most empowering things you will ever do.

GETTING HELP

If you have a long-lasting or recurring health problem, it is worthwhile considering if there are any underlying emotional conditions which may be contributing to it.

You may need help with emotional challenges or in identifying and then dealing with the psychological issues behind an illness. This help may come through informal discussions with friends, relatives or a respected figure such as a teacher, doctor or religious leader. Or you may seek the services of a professional counsellor — your health practitioners, doctor, local health centre or hospital may be able to refer you.

Good counsellors will allow you to talk; they will then help you gain some insight into your difficulties. The best counsellors are non-judgmental, which means they will suspend their own beliefs while they help you work out what is best for you.

Make sure you find a counsellor with whom you feel comfortable and be prepared to continue the counselling sessions for the period of time your situation requires. You may need to attend a number of sessions before you feel any obvious results, so rather than seeking a quick "cure", try to view your sessions as a voyage of self-discovery. It is often a good idea to make a personal promise to continue for, say, eight weeks. This is important because sometimes a counselling session can feel uncomfortable, or even threatening, as you come to terms with your feelings or the consequences of your actions. These feelings of discomfort are an indication you are getting to the source of your problems, so it is essential you stay with it.

If examining a health problem, your counsellor is likely to be interested in the onset of the condition, what was happening in your life at the time and, more importantly, how you felt about it.

SOME COUNSELLING APPROACHES

Many professionals advertising themselves as counsellors or psychotherapists will not necessarily be psychiatrists or psychologists. They come from a variety of backgrounds including, for example, nursing, social work or education. They may then have acquired further qualifications in counselling and/or psychotherapy.

Counsellors are trained to deal with here-and-now situations that arise in a person's life and may have an area of specialty such as crisis counselling. Psychotherapists have undergone further training in the formation of the personality from childhood and are therefore equipped to enable a client to look further back for the cause of their problem.

ONE CONTEMPORARY APPROACH

In the early 1980s an American woman named Louise L. Hay published a booklet called *Heal Your Body*, chronicling her recovery from vaginal cancer.

Hay had undergone several nutritional and physical therapies which had contributed to her recovery, but she believes that an important aspect involved dealing with her long suppressed emotions stemming from incidences of physical, mental and sexual abuse during her childhood. This personal experience and her work as a counsellor with the Church of Religious Science led her to formulate a theory of the metaphysical causes for physical illnesses. She has authored a number of books and audio-tapes aimed at self-help and her ideas have become popular in the general community and among many holistic health counsellors.

Hay believes that different parts of the body are associated with certain dominant emotions that she believes to be the root cause of problems in that particular area of the body. For example, Hay believes the eyes represent the capacity to see. "When there is a problem with the eyes, it usually means there is something we do not want to see, either about ourselves or about life, past, present or future," she says.

To help you change the underlying psychological cause, and improve the health of your eyes, Hay recommends you work with an affirmation, such as "I see with love and joy".

Following these lines, a holistic counsellor may help you look at and deal with the emotional component of your health condition. Techniques used may range from simple Louise Hay-style affirmations (see also page 50) to major psychotherapy, depending on the therapist and your particular problem.

A psychotherapist will look to the person's family and origin and perhaps to patterns and ways of functioning learnt in childhood. Both counsellors and psychotherapists will be listening for the client's feelings and encouraging these to be expressed and released in ways that will be beneficial to the client.

The theoretical base of much of this kind of work is known as humanistic psychology. This theory is based on the assumptions that human beings are born good and lovable and that if they end up feeling and behaving otherwise as adults something detrimental has happened to them. Humanistic psychology works on the assumption that human beings naturally want to grow and better themselves and will be trying, in the ways they know how, to achieve this.

Most counsellors will also understand that people function in the context of a society that has certain beliefs which may or may not be helpful and that, in some instances, the society will create or add to the problems — the case of eating disorders is an example prevalent in our society.

Generally in our culture health and well-being are thought of as physical issues, perhaps encompassing a positive mental attitude. People would seek support from a counsellor when they come to the awareness, perhaps as a result of a physical illness, that their feelings are preventing them from having a positive mental outlook.

There are many different types of counselling and therapy that you may see advertised, for example: Gestalt therapy, voice dialogue, rebirthing, transactional analysis. These are all ways to describe different ways of working according to different techniques and would all be described as humanistic.

A holistic counsellor will probably also base their work on humanistic ideas and will also consider other aspects of the person — physical and spiritual as well as emotional and intellectual.

But rather than having to understand the ins and outs of each method, it is more important that prospective clients look for a person they can trust and a way of working they feel comfortable with. It is advisable to shop around and have a chat with several different people. Be sure you feel your chosen practitioner will treat you with dignity and respect, for without that, any method of counselling or therapy is open to abuse.

WHAT YOU CAN EXPECT

An individual counsellor will usually suggest a minimum of four to six sessions to get to know you properly and give you sufficient time to talk over what's bothering you. A psychotherapist will expect to see you for considerably longer in order to fully understand your background.

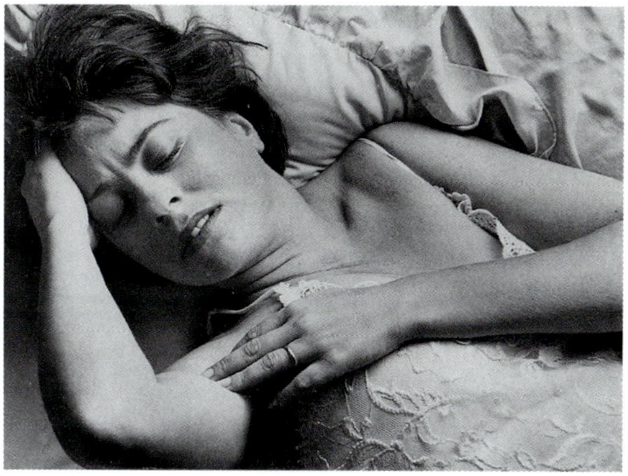

Stress-related insomnia and troubled sleep is just one way that unresolved emotions can affect your health.

Couples counselling is where a counsellor has undertaken specific training in the dynamics of relationships and how to work with them. Individual sessions may also be part of this process.

Family therapy is usually recommended if there is a child with a problem as it is understood that a child's difficulties will usually relate to the dynamics of the family as a whole. Family therapists have to undergo intensive training in families and their dynamics and will usually be professionally trained in this area.

Group counselling or therapy can be very useful to share with others with a common problem, e.g. cancer support groups or as an adjunct to individual work, where people can learn from listening to and sharing with others in a supportive and challenging situation.

LISTEN TO YOUR LANGUAGE

You only have to listen to our everyday language to see how closely our feelings and our bodies are linked.

For example:

She is a pain in the neck.

He makes me sick.

I feel sick to the stomach.

I don't want to hear that.

It gets under my skin.

They get right up my nose.

That makes my blood boil.

THE FELDENKRAIS METHOD

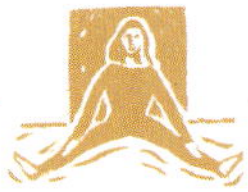

THE FELDENKRAIS METHOD IS A SYSTEM FOR LEARNING THROUGH MOVEMENT. THE PROCESS INVOLVES CONSCIOUS THINKING, MOVING, SENSING AND FEELING. THE AWARENESS GAINED FROM THIS EXPLORATION ALLOWS YOU TO FUNCTION AT YOUR OPTIMUM.

An explanation of how the Feldenkrais Method works lies in understanding how the human nervous system operates. As yet this is not understood and can only be observed.

Dr Moshe Feldenkrais was born in Russia in 1904 and spent more than 40 years developing this method of movement education. He received a doctorate in physics from the Sorbonne in Paris and is recognised as the person who introduced judo to the West.

During his youth Feldenkrais suffered a knee injury. It troubled him as he grew older and he found conventional treatment was not able to help him. This led to a lifetime of study of the structure and function of the nervous system and the relationship between human development, learning and movement. He died in 1984.

Feldenkrais guilds have been established in the United States, Scandinavia, Germany, France, Italy, Britain, Israel and Australia.

HOW THIS METHOD CAN HELP

If you have aches and pains, the Feldenkrais Method can help you. It can help athletes and dancers with recurring injuries, people with breathing disorders, or chronic anxiety. People who have had strokes, paralysis and chronic pain have benefited from this method.

The Feldenkrais Method is particularly useful for the elderly because it does not require physical exertion. It is a physical training, but it is gentle, not strenuous, and not actually a form of exercise; training of the mind is a significant aspect of this method.

The Feldenkrais Method can assist you by:

- improving the way you function in everyday life
- expanding your repertoire of movements
- allowing you to move more comfortably and efficiently

- teaching you how to observe and monitor your patterns of movement and to notice the cooperation your whole body gives to any action
- helping you develop an awareness of yourself and your movements in relation to your physical and social environment.

A VEHICLE FOR DEEPER LEARNING

While the Feldenkrais Method will teach you about how you move, the movements are a vehicle for a deeper learning. They will help you to expand your understanding of what you can do.

Feldenkrais talked about four states of being:

- asleep
- awake
- conscious
- aware.

He understood awareness as consciousness linked to knowledge. Feldenkrais often quoted the Chinese proverb:

"I hear and I forget

I see and remember

I do and understand."

HOW FELDENKRAIS IS TAUGHT

The method is taught in two parallel forms.

1. AWARENESS THROUGH MOVEMENT

In these lessons, a teacher talks you through a series of movement sequences. The lessons are given to groups and are suited to people at all levels of activity. They are precisely structured "movement explorations" based on developmental movements, functional activities and the investigation of joint, muscle and postural relationships.

In the lessons you learn to:

- direct attention to subtle differences in movement
- perceive interconnections within your total body movements
- explore your actions through a process of thinking, feeling, sensing and imaging.

The desired result of these lessons is that you become aware of your habitual patterns, expand your movement options, and choose more efficient and appropriate ways to move.

2. FUNCTIONAL INTEGRATION

The second form of Feldenkrais lesson is called Functional Integration. This is conducted on a one to one basis. These lessons are designed according to specific needs. The teacher will create a learning environment based on rapport and respect for your abilities, and communicate through touch and speech.

Comfort, pleasure and ease of movement are usually experienced during these lessons while you learn how to reorganise your body and behaviour in new and more efficient ways. As a result you may expand your functional abilities and restore functional motor patterns which have been disrupted, often as the result of an injury or operation.

For example, after a person has broken a leg they often find it difficult to stand on the leg or bear weight on it, which makes walking difficult. This is a result of fear as well as the physical problem and the Feldenkrais Method can help with this.

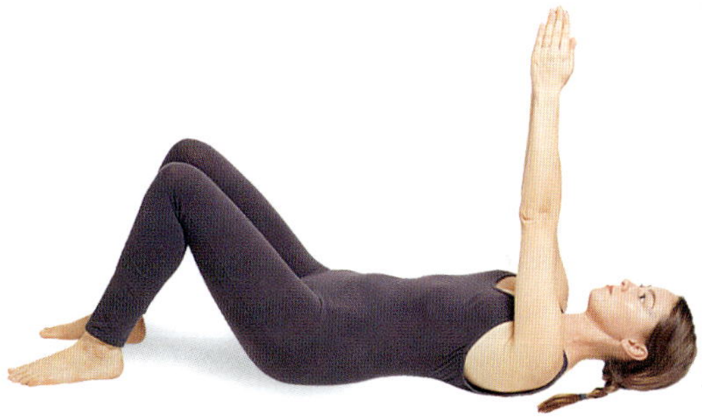

The Feldenkrais Method cannot just be described in a series of exercises. It is experiential and much depends on the quality of the movement.

A DIFFERENT APPROACH TO LEARNING

Often it is pain that draws attention to our body. Until our back begins to ache, for example, it's just there. Feldenkrais is about developing an awareness of how your body works, and distinguishing between what feels comfortable or uncomfortable and not feeling much at all. As the experience is a learning one, you can learn to be independent by organising yourself in more comfortable ways. This can break the cycle of dependence on support from professionals. You become an expert yourself.

Feldenkrais regarded all who came to him as students, not patients. He encouraged his students to explore ideas and think for themselves. Rigid concepts of "right" and "wrong" are constantly questioned by Feldenkrais teachers. Students are encouraged to trust their instincts, to trust what they feel both physically and mentally.

Feldenkrais believed that any authoritarian method of teaching creates anxiety and results in learning by rote instead of by thought. He encouraged his students to go back to learning in the way we all did as infants when we experienced a delightful exploration of our bodies and minds. He taught through experience so that your body can replace the old, inefficient methods of movement with freer, easier movements which require less energy and create more flexibility.

Physical struggle is not part of the Feldenkrais way. If there is a struggle it is in learning to think in a different way; as well, you need to keep questioning your habitual notions. For example, if you have back pain a Feldenkrais teacher will look at the way you stand, sit, walk, lift and perform other activities. The lesson will be based on your experiencing different movement options so that you learn alternatives to those habitual movement patterns that have caused you discomfort.

MOVEMENT IS THE KEY

Feldenkrais saw movement as the key. Every thought a person has is communicated in a movement of some type, even if it is only a slight dilation of the pupil.

Consider how you use movement to express emotions — anger stiffens your muscles sometimes to rigidity, fear will tense your shoulders and your head will droop when you are depressed. When these movements are habitual, the state of mind will be reflected in body movement. For example, you may have constantly tense shoulders and low-level associated anger or fear. This pattern then becomes normal for you.

The Feldenkrais Method helps to develop body awareness, which in turn enables you to change the brain's signals and find a new freedom in movement and feelings. Over time you will learn how to dissolve not just rigid patterns of movement but rigid patterns of thought and behaviour.

Feldenkrais lessons can make you more sensitive to the differences in movement. This means that your awareness of the moment between when you mobilise yourself for movement and when you actually perform the movement is increased. During that moment — that point of choice — you can change from the habitual way, to the new, freer way of moving.

For a long-term benefit, the Feldenkrais Method requires you to experience many different movement options. While the process is not instant, most people do experience a difference in a single lesson. Your pain or problem may not instantly disappear but you do have the realisation that change is possible.

Feldenkrais spoke not of disease but of faulty learning.

"People are not a bunch of properties, they are a process," he said. "All life is a process. Improve the quality of the process and the rest will take care of itself."

FELDENKRAIS MOVEMENTS — SITTING SPINE MOVEMENT

All movements should be done slowly, smoothly, and without effort. Remember to breathe easily. Do each movement a few times and notice the ways — significant or small — in which your *entire* body participates.

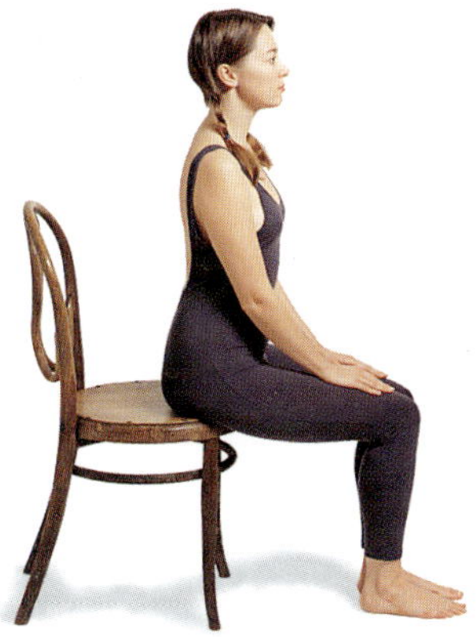

FIRST sit on the front of a firm chair and rest your hands on your thighs. Place your feet flat on the floor, directly below your knees which should be shoulder width apart.

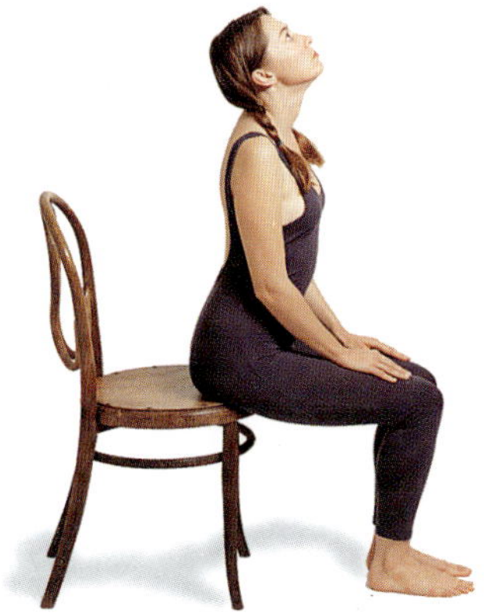

SLOWLY look toward the ceiling, arching your back. Take note of how far you can see without straining. Return to the start position.

REPEAT the previous movement, looking towards the ceiling again. Is your back arching further and more easily?

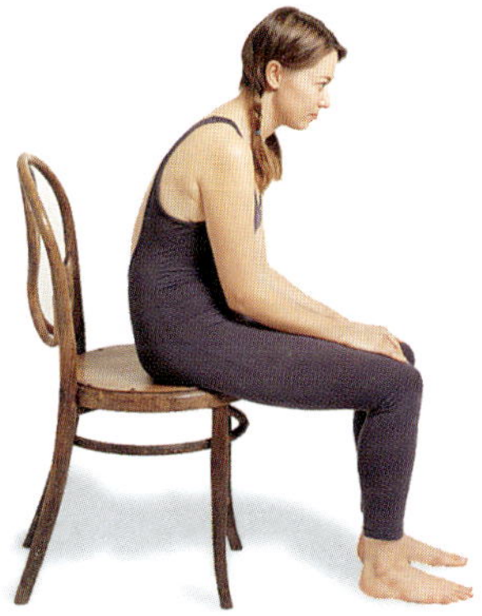

SLOWLY look toward the floor, allowing your back to round. Your shoulders, chest and neck should be relaxed.

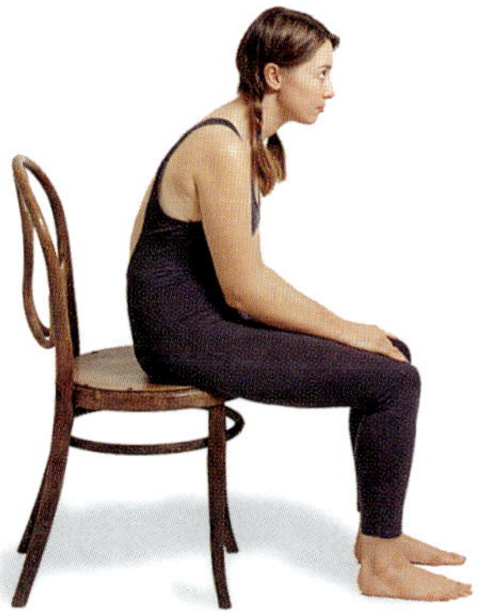

NOW slowly lower your head further, letting your back stay round while you look toward the ceiling using your eyes only. Your movement will be restricted because your eyes and head are moving in opposite directions.

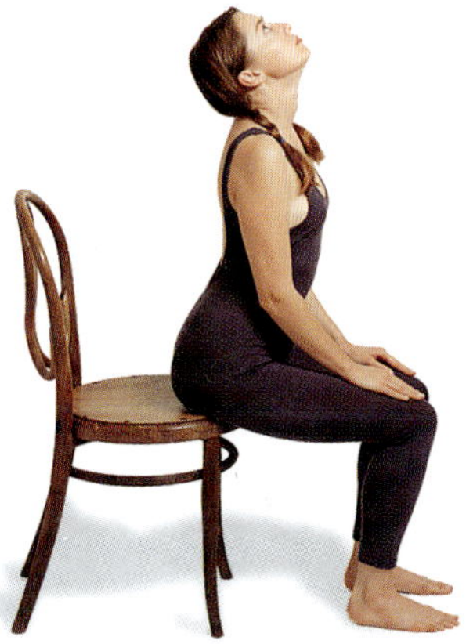

NOW let your head and eyes move together, looking toward the ceiling. Feel the middle and upper part of your back arching. Can you see further and more easily than at the start?

HEALING ENERGIES

THE SUBTLE PROCESS OF USING HEALING ENERGY CAN BE FOUND IN MANY FORMS – SPIRITUAL HEALING AND CHAKRA BALANCING ARE JUST TWO BROAD CATEGORIES WHICH, IN TURN, INCORPORATE VARIOUS TECHNIQUES SUCH AS REIKI. THE ESSENTIAL PURPOSE OF EACH TECHNIQUE IS TO TRANSFER HEALING ENERGY FROM ONE PERSON TO ANOTHER.

Healing methods have been taught for centuries and people with an innate ability to heal have naturally attracted students. The methods used may differ. Often rituals are developed to aid concentration and the opening of psychic centres; they also give students a framework in which to learn and then practise. In some cultures, techniques are handed down along family lines.

The ability to heal gives the healer a great deal of power and the techniques may be shrouded in mysticism. Some teachers require their students to go through rigorous training and initiations. This is true even in Western society where doctors are often held in awe by their patients and spend long years of medical study in universities and hospitals.

Healing energy, however, is available to everyone. We all have the ability to heal and to be healed. Many people channel healing energy without consciously realising it. These are the people who we like to be around — they have a strengthening or calming influence. That in itself can be a form of healing.

HOW DOES HEALING ENERGY WORK?

Although a human body appears solid, it is made up of subatomic particles surrounded by electromagnetic energy. One theory is that this energy field is part of a current that runs through all living things and the cosmos. It is this energy which is central to therapies such as MEDITATION and ACUPUNCTURE. It is timeless and limitless and is called many names including Qi, Ch'i, Ki and prana (see pages 178 and 182) or the life force.

When you are ill, stressed or tired, your ability to draw on the life force is impaired. But this can also be seen as a chicken and egg situation, because many therapists conclude that illness manifests in your body as a result of a weakening in your life force.

In any event, healing energy can be absorbed by your body to help you regain a balance in your life force. You can learn to channel the energy to yourself or you can have a healer or friend channel it to you.

The person channelling this energy can be touching you or the channelling can occur from a distance. Absent healing, as it is often called, involves the healer opening themselves to the healing life force and then sending that energy to you, usually by a process of visualisation.

The experience of this energy has been described as a variety of sensations, such as heat, tingling, cold, warm feelings of love or peace. But, while some claim to have recovered from physical and emotional problems as a result of this process, the existence of healing energy has not yet been fully documented and proven beyond doubt.

Scientific studies have shown, however, that there is something going on. This research includes experiments on healers such as the Hungarian, Oscar Estebany in the 1970s. The experiments showed that when Estebany touched people who were ill, the levels of haemoglobin in their blood increased and they reported an improvement in their symptoms.

The British psychic healer, Matthew Manning also underwent a series of tests in the 1970s. From these, the Toronto Society for Psychical Research concluded that Manning's abilities were associated with an unknown form of electromagnetic phenomena which was accompanied by changes in Manning's brainwave patterns.

KIRLIAN PHOTOGRAPHY

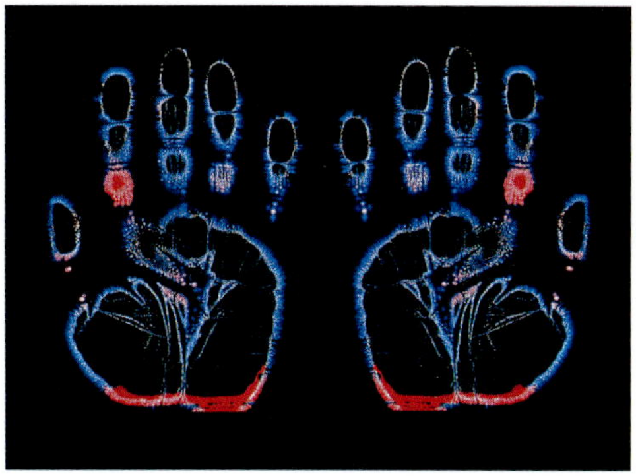

There have long been claims about the existence of auras, a luminous energy that surrounds people and all animate and inanimate things. One possible support comes from Kirlian photography, a special technique that seems to photograph the body's energy. It is claimed that ill-health will affect the colour and density of a person's aura, and that careful examination of Kirlian photographs will reveal the nature of the illness, thereby enabling the possibility of a cure. The reading of auras can form part of the diagnostic procedure in the practice of healing energy channelling and colour therapy (see page 207) among other therapies.

FINDING A HEALER

Healing energy can be delivered by someone who has studied a technique for several years and been "initiated" through various levels, but you may be content to accept the loving ministrations from a friend who has "the gift" or who has just completed a one-day workshop on healing. (If you are interested in learning how to heal or to receive healing, you will find there are a range of books, tapes and workshops available.)

While there have been reported cases where people with serious health problems have sought healing from a psychic healer and have experienced remarkable recoveries, healing will not necessarily provide you with a miracle cure, although it can be a valuable addition to your health regime.

Because healing energy is healing at its most subtle level and the process itself can be largely invisible, this area has been open to exploitation by charlatans. Care and astuteness are required when locating a healer. It is important to find one who is honourable, genuine, sensitive to your needs and with whom you feel comfortable. A recommendation from someone you know can be a good way to locate a healer; or a holistic health centre may be able to refer you.

When deciding upon a healer you should ask yourself if the healer is:

- in good health
- humble about their successes or could they possibly be exaggerating their record

- asking a reasonable fee
- "grounded" and down to earth
- non-judgmental.

The last question is important. When you receive healing you are opening yourself to energy. What you want to receive is the nourishment of the life force. You don't want your healer to be chattering away about how dreadful their neighbour is or making assertions about why your digestion is poor. Healing energy is often connected to other psychic abilities so that skilled healers may pick up certain information about you. This does not mean they will know the details of your sex life, but they can tune into you and sense what could be at the base of your problems. If they do pick up information, a sensitive healer will ask questions rather than make bold statements.

For example, if you did have poor digestion, a sensitive healer might ask: "is your digestion worse if you have had a stressful day at work?" An inexperienced healer might say: "I'm sensing that your poor digestion is caused by unexpressed anger at your boss." In the first example, the question allows you to explore what may be causing your anger. A sensitive healer will keep asking questions until you come up with your own answers. The statement made by the inexperienced healer leaves you no room to move. If the healer is right then you can feel disempowered, even impinged on. If the healer is wrong, you can be left searching along the wrong path or feeling uneasy, even a little depressed.

REIKI

Reiki is one of the better known schools of healing by energy. It was founded by Japanese Christian minister Dr Mikao Usui, who studied a variety of healing methods last century. He was particularly impressed by some Tibetan teachings which he named Reiki from the Japanese words *rei*, meaning "boundless and universal", and *ki*, meaning "life force energy".

Usui passed his knowledge on to several students and there are now two internationally known Reiki schools. One teaches a technique called the "Radiance Technique" and the other teaches a technique known as the "traditional Usui system" of healing. To learn Reiki a student is attuned to the energy by a Reiki master through a number of initiations and then instructed in the basic hand positions for treatment and the ways in which to use Reiki in their own life and in service to others.

Reiki practitioners draw in the Ki energy and then send it out through their hands. They believe that the energy is modulated by a higher power who decides how much energy the person receiving it needs. Most sessions usually last an hour, although they may range from just a few minutes to a few hours. During this time you lie comfortably and the practitioner will channel energy to you, moving around to hold various parts of your body. It is believed that the energy will flow to the areas where it is needed, not necessarily where you or the healer think it is required.

As with other forms of healing, it is not fully understood how or why Reiki works. The experience can differ from person to person, session to session. Some people feel more relaxed, others feel more energised.

While it can be used on anyone or for any condition, therapists say that Reiki does not require any belief system or religious conviction for the healing energy to work. Practitioners do not promise miracle cures and will not lead you to expect any more than a feeling of being relaxed.

BODY HARMONY

This form of healing was developed by Don McFarland, a Californian chiropractor who also studied rolfing (see page 139) and had an interest in dance and sports medicine.

During a session — which usually lasts around an hour — the therapist will channel healing energy to you and at the same time assist your body to move in a manner natural to it. This may involve the gentle, almost involuntary rotating of your neck or the lifting of your knee. The therapist is careful to "listen" to your body and follow its direction, to assist your body, not direct it.

The therapy is based on the notion that your body knows how it wants to move and will create the correct "energy circuit". This is turn encourages the release of stressful memories locked in your bodycells. Often these can be consciously linked with

SELF HEALING: FEELING THE ENERGY

To give you some experience of electromagnetic energy, try this exercise:

Sit or lie comfortably and still your mind by taking three deep breaths. While you breathe, feel your body relax. Now hold your hands in front of you and slowly bring them together, palms facing.

As you move your hands towards each other, try to feel the sensations within them. At some stage you may feel either a slight resistance or a slight drawing together. If you have ever played with magnets, putting the poles together, you will be familiar with this sensation.

When you feel the resistance or attraction, move your palms around as if you were massaging an invisible ball. This will help you develop a better sense of the energy.

When you have felt the energy, check to see if you feel any other sensation — heat, cold, tingling; perhaps you see a colour.

Relax. Now try the following energy channelling exercise, but first familiarise yourself with the chakra diagram on page 124.

Sit comfortably and ensure that your body is relaxed. Take three deep breaths, slowly inhaling and exhaling.

Now imagine that healing energy — you can visualise it as blue light — is entering your body through your crown chakra at the top of your head. See the energy moving down your spine, lighting up each of your chakra centres, and then spreading out through your body, filling each cell until every cell in your body is vibrating with blue healing light.

Keep breathing and pulling the energy from outside your body down through your crown chakra. Do you feel different — hotter, colder, a tingling sensation or spreading warmth?

When you feel that your whole body is filled with the healing energy, focus your attention on your palms. In the centre of each palm visualise a blossom opening, through which the blue energy is able to flow out into the atmosphere.

Continue to bring the energy down through your crown chakra then out through your palms, and slowly bring your hands together, palms facing. While keeping the energy flowing, focus on your palms. When you feel the sensation of resistance or attraction, hold your palms in that position and visualise a ball of blue healing energy building between your hands.

You can move your hands to shape and massage this ball of energy. Keep bringing the energy down and visualising the ball taking shape until you can feel or sense it. After a time, it will feel increasingly solid.

You can keep bringing this energy down through your crown chakra and use it for healing. Place your hands on a part of your body that is out of balance, or just rest them on your thighs, or if you are lying down, your stomach.

Keep the energy flowing and see if you can feel it re-entering your body through your palms. This may be experienced as a feeling of warmth or coolness or a tingling sensation.

When you have finished, see the blue light retreat out of your body. Visualise closing the points on your palms (the blooms return to buds), and do the same with each of your chakras, ending with your crown chakra. It is important to close your chakras at the end of every session. Many teachers of healing also believe in ending a visualisation with thanks to the energy or life force. This is a personal choice.

Now that you have felt this energy, try using it whenever you want. You don't need to open the points on your palms, just visualise the healing energy filling you so that every cell is revitalised.

past experiences of physical or emotional pain.

People who have experienced body harmony report feeling deeply relaxed; they describe the sensation as if the body had opened up and expanded during the session. Sometimes they will also recall traumatic events, forgotten prior to the session.

CHARISMATIC HEALING

Recently there has been a return to charismatic healing in some Christian churches. Charismatic healing involves praying for the health of yourself and others. The sessions can last hours or just a few minutes. The aim is to appeal to the Holy Spirit to direct healing energy to the sick. The idea stems from the healing miracles performed by Jesus Christ. Some church groups will meet purely for this purpose; others incorporate their prayers into normal services.

FAITH AND SPIRITUAL HEALING

These two forms of healing, found among Christian groups and spiritualist churches, are similar to charismatic healing and involve the use of prayer, faith, meditation and the laying on of hands to activate the body's own healing force. In essence, the minister or healer will pray and ask God or the life force to channel healing energy through them. While they do this, they place their hands on the person requesting healing, often at head or shoulder level.

PSYCHIC SURGERY

Psychic surgeons claim to be able to part the skin and extract tissue and other matter then heal the incision without leaving a scar. Psychic surgery can be found among the faith healers of the Philippines and Brazil.

CHAKRA

CHAKRA	LOCATION	COLOUR	FUNCTION	PHYSICAL PARTS AND ORGANS GOVERNED
Base	Base of spine	Red	Expectations, physical energy, physical restrictions	Legs; feet; genitals; anus; coccyx; kidneys
Spleen	Just below the navel	Orange	Trauma, shock, recall	Pelvis; genitals; reproductive system; belly; sacrum; lumbar vertebrae
Solar plexus	Just above the navel	Yellow	Subconscious thoughts	Lumbar vertebrae; stomach; gall bladder; liver; diaphragm; nervous system
Heart	Centre of chest	Green	Empathy, emotion, unconditional love	Heart, blood, cirulatory system
Throat	Base of skull	Blue	Communication	Arms; hands; throat; mouth; voice; lungs; cervical vertebrae; respiratory system
Third eye	Brow or centre of forehead	Indigo	Higher consciousness, intuition, awareness	Forehead; ears; nose; left eye; base of skull; medulla; nervous system
Crown	Top centre of head	Violet	Spirituality	Cranium; cerebral cortex; right eye

GIVING HEALING TO OTHERS

If you want to give another person healing energy, follow the instructions for self healing on page 123 and then place your hands on or near your friend — whatever or wherever your intuition tells you is appropriate. If you are not sure where to start, begin at their shoulders and then follow your intuition.

See the blue healing energy entering your body and then moving through your palms to fill your partner's body. You may notice some sensation in your palms and often the other person will feel warmth, cold or tingling. As you become more familiar with the energy, you will be able to feel it switch on and then off. When the energy switches off, the session is over — complete it as you would a self healing.

ABSENT HEALING

Absent healing can be given to anyone over any distance.

See blue healing energy filling your body via the crown chakra and then think of the person to whom you want to send healing.

You don't need a name but if you know what the person looks like, visualise the energy filling their body. If you have never met them, just think of them and visualise a body filling with blue energy.

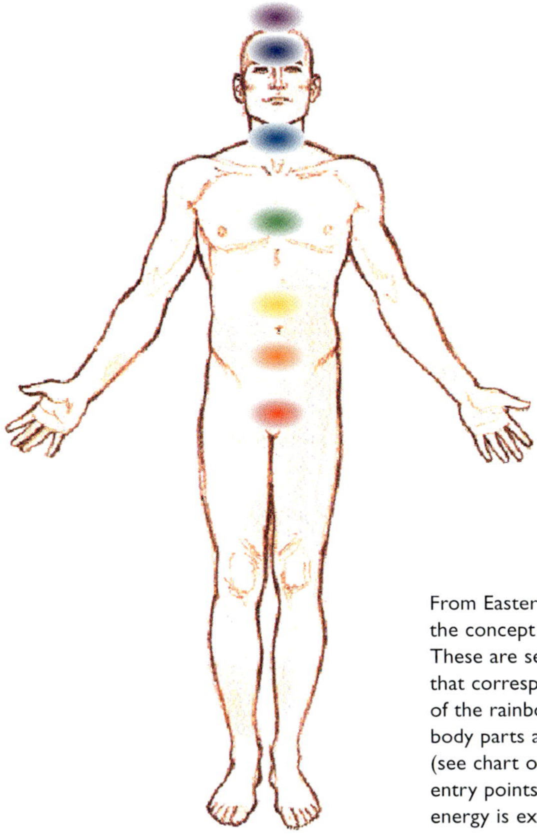

From Eastern teaching comes the concept of chakras. These are seven energy centres that correspond to the colours of the rainbow and to particular body parts and emotional states (see chart opposite). They are entry points to the body where energy is exchanged.

HERBALISM

HERBAL MEDICINE IS PART OF A WAY OF LIVING. IT IS THIS "DOMESTIC" QUALITY IN HERBALISM WHICH HAS ENSURED ITS SURVIVAL OVER THE CENTURIES. IT USES APPROPRIATE HERBS TO EASE SYMPTOMS OF ILLNESS AND EFFECT AN UNDERLYING HEALING; IT CONSIDERS DIET AND EXERCISE, AND MAY INCORPORATE OTHER NATURAL DISCIPLINES.

In matters of healing, Western medicine relies primarily on medications made in laboratories from chemicals, some of which have uncomfortable or dangerous side effects. Herbal medicine provides a safe, effective alternative.

CONSULTING A HERBALIST

Before prescribing herbal remedies, a herbalist will build up a comprehensive picture of your total condition, including your diet, lifestyle and exercise practice and, in particular, the amount of stress you are carrying.

The interview begins before you sit down; the herbalist checks your posture, the colouring of your skin, the colouring of your face, especially around the eyes, the ridges in your nails, your gait and your overall energy.

You may be asked to fill out a questionnaire for details of family history of disease, past illnesses and infections, accidents, physical and psychological trauma, vaccinations, known allergies, diet, vitamins you might be taking, medications, exposure to chemicals, and your presenting symptoms.

The herbalist may palpate lymph nodes for any swelling, check blood pressure or listen to lung and heart sounds for anomalies. They may also do a test using a urine sample to determine the health of bacteria in the gut. Iridology (see page 209) can also play an important part in verifying any suspected weaknesses.

While a herbal formula designed for your individual symptom pattern may be all you require, a herbalist may advise a special diet: one where salicylates and solanine chemicals are not ingested, or a cleansing regime free of yeast, moulds and fungus in which dairy products, sugars and chemicals are eliminated.

Herbalists work with other natural health professionals as well as referring to medical doctors for specialist tests such as blood and allergy testing.

WHAT CONDITIONS CAN BE TREATED?

Conditions that a herbalist may be most useful in treating include:

- Arthritis
- Bladder Problems
- Blood Pressure Problems
- chemical toxicity
- Chronic Fatigue Syndrome
- Digestive Problems
- Eczema
- female reproductive disorders
- Headache
- Infertility problems
- Shingles
- stomach Ulcers.

While herbalists may not treat life-threatening disease, they can — in consultation with a doctor — help support the well-being of people with such conditions.

USING HERBS

Generally, herbs aid healing by assisting the body to remove toxic or waste products; to ease symptoms and trigger the body's own healing mechanisms, or to build healthy organs, blood and tissues.

Herbs can give instant relief but often they differ from medical drugs in that their effects are gentle and slow acting. If you have a chronic health problem, you may need to take a course of herbs over some months before your condition will improve. And you'll need to do it with the guidance of a trained herbalist.

In their pure form herbs are generally prescribed on their own or as part of a herbal formulae. They can be used either internally or externally.

For acute or chronic ailments, you should consult a herbalist for a tailored prescription. However, one advantage of the more simple herbal treatments, particularly when used for less complex health conditions, is that you can purchase over-the-counter remedies for use at home, or you can safely prepare many of them yourself. These treatments include:

- **Teas** — made by steeping soft plant material in boiling water. Teas can be used internally as a drink or externally as a skin wash or in a bath.
- **Infusions** — similar to teas but stronger; the herbs are steeped for greater periods of time. Hot or cold oil infusions can be used for massage.
- **Decoctions** — usually made from harder plant material such as roots and bark, decoctions involve bringing herbs and water to the boil and simmering slowly.
- **Tinctures** — usually bought commercially, they are made by steeping the herb in alcohol or apple cider vinegar.
- **Compresses** — soft cotton cloth is soaked in tea, decoction, or diluted tincture (either hot or cold, depending on the condition). The excess liquid is squeezed out and then the cloth is applied to the affected area.
- **Poultices** — the direct application of crushed, ground, heated, soaked or boiled herbs to the skin.
- **Inhalations** — boiling water is poured over herbs and the steam is breathed in.

There are also a number of ready-made herbal preparations that can be found commercially. In addition to herbal tablets or capsules and concentrated liquid medication, herbs may be incorporated into ointments, oils, liniments, embrocations, salves, creams, balms and lotions.

SELF-TREATMENT

The many remedies outlined in the A–Z section of this book provide a starting point for using herbal medicine at home. Keep in mind that herbs act differently on different people, and the method by which a herb has been cultivated and stored will impact on its strength. Whatever your chosen form of self-treatment, if your condition does not start to improve gradually after a few days or weeks, consult a herbalist.

Many herbs have a variety of popular names. The list of botanical names on pages 403 and 404 should clarify any confusion. In addition, the healing properties of some plants are listed in the chapter on AROMATHERAPY.

IMPORTANT

It is best to use herbs under the consultation of a herbalist. Just as with chemical drugs, there can be a level of dosage where a herb is most effective (this varies from individual to individual) but there is also the possibility of overdose by over-use or, in a few cases, because the therapeutic dose is close in level to a toxic dose.

Working with herbs can be used to a patient's advantage, either by reducing medication or eliminating medication forever. However, some herbs have opposing or parallel interactions with drugs and should be monitored carefully by both a medical doctor and the herbalist when taken together. See page 65 for advice on pregnancy and herbs.

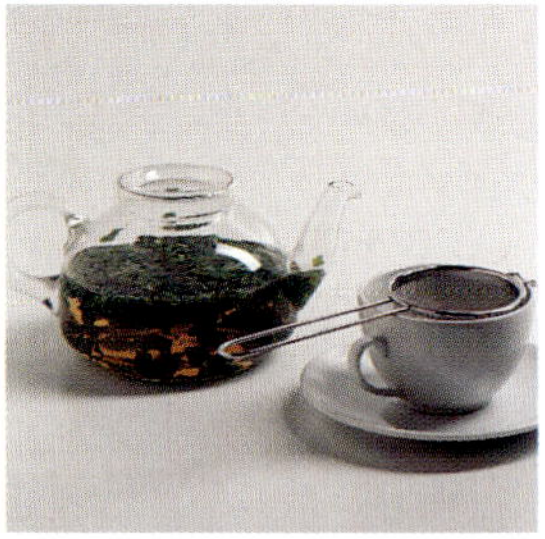

INFUSIONS AND TEAS
For a weak tea, use 1 to 3 teaspoons of herb for every cup of water and steep for up to 1 minute.

For a stronger tea, use about 90 g (3 oz) herbs in 500 ml (16 fl oz) water and let stand for 3 minutes.

Teas and infusions should be made fresh daily, but can be kept in the refrigerator for up to 2 days.

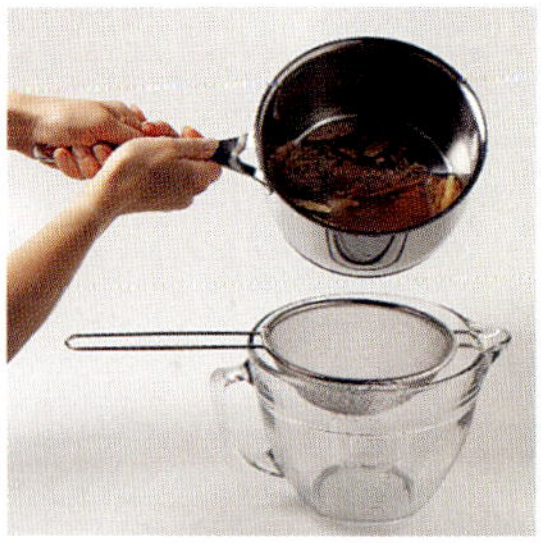

DECOCTIONS
These are made in roughly the same proportions as strong teas but require longer, hotter steeping. Water and herbs should be brought to boil in a pan, then covered and simmered for 10 minutes. Strain liquid before using.

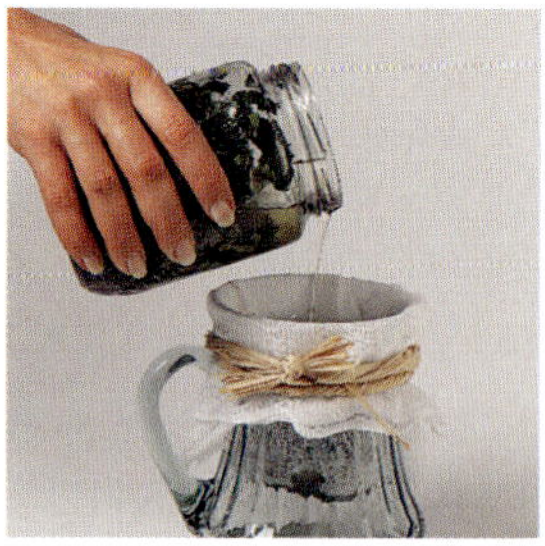

COLD OIL INFUSION
Pack 250 g (8 oz) dried herbs or 750 g (24 oz) fresh into a large jar and cover completely with cold-pressed vegetable oil. Seal and leave in a sunny place for two to three weeks. Strain the mixture through muslin, cheesecloth or coffee filter paper, squeezing out as much liquid as possible. Pour this oil back into the jar with more herbs and repeat the entire process three times. Finally, transfer the infused oil to clean, airtight, dark glass bottles and store in a cool, dark place.

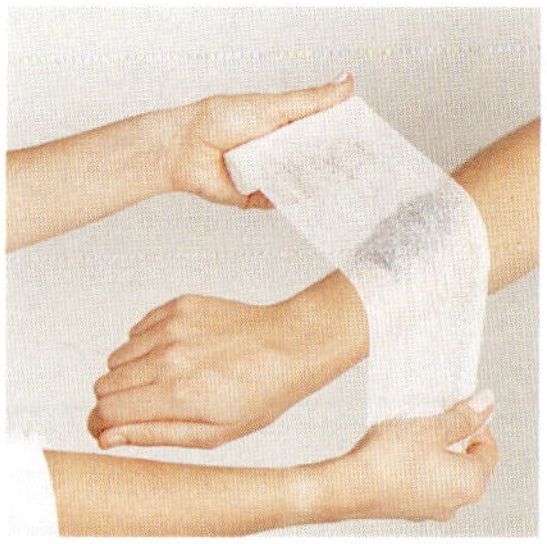

POULTICE
Herbs are first steeped in boiling water for 1 minute, then allowed to cool slightly. The wet herbs are applied directly to the skin for at least 30 minutes. A thin layer of oil may be applied first to prevent sticking, and the herbs can be covered by a dressing. The poultice should never be applied to broken skin as the moist conditions may encourage bacteria in the wound.

A HISTORY OF HERBALISM

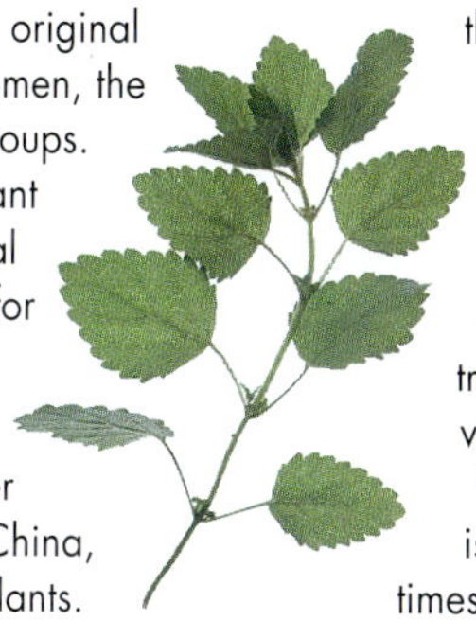

In the beginning, all medicine was herbal. The original practitioners of herbal medicine were usually women, the predominant gatherers of food in early tribal groups. Tribal women herbalists experimented with plant life native to their territory, and generations of trial and error taught them which plants were good for treating illness, which were good to eat, and which would cause poisoning and death.

Written records of herbal study date back over 5000 years to the Sumerians. A herbal from China, dating around 2700 BC lists 365 medicinal plants. The earliest Ayurvedic texts from India date from around 2500 BC (see page 206).

Among the earliest successes of herbal medicine are those recorded in the medical papyri compiled in Ancient Egypt. Many of the plants recorded have medicinal properties recognised in modern herbal medicine. One myth tells of a remedy for headache made by the goddess Isis for the god Ea. It included coriander, juniper berries, wormwood and honey, administered as a poultice.

Modern Western medicine, as well as herbal medicine, has a basis in early Greek and Roman writings, especially those of Hippocrates (460–380 BC) and Galen (AD 130–200). Hippocrates placed emphasis on careful diagnosis and minimal intervention, and advocated the use of simple herbal drugs (see page 157). Galen won renown for his complex plant, animal and mineral concoctions known as galenicals.

Knowledge of herbs was precious, and was entered in great books known as herbals. Diosorides' *De Materia Medica*, for example, covered about 600 plants and was the most widely used physicians' textbook for several centuries.

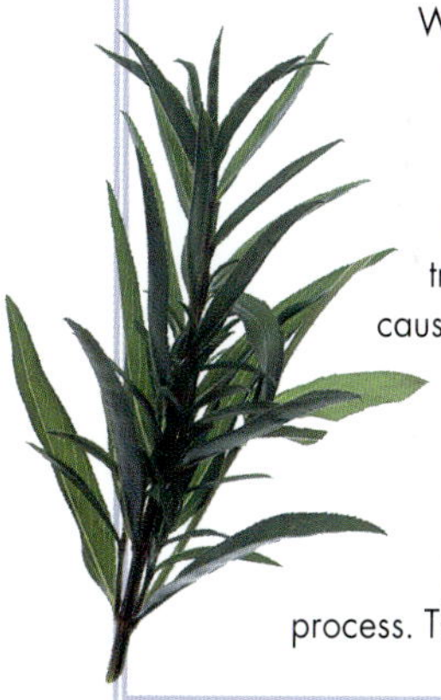

While these academic studies developed, the domestic art of herbalism — largely practised by women — flourished. All over the world, from time immemorial, herbalists worked in villages and within tribal groups. Because diseases and their causes were largely mysteries to these ancient cultures, religious explanations were often given for both the illness and any healing that took place. Prayers and rituals could be just as important as the herbs and remedies in the healing process. The mystical overtones of this process meant that successful healers often held a significant amount of respect and power within their communities. In some cultures, this was institutionalised with healers also in the roles of priestesses.

When the Church began its suppression of traditional beliefs in Europe it competed with the village herbalists by making churches centres of healing. In the rivalry which followed, herbalism, superstition, magic and Christianity did at times become interconnected, even by those in the educated ruling classes.

By the end of the 6th century most medical practitioners were monks, their monastery gardens providing the raw ingredients for their medicines. The monks preserved many Greek and Roman writings on medicine and herbal lore in the libraries of the great monasteries. As well, they produced several treatises of their own.

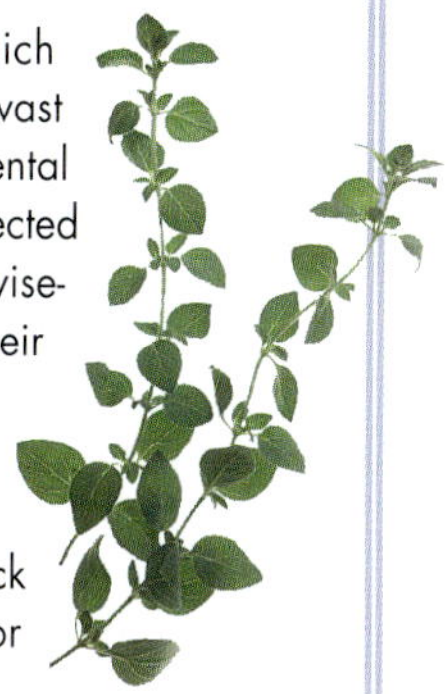

During the Christian Inquisitions which plagued the 13th to the 18th centuries, vast numbers of women healers in continental Europe were slain. When cures were effected and when the village flourished, the wise-women were usually thought to be using their powers for good (although this sometimes resulted in persecution by the medical establishment). If anything went wrong, they were often accused of black magic and either arrested for trial or murdered by an enraged mob.

The preservation of herbal lore during the European Dark Ages owes much to the Arab empire which spread quickly east towards India and west into Spain. In Baghdad, a huge library housed an extraordinary collection of mainly Greek writings. During this period, Arab writers on medicine and pharmacy, including Rhazes and Avicenna, were also active. Rhazes urged healers to prefer diet to drugs, simple remedies to complex ones.

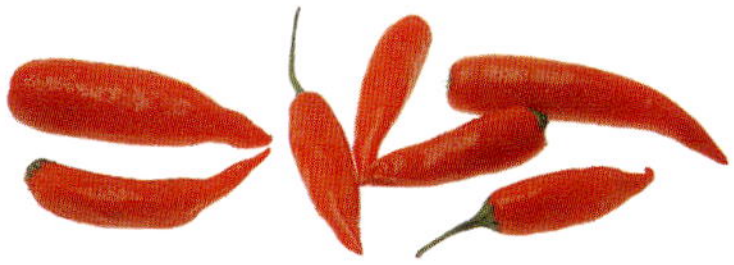

A HISTORY OF HERBALISM

Following the invention of printing in the 15th century, hundreds of herbals were published. One of the most renowned was Nicholas Culpeper's *The English Physician Enlarged*, with "369 Medicines made of English Herbs" — a blend of traditional herbal medicine, astrology and magic.

The science of chemistry developed rapidly in the 18th and 19th centuries, along with a significant change in the way in which patients and their illnesses were considered (see MODERN MEDICINE). The first scientific treatise on the use of a folk medicine was published in the late 18th century. Within it, William Withering presented the idea that the detailed examination and assessment of individuals and their case histories formed a sound basis of knowledge for the use of herbs. This premise remains in line with modern herbal treatment but was at odds with developments in medical practice at the time.

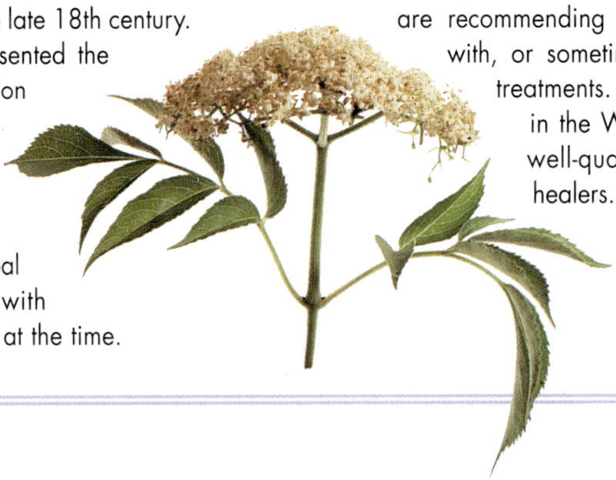

The 19th century saw the development of HOMOEOPATHY and NATUROPATHY. By the turn of the 20th century, the synthetic drug aspirin was produced, based on a herbal remedy. Many of the drugs we use today originally came from plants or are synthetic versions of plant substances.

Among medical consumers concerned about the side effects of various drug therapies or medicine's approach to the individual, herbalism has come back into its own. The interest has spread to the medical profession, many of whom are recommending herbal remedies in conjunction with, or sometimes in place of, chemical drug treatments. As well, almost every community in the Western world now has access to well-qualified herbalists and natural healers. Herbalism survives and prospers, its emphasis on the healer's sympathy with the human condition now recognised as essentially good medicine.

HOMOEOPATHY

HOMOEOPATHY IS A SYSTEM OF MEDICINE BASED ON THE PRINCIPLE OF "LIKE CURES LIKE". IT HAS BEEN OBSERVED THAT ANY SUBSTANCE THAT CAN CAUSE A SET OF SYMPTOMS IN A HEALTHY PERSON, CAN ALSO CURE A SIMILAR SET OF SYMPTOMS IN A SICK PERSON WHEN GIVEN IN MINIMAL DOSES.

Homoeopathic medicines work gently yet powerfully on the vital energy of the patient. All the remedies are made from naturally occurring sources such as plants and minerals.

Homoeopathy aims to treat the whole person. To a homoeopath, symptoms of an illness are seen as the body's natural healing process in operation. Symptoms such as diarrhoea, headache and cough are outward signs of the body attempting a healing response — they are not part of the disease itself. While many conventional medicines suppress the symptoms of illness, the homoeopath uses natural remedies that support and boost the body's own healing ability, as well as addressing the actual cause of the problem.

A HISTORY OF HOMOEOPATHY

Homoeopathy is the work of the German doctor Samuel Hahnemann (1755–1843). Hahnemann trained as a doctor but became disheartened by the inadequacy of the principles and techniques used. He gave up medicine to translate medical texts and become involved in chemical research.

While Hahnemann was translating William Cullen's *Materia Medica*, he came across something which changed his life. Cullen wrote about the use of cinchona bark to cure malaria (quinine would later be extracted from the same plant source). Hahnemann was critical of Cullen's rationale, so began taking doses of the bark himself to observe its effects. To his surprise, he found that he developed malaria-like symptoms: drowsiness, trembling, heart palpitations, flushed cheeks, fever and thirst.

The outcome of Hahnemann's experiment suggested that the same substance which was being used to treat malaria in the sick (cinchona bark), would also produce the symptoms of malaria in the healthy. Conversely, and more importantly, the same substance which produced

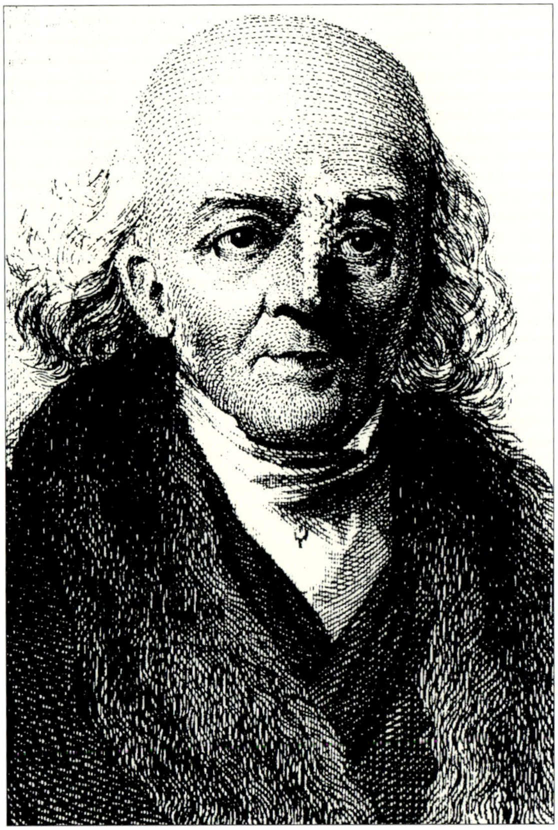

Samuel Hahnemann was the founder of homoeopathy. The first edition of his major work, *The Organon Of The Healing Art*, was published in 1810. Five more editions were published, although the last did not appear until 1920, after his death.

"illness" in the healthy could be used to cure the sick. Hahnemann had read in the ancient literature of Hippocrates reference to a medicine of "similars" — substances which could both cause and cure illness. Now, he had witnessed it to be so. He developed this idea into a theory called the "law of similars" and called his new form of medicine "homoeopathy" meaning "similar suffering" in the Greek.

A few years later, Edward Jenner discovered smallpox could be prevented by vaccinating with a similar disease, cowpox. While most doctors treated Jenner as a quack, Hahnemann supported his endeavours.

Hahnemann then began researching plants, herbs, animal and mineral matter and the effects they produced on a healthy person in general. He tested the substances on himself and cooperative colleagues. He would make a safe preparation, administer it, then observe and carefully record every effect on the physical body, emotions and mind. After being tested on many people, the results were collated and a "picture" of the remedy was created. This process is called "proving a remedy".

Hahnemann and his colleagues then began testing the remedies in their clinics. They would match the remedy picture with that of the sick patient, i.e. the patient would be exhibiting symptoms very close to those produced by the chosen remedy in its proving. It was found the remedies worked, and patients were being cured by this application of a "medicine of similars".

However, it was observed that patients would sometimes suffer aggravations from the remedy before the condition was alleviated. For this reason, Hahnemann decided to try diluting the substances for a gentler effect. This seemed to work and aggravations were diminished. But, with continued dilution alone, the effectiveness was diminished as well.

After further experiments, Hahnemann discovered that if the substance was not only diluted to make it milder but also shaken vigorously (or "succussed") during the preparation process, the complications were reduced and also the power to heal was increased.

The succussion appears to make the remedy more potent by revealing curative energy. It is this energy which resonates on the same level as the patient's to facilitate the body's own healing process.

HOW REMEDIES ARE MADE

During his lifetime, Hahnemann was able to "prove" about 100 remedies. The method of preparation of remedies by dilution and succussion is called "dynamisation" or "potentisation".

Remedies have a potency scale. For example, one part of the original substance or "mother tincture" when diluted in 99 parts of strong alcohol and succussed 10 times is written as 1C.

In health food stores you will often see remedies already made up to the 6C strength. This is when one part of the mother tincture is diluted in 99 parts of strong alcohol and successed ten times. This is done six times so, in total, the tincture is successed 60 times and diluted to one part in a million.

Remember that in homoeopathy the ideal is the minimum dose necessary to stimulate self healing. Less of the mother substance when potentised or dynamised reduces its toxicology, not its effectiveness.

New homoeopathic remedies continue to be developed in the same way. They are tested on volunteers, and their effects closely monitored until the "picture" is established.

THE CONSULTATION

The process to ascertain which remedy is appropriate to treat a person is potentially complex, although some over-the-counter remedies can be used at home as a first-aid application in simple situations.

A properly trained homoeopath will have developed astute powers of observation as it is the individual's unique physical and psychological make-up that interests a homoeopath. It is this that determines the likelihood of illness and what symptoms are displayed. It also determines which remedies are required. Different people may be treated with different remedies for the same illness, and the one remedy may be prescribed for many different illnesses depending on the individuals who are displaying the illness.

A homoeopath requires a personal history which may include details of how you live, your emotional reactions to various situations, medical history, likes and dislikes in food, reactions to weather and how you fare socially. They will also try to assess through observation and discussion, your state of mind, concerns, emotional responses and beliefs.

Once the homoeopath has worked out which is the best remedy for you, take it as directed then wait the appropriate interval before your condition is reviewed at a second consultation.

THE HEALING PROCESS

The healing process can be fast or slow, because with each ailment, compounded problems are removed layer by layer — much like peeling away the layers of an onion. Your symptoms may change as the body deals with each of these layers. For example, you may attend a homoeopath because you have a digestion problem; as you go through treatment, there may be a stage in which you develop a skin rash.

Symptoms are ranked in order by a homoeopath, depending on severity and how they impact on a person's ability to function. Unusual symptoms are given great significance, as are mental and emotional symptoms. Thus, you may find that when you consult a homoeopath for one problem, a number of other seemingly unrelated problems are treated first.

One of the pioneer homoeopaths to follow Hahnemann was Constantine Hering (1800–80). The German-born American explained that symptoms disappear first from "the most important organs to the least important organs" — superior to inferior, in reverse chronological order of the unresolved acquired problems.

This may explain why you can even experience what homoeopaths call a "healing crisis" when your symptoms become initially worse. To a homoeopath, the symptoms are a sign of healing and any temporary worsening is an indication that the body is in the process of healing itself and that an improvement will soon be evident.

So it is essential when you attend a homoeopath that you give the healing process a chance to work properly.

It should be stated, however, that the healing crisis should not be too severe. Monitor your symptoms and contact your practitioner if you are concerned.

Often a homoeopath will have a background in general medical practice; many are also involved in NATUROPATHY.

Homoeopathic remedies may be incorporated into other health treatments, but this should always be under the guidance of health professionals.

USING HOMOEOPATHIC REMEDIES AT HOME

In most cases it is advisable to see a homoeopath for a homoeopathic treatment, but for minor ailments, you may choose to try the remedy recommended for your health condition in the A–Z OF HEALTH CONDITIONS.

Take the dosage recommended for the ailment, and stop taking the remedy as soon as you feel better (unlike antibiotics, you do not take a whole course).

For maximum effect, take the remedy at least half an hour before or after eating or drinking any substance apart from water, or cleaning your teeth. This is because homoeopathic remedies are easily affected by other substances on your tongue.

If the remedy is in pill form, suck it rather than swallow it, or dissolve the pill in a teaspoon of water. Don't handle the pills with your fingers as they may lose their potency if in contact with skin — use a spoon.

If the remedy comes in liquid form, shake the bottle well before you take the dosage as this will increase its effectiveness. The remedy can be taken undiluted or mixed into fruit juice. (The remedies available from health food stores usually come in liquid form.)

Use only one remedy at a time. This enables you to find out what works best for your condition. If the remedy has not taken effect after a day, you may need a different remedy. If you have any doubt about a home remedy or prescribed treatment, consult a homoeopath for a full assessment.

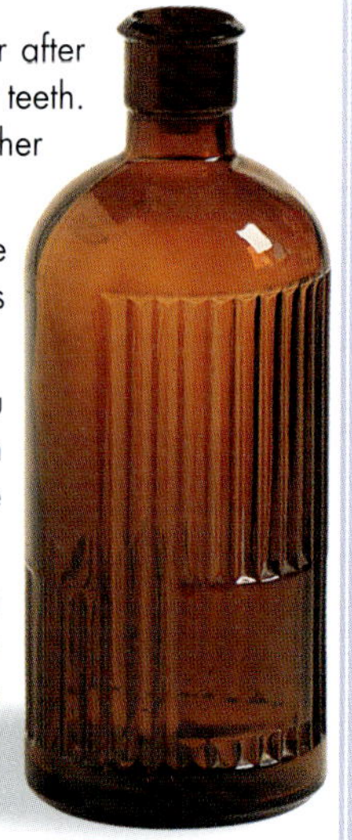

MASSAGE

A MASSAGE IS A SYSTEMATIC PROCESS OF TOUCH COMBINING A NUMBER OF TECHNIQUES SUCH AS STROKING AND KNEADING. THERE IS A VARIETY OF MASSAGE THERAPIES RANGING FROM DEEP TISSUE TO GENTLE AROMATHERAPY MASSAGE. MASSAGE IS ALSO USED IN CONJUNCTION WITH OTHER THERAPIES SUCH AS OSTEOPATHY AND CHIROPRACTIC.

Of all the healing arts, massage is one of the oldest and the simplest. Every day we unconsciously employ massage techniques because the desire and need to touch, and the action of touching, is instinctive. We stroke our temples to soothe a headache, we hold a friend's hand to comfort them, we "rub away" a child's knocks and bumps, and if there is an injury we "kiss it better".

The benefits of regular or even occasional massage therapy are extensive. The physical benefits — when combined with the psychological benefits of conveyed warmth, understanding and reassurance — can very quickly produce a heightened, uplifted sense of well-being.

THE BENEFITS OF MASSAGE

On a physical level:

- relaxes the central nervous system
- soothes tight, tense or overworked muscles
- removes toxins from the body
- improves circulation of both blood and lymphatic fluid
- increases healing
- softens skin where scar tissue has formed
- breaks down fibrous tissue around joints
- prepares healthy muscle for demanding activity and aids recovery from this activity.

On an emotional level:

- calms the mind
- reduces stress
- relaxes or stimulates thought processes
- increases energy levels
- reduces apathy and depression
- soothes emotions.

IMPORTANT

It may not be appropriate to be massaged if you have any of the following conditions:

- recent trauma — fractured bones, whiplash, sprains etc
- an acute inflammatory condition — signs include redness, swelling, pain or loss of function
- recent damage to ligaments, tendons or muscles
- skin problems, burns, sores, etc
- thrombosis
- tumours or cancers
- recent surgery.

Care should be taken with the following conditions. Check with a doctor or therapist if you have:

- high blood pressure or a heart condition
- loose joints and joint replacements
- osteoporosis or brittle bones
- multiple sclerosis
- diabetes
- varicose veins
- or are pregnant.

THE HISTORY OF MASSAGE

Massage is most likely the oldest form of medical treatment. Evidence of its use can be found throughout history and across all cultures, from ancient times to the present.

Historical artefacts show that the Chinese were using massage techniques as early as 3000 years before the birth of Christ. The Ayurveda, an Indian medical treatise written about 1800 BC, describes a process of rubbing and "shampooing" the body as a means of promoting recovery and healing of the body after injury. In both the art and literature of ancient Egypt, Persia and Japan, many references are made to physicians employing the benefits of massage in an effort to counteract and heal many illnesses.

To ancient Greek and Roman physicians, massage was the first and principal method for treating and healing ailments and physical pain. Hippocrates, considered "the father of medicine", wrote in the 5th century BC: "The physician must be experienced in many things, but assuredly in rubbing ... for rubbing can bind a joint that is loose and loosen a joint that is too rigid". Julius Caesar, an epileptic, was daily pinched all over to relieve recurring headaches and neuralgia, and Pliny, the renowned Roman naturalist, regularly received a "rub" to alleviate chronic asthma.

After the collapse of the Roman empire in the 5th century AD, massage fell in status, and during the Middle Ages in Europe, it came to be identified with the sinful pleasures of the flesh. The Renaissance of the 16th century, however, revived the therapeutic art. The work of two physicians — one a French doctor, Ambroise Pare, and the other an Italian, Mercurialis — became fashionable, firmly re-establishing massage therapy as a legitimate and effective, albeit relatively elite, medical practice.

It was in the early 19th century, due to the developments by a Swede, Per Henrick Ling, that massage took another leap forward and became commonly available. Ling was a fencing master and gymnastics instructor who cured himself of rheumatism in the arm by using a series of percussions.

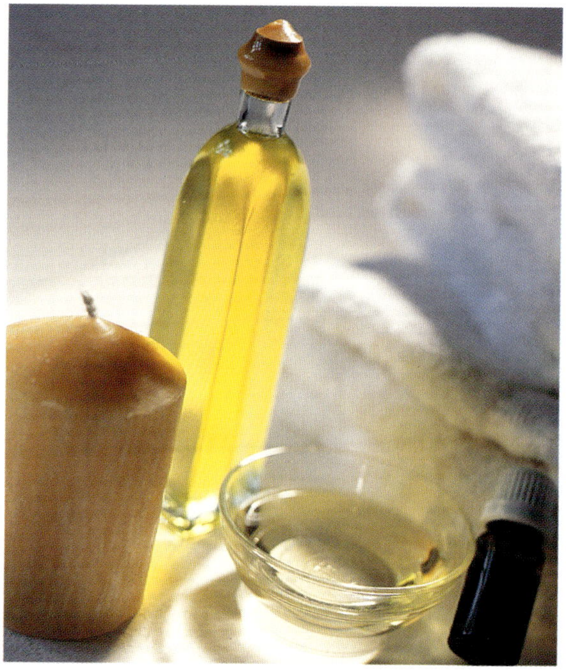

Oils and lighting are important to a relaxing massage.

After travelling to the Orient as well as studying ancient Egyptian, Roman and Greek techniques, Ling assembled a system of massage therapy known today as Swedish massage. In 1813 the first college to offer massage as part of the curriculum was established in Stockholm.

Most of Ling's knowledge about massage came from studying Eastern methods. In the East, massage therapies have always held a highly respected position where their use has continued in an unbroken line since prehistory. This positive attitude provided the perfect environment for experimentation which, over the centuries, has produced several different types of massage therapy.

DIFFERENT STYLES OF MASSAGE

The style of massage which best suits you depends on your personality and what you require from the massage. Massages can vary from a sensuous experience which leaves you feeling relaxed to a vigorous pummelling which stimulates and energises you.

Western massage techniques consist of several strokes performed on the body in a variety of ways — the strokes can be gentle and reassuring, percussive and stimulating, or work more deeply into the body. See page 141. A relaxation massage is likely to involve more gentle strokes.

Kneading, pulling, wringing and pressure strokes are more common in a therapeutic or deep tissue massage. During this type of massage the therapist will use the pressure of the heel of the hands, fingertips or thumbs to stimulate blood supply and lymph drainage. The masseur also aims to break-down any congestion or crystalline deposits of lactic acids in the tissues. This deeper, more penetrating massage can be painful at times. This type of massage might, however, be more effective if you have specific aches or pains.

A massage aimed at preparing you for a sporting event or stimulating you, will have an emphasis on what are called percussion strokes. This is a range of brisk, rhythmic strokes performed by repeatedly alternating hands. It is similar to playing the drums. The strokes involve such movements as plucking or pinching small bundles of flesh or pummelling the flesh with loosely closed fists.

SELF-MASSAGE OF THE ABDOMEN

Massage can be invaluable in relieving abdominal discomfort. Attention should be given to the large intestine (colon) which runs in the shape of an inverted "U" up the right side of the abdomen, across and down the left side.

1. Lie on your back, with a pillow or rolled towel under your knees and head if you wish.

2. With the fingers of the right hand, pull up from the groin area to the ribcage, push across the abdomen to the left side, then stroke down with the heel of the left hand from the ribs to the groin area.

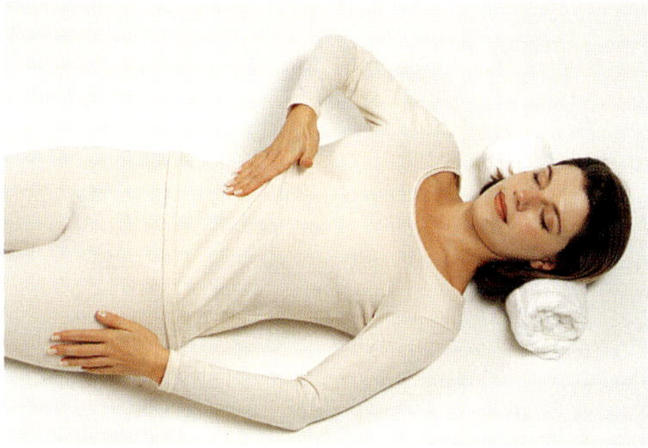

These strokes stimulate the soft tissue area, improve circulation and increase your energy.

The positional release technique was designed to alleviate and release painful muscle spasms in the body. The body has a number of surface "trigger points" which may suggest deeper muscular problems. The body is moved into various positions to reduce stress on the muscles, helping them to unwind and relax. This technique is very useful for headaches, muscle pain, poor posture and fatigue.

Chinese massage and Japanese SHIATSU differ from the Western massage methods. The Chinese massage therapist uses strokes that are similar to Western massage but utilises a knowledge of the energy meridians of the body which are stimulated in ACUPUNCTURE or ACUPRESSURE. A shiatsu massage is very different from a Western massage. Rather than strokes and kneading, the shiatsu therapist uses pressure and stretching. See page 178.

MASSAGE CHART

DEEP TISSUE MASSAGE

SYNOPSIS/HISTORY

This technique grew out of remedial massage. Deep pressure is used to release long-held stress to help your body realign itself and return to its natural posture. Two therapies associated with this idea include rolfing and ka-tone. Both are popular in the United States.

TECHNIQUE

Involves working on areas where stress, misuse or injury has altered your natural posture, often leading to pain or misuse of your body.

BENEFITS

Can reduce muscle tightness and pain, improve flexibility and emotional well-being.

KINESIOLOGY

SYNOPSIS/HISTORY

Related to another therapy called touch for health, kinesiology was developed by an American chiropractor, Dr George Goodheart, in 1965. It is based on the notion that each muscle group in the body is related to other body functions such as organs, glands, circulation and the digestive system.

TECHNIQUE

A technique called muscle testing is used as a diagnostic tool. It draws on a combination of Western and Eastern principles, relating certain muscles to particular energy meridians. It also relies on the idea that muscles will respond in a strong or weak manner when touched in a particular way. A weak response in a certain area can indicate poor functioning of a related area of your body. For example, if you hold your arm away from your body and your shoulder strength is tested, a muscular weakness may indicate low liver energy. This is believed to be so because the shoulder muscles lie on the liver meridian. Correspondingly, if your muscle tone is strengthened, it is believed this will in turn tone the meridian and improve the function of your liver.

A treatment involves finger massaging of reflex points combined with specific body movements.

BENEFITS

Kinesiologists believe this relationship between your muscles and your meridians can help to diagnose conditions which could otherwise be difficult to detect. This therapy has therefore been successful in helping to trace allergies, especially food allergies, and to treat conditions such as fatigue, depression and headaches.

LOMILOMI

SYNOPSIS/HISTORY

Based on a traditional Hawaiian form of massage.

TECHNIQUE

Generally the massage lasts two hours and the strokes are rhythmic and flowing. The therapist will work on deep tissue and often the massage is performed to music.

BENEFITS

Aimed at restoring balance to your body's energy system to improve your physical and emotional well-being and increase your energy levels.

LYMPHATIC DRAINAGE

SYNOPSIS/HISTORY

The goal is to assist your lymphatic system in ridding the body of toxins and mucus.

TECHNIQUES

Often incorporated into other forms of massage such as Swedish, aromatherapy or remedial. The technique includes deep muscular massage and stimulation of lymphatic points which can become tender if the body is overloaded with toxins.

BENEFITS

Used for achieving balance within your body and for specific conditions such as allergies or migraines where poor lymphatic drainage may be a contributing factor. Note, however, that stimulating the lymph system is not advised in some cases, so ensure your therapist is properly qualified.

REMEDIAL MASSAGE

SYNOPSIS/HISTORY

In lay terms, this form of massage is a combination of Swedish massage techniques with a sound knowledge of anatomy and physiology.

TECHNIQUES

May include soft tissue and deep tissue work with stretches, therapeutic exercises and even some acupressure.

BENEFITS

Often used to treat specific problems such as back, neck and shoulder pain, sprains, strains and sciatica.

MASSAGE CHART

ROLFING

SYNOPSIS/HISTORY

Developed by American biochemist Ida Rolf who studied a range of holistic therapies including OSTEOPATHY and the ALEXANDER TECHNIQUE.

TECHNIQUES

Hands, elbows and knees are used to apply deep pressure on the soft tissues. The aim is to help your body return to its natural balance and alignment. The technique is carried out across ten sessions and each session looks at a different area of your body. For example, the first session may concentrate on opening up your breathing while the second may focus on your feet and lower legs. The final sessions look at integrating your body as a whole. Since this therapy can sometimes be painful, it is best to consult a certified rolfing therapist.

BENEFITS

Can help your body realign, aid the release of blocked emotions, assist in pain relief and improve overall functioning.

SPORTS MASSAGE

SYNOPSIS/HISTORY

A form of remedial massage specifically aimed at athletes. Has become an important part of sports medicine.

TECHNIQUE

Used before a sports event to warm and tone muscles or after the event to treat pain and injury. The emphasis is usually on prevention, and the masseur will look for knotted muscles which can prevent maximum efficiency and lead to more serious problems.

BENEFITS

A good massage before a sporting event is thought to aid in the prevention of injury. Massage following an event is aimed at assisting the body remove waste products produced as a result of the exertion and to minimise tightness and spasm which come from stiff and sore muscles.

SWEDISH MASSAGE

SYNOPSIS/HISTORY

Per Henrik Ling of Sweden developed this therapy in the early 1800s and it has become the standard form of massage. It is also easy to learn through courses, books, vidoes etc for home use.

TECHNIQUE

Includes a range of techniques include stroking, effleurage, petrissage, kneading, tapotement, vibrations and passive movements.

BENEFITS

This method can be used to relax or to stimulate muscles. It also increases circulation, aids the elimination of waste products and improves digestion.

TOUCH FOR HEALTH

SYNOPSIS/HISTORY

This is a simple form of kinesiology that can be used by the lay person.

TECHNIQUE

It combines muscle testing with acupressure, massage and touch.

BENEFITS

It can assist a variety of conditions including fatigue, allergies, headaches and digestive problems.

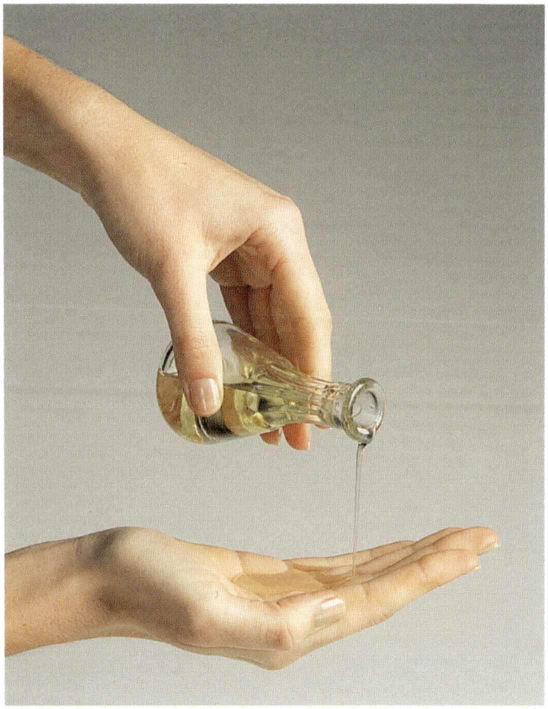

SELECTING A THERAPIST

It is best to decide whether you want a relaxing or a therapeutic massage before you decide on your therapist.

Some will perform both varieties of massage but many have a preference for one style only.

The therapist who specialises in the relaxing massage usually has all the necessary atmosphere provoking tools such as aromatherapy oils, soft music and dim lighting.

If you decide on this type of massage it is desirable to avoid doing anything after it. Arrange your day so you can go home or sit in a park — anything that will allow you to retain the calm and peace for as long as possible. The purpose is defeated if you cram a relaxing massage into your lunch hour then rush back to work. Massages designed to relieve tense muscles, however, can be performed under noisy conditions such as you would find at your local gymnasium and still be satisfying. But it is wise to keep calm both physically and mentally immediately after a massage. Often your sore areas will recover more quickly if you allow them a chance to relax and rest.

When you telephone to make your booking ask to speak to the therapist. Discuss the style of massage you want to ensure you choose the masseur to suit your needs.

Also when you are being worked on, it is acceptable to direct the masseur to the area of your body you consider needs the most work. Likewise if you are experiencing pain and want a more gentle approach then express that too.

But most importantly, do not wait until you are ill or have sore muscles before treating yourself to a massage.

GIVING A MASSAGE

Unless you have a professional massage table, the best place to massage at home is on the floor on a thin foam mat or folded blankets covered by a sheet. A thick soft mattress or futon is not recommended as it will counteract much of the pressure applied by the masseuse.

You will also need to have on hand two pillows, several towels (bath and hand size), a blanket for covering the body, and possibly a hot water bottle for the feet. The massage oil can be a commercial preparation, an essential oil blend (see page 99), or even common olive oil.

CREATING A SUITABLE ENVIRONMENT

Ensure you have privacy and won't be interrupted. Play soft, soothing music if you find it helps you to relax, and keep the lighting soft and subtle (candlelight is ideal). An eye patch is handy when lying on the back. The room should be comfortably warm and free of draughts. An oil burner can be used to scent the room with suitable essential oils (see page 99).

You should be relaxed and comfortable as any tension will be communicated to your partner. Clean your hands and stretch them to increase sensitivity and flexibility. Wear loose clothing and watch your posture. If you are not comfortable in your assumed position, change it until you are. Remember to use the weight of your body when applying any pressure to lessen strain on yourself.

THE BASIC MASSAGE MOVEMENTS

In Swedish massage there are a number of basic techniques which are very useful to learn, as they are frequently repeated throughout the massage.

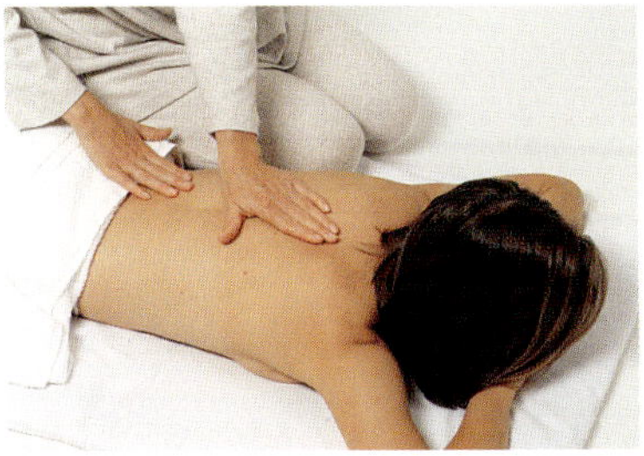

STROKING

Stroking is very important as it establishes the first contact with the patient. It will also help you locate areas of muscle tightness or pain. Long, gentle strokes are used to spread oil over the area being massaged. Both hands may stroke at one time, or alternate.

On the legs or hands, stroking is usually in the direction of the feet or hands. Stroking should always be soothing and comforting — use a light touch.

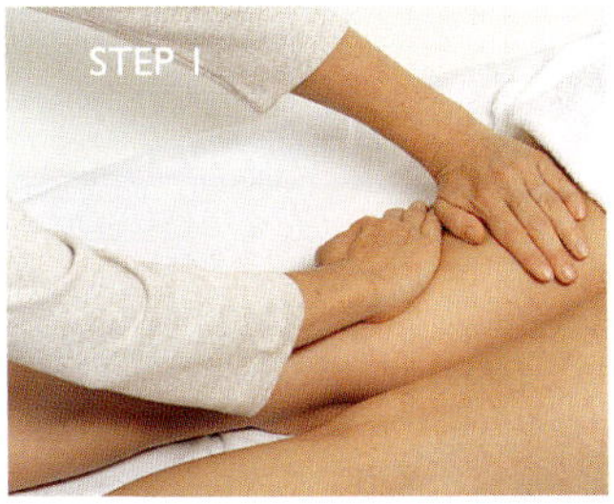

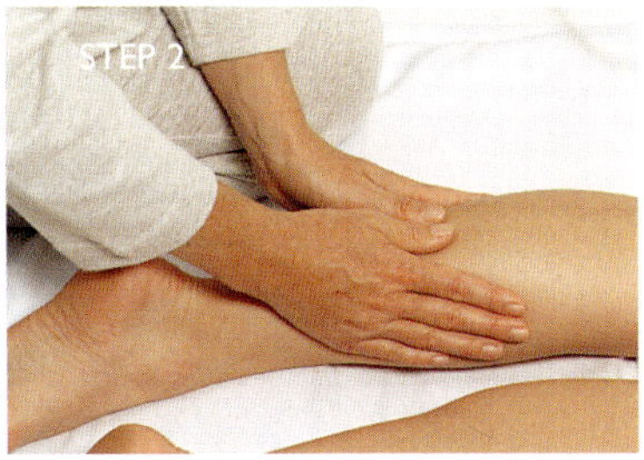

EFFLEURAGE

Effleurage warms the area being massaged and promotes circulation. It also has a relaxing effect on tight, tense muscles.

Effleurage is generally a long, even stroke applied with firm pressure. It is a movement that has two parts.

First, slide your hands forward. Generally, both hands work at the same time, either side by side with thumbs touching, or one below the other as illustrated in the first picture. When used on the limbs, the movement should always be in the direction of the heart — this is the opposite to stroking.

Second, after sliding hands forward, draw them back lightly in the opposite direction, as in the second picture.

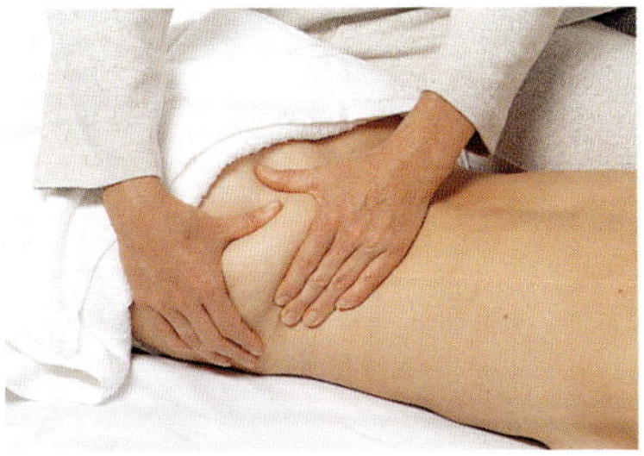

PETRISSAGE

Petrissage helps to relieve muscle fatigue and eliminate the build up of toxins. It includes a range of movements, such as kneading, rolling, wringing and squeezing. While stroking and effleurage are long, gliding movements, petrissage concentrates more on specific muscle areas to soften them up for deeper massage.

Kneading is just like kneading bread. Use each hand alternately to hold and squeeze flesh between your fingers.

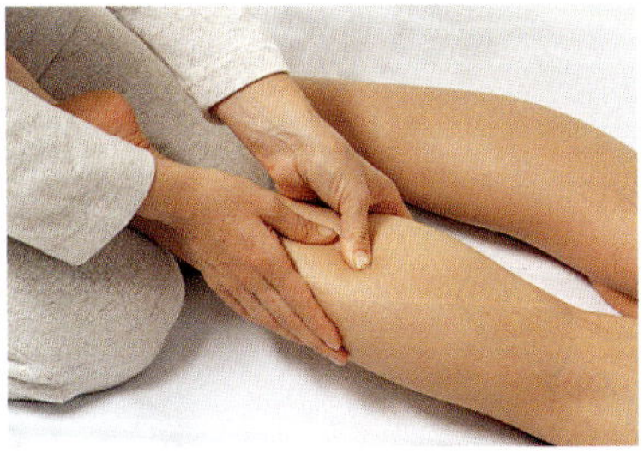

FRICTIONS

Frictions work at a deeper level, concentrating on just a small section of the body at one time. This movement is designed to penetrate problem areas of tension build up.

Generally the pads of the thumbs or fingers are used to create small circular movements. It is also possible to use the heel of the hand. Work slowly and carefully into the area — start gently and increase pressure as you feel the tissue relaxing beneath your fingers.

PERCUSSION

If the aim of the massage is to quietly soothe your partner, percussion may be too vigorous. However, it can be a great stress reducer and very uplifting.

The most common percussion movements are featured on this page. They are:

- flicking
- cupping
- plucking
- pounding

If you do decide to use them, make sure to keep your wrists loose. Always follow them with flowing movements such as stroking or effleurage.

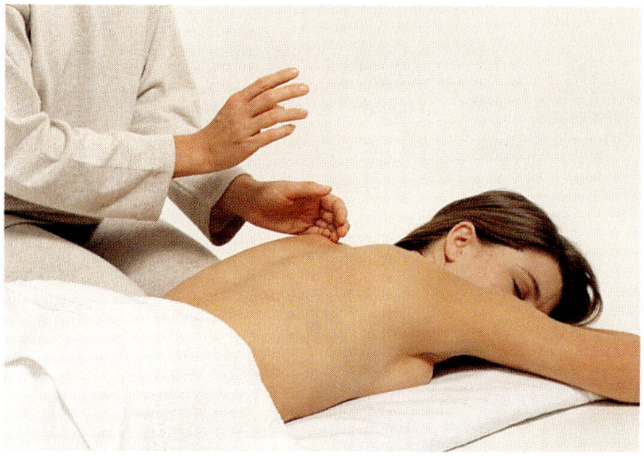

Flicking

Also known as hacking. In this movement the hands are relaxed, with palms facing one another. Use the little finger side of the hands and gently flick the surface of the skin with one hand and then the other. Keep the hands close together and try to form an even rhythm. The hands should be loose, bouncing easily off your partner's skin.

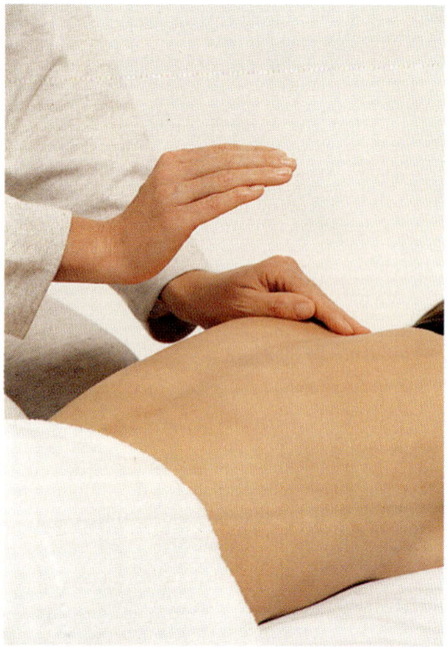

Cupping

Once again, keep wrists loose but form the hands into a cupped position, fingers touching lightly. The hands should be arched at the knuckles, forming a cavity. Each hand cups the surface of the skin alternately, keeping an even beat.

This movement should create a loud, hollow sound.

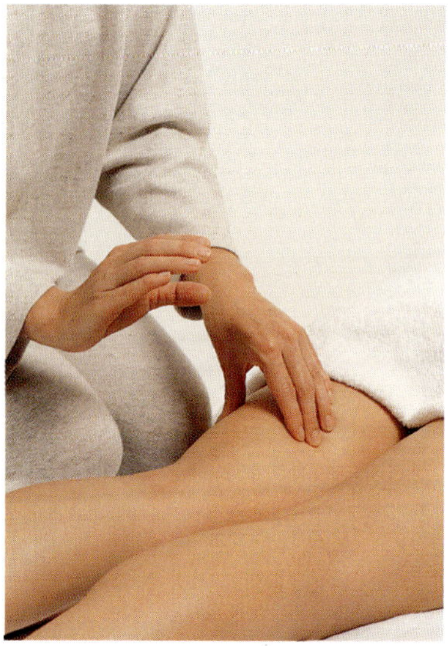

Plucking

This is a gentle and fairly rapid movement. Pick up the flesh between the thumb and fingers and then release, creating a plucking movement. Alternate the plucking from hand to hand to form a smooth rhythm.

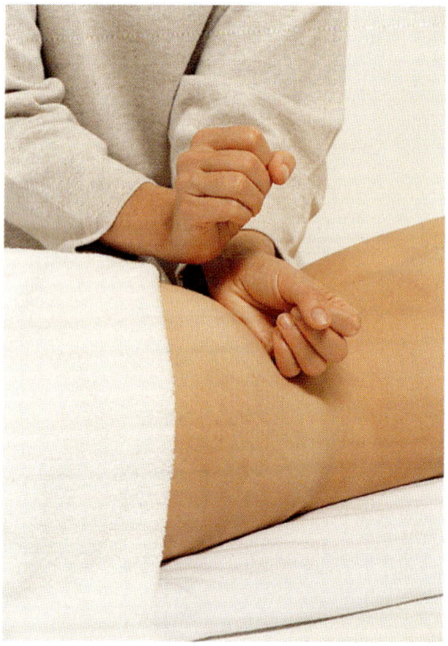

Pounding

Also known as pummelling, in this movement the hand is held in a loose fist.

Use the little finger side of the fist, one hand after the other, to gently pound the muscle mass. Lift your fist off the skin straight away, creating a light, springy motion.

A FULL-BODY MASSAGE

A few tips to keep in mind

- Try to maintain contact with your partner's body at all times during the massage; even when moving into a new position, try to keep one hand on the body.
- When massaging different parts of the body, keep the rest of the body covered with a large towel or blanket. This will keep your partner warm — this warmth will not only be soothing but will also assist the therapeutic benefits of the massage and increase the absorption of oils used.
- Try not to talk too much throughout the massage as it will interrupt the process, but do encourage your partner to let you know if there is any discomfort or a particular need.
- Always ensure your hands are warm before placing them anywhere near your partner — rub briskly together if they are at all cold.

A full body massage can be performed in any order. It is common to begin with the back or back of the legs, progressing to the front of legs, arms, abdomen, chest and finishing with the neck and face. However, this can be varied depending on preference.

CONNECTING

The most important parts of a massage are the beginning and the end. The initial touch will set the mood of the massage for you both. Once your partner is comfortable and covered by a blanket or towel, gently place your hands on their body — one hand on the nape of the neck and the other on the small of the back, for example. Breathe slowly and deeply, close your eyes and let the energy flow between you. Very softly rock your partner's body from side to side. Focus in this position for several minutes before allowing your hands to lift from the body. Now you are ready to fold back the covering and begin massaging.

THE BACK

Your partner should be lying face down with the head turned to one side — changing the direction of the head from time to time will help prevent a stiff neck. Position the arms where they are comfortable. A pillow under the ankles will add extra support.

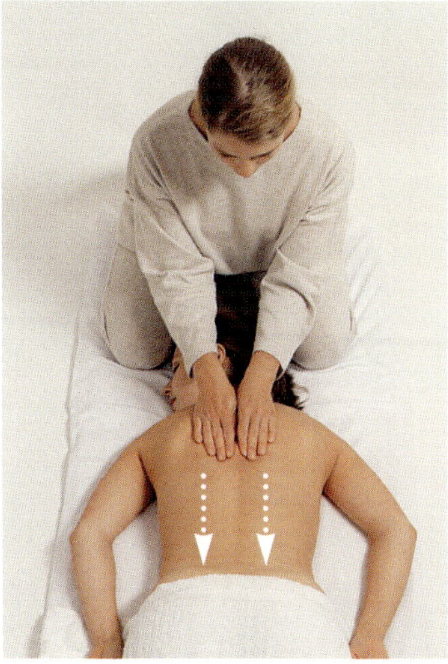

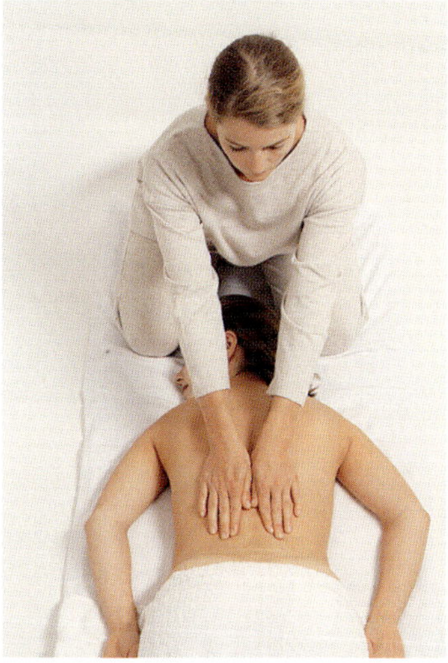

1. Kneel near the head of your partner and apply a light coating of oil with long gentle stroking movements over the entire back and shoulders.

Using the effleurage stroke, glide your hands down each side of the spine then slide them back up the side of the body. Let your body lean into each movement as you work down the body and then back up. Repeat several times.

2. Work the muscles that run each side of the spine. Using the friction movement, move your thumbs in circles from the top of the spine to the base — then return up the sides of body.

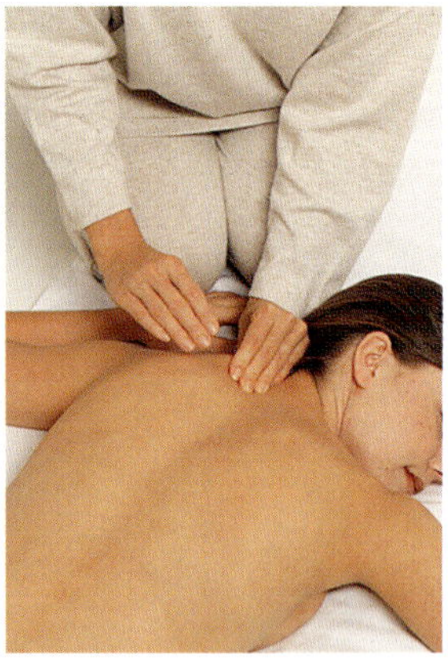

3. Moving on to the shoulders, knead the upper shoulder muscles. Gently squeeze and release around the whole shoulder area.

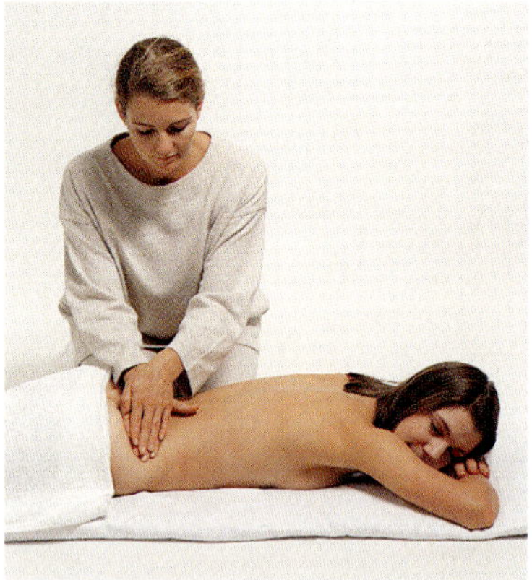

4. Move to one side of your partner, kneeling near their ribs. You will be massaging the side of the back opposite you. Place both hands on the buttock area, one hand on top of the other. Circle with the hands in wide, sweeping movements from the buttocks towards the head, covering the entire side up to the shoulders. Return, running your fingers lightly down the spine.

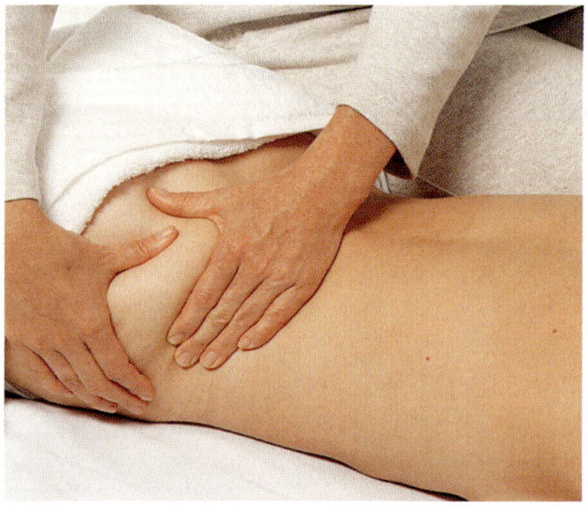

5. Knead the buttock area on the side opposite you, using squeezing and releasing movements.

6. Work a little deeper with frictions over the buttocks and base of spine. Use the pads of fingers to locate and work tight muscle areas.

7. Move to the other side of your partner and repeat movements 4 to 6.

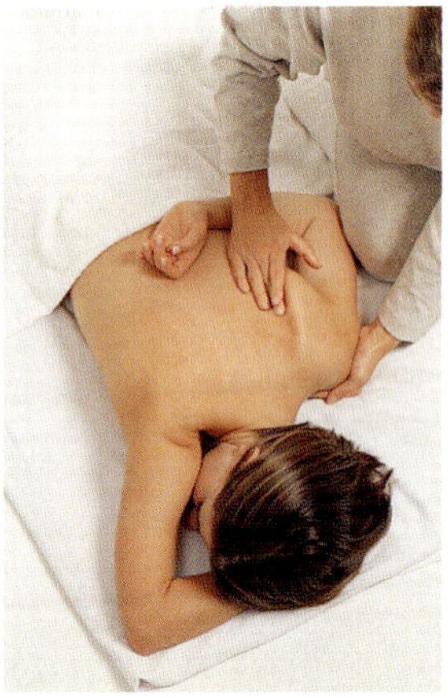

8. Kneel near the shoulder of your partner. It may be easiest if you lift your partner's arm and place their forearm on their lower back as shown. Slide your hand under their shoulder for support. Use your fingertips and the circular friction movement to massage the shoulder blade. Change sides and repeat.

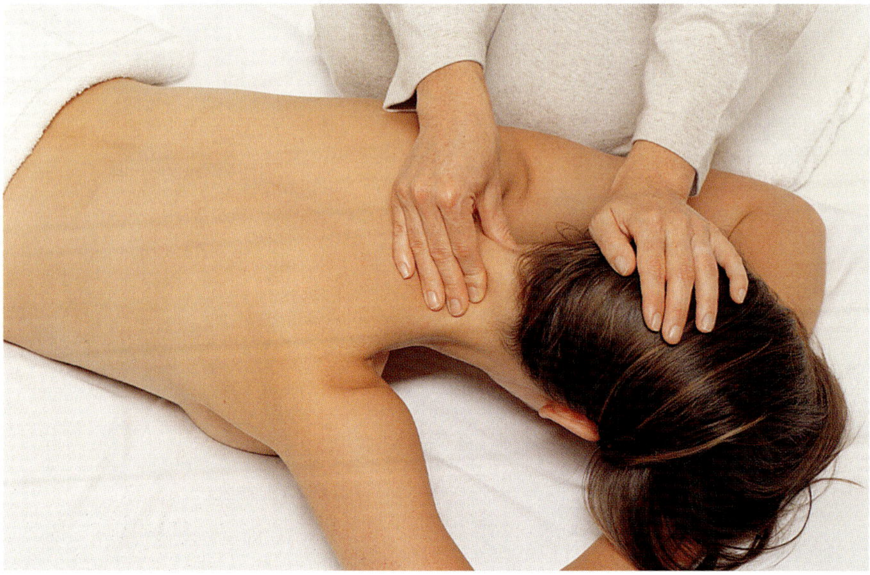

9. Move to the head of your partner, and gently stroke from base of spine to neck. Cover the back with a towel and pat or rock gently.

THE LEGS

Uncover one leg, keeping the remainder of the body covered and warm. Try placing a pillow under the shin as it relieves pressure from the lower back.

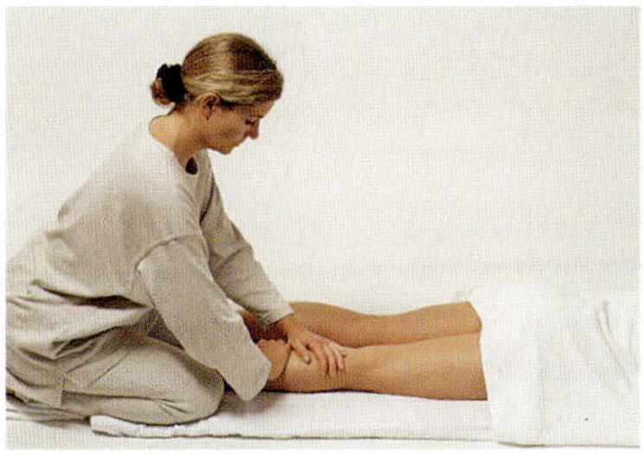

1. Kneeling near the foot of your partner, apply oil with gentle stroking movements covering the entire leg, from thigh to ankle.

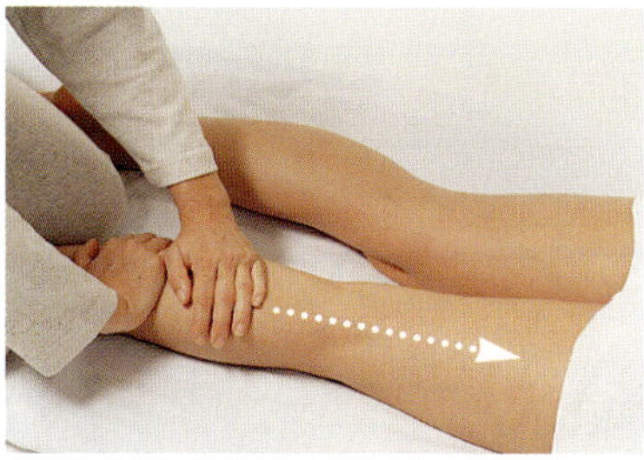

2. Using the effleurage movement, firmly glide both hands up the middle of the leg from ankle to the top of thigh. Return very gently down the sides of the leg to the ankle.

3. Kneel or sit cross-legged near your partner's toes and cradle the foot in one hand. Stroke the foot firmly with the other hand.

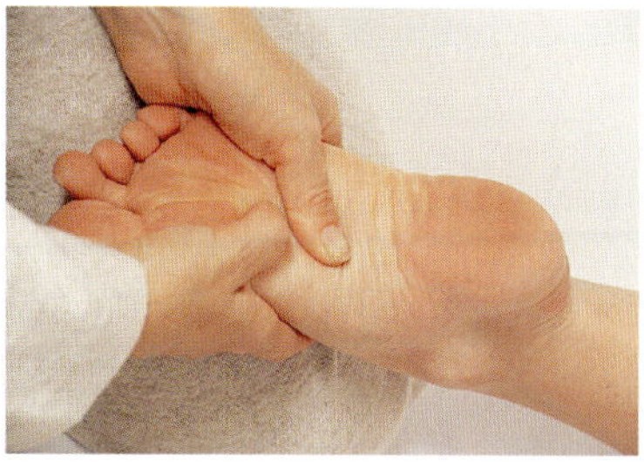

4. Rest the foot on your knee or in your lap and use your thumb in the friction movement to massage in small circles over the entire sole.

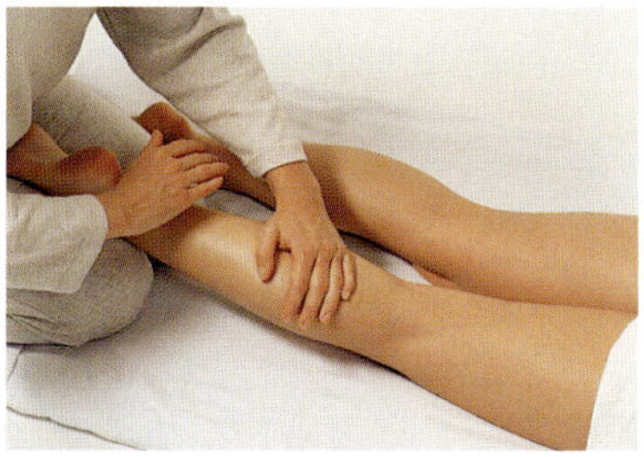

5. Now work on the calf of the leg — you may find it comfortable to place your partner's leg on your knee. The movement is a firm effleurage stroke, using only one hand at a time. Cupping your hands, stroke up the calf muscle with one hand — as it reaches the top of the calf, the other hand begins with the same movement from the ankle to form a rhythmic, flowing motion.

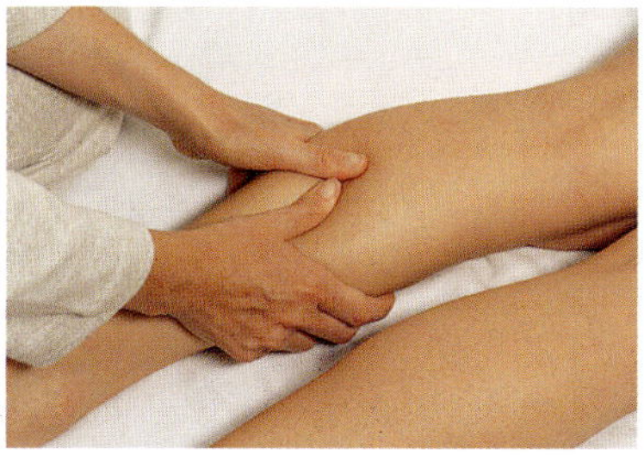

6. Having relaxed the area, now work more deeply into the muscle mass using circular thumb frictions. It is best to work up the calf, stroking upwards and outwards with the thumbs. Begin gently, increasing pressure gradually — many people are very sensitive in this area.

7. Move up to the thigh, repeating the same effleurage and friction movements.

8. You may now like to reposition yourself beside your partner's leg and try a series of kneading and percussion movements. Avoid the area around the back of the knee when using percussive movements.

9. Finish the leg massage with effleurage to the entire leg. End by softly drawing your fingers over the foot and off the edge of the toes.

10. Cover the leg with a towel and pat entire area. Then repeat the entire process on the back of the other leg.

11. Ask your partner to roll over onto their back. Cover again with towels and place a pillow under the knees for support. Repeat the same process on the front of the legs but concentrate on the upper thigh. Remember there is no real muscle mass on the front of the lower legs so stroking and gentle kneading is all that is required.

THE ARMS

Cover the legs and reposition yourself so that you are kneeling beside your partner's arm. Apply oil with stroking movements to the whole arm.

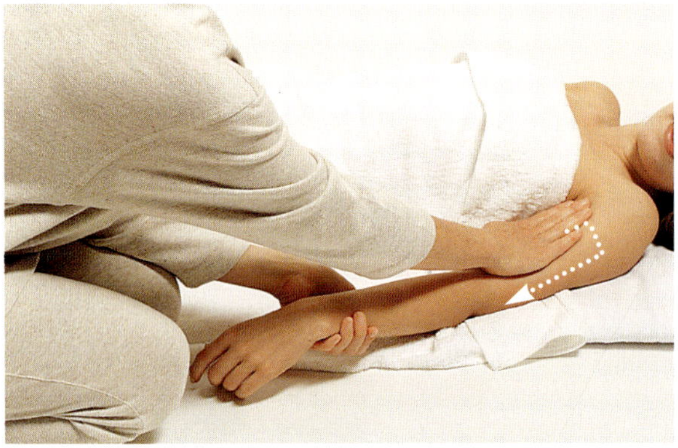

1. Hold the arm softly at the wrist with one hand, while effleuraging with the other. Stroke from the lower arm to upper arm, glide around the shoulder and slide back down to the hand.

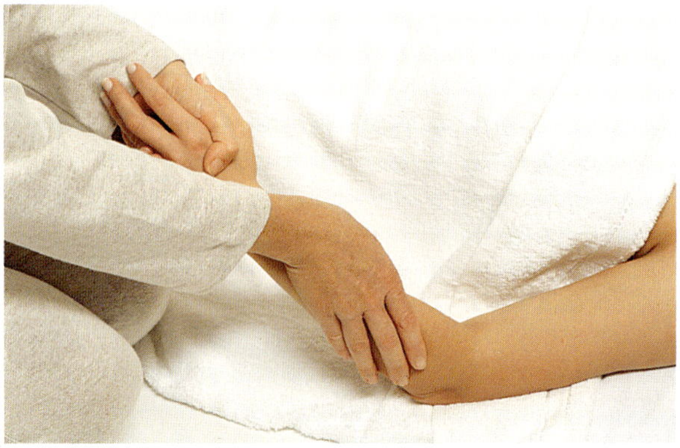

2. Concentrate the same movements to the forearm.

Next try circular friction movements to the area, on the front and then the back.

3. Now work on the upper arm, first with effleurage then with friction movements.

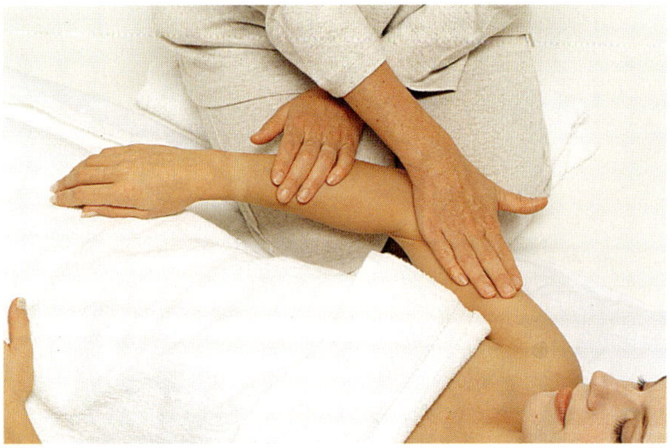

4. Follow with effleurage to the entire arm.

5. Hold your partner's hand in yours and rub the palm with your thumb. Stroke the upper surface of the hand. Gently rotate the wrist; rotate the fingers and very softly pull them away from the hand.

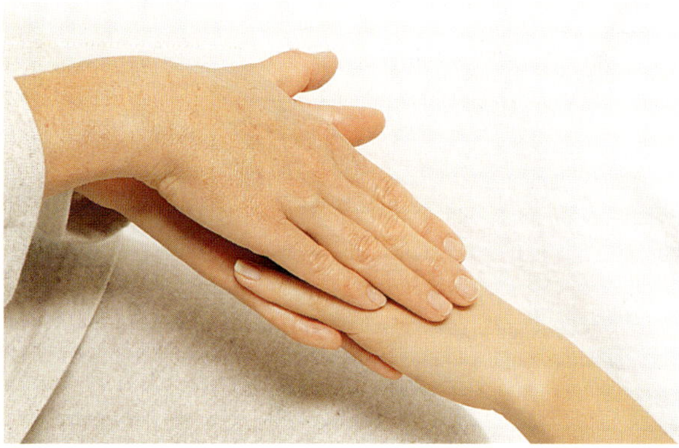

6. Conclude the arm massage by gently stroking from shoulders to hands; on the final stroke let your hands glide lightly off your partner's. Cover the arm with a towel and pat gently.

7. Repeat process on the other arm.

THE ABDOMEN AND CHEST

Arrange towels so only the area from the rib cage to the pelvis is exposed.

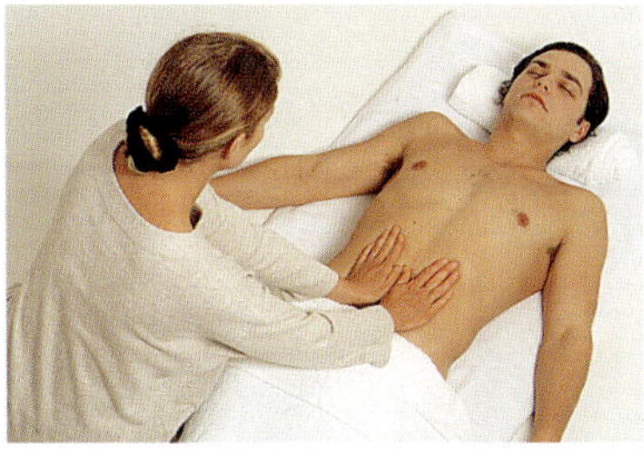

1. Kneel on one side of your partner near the waist. Apply oil to the whole area with gentle, stroking movements. Effleurage up the middle of the abdomen, out over the lower ribs and down towards the waist. Pull back down to the lower abdomen, and repeat the whole movement.

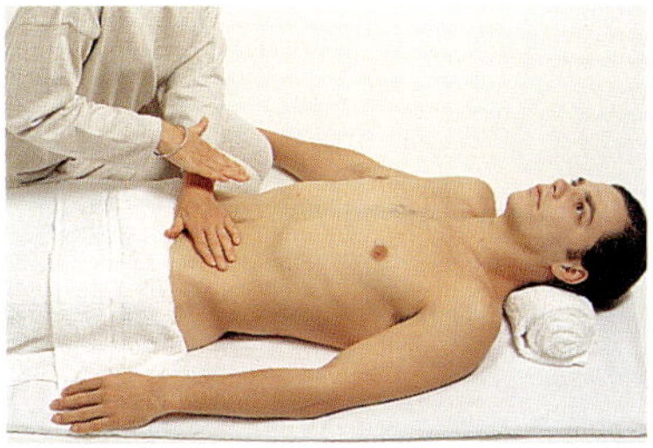

2. Soothe the area with circular effleurage, alternating one hand with the other. Cover the area with a towel, and place both your hands on the abdomen, applying gentle pressure, before allowing the hands to lift from the area.

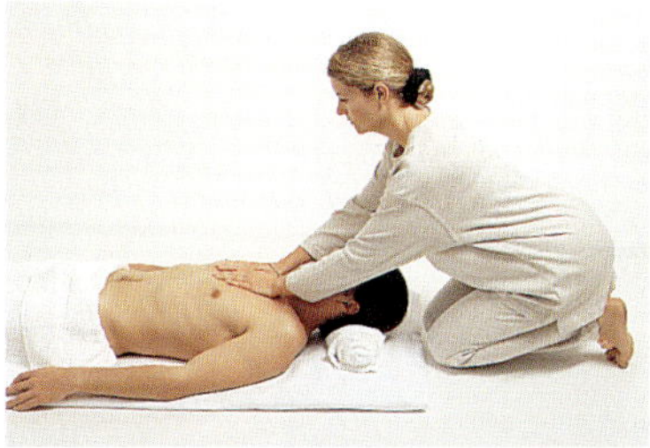

3. Follow with massage to the chest area. You can cover the breasts if you wish, leaving the upper chest area and shoulders exposed.

4. Kneel at the head of your partner and apply the oil by gliding hands down the middle of chest. Separate the hands, go around the breast area and return up the sides of body.

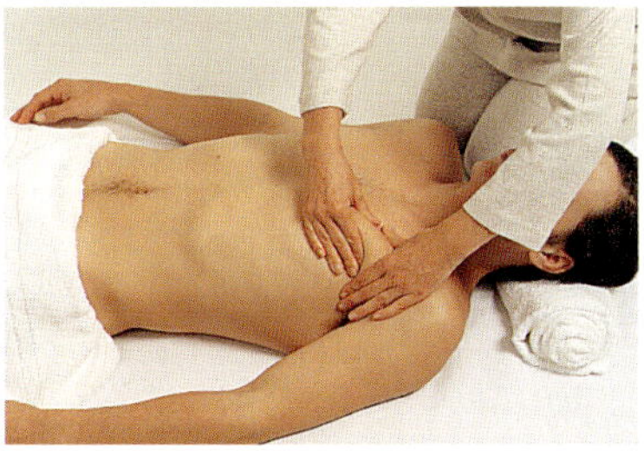

5. Knead the upper pectoral area — the fleshy area below the collarbone.

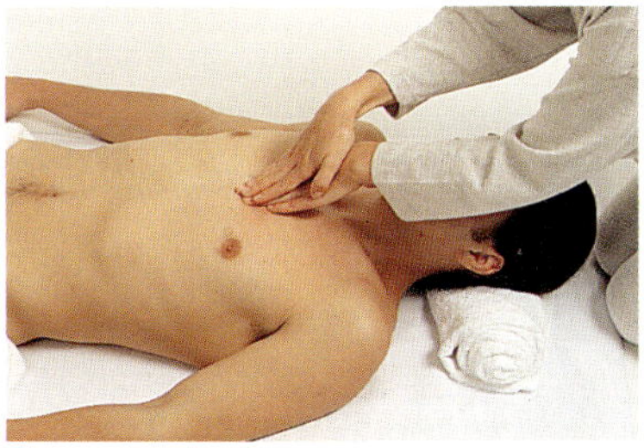

6. Using the pads of the fingers and light pressure only, work with friction movements over the breastbone.

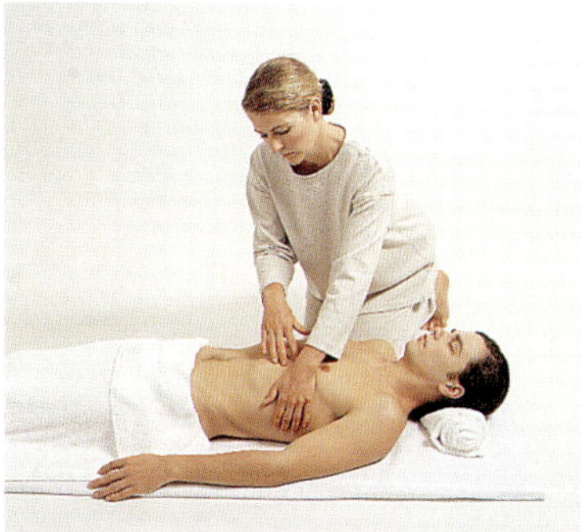

7. Move to the side of your partner, and with the palms of your hands alternately stroke over the ribs opposite you, towards the middle of your partner's body. Repeat on the other side.

8. Finish by repeating the movements in step 4, then cover the area with a towel.

THE NECK

This is a very important area, as most of us store a lot of tension in the neck and upper shoulders.

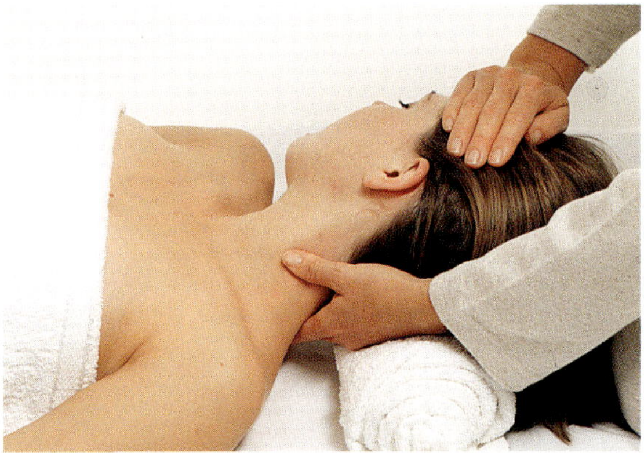

1. Place a rolled towel under your partner's head. Turn the head to one side and gently stroke with your thumb from the base of the skull to the collarbone. While the head is in this position, knead the upper shoulder muscle. Turn the head to the other side, and repeat.

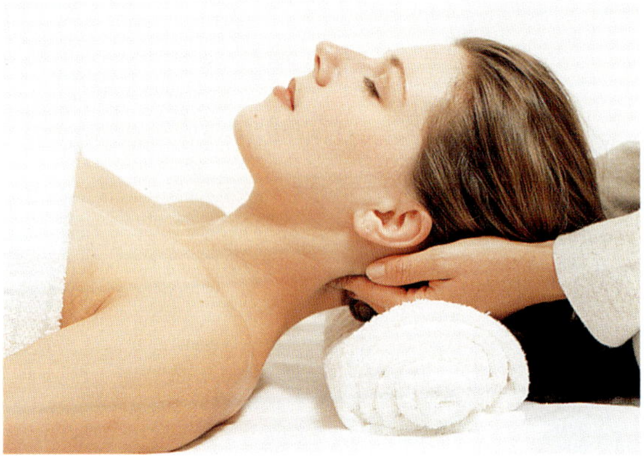

2. With the head facing straight up, place both your hands under the base of the neck, and using the pads of the fingers, create circular movements up the neck to the base of the skull. The circles should be quite large.

3. Use small friction movements with the pads of the fingers along the base of the skull — work out to the ears and back. This area, where the head joins the neck, is often very tender.

4. Finish by stroking with both hands from shoulders to back of scalp.

THE FACE AND SCALP

It is very relaxing to conclude a massage with the face and scalp. This will gently soothe away any remnants of tension and leave your partner in a state of blissful calm.

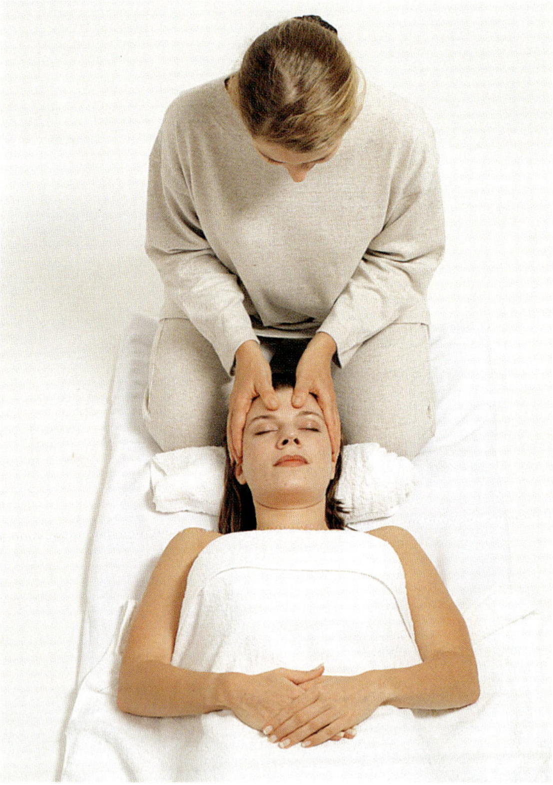

1. Sit at the head of your partner and begin with stroking the forehead from the middle to the temple area.

2. Facial massage can be very intuitive. You may like to incorporate some of the following movements:

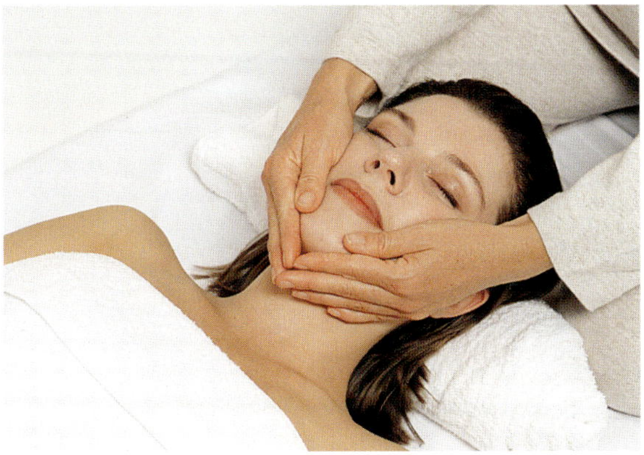

• stroke along the jaw line from chin out to ears

• knead the chin area by gently squeezing and releasing along jaw line

• smooth your fingers across the cheeks and out to the ears

• stroke over the eyebrows with your fingers

• squeeze along the edge of the ears

• use small circular friction movements around the mouth and cheek area, and along the sides of the nose

• use the index or middle finger to press each side of the eye socket and hold for a few seconds.

3. Don't forget to incorporate a scalp massage, using a "shampooing" motion over the entire area.

4. Finish by gently stroking over the forehead with the heels of the thumbs and the side of face with the fingers.

5. Finally, rub hands together till they are very warm, and hold just touching, and completely covering, your partner's face. Hold for several minutes, allowing your partner to drink in the warmth.

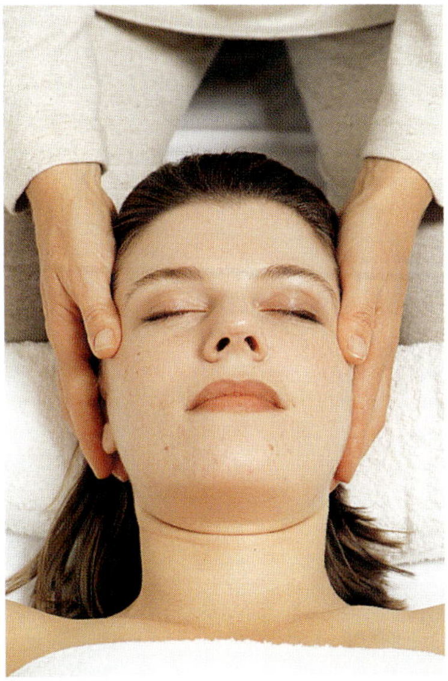

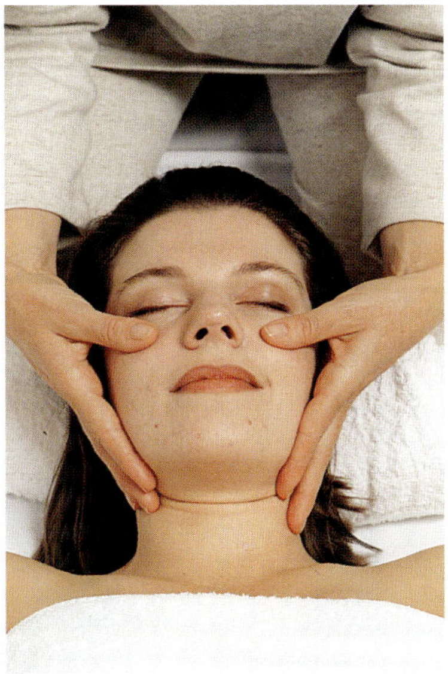

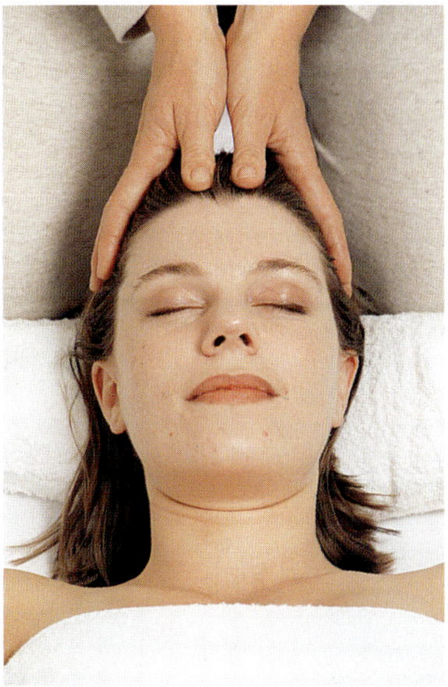

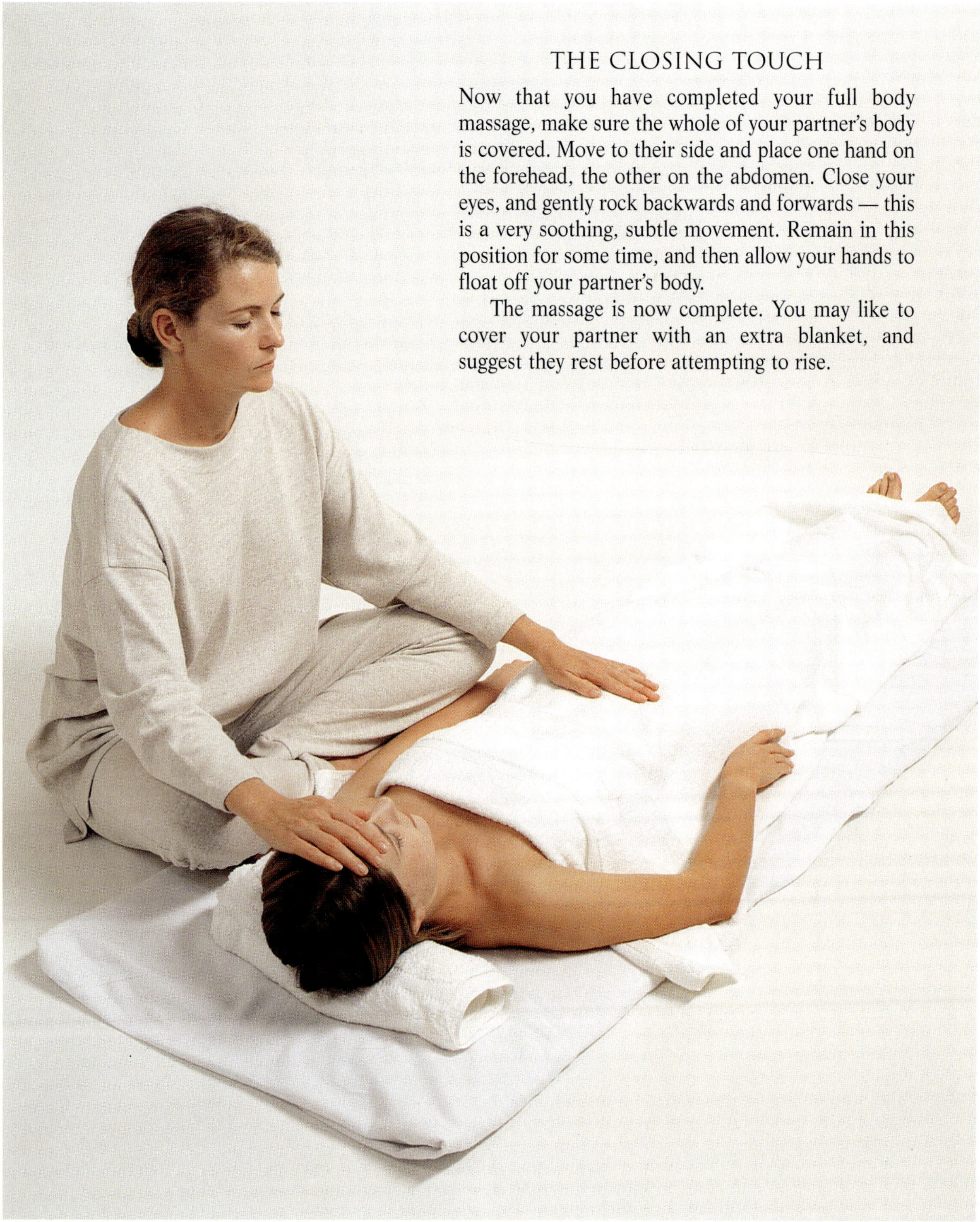

THE CLOSING TOUCH

Now that you have completed your full body massage, make sure the whole of your partner's body is covered. Move to their side and place one hand on the forehead, the other on the abdomen. Close your eyes, and gently rock backwards and forwards — this is a very soothing, subtle movement. Remain in this position for some time, and then allow your hands to float off your partner's body.

The massage is now complete. You may like to cover your partner with an extra blanket, and suggest they rest before attempting to rise.

THE QUICK, DO-ANYWHERE MASSAGE

With the quick, do-anywhere massage, the person getting the massage is seated and can remain fully-clothed. They should sit astride a chair, with arms folded and head resting on their arms. The following instructions are for the person doing the massage.

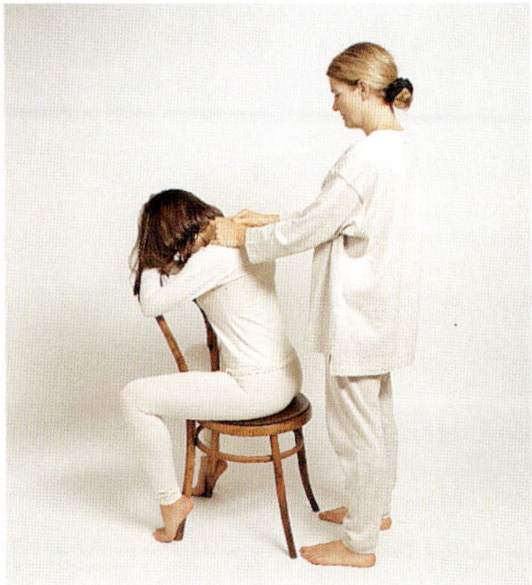

1. Work the whole shoulder area, using kneading movements, squeezing and releasing with both hands at the same time. Continue down the upper arms.

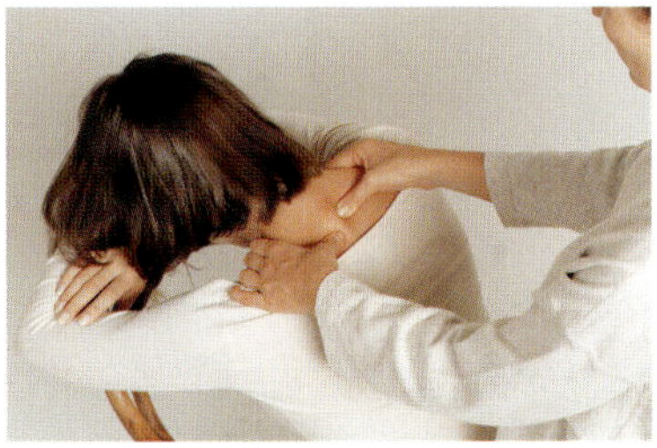

2. Using small, deep friction movements with your thumbs, work the shoulder area and base of the neck.

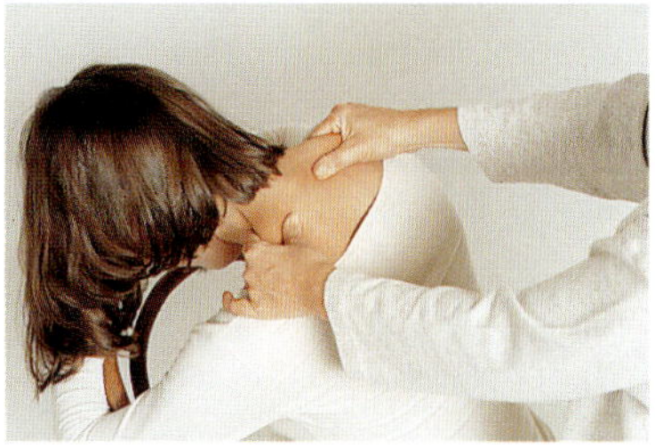

3. Place one thumb on each side of the base of the neck and apply firm pressure, using your body weight. Move your thumbs down the spine a little and reapply pressure. Continue like this down the spine until you are parallel with the end of the shoulder blade.

4. With the same movement, work along the inside edge of the shoulder blade, moving upwards toward the top of the shoulder.

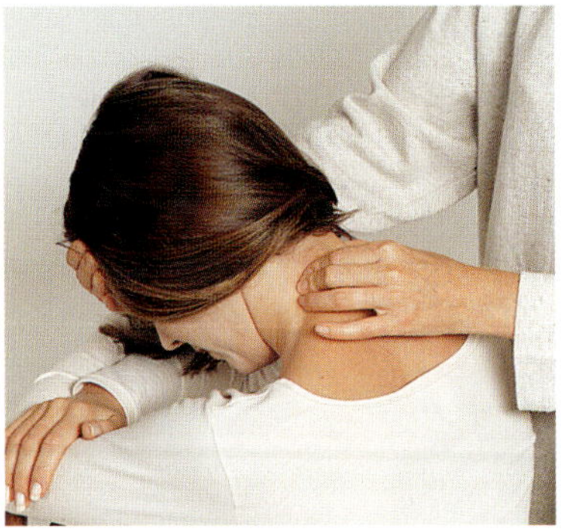

5. Place the palm of your hand on your partner's forehead for support, and knead the base of the neck with the other hand. Continue kneading up the neck to the base of the skull.

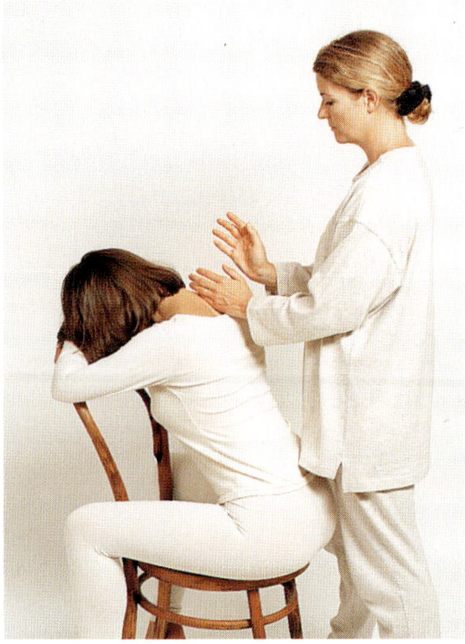

6. Apply gentle flicking movements to the whole of the upper back, avoiding bony areas. Your hands should be relaxed, with wrists soft and palms facing each other. Create a light, fast bouncy movement using your little fingers.

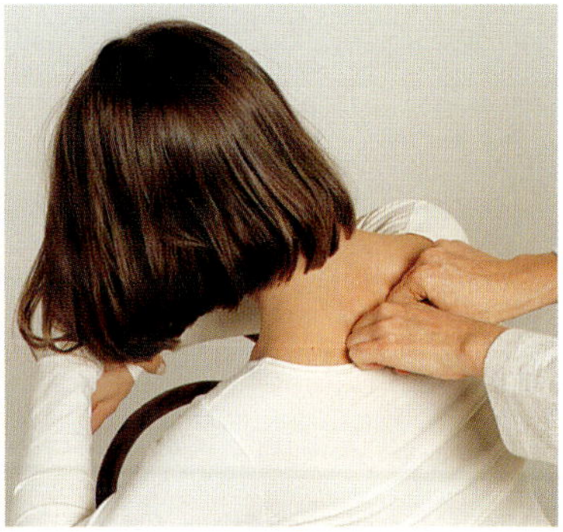

7. With closed fists, gently press in with knuckles each side of the spine from the base of the neck to below the shoulder blades.

8. Soothe the area with more kneading to the arms and shoulders, and conclude with more stroking to the whole area.

MEDITATION

EVERY MOMENT OF EVERY DAY YOUR BODY HAS TO COPE WITH A MYRIAD OF SENSORY INPUTS: SOUNDS, SMELLS, SIGHTS AND INFORMATION. THE DEMAND THIS PLACES ON YOUR MIND IS ENORMOUS. THE STILLNESS MEDITATION BRINGS GIVES THE MIND A CHANCE TO REST.

Meditation is a term which covers a number of techniques aimed at creating a sense of calm within the mind. For thousands of years, one of its uses has been as a way of achieving spiritual enlightenment. Buddhism, Hinduism, Sufism, Shintoism, the Cabbalistic tradition, Jewish mysticism and Christianity all practise some form of meditation.

However, in modern times, within Western culture, many people are more concerned with the enhancement to lifestyle and health which can come with practising meditation on a regular basis than its more spiritual benefits.

Meditation has the effect of gradually slowing respiration and decreasing the heart rate, thus lowering blood pressure. Because it creates a state of deep relaxation, meditation is believed to have several health benefits including strengthening the immune system and improving circulation, as well as increasing perceptual ability and decreasing anxiety.

Today, meditation is encouraged by a variety of health professionals for many reasons:

- if you are healthy, it can help you stay that way
- if you are stressed, it can help you relax and cope with life's pressures
- if you are dealing with a health crisis, it can "nourish" you both physically and spiritually.

Meditation is particularly effective in managing ailments aggravated by tension, e.g. insomnia, pain, and breathing difficulties.

DIFFERENT FORMS OF MEDITATION

Because meditation has developed in many dissimilar cultures at various times, there is a diversity of techniques based on different principles. These principles include:

- working with body control to attain immobility
- focusing attention on a single item e.g. an object, a symbol or word, a visualisation, your pattern of breathing

- "letting go" of the mind so that it is passive and open to insight
- the deliberate and systematic process of releasing muscular tension.

TRANSCENDENTAL MEDITATION

The relationship between meditation and health has been highlighted in recent decades by studies initiated by the Maharishi Mahesh Yogi.

The Maharishi came to the public's attention in the 1960s as "guru" to The Beatles and since that time millions of people have learnt Transcendental Meditation (TM), the form of yoga that he advocates.

TM involves a secret personal mantra — a sacred word or syllable — that is given to each individual by their teacher. This mantra is repeated while the person is in a deeply relaxed state (see page 154).

LEARNING HOW TO MEDITATE

Meditation is a self-help technique and there are dozens of tapes and books outlining various meditation methods.

While it is possible to learn to meditate on your own, it may help to be in contact with other people who practise meditation. If you lack self-discipline, joining a meditation group can be a good way to get started. Your local health clinic, community centre, church, yoga school or Buddhist organisation may have information about such groups in your area. Many hold courses in meditation and organise weekend retreats outside urban centres.

As well as ensuring you meditate regularly, meditating with a group of people can give you the opportunity to discuss your experiences and hear about the experiences of others.

If you are uncomfortable with religious associations involved with one form of meditation or meditation group, try another. Meditation should not be hard work. Experiment until you find a technique that brings you a sense of tranquillity.

Some people meditate for 20 minutes each morning and each night. Others meditate when they feel the need and for as long as they require. Daily meditation is recommended, even if it is only one 10-minute session per day.

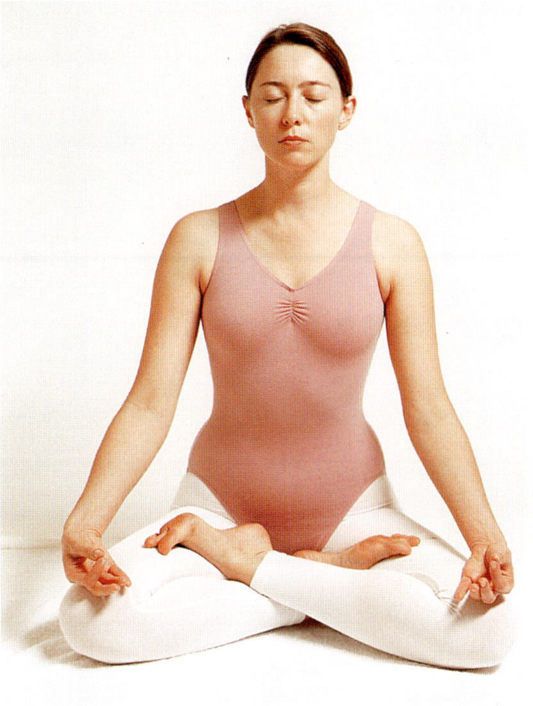

Meditation poses range from the lotus position to sitting in a chair or lying down.

RELAXATION — THE FIRST STEP

Most of us think all the time, many of us are constantly talking to ourselves — with some people it is a compulsion which interferes with their day-to-day living. There are dozens of ways of dealing with obsessive or unwanted thoughts. They range from counting breaths to complex visualisations. This chapter contains some popular methods you may wish to try. You may also like to incorporate the techniques described in AFFIRMATIONS AND VISUALISATIONS.

To begin meditating, try to find a quiet space where you will not be disturbed. Either lie down or sit comfortably with your back straight — a chair may be more suitable than sitting cross-legged on the floor. Let your hands rest comfortably with your palms open.

When you are comfortable, take your attention to your feet and check they are relaxed. Do the same as you move your attention up through your body to your ankles, calves, knees, thighs, buttocks, back, chest, shoulders, arms, hands, neck, scalp and face. (For more detail on how to relax your body, see Relaxation and Dealing with Stress.)

Once relaxed, focus on whichever meditation exercise you choose and allow your mind to open. If you wish you can write down your experiences at the end of each meditation session. This can be useful in giving you a record of your progress.

EXAMPLE 1: COUNTING YOUR BREATH

Now you are prepared for meditation turn your attention to your breath. Feel the air move into your nose and fill your lungs; be aware of how the air causes your chest to rise; then feel your chest contract as the air leaves your lungs, exiting your body through your mouth or nose. Be careful not to alter your normal pattern of breathing.

When you concentrate on your breath, the automatic response is for your breathing to slow and deepen and become regular. Try to avoid this. Watch your breath with a "lightness" of being. Don't focus on it. Just quietly observe it, allowing your body to do the breathing as it does while you are busy with other concerns.

Now that you are observing your breath, increase your focus — but again with the same "lightness" by counting the breaths. Count one beat for the inhalation and one beat for each exhalation — in/one out/one, in/two out/two, in/three out/three and so on.

Try and keep your mind focused on the breath and the counting. If it wanders bring it back to counting and your light observation of how each breath feels in your body. If you are observing with the optimum "lightness", your breath may be uneven. If your breathing becomes mechanical, just relax for a moment, let go and become a more passive observer.

If you lose count of your breaths at any time, begin again from one.

Aim to count 20 breaths. This is much harder than it seems. Then increase your goal each meditation. If you achieve 50 breaths, you are doing extremely well.

SPIRITUAL ASPECT OF MEDITATION

In an holistic approach to health, your spirit and your ability to nourish it is just as important as taking care of your body. Meditation decreases negative emotions and assists in creating a sense of inner peace. It helps you increase your self-awareness and gives you an experience of your true self. It also helps loosen your preconceptions of the "real world" and can put you in touch with the spiritual nature of your being. Facing a serious health problem can leave you feeling frustrated, angry and powerless. Spiritual meditation can help turn these feelings of powerlessness around.

EXAMPLE 2: MANTRA MEDITATION

Many forms of meditation recommend using a mantra or a sound to give your mind a point of focus.

The classic mantra is Aum (or OM), pronounced Aummmmmmm. This sound is said to represent the total energy of the universe. It's used because it runs from the back of your throat to your lips and contains your full voice range. You can vary it — emphasising the aaaaa or mmmmmm, sections of the sound. The other part of the mantra is Aum Mani Padme Hum.

Other classic mantras are:

- OM Nama Shivaya
- Hari Krishna Hari Krishna Krishna Krishna Hari Hari (Krishna is an Indian deity)
- Hallelujah Hallelujah Hallelujah.

You can also make your own mantra, perhaps a saying that appeals to you. Just keep repeating it to yourself until the words lose their meaning. If you chant any mantra long enough you'll find the words become pure sound.

To begin, relax yourself (see above) and then start your mantra. Immerse yourself in the sound. Notice how it feels in your body. It helps to say it out loud but if you find that makes you self-conscious just sound the mantra in your mind. If your concentration flickers to other thoughts gently bring it back to the mantra and the purity of the sound. You can vary the rhythm as you go, making it faster or slower or emphasising various syllables to suit your mood.

EXAMPLE 3: KEY THOUGHT MEDITATION

This is slightly similar to mantra meditation in that you begin with a particular phrase — your "key thought". You can make up your own or select a profound quote which appeals to you.

When you are in the relaxed state bring your awareness to the key thought. Passively and dispassionately notice what other thoughts this triggers and the next thought and the next and so on. Let the thoughts arise until such time as it becomes obvious your current thought has no connection to your original thought. Then take your attention back to the original key thought and let the process begin again.

This method is useful if you are confused about something and want quiet time to "think" the matter through. Remember not to get too involved in the thinking process and try to remain the passive observer. The aim is to calm your mind, not upset it; so it is preferable not to involve your emotions. But at the same time don't suppress them. If you are moved to tears, let them run. If you feel anger, let it move through you. The aim is neither to suppress nor inflame emotions but simply to observe your own conscious thoughts.

EXAMPLE 4: HEALING MEDITATION

This meditation technique, which is inspired by the Chinese system of health, is particularly useful for calming the mind. It works best in a sitting position and you will need to visualise.

OPENING AND CLOSING RITUALS

How you choose to meditate is a personal preference, whether it involves focusing on an object or repeating a mantra. However, whatever form of meditation you choose to do, it is a good idea to include an opening and closing ritual at the beginning and end of each meditation session.

Including an opening ritual helps you to part the "curtains" between the physical plane and the meditative state.

At the end of each meditation close these curtains again by going through a closing ritual. This helps to bring you back down to "earth".

You can design your own ritual. This can be a matter of going through the same physical steps each time in preparation for starting meditation or resuming normal activities. Or it may be a mental clearing process. Some people like to thank God or the life force.

Begin with an opening ritual. When you are sitting or lying comfortably, imagine a pyramid of white light descending over you, surrounding you and filling your body.

Next begin the relaxation process described above. When your body is completely relaxed, take your attention to your crown chakra (see page 124) and visualise a white glowing ball of light. Breathe in and see this ball of light glow brighter, breathe out while keeping your attention on the ball.

Keep breathing and when you have the ball glowing brightly switch your attention to a point between your genitals and anus, at the base of your body. See a ball of white light form there.

Breathe in and see this ball move up through the centre of your body to your heart chakra. See the ball at your heart centre. As you breathe out see it move back down to the base of your body.

Breathe in and allow it to move up again, breathe out and watch it float down. Do this several times.

Meanwhile, the ball of light at the top of your head should still be in place.

When the second ball has moved down to the base of your body breathe in and see it move up your spine until it reaches the ball at the top of your head. See the two balls merge, and then on your exhalation see it move down the front of your body to the base of your body. With the next inhalation see it move up the spine to your head again, and continue breathing while moving the ball of light down the front of your body. Do this cycle several times.

When the ball of light is at the base of your body, move it up to the heart on the inhalation and down on the exhalation.

If your ball of light keeps turning a colour other than white, perhaps blue or pink, and that colour feels right to you, allow it to remain. Black, brown or muddy colours, however, are unlikely to contain healing vibrations — if you think the colour is the result of your imagination, bring your visualisation back to white light.

You may wish to end the exercise with a prayer or a giving of thanks. After this, try imagining that each of your chakra centres is a different coloured rose. Start from the bottom and see each rose close into a tight bud.

When each of your chakra centres is closed, see a cloud of white light swirling over the top of your head, moving down and around your body to enclose your feet.

As this cloud of white light swirls around you, see it melt away, leaving you enclosed in protective energy — imagine it as a bubble of clear glass if that assists you.

TO SLEEP OR NOT TO SLEEP

Sometimes during meditation it is difficult to remain alert. Many meditation teachers believe that falling asleep is one way to avoid the discipline of meditation. However, others contend that the act of truly meditating is to be present, and if sleep is part of your "present" so be it. Certainly if you are ill, your body will require more rest, so if you fall asleep while meditating it probably isn't of concern. If, however, you routinely fall asleep instead of meditating, perhaps you need to change the time of day you meditate. It may be easier for you to meditate at midday or in the early morning. Experiment until you find the time that best suits you, and if you fall asleep on occasions don't berate yourself. Go with what happens and gently observe yourself.

WORKING MEDITATION

One of the rewards of meditating regularly is that you learn to live more in the present. If you live in the present there is no space for fear because fear can only exist if you take an event from the past (a dog once bit me) and project it into the future (the dog which is currently barking at me is going to bite me). If you are totally in the present then all your attention is on observing the barking dog — there are no thoughts of past dogs or future dog bites.

Working meditation brings you into the present. It sounds simple but this form of meditation can be the most difficult. It is where everything you do becomes a meditation. For this reason you have no need for the opening, closing or relaxation rituals associated with the other meditations. This discipline is best explored under the guidance of a teacher, after you are familiar with other forms of meditation.

MODERN MEDICINE

MODERN MEDICINE IS AN INCREASINGLY SUCCESSFUL SCIENCE. THROUGH TECHNOLOGY WE CONTINUE TO GAIN KNOWLEDGE OF THE HUMAN BODY, AND HAVE DEVELOPED TREATMENTS THAT WILL HALT, AND SOMETIMES REVERSE, THE PROGRESSION OF MANY DISEASES.

Once, huge numbers of young children died of diphtheria, whooping cough and scarlet fever. Now, drugs will neutralise toxins and poisonous microbes, and kill parasites. Severe injuries, which once would have meant amputation or even death, can be repaired; and diseased tissue can be isolated and removed without damaging healthy tissue.

Recent advances have made it possible to determine the likelihood of a person contracting heart disease, cancer and many other life-threatening illnesses according to their genetic heritage, enabling them to take preventative action.

Advances in medicine have become intrinsic to our culture and are sometimes taken for granted — we expect cures to be just around the corner, and sometimes they are. Treatments at first considered remarkable quickly become the expected norm. Heart bypass surgery is now performed on suitable candidates from all walks of life. Few women die in childbirth these days and no woman expects to. Yet only decades ago, pregnancy and childbirth were life-threatening experiences.

THE DEVELOPMENT OF MODERN MEDICINE

The system of modern medicine we have today is largely scientific and technological. However, the approach to health practised by Hippocrates, the man claimed as the founder of scientific medicine, was quite different to that practised by many doctors today.

Hippocrates was born about 460 BC on the island of Cos, off the coast of Asia Minor. Like the physicians who came before him and those who followed, Hippocrates focused on the individual. There were no disease groups, no names for conditions. Each person with their set of symptoms was treated individually. Hippocrates believed in detailed observation and asked his patients many questions. As well as being interested in a person's symptoms, he was also interested in their nutrition and their environment. He believed in relying on his powers of empathy, understanding and intuition. Regarding treatment, he was in favour of relying on "the healing power of nature". Often he prescribed plenty of rest and a specific diet to aid recovery.

Even as the inner workings of the body were revealed over the next centuries, the individual remained the focus for medical treatment until the 17th century. Then, in the 1600s, the view shifted from the individual to the illness as specific conditions such as dysentery, syphilis and gout were identified, and specific medicines were used to treat particular disorders, such as quinine for malaria. Illness came to be seen as a conflict between the body and an injury or malady.

In the same century, the philosopher Rene Descartes taught that the body was like any other physical object and that the mind, with its emotions and feelings, was the "ghost in the machine". This separation of the mind and body was to have a lasting impact on medical science. Henceforth, the approach to disease and healing became more "mechanical". In general terms, the focus shifted from the whole person to the disease, its symptoms, and how it altered the physical functions of the body.

Over the next centuries, the work of Edward Jenner, Louis Pasteur, Joseph Lister, Ferdinand Cohn, Robert Koch and other medical scientists isolated and classified microbes and developed vaccinations. This provided a framework for specific aetiology, the idea that certain diseases have certain causes. There was an optimism that if the germs and viruses could be identified then chemicals could be developed to combat them. For many, it appeared that science had all the answers, and consideration for other components such as a person's emotional well-being, their nutritional status, their levels of poverty or hygiene were obscured.

With the development of penicillin and other powerful drugs, killer diseases like tuberculosis and typhoid fever were defeated. These chemical solutions seemed almost miraculous and the medical profession took on an almost priest-like status.

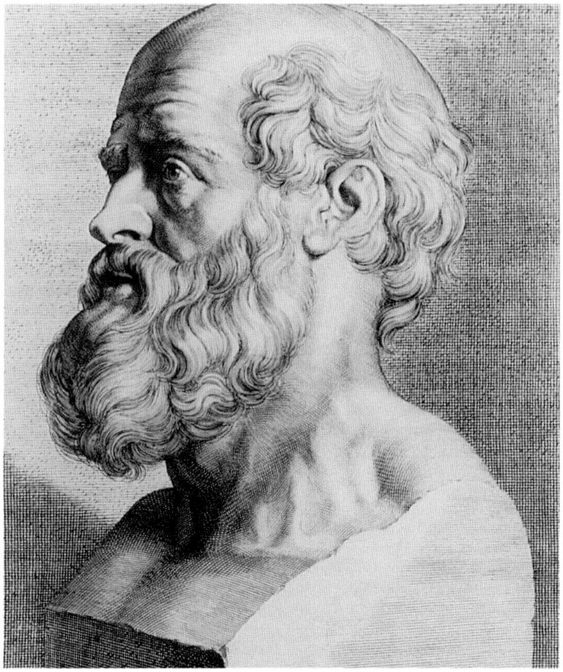

Hippocrates is seen to be the father of modern medicine. The Hippocratic Oath, sworn by doctors, takes its name from him.

People who would have otherwise died, recovered and lived. The idea that a doctor could prescribe a specific drug or "magic bullet" as the cure for all ills became entrenched in our culture. Drug companies grew into multinational empires, and millions of dollars were funnelled into scientific research.

LIMITATIONS OF MODERN MEDICINE

In recent decades there has been a subtle turn in the tide of medical science. Despite the funds and the research, many illnesses from cancer to the common cold continue without a cure, and the side effects of some drugs are emerging. While modern medicine has had success in a variety of areas, there is also a growing recognition that the pairing of disease and "cure" is no longer adequate.

The health of each individual is constantly influenced by events within and outside the body. These can range from genetic inheritance to personal body chemistry, emotions, relationships with other people, work factors, the weather, food, the quality of the air, and the water a person drinks or washes in.

Illness cannot be isolated from all these influences. Any healing which takes place has to work within this framework and this framework constantly changes.

Many people have been disillusioned by brief appointments with doctors who view only the diseased organ or system rather than the human being. The best doctors, however, have always combined empathy and understanding, intuition and sympathy with their technical knowledge, and even more practitioners are doing so now.

There is a new movement to encourage individuals to take responsibility for their health and well-being under the guidance of a medical practitioner. Ultimately it is you, not your doctor, who has the illness and the power to move towards good health — it is you who must change your diet, decrease the stress, or take whatever action is required to improve the conditions of your life.

CONSULTING A DOCTOR

Before visiting your doctor, make sure you have worked out a list of your symptoms. Write down all your symptoms, indeed anything at all that is unusual — just because something seems trivial to you, does not mean it is. The more information you can give the doctor, the better equipped he or she is to form opinions on possible diagnoses.

It is most important you inform your doctor of any allergies you may have. If you are scheduled for tests, but feel apprehensive, then tell your doctor: anxiety can cause tensing of muscles, it can even affect some body processes.

Often when you are consulting your doctor, you may feel too ill or embarrassed to ask questions, or you may forget your questions, like the side effects of medication, when confronted with theirs. So before you visit your doctor it is a good idea to also make a list of questions you want answered (see page 160). Sometimes people are concerned about taking up a doctor's valuable time, but keep in mind that you are paying the doctor for his or her time, that you are there for matters of your health — your most valuable asset — and that all questions you have should be asked both for practical reasons and for your peace of mind.

VACCINATIONS

Vaccines, as an injection or in tablet or liquid form, are designed to induce immunity against a particular bacterial or viral disease. There are both benefits and hazards associated with them—ask a range of health practitioners for advice and literature before making your choice. New vaccines are constantly being developed. Among those conditions that have vaccines currently available are:

• cholera • diphtheria • hepatitis A and B
• haemophilus influenza B • influenza
• Japanese B encephalitis • measles • meningitis
• mumps • plague • pneumococcus • polio • rabies
• rubella (German measles) • tetanus • tuberculosis
• typhoid • typhus • whooping cough • yellow fever.

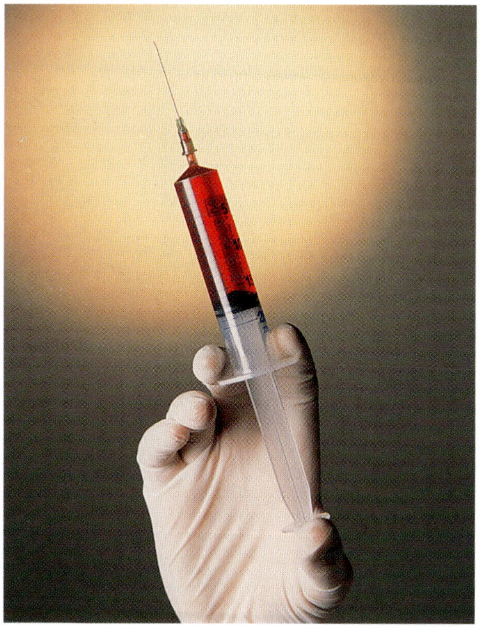

Sometimes when you do ask the right questions, your doctor might answer using obscure or difficult terms. If this should happen, do not be embarrassed about asking your doctor to explain using plain language. These days, most doctors are happy to comply because they realise people want to understand more about their bodies and their health. If your doctor is reluctant to discuss these matters with you then consider changing doctors.

And if you should feel self-conscious about intimate examinations, try to remember your doctor conducts such examinations many times a day, every day, every week throughout their career — they are accustomed to examining the human body and feel no embarrassment; there is no reason why you should either. Remember that you can ask for a second opinion or bring a chaperone, especially if you feel compromised.

It is important to feel comfortable with your doctor as good communication will ensure you get the best possible care. Shop around until you find a practitioner who suits you.

QUESTIONS TO ASK YOUR DOCTOR

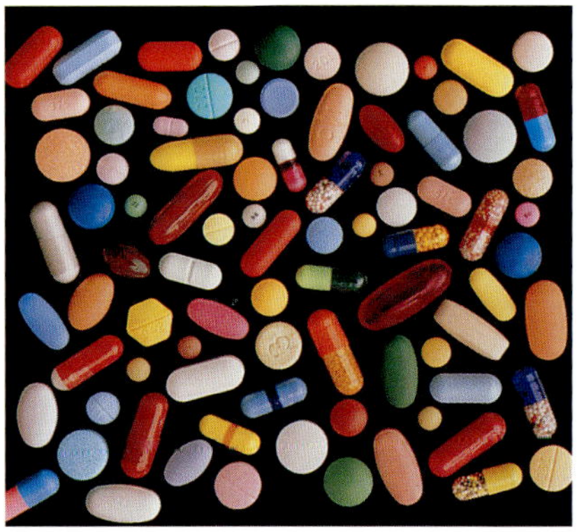

What is causing my symptoms?

Am I infectious? If so, for how long?

What are my options for treatment?

What are the side effects of each one?

Which treatment is best suited to me?

How long can I expect to feel like this?

What other symptoms am I likely to develop?

How long will it be before I feel well again?

Should I be off work and for how long?

What is my long-term prognosis?

USING ALTERNATIVE THERAPIES WITH MODERN MEDICINE

Alternative therapies can be most effective for many illnesses but the strength of modern medicine is in crisis intervention, treating serious illnesses, and in its diagnostic equipment. Many alternative health practitioners have good working relationships with doctors. Doctors will authorise pathology tests required by naturopaths to identify certain conditions, and arrange X-rays for a client with spine or joint problems who is consulting a chiropractor or osteopath.

It is not unusual these days for doctors to be tolerant, if not supportive, of clients combining modern medical treatment with other approaches such as massage, yoga, aromatherapy and acupuncture. The number of doctors who take a holistic approach is slowly increasing. Your local alternative health professionals will know if there are any general practitioners in your area sympathetic to this approach.

TESTS: THE TOOLS OF DIAGNOSIS

It is always useful to see a doctor for a diagnosis of your condition. Following initial questioning and observation, your doctor may conduct basic testing, like taking blood pressure and checking respiration, in the surgery. If additional testing is required, you may have to go to a pathology laboratory or to a hospital where specialist equipment and technicians are available. Diagnostic testing ranges from taking blood and urine samples to X-rays to scanning with sophisticated machinery to undergoing exploratory surgery. The tests will be carried out by people trained for that specific task; the results will be interpreted by specialists in the appropriate field.

Pathology tests provide important information on how your body is working — for example, blood iron levels and the effectiveness of your various organs such as kidneys and liver. But don't be afraid to seek a second opinion or a second lot of pathology tests. (It has been revealed recently that some pathology laboratories are not as accurate as others so often a second test for such things as cervical cancer is worth considering.)

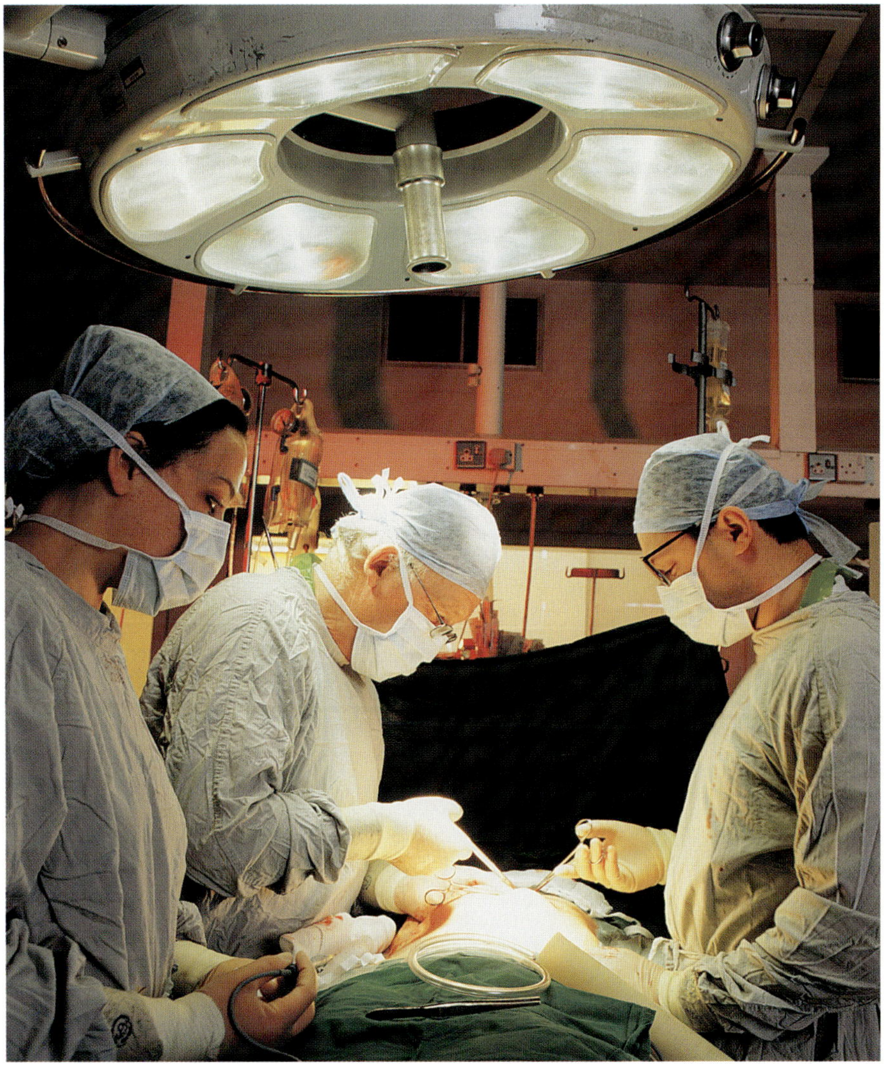

Modern surgery in sterile conditions using an anaesthetic is one of the great advances of Western medicine.

COMMONLY USED DRUGS

TYPE	DESCRIPTION	SIDE EFFECTS
anaesthetics	Substance or drug that causes loss of sensation, especially pain. There are two main types: local, which removes pain from one point in the body, and general, used for surgical procedures, which removes all sensation from the body.	Side effects are rare in local anaesthetics, but vary greatly with general anaesthetics.
analgesics	Drugs that block pain, including narcotics (see entry), paracetamol, and salicylates — a subgroup of NSAIDS (see entry) which includes aspirin.	Side effects are rare in paracetamol and aspirin but overdose is possible and has severe consequences, especially in children.
antacids	Substances used to treat acidity, especially in the stomach.	Should be used with care in patients with kidney disease.
antibiotics	Substances extracted from a mould, or other living structure, that kill bacteria – not effective against viral infections.	There are several groups of antibiotics, and some people may be allergic to one or two of these but not to others. Full course must be taken to avoid a rebound reaction.
antidepressants	Drugs used to control depression.	Expect minor and major side effects.
antihistamine	Drug that neutralises the effect of histamine, used especially in treatment of allergies. People who suffer from epilepsy or asthma, or who are breastfeeding should avoid these drugs.	Side effects may include dizziness and drowsiness; use with care when driving or undertaking other activities requiring alertness. Do not use with alcohol.
antiseptics	Destroy undesirable micro-organisms, such as those that cause disease or putrefaction.	Minimal side effects, but may cause allergic reactions in some people.
antivirals	Drugs that kill viruses and cure viral infections.	Side effects are uncommon.
benzodiazepines	Group of tranquillising drugs used to treat anxiety, stress and insomnia.	If used inappropriately, these drugs may become habit-forming. They should not be used with alcohol or while driving or using machinery.
barbiturates	Derivatives of barbituric acid used in medicine to control convulsions and before operations.	Inappropriate use may lead to serious addiction. Overdose is dangerous.

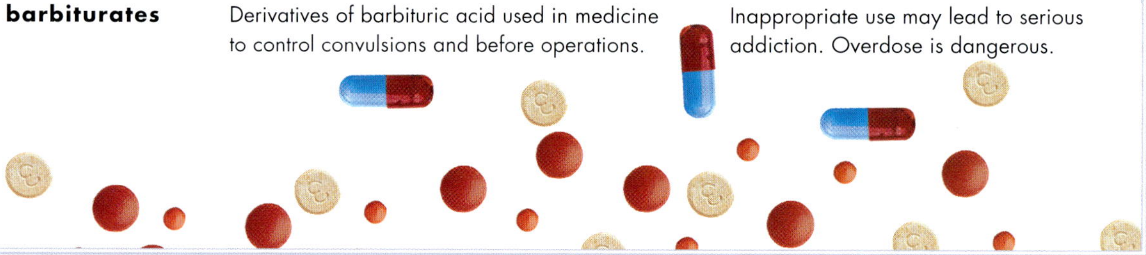

COMMONLY USED DRUGS

TYPE	DESCRIPTION	SIDE EFFECTS
beta-blocker	Type of drug prescribed to treat heart conditions, raised blood pressure and the symptoms of anxiety.	Side effects include low blood pressure, dizziness and insomnia.
hormones	Chemical substances produced by the body in many different glands and transported in the blood to certain tissues on which they exert specific effects.	Hormone replacement therapy is a treatment to replace hormones used on women who have had their ovaries surgically removed or who are going through menopause.
hypnotic	A drug or agent that induces sleep.	Safe if used according to directions, otherwise dependency may occur.
muscle relaxants	Used to relieve muscle cramps and spasms.	There may be some side effects in some patients.
narcotic	Any of a group of drugs, such as opium and morphine, that produces numbness and stupor; they are a strong and effective painkiller	Extremely addictive.
NSAIDS (non-steroidal anti-inflammatory drugs)	Reduce inflammation in tissue. Used mainly in treatment of rheumatoid and osteoarthritis, sporting injuries and menstrual pain.	Can cause peptic ulcers in stomach and small intestine.
sedative	A drug or agent that has a soothing or calming effect.	Safe when taken according to directions, otherwise dependency may occur.
steroids	Corticosteroid hormones are powerful reducers of inflammation in damaged tissue. Anabolic steroids are synthetic hormones used to stimulate muscle and bone growth and thus to treat some blood diseases and cancers, osteoporosis and kidney failure.	When used on skin or surface areas, side effects are mild. When taken as tablets in high doses over a long period, serious side effects may occur including brittle bones, diabetes, heart failure, high blood pressure and weight gain. Serious side effects of anabolic steriods include liver disease, infertility and personality changes.

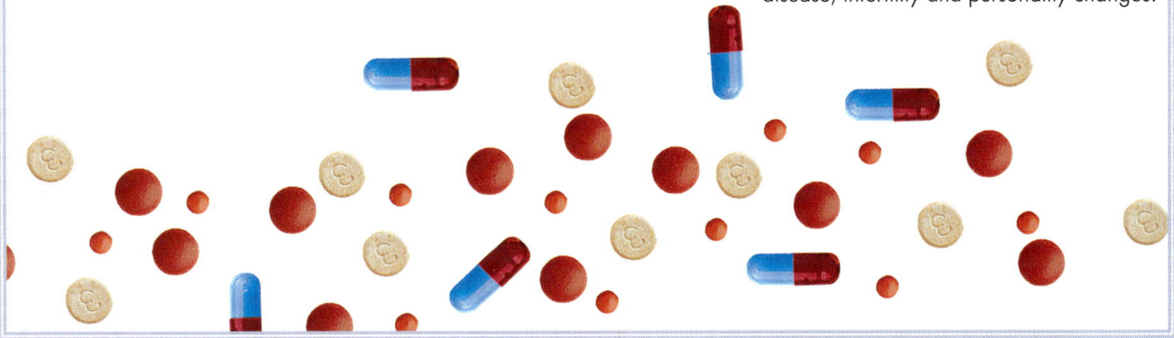

NATUROPATHY

MOST NATUROPATHS USE A COMBINATION OF THERAPIES TO TREAT CLIENTS. AS WELL AS THEIR NATUROPATHIC TRAINING, THEY MIGHT PRESCRIBE FLOWER REMEDIES, HOMOEOPATHIC REMEDIES, GIVE YOU A MASSAGE, OR SUGGEST YOU ADD ESSENTIAL OILS TO YOUR BATH. HERE, HOWEVER, WE WILL EXAMINE NATUROPATHIC MEDICINE IN ITS BASIC FORM.

Naturopathy, like HERBALISM, has been developing for as long as human beings have sought relief from illness. In essence, naturopathy harnesses the healing power of nature. It draws its "medicines" from foods and its therapies from heat and water.

Naturopathy as we know it today was pioneered in Germany in the early 19th century by therapists like Vincent Preissnitz (1799–1851) who founded hydrotherapy (see page 208). Towards the end of the century the German physician-monk, Father Sebastian Kneipp, successfully treated an American named Benedict Lust with his combination of herbal treatments and water cures. Lust returned to the USA, and in 1896 opened America's first health food store which he affiliated with two Yungborn Sanitariums. He founded the American School of Naturopathy, which granted degrees in the art of natural healing. Today there are numerous schools of naturopathy all over the world, and well-qualified naturopaths can be found in most communities throughout the Western world.

WHAT IS NATUROPATHY

Naturopaths believe that any disease comes from a biochemical or metabolic imbalance that is trigged by prolonged stress — either physical or emotional. These stressors include poor nutrition, overeating, lack of exercise, too many toxins (from your environment or from consuming tobacco, alcohol or medical drugs), lack of rest or living in a "toxic emotional" environment.

Over time, all or any of these conditions can negatively influence the functions of your body and ultimately inhibit your immune system.

Naturopaths believe that when your immune system is impinged on, disease shows up, not as a cause of illness but as the end result — a symptom that all is not well. To a naturopath, a bout of the flu indicates that your body needs some maintenance work and the symptoms are indications of what needs to be worked on. If the underlying causes of the illness are repaired, the symptoms will disappear.

The naturopath sees the symptoms as the body's defence mechanism attempting to move you back to a state of health. They will try to work in conjunction with this process, rather than suppressing the symptoms, such as fever, diarrhoea or loss of appetite. Naturopaths believe in allowing the body time to heal itself. They warn that our modern-day concept of suppressing the symptoms and "soldiering on" when we are feeling unwell can break down the body's healing process and lead to long-term damage.

To help your body recover and to move back into balance, your naturopath will take a serious look at all aspects of your life.

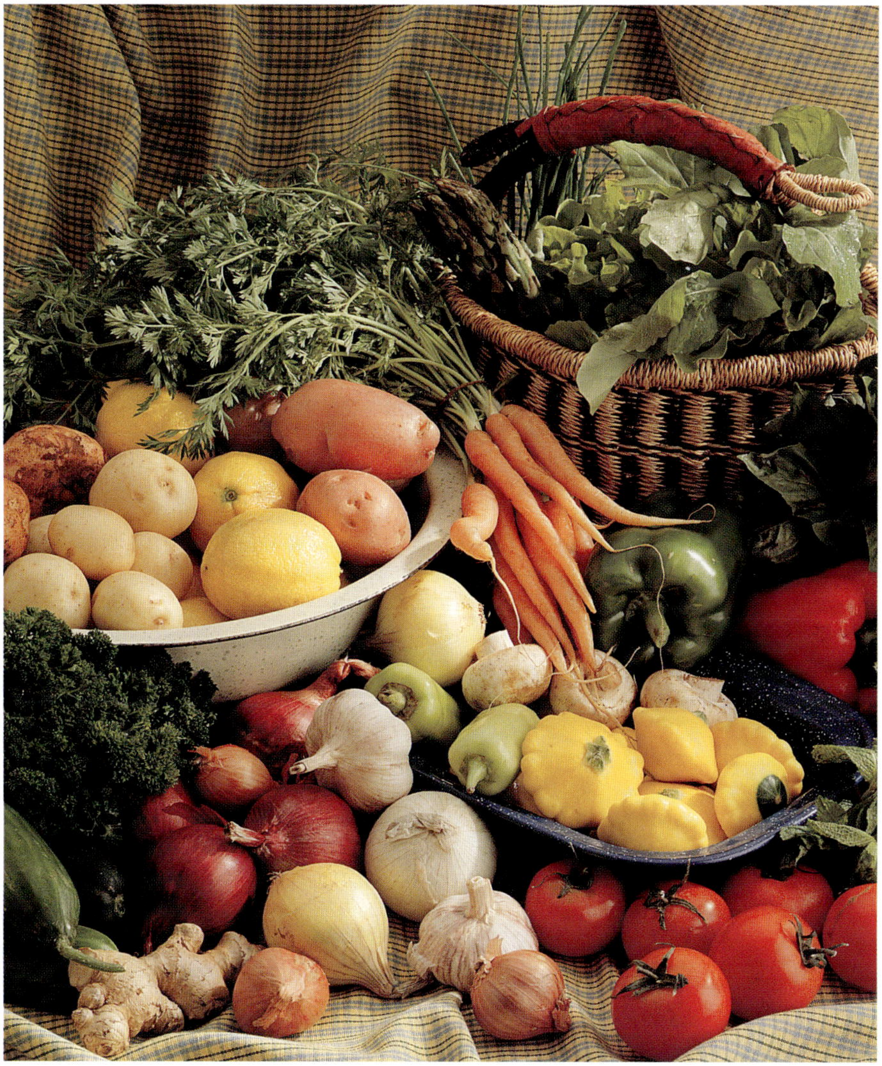

Food is medicine to a naturopath. Not only does your diet have a significant impact on your health, but specific foods can be eaten to benefit particular conditions.

THE VALUE OF FRESH JUICES

Naturopaths often prescribe fruit or vegetable juices as a medicine. This is because raw juices are:

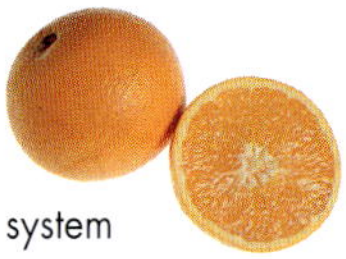

- rich in vitamins, minerals, trace elements and natural sugars
- assimilated easily into the bloodstream without straining the digestive system
- alkaline, which helps bring the body's acid–alkaline ratio back into balance
- natural medicines, because they contain special substances (for example, radish, tomato, onion and garlic juice contains natural antibiotics) that you can consume in greater quantities than if you were to eat the whole food.

It is best to drink the juice immediately as valuable vitamins and minerals are lost when left standing for any time.

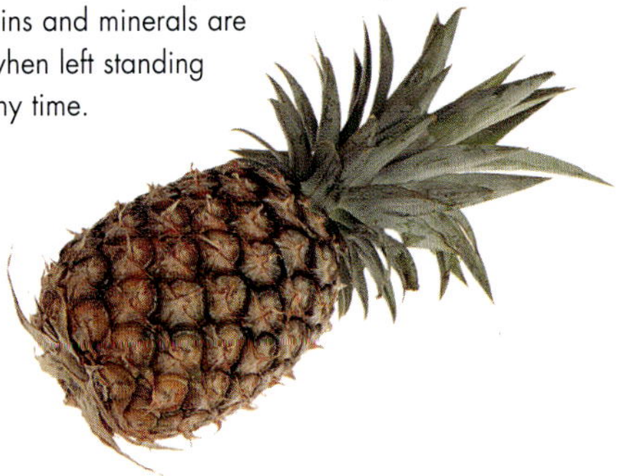

CONSULTING A NATUROPATH

During the first consultation, the naturopath will take down your medical history in detail, ask about your work, home and emotional life, and have you list the foods you have eaten during the past few days. This examination of your diet will give them an indication of your nutritional status, so don't distort the details. If you have eaten doughnuts for breakfast for the past three days, be honest about it. To a naturopath this information provides a valuable insight into such things as the state of your blood sugar levels or your need for carbohydrates.

Many naturopaths will use pathology tests to gain an insight into your health status. It is not uncommon for them to ask you to have your doctor test for such things as allergies, glandular fever, blood iron levels, and thyroid or liver function.

NATUROPATHIC TREATMENT

A naturopath will approach your condition and treatment from several angles.

Firstly, they will advise you on how to remove the underlying causes of the stress. This could involve recommending dietary changes, encouraging you to increase your levels of relaxation, or suggesting you do something as life changing as reconsidering your job.

They will then approach treating your body in two ways — they will nourish it and then cleanse it. Nourishing your body involves specific dietary considerations plus ensuring you receive pure food and water. The dietary changes could involve avoiding certain foods, eating certain foods, taking various vitamin and mineral supplements, or drinking fruit and vegetable juices as a form of natural medicine. Generally, your naturopath will recommend a diet high in fresh, raw fruits, vegetables, seeds, nuts and grains.

Naturopaths are also concerned about toxins. They believe that an accumulation of toxins in the body, either from ingesting them or from poor elimination, undermines the body. Accordingly, most naturopaths advise against tea, coffee, tobacco, alcohol, and pharmaceuticals. They also believe that our bodies are stressed by polluted water, air, and toxic substances either sprayed on or incorporated into the food we eat. Many naturopaths recommend cleansing diets.

A HEALING CRISIS

Many naturopaths talk about a "healing crisis". They say that changes in your diet or fasting and cleansing diets can sometimes trigger a worsening of your symptoms. This healing crisis happens particularly in people who have accumulated a large amount of toxic waste in their body tissues. The dietary changes can dissolve accumulated toxins and release them into the bloodstream to be eliminated. As a result, the kidneys, liver, lungs and skin can be overloaded.

This healing crisis can lead to a worsening of your original condition, plus such symptoms as headaches, bad breath, skin eruptions, and aches and pains. But usually this crisis is short-lived, lasting only a day or two.

If you do experience a worsening in your condition, discuss it with your naturopath.

Most naturopaths are in favour of rest and relaxation as a means for the body to recover. They will urge you to incorporate plenty of fresh air and exercise into your health maintenance program. It is common for a naturopath to prescribe something as simple as a daily walk.

In addition, they will look at your emotional state. Naturopaths believe peace of mind is as vital to sound health as anything else. They will encourage you to look at ways in which you can improve your internal emotional state.

Coupled with this general approach may be some specific symptom-related therapies. This could include various remedies such as intermittent hot and cold showers, skin brushing, afternoon naps, hot sitz baths with specific herbs or herbal compresses. Generally, naturopaths do not talk about "cures". They see healing as a process rather than a "quick fix".

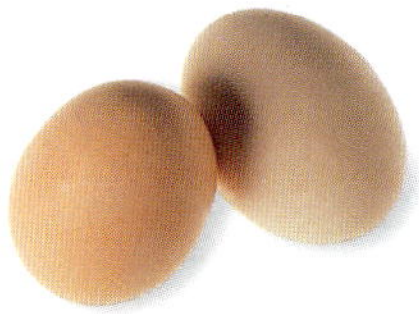

Naturopathy can be used to treat a wide range of disorders — practically all illnesses except those resulting from accidents, acute infections, broken limbs etc which require immediate intervention and are best treated by a doctor.

To achieve results with naturopathy you have to be prepared to make some changes in your life and work in conjunction with your naturopath.

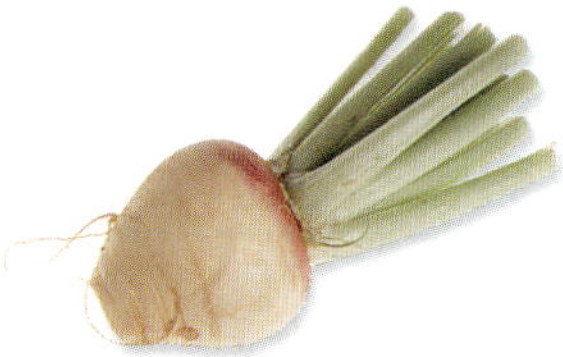

A WORD OF CAUTION

- There are many cautions for vitamin E. Be careful taking it if you have high blood pressure because it can make the condition worse. Start with 100 iu per day and then gradually increase it to 500 iu over a few weeks. Take a low does of vitamin E (100 iu per day only) if you have diabetes and stay on this low dose. Also, if you have rheumatic fever or rheumatic heart disease, don't take more than 100 iu per day; higher doses can cause a recurrence of symptoms.
- Fish oil should not be taken if you are using strong anti-clotting agents such as warfarin.

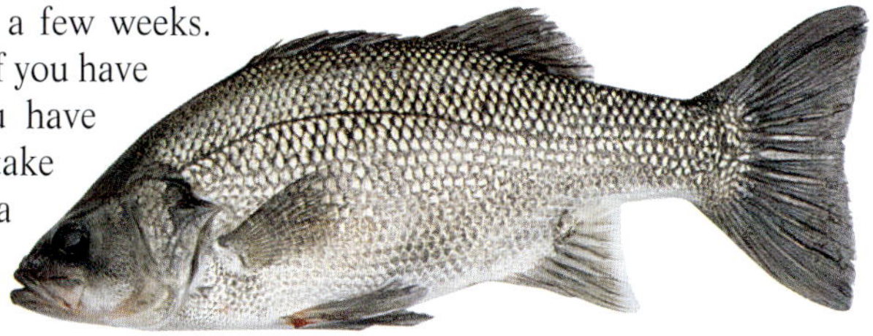

WHY WE NEED SUPPLEMENTS

There is a great deal of debate about the value of taking vitamin and mineral supplements. From a naturopathic point of view, supplements are essential to our well-being.

Ideally, we should receive all our nutrients from the foods we eat. As a result of modern agriculture, however, our soils are now so depleted that much of the food we eat is empty of essential vitamins and minerals.

Naturopaths prescribe supplements in two ways: firstly, to correct deficiencies in our diets; and secondly to use as a natural drug.

When naturopaths prescribe vitamins or minerals as a natural drug, they will usually give them in large amounts. For example, your naturopath could recommend you take supplements of vitamin C in megadoses. The usual daily dose is around 200 mg, while a megadose could be upwards of 2000 mg a day. When vitamin C is taken in a megadose it will act as a natural antibiotic, speeding up the healing process and neutralising various toxins.

Generally, naturopaths will recommend you take the supplements found in health food stores, which are natural vitamins rather than synthetic ones. If you are in doubt as to which type of supplement to buy, ask your naturopath to recommend a brand.

In the A–Z OF HEALTH CONDITIONS you will notice quantities of vitamins A and E given in international units — iu. This is the way these vitamins are measured.

OSTEOPATHY

OSTEOPATHY IS A SYSTEM OF HEALTH CARE THAT FOCUSES ON THE TREATMENT OF THE BODY FRAMEWORK – THE NEURO-MUSCULO-SKELETAL SYSTEM. THE NAME OSTEOPATHY IS THE COMBINATION OF THE GREEK WORD OSTEO, MEANING BONE AND PATHOS, MEANING SUFFERING.

WHAT IS OSTEOPATHY?

While it can help reverse some long-standing conditions, osteopathy is not about "changing" your body structure completely, but rather helping it to function at its best so you can deal more easily with the demands of daily life, strengthen your body against illness, and prevent further deterioration. By using hands-on techniques, osteopaths aim to:

- restore the body's proper structure, good muscle tone and movement in the joints
- enhance the circulation of blood and lymph
- and balance the function of the nervous system.

The principle is that the structure and function of the body are inter-related and depend on each other.

OSTEOPATHY VERSUS CHIROPRACTIC

While osteopathic and chiropractic techniques overlap, there are fundamental differences in the underlying philosophical and treatment approaches. Chiropractic focuses on mechanical disorders of the spine. Osteopathy is concerned with the person's whole skeletal framework, their soft tissues, their nervous system and the enhancement of a healthy blood supply so that all the body systems can function at their best. Although much attention may be paid to the spine, osteopathic care encompasses the whole person.

Chiropractic uses less leverage than osteopathy, but has closer contact and thrust on the vertebra needing treatment. Nevertheless, the difference between the two is diminishing as chiropractors and osteopaths exchange knowledge and techniques.

A HISTORY OF OSTEOPATHY

The relationship between structural problems and disease was observed by the Ancient Chinese, Greeks and Egyptians; and the Aztec and Mayan tribes of South America are reported to have used massage and manipulation in their healing arts. The Greek physician Hippocrates, the father of MODERN MEDICINE, also understood the connection between spinal problems and the onset of various illnesses and acknowledged that the body had inherent self-healing, self-corrective and self-regulatory mechanisms. But it wasn't until the late 1800s that osteopathy was developed.

American physician Dr Andrew Still (1828–1917) became disillusioned with the medical practices of his time when his three sons died of spinal meningitis. He was a deeply religious man who sought to understand disease from a different angle. Dr Still believed the body was created as a perfect harmonious whole and contained the basics for its own self-healing, which it would do naturally if not prevented by any mechanical stresses. He realised there was a profound link between the structure of the body and the ways in which it functioned.

Dr Still discovered that dysfunctions of the body structure — the muscles, joints and skeleton — can affect the nervous and circulatory systems, causing difficulties in the way the body works, e.g. the way we move, breathe or digest food. For example, a problem in the spine will affect the muscles and nerves around it. This may, in turn, affect other muscles and nerves and lead to problems in another part of the body.

Dr Still found that he could diagnose various health conditions by feeling changes in the position and movement of the skeleton, joints and connective tissues because these related to changes in the blood supply, lymphatic system and nervous system. He noticed that the spine, in particular, and the function of the nervous system are closely related.

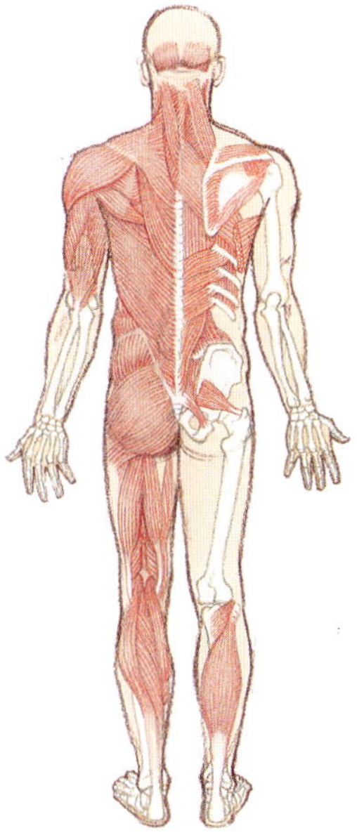

musculo-skeletal framework

Dr Still recognised that changes in the position or motion of the soma (physical body) could have far-reaching effects on the blood flow to related regions and organs. This could set up the conditions for potential problems. This is defined today as "somatic dysfunction". Dr Still found that by manually correcting these changes of position and moving the musculo-skeletal framework, he could relieve the dysfunctions and give the body a better chance to heal itself.

Dr Still began his work in the 1870s, founding a college of osteopathy some 20 years later.

THE OSTEOPATHIC APPROACH

Pain is a signal your body may be out of balance. If the pain has been triggered by stress, a fall, injury or some other obvious structural damage, a visit to an osteopath is well worthwhile. The practitioner will probably be able to relieve the pain, and prevent long-term damage through early intervention. For example, perhaps you recently suffered a sprained ankle. This, in itself, is not too serious but if not corrected you may find it could trigger other structural problems.

During the time it takes your ankle to recover, you may compensate by shifting your weight onto the other side of your body when walking. This places strain on the vertebrae, hip, knee and muscles and can develop into a pattern which will lead to long-term problems. An osteopath can help you become conscious of how you are compensating, relieve the tension, and ensure you recover fully.

There is a wide range of treatment approaches available to osteopaths, which they will use according to your need. These include soft tissue stretching, joint articulation and manipulation, and deep tactile pressure. Osteopathic treatment is gentle and uses minimum force, because it is governed by the forces and tensions within your own body. Techniques are adapted to suit the needs of each patient from the newborn to mature-aged.

A practitioner can assess your suitability for osteopathic care through a physical examination and by considering your history. Osteopaths are most frequently consulted for problems with posture and movement and to relieve the pain of injuries to the spine or joints, e.g. from accidents, wear and tear, pregnancy etc. Osteopathy may also relieve some types of headaches and gynaecological conditions as well as breathing problems and digestive difficulties. It can aid your immune response to illness or allergy.

Osteopathy may be applied preventively and can give asssistance to other therapies in the treatment of many diseases. It does not claim to cure but to provide the body with a better opportunity for self-correction.

CRANIAL OSTEOPATHY

Cranial osteopathy is a type of treatment approach practised by many osteopaths. It involves treatment of the head as well as the rest of the musculo-skeletal framework.

The skull or cranium is made of several bones. Membranes join these bones together and also link the cranium to the rest of the body. Dr William Garner Sutherland, a student of Dr Still, recognised that these joints in the skull are designed for movement. He also proposed that the cerebrospinal fluid is connected with the nervous and muscular system. The doctor then developed a system of gentle techniques, working with the fluid fluctuations in the cranium and body tissues. He worked with the bones of the skull, face and mouth, and the spinal cord to improve the whole body.

This approach is especially applicable to the treatment of children, although it can be used throughout life. It is particularly effective in treating old or recent injuries to the head, neck or back and relieving headaches, migraine and neuralgia.

THE CONSULTATION

Regardless of the approach, touch and observation are particularly important to osteopaths when they are treating you.

At your first consultation, an osteopath will take a comprehensive history, including details about your present complaint, your past medical history and any illness, accidents or surgery. They will also explore your lifestyle including diet, occupation and exercise. An examination will be performed, involving medical tests if necessary but also specifically examining your body structure. They will ask you to undress to your underwear and put on a loose robe then observe you standing, sitting, moving and lying, noting your posture and use of your body. If appropriate, they may request further tests such as X-rays, scans or other procedures — perhaps in conjunction with your general practitioner.

A specific way of touching your body known as hands-on palpation will indicate areas of dysfunction. The osteopath will be looking for changes in joint position and movement (particularly throughout the spine) and observing muscle tone and other connective tissues, including the health of your skin. They will decide whether you are a suitable candidate for osteopathic care and then proceed with treatment or refer you to an appropriate care-giver. The osteopath may also give you advice on diet, exercise, posture and lifestyle changes to assist your body's return to balance.

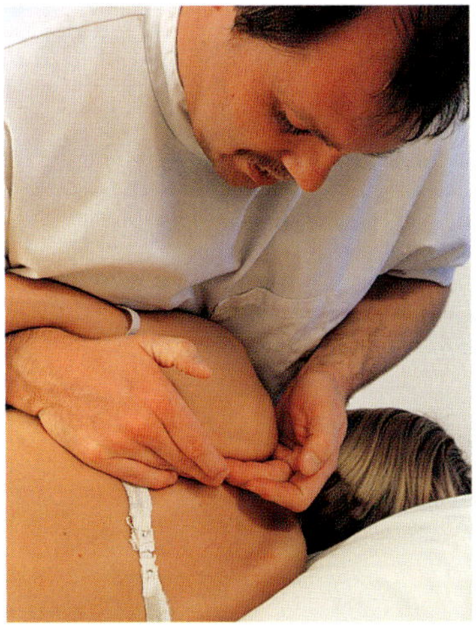
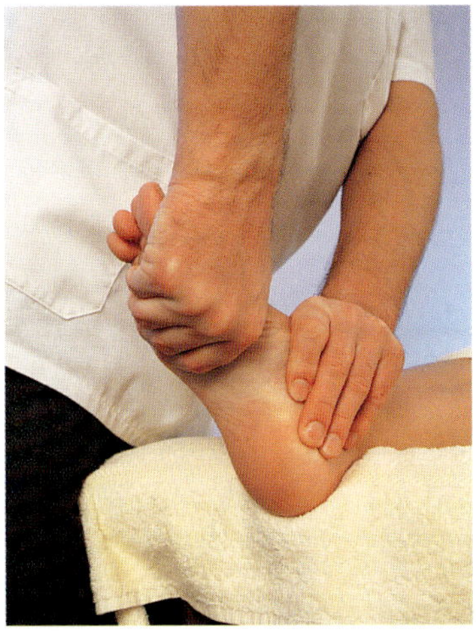
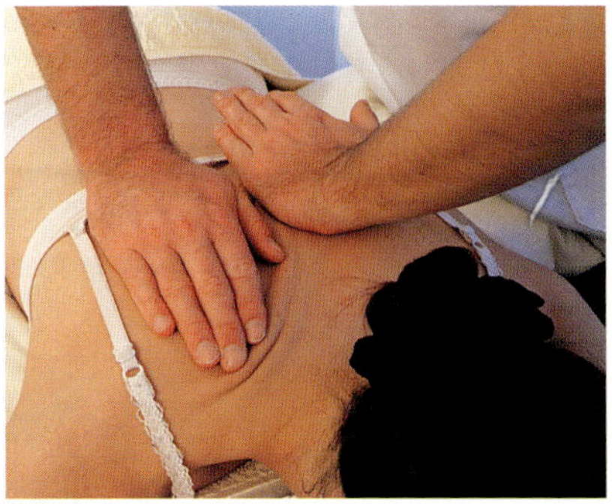

Osteopathy is a hands-on treatment approach. Different techniques are used depending on the specific condition and the individual practitioner. As a therapy, it involves treatment of the whole body framework of muscle and skeleton.

The details of treatment will depend on the patient's requirements and suitability and the practitioner's own particular technique preferences. Manipulations that "click" or cavitate the intervertebral joints do not always take place; many other techniques may be chosen. Some practitioners may use oils, others may be trained in the use of ultrasound, but this is not standard to all practices. Most practitioners will just use their hands.

While some problems can be relieved by a single treatment, others will need further visits. On average, the first consultation may range from 30–60 minutes, while follow-up treatments and consultations will vary from 20–40 minutes.

IMPORTANT

Treatment should only be given by a professional, experienced osteopath.

The therapy involves pushing and pulling bones and muscles. It is quite safe, and hugely beneficial, if performed by a fully-trained expert. However, if the person is not qualified, such activity may cause serious injury.

If you are seeking an osteopath, ask for recommendations or contact the association in your area for a referral.

Osteopaths undergo years of training in a degree course that incorporates the medical sciences and specific osteopathic subjects, gaining the skills of palpation (specific touch), observation, diagnosis and treatment. They achieve a double degree in science and applied science, majoring in osteopathy. In some countries such as Australia, there are government registers of practitioners.

Osteopaths are trained to diagnose and recognise situations where the use of particular osteopathic techniques is best avoided, or where referral to another type of health practitioner is called for, e.g. cases of critical illness, recent head trauma, fractures and haemorrhages.

REFLEXOLOGY

REFLEXOLOGY IS A UNIQUE METHOD OF HELPING TO ACTIVATE THE BODY'S NATURAL HEALING POWERS. IT IS BASED ON THE PRINCIPLE THAT THE BODY HAS AN ENERGY SYSTEM THAT RUNS IN VERTICAL "ZONES" WHICH TRAVEL THE LENGTH AND BREADTH OF THE BODY. AS A RESULT, THERE ARE AREAS OR POINTS IN THE FEET AND THE HANDS WHICH RELATE TO ALL THE ORGANS, GLANDS AND THE STRUCTURE OF THE BODY.

For centuries, Chinese medicine has used finger pressure to stimulate these points. The Chinese believed specific points on the feet could have a powerful effect on the overall functioning of the body. The ancient Egyptians also seemed to practise a similar kind of foot massage.

Although reflexology was recognised in Europe in the Middle Ages, it wasn't fully explored until the early 1900s when an American doctor, William Fitzgerald, theorised that the body could be divided into ten vertical zones. He discovered that if pressure was applied to a particular finger, for example, an analgesic effect would be produced in another corresponding body part that lay within the same zone as that finger.

Then another American, Eunice D. Ingham, took this theory and refined it further. Working in the 1930s until her death in the early 1970s, Ingham taught that the feet were the most important focus of this therapy.

She also discovered that the use of alternating pressure was far superior to the constant pressure used in Fitzgerald's zone therapy. Thus, reflexology as we know it today was born.

WHAT IS REFLEXOLOGY?

Reflexology is based on the idea that by "massaging" specific points in the feet or the hands, the related organ, body structure or system is stimulated. The improved performance of glands and organs brings the body back to a state of balance and health.

A person applying pressure to these points can stimulate and relax various parts of the body in a "reflex" action. Reflexologists use the term "working" to describe the alternating pressure used. If you "work" your own feet you may feel little crystals beneath the surface of the skin. It is believed that these are sediment deposits that settle in the body. Working these deposits will break them up making reabsorption into the body and thus elimination possible.

Within each session, care should be taken not to overstimulate particularly sensitive areas as this could then cause added stress for the recipient.

During a session, the client may become conscious of spots sensitive to the touch. If a tender spot is touched, and keeping the aim of relaxation in mind, it is important the client informs the therapist. To a reflexologist, this indicates the energy relating to that area is out of balance.

A TYPICAL SESSION

Most sessions will take between 45 to 60 minutes and you will be invited to be seated or to lie down and remove your shoes and socks. Some reflexologists may use powder to make working the feet easier; massage oils are not used as they are too slippery.

The main aim of reflexology is to increase the body's overall state of relaxation. If the tension in the body is reduced, blood and energy circulation improves.

Usually the reflexologist will pay special attention to the tender points but this pressure should be firm, not uncomfortable, nor should it tickle, otherwise you will tense up and lose the benefits of relaxation.

The therapist will mainly work with their thumbs or fingers, stroking, pressing and rubbing pressure points on your feet.

Therapists have their preferred routines and most will work on toes, ankles and the top of the foot as well as the soles.

Although the feet usually form the focus of a treatment, the same principles are applied to the hands. The positions of some of these reflex points are different, however, and are usually deeper, making them more difficult to locate.

It may take a few sessions before tenderness in the hands or feet is eliminated. It is wiser to take time with tender points over several sessions than to create stress by overworking them in one or two intensive workouts.

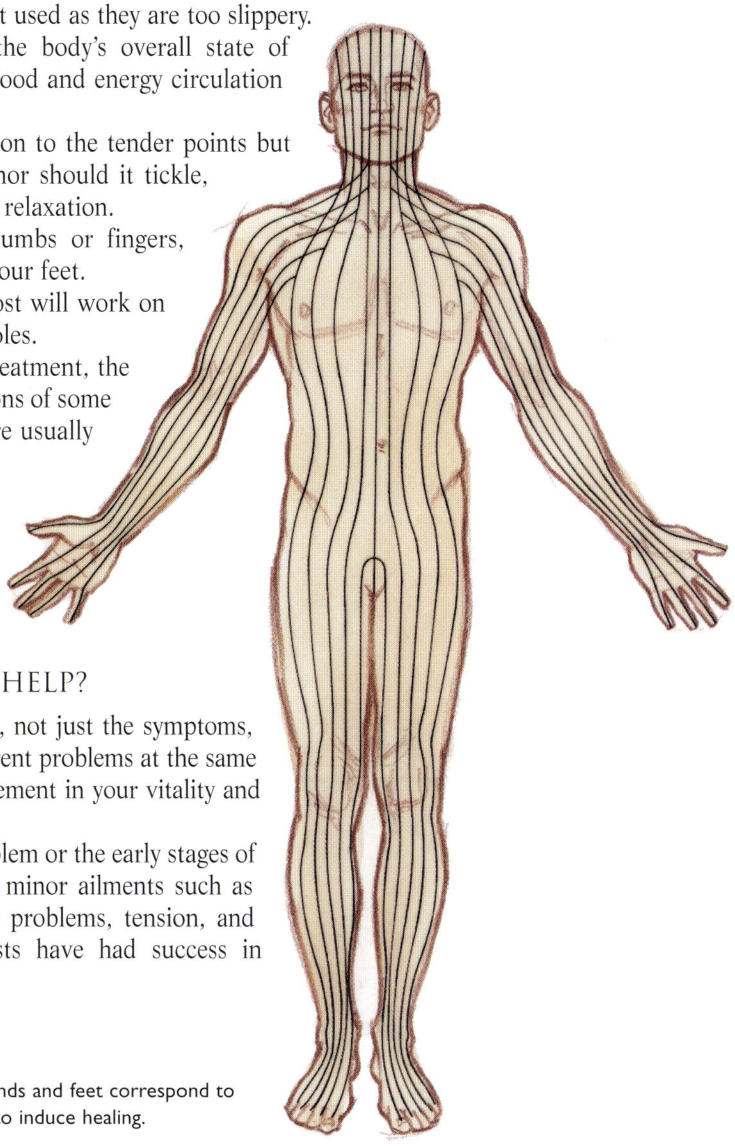

WHO CAN REFLEXOLOGY HELP?

Reflexology helps deal with the cause of an ailment, not just the symptoms, and it can work on many parts of the body and different problems at the same time. With regular use you should notice an improvement in your vitality and feelings of well-being.

Reflexology may also help detect a potential problem or the early stages of illness. It can be used at home to give relief from minor ailments such as period pain, neck and back pain, headache, sinus problems, tension, and problems with digestion. Professional reflexologists have had success in helping with more serious conditions.

In reflexology, the body is divided into zones. Areas on the hands and feet correspond to other parts of the body within a zone and can be stimulated to induce healing.

REFLEXOLOGY CHARTS

A REFLEXOLOGY "FOOTPRINT"

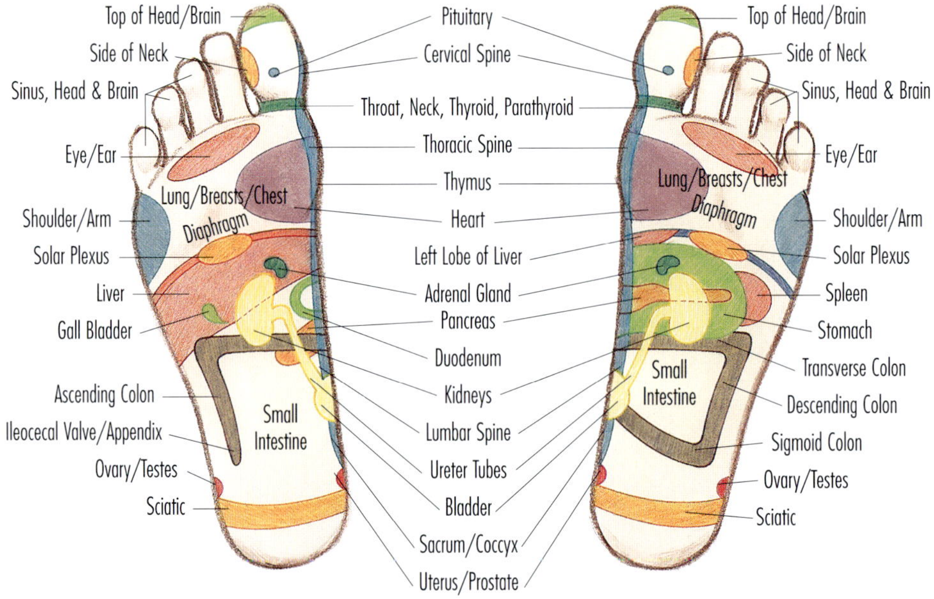

A REFLEXOLOGY "HANDPRINT"

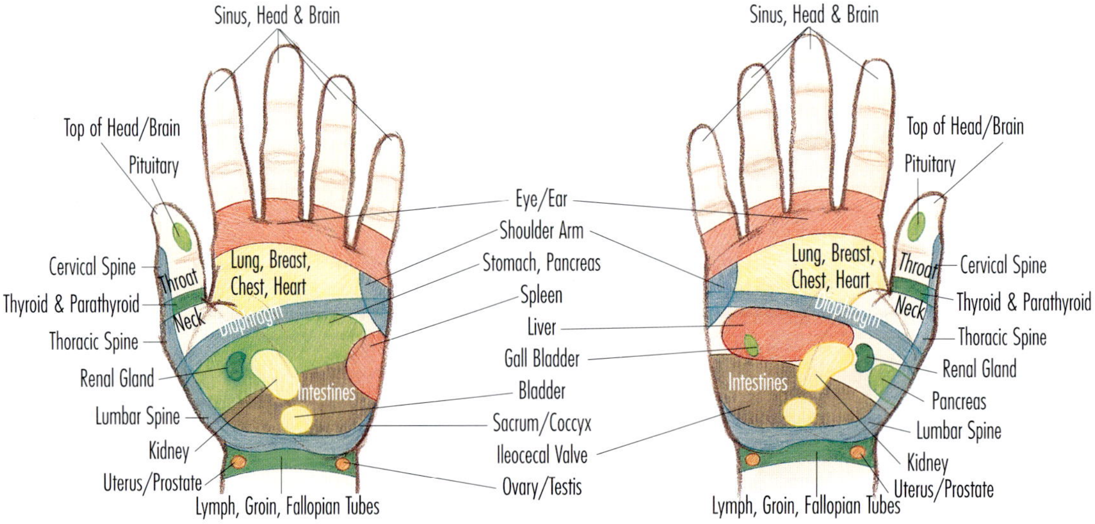

SELF MASSAGE

Feet are often neglected. That's why most people find a reflexology session so soothing.

It can be interesting to check which part of your body any tender spot corresponds to, but be wary of jumping to conclusions and self diagnosing. For example, tenderness at the point relating to your stomach may indicate overeating the night before, rather than a sign of impending illness. On the other hand, if you find the same spot is consistently tender, take notice of the message your body is sending you, and seek professional assistance.

Reflexology is a treatment you can learn to give yourself or your friends. To begin, try the basic steps illustrated on the next page but to learn correct techniques, consider attending a reflexology course.

BEFORE YOU BEGIN

A footbath with warm water and a few drops of essential oil (see page 99) can be a delightful way to begin a reflexology treatment. Make sure you dry the feet thoroughly.

Have the person receiving the reflexology treatment sit or lie down. Position yourself so that their foot is about level with your chest — sitting cross-legged or kneeling is often most comfortable. You may wish to support their leg with a cushion and to prop their foot on your leg.

Your first concern is to make the person feel comfortable and secure.

You may wish to dust the feet with powder. Begin by laying your hands gently on one of their feet, then encircle that foot with your hands.

Start every reflexology treatment with some relaxing "passive" movements. Support and steady the ankle area firmly with one hand, and hold the instep of the foot with the other hand. Now gently rotate the foot several times first clockwise then anti-clockwise.

Slowly stretch the foot back and forth to warm and loosen the Achilles tendon. This should be a relaxing movement — not vigorous.

UPPER FOOT

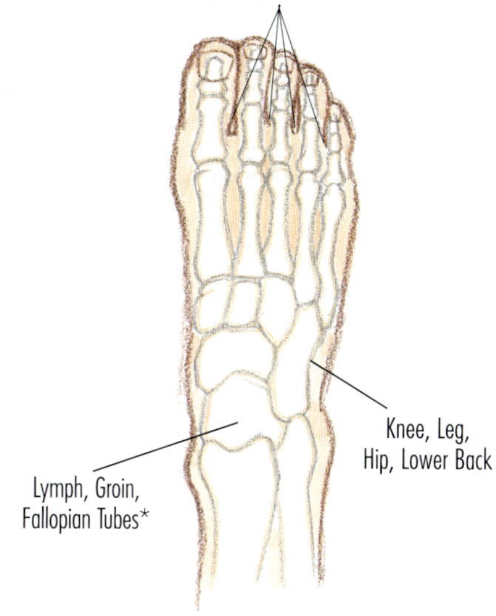

* Note: this reflex can also be found at the hollow "groove" around the back of the ankle where the ankle meets the foot.

GROUPS OF POINTS

COLON	transverse colon, descending colon, sigmoid colon, ascending colon
LOWER SPINE	lumbar spine, sacrum/coccyx
WHOLE SPINE	cervical spine, thoracic spine, lumbar spine, sacrum/coccyx
REPRODUCTIVE SYSTEM	ovary/testis, uterus/prostate, Fallopian tubes
ALL GLANDS	pituitary, thyroid, adrenal glands, pancreas, ovary/testes

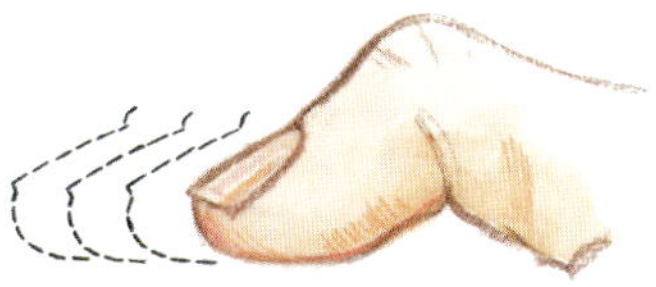

To work a point: flex and unflex the first joint of your thumb or finger to make small "walking" movements. Use the outer edge of the ball — do not use the tip as it applies too much pressure and injury may be caused by the fingernail.

REFLEXOLOGY HOME-TREATMENT

1. Support the foot by overlapping the hands behind the foot, just below the toes. Press along the "diaphragm line" — from left to right under the ball of the foot. Repeat several times.

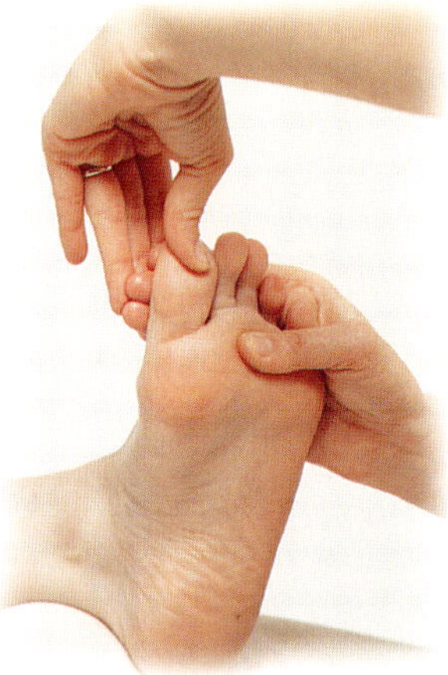

2. Firmly hold the foot with one hand, ensuring the toes are well supported to limit movement. Now, with the thumb of the other hand, work all over the front, top and sides of the big toe. This area corresponds to the head. Then work over the other toes in the same manner for the sinus area.

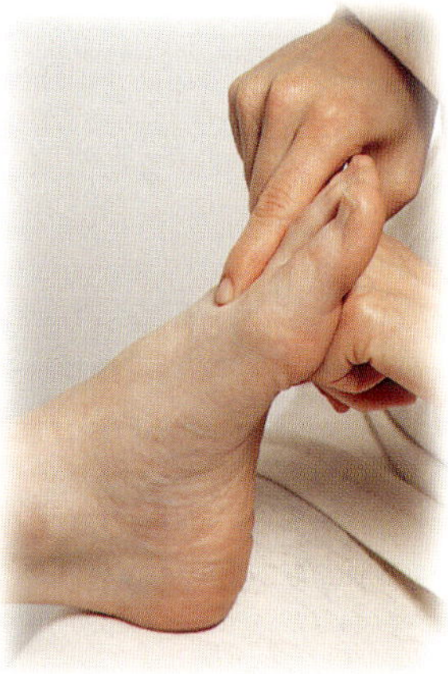

3. Using your index finger, apply a line of pressure between each of the tendons on the top of the foot. Working from the base of the toes to half way down the foot releases tension in the chest. To provide support during this movement, place the clenched fist of your other hand on the ball of the foot.

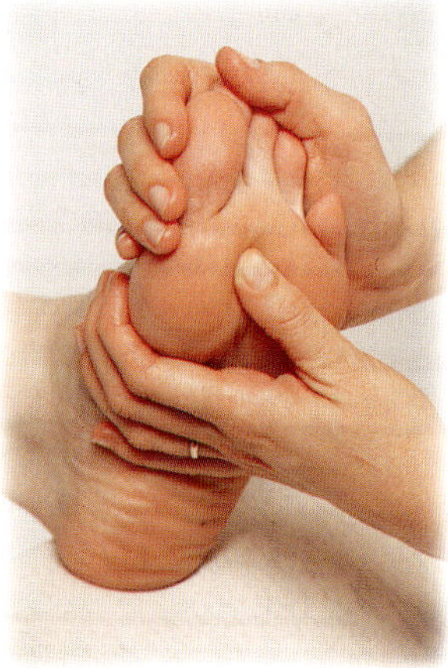

4. Using the pad of your thumb, apply pressure over the ball of the foot underneath the big toe. This will work the lung and chest area.

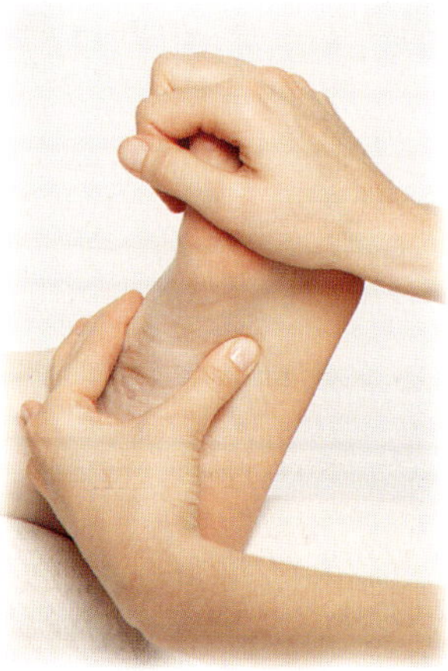

5. Holding the ball of the foot in one hand, and with the thumb of the other hand pointing towards the little toe, work in diagonal lines from the waist line (or middle) to the diaphragm line to tone the liver, gall bladder and stomach.

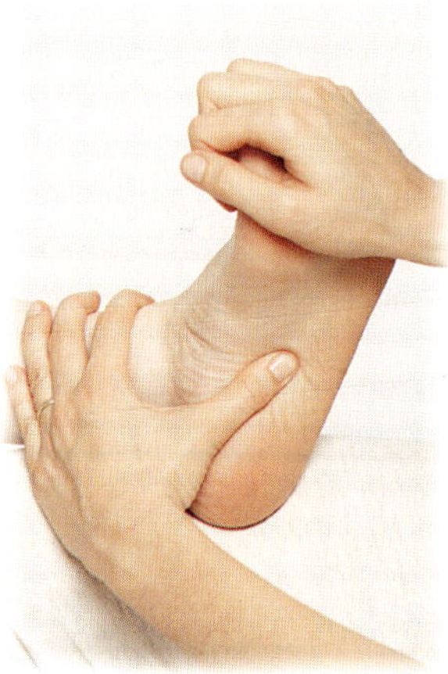

6. Working from the heel to the waist line, continue the diagonal line of pressure. This will work the digestive system, especially the small and large intestines.

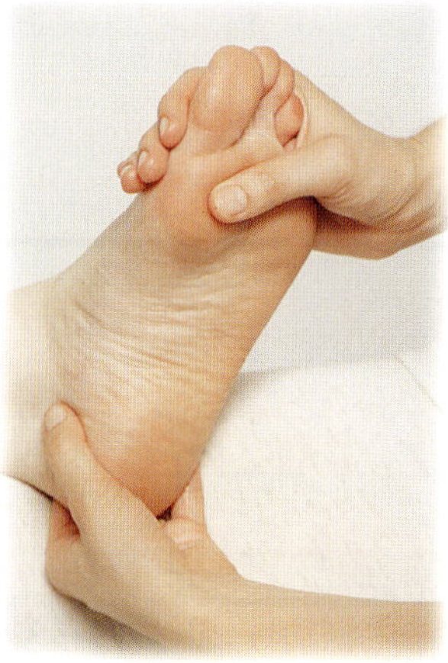

7. Applying gentle pressure all around the ankle and Achilles area will address the lower back, legs and the reproductive organs. Working all over the heel with the soft pad of the thumb will help prevent or relieve lower back pain.

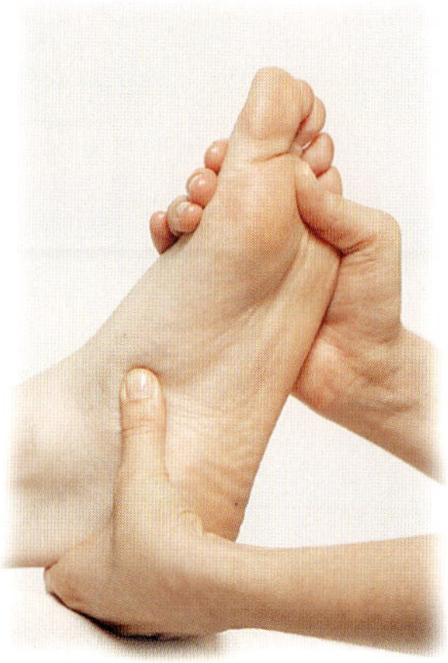

8. Work upwards from heel to big toe, tracing the main arch of the foot. This stimulates the spinal column. The same movement repeated on an arc about a finger-width inwards, will work the urinary system. Press gently as the kidney area is often tender.

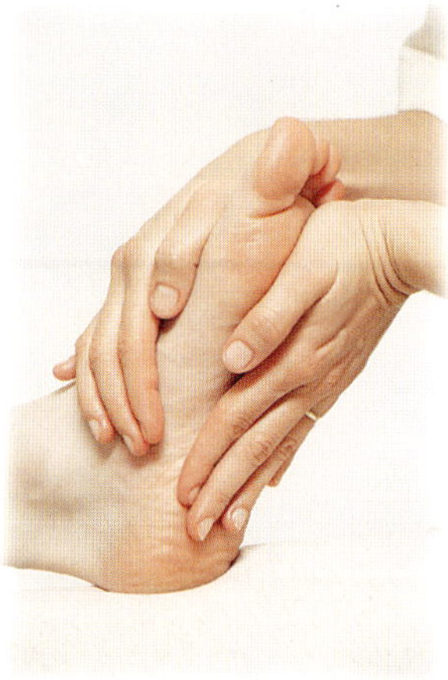

9. Finish the treatment by gently and smoothly stroking the foot from ankle to toes. This will calm, relax and soothe the whole area.

WHEN TO AVOID REFLEXOLOGY

It is best to be particularly careful about reflexology, if you:

- are in your first trimester of pregnancy
- have a history of unstable pregnancies
- have lymphoma
- there is the possibility of unstable blood pressure
- have heart disease
- have deep vein thrombosis
- are undergoing substantial drug treatments
- have varicose veins on your feet and ankles.

If you have any of the conditions described or are in doubt about using reflexology, check with your health practitioner. If you do have a treatment make sure it is with a properly trained reflexologist and the treatment is extremely gentle and relaxing

SHIATSU

SHIATSU IS STRICTLY TRANSLATED FROM JAPANESE AS "FINGER PRESSURE". HOWEVER, OTHER PARTS OF THE BODY – KNEES, ELBOWS, KNUCKLES, PALMS AND FEET – MAY ALSO BE USED BY THE SHIATSU THERAPIST TO RELEASE ANY BLOCKAGES IN THE FULL FLOW OF YOUR VITALITY OR LIFE FORCE.

The notion of life force or Ki (known as Qi or Ch'i to the Chinese) flowing through a meridian system in the body has its origins in TRADITIONAL CHINESE MEDICINE, of which ACUPUNCTURE and ACUPRESSURE are branches. The Japanese combined this meridian system with their own massage known as anma and a system of breathing and stretching exercises known as Do-in, to form the basis of shiatsu.

Traditionally anma was practised by blind people as relaxation massage. It went through further development in the early part of this century as a therapy for medical treatment. It changed its name to shiatsu to distinguish it from traditional anma, and to represent more authentically the shiatsu practised today.

There are different styles of shiatsu. Two of the most popular in the West are the Namikoshi style which is based on the traditional anma system combined with Western anatomy and physiology and developed by Tokujiro Namikoshi (1905–) and Zen Shiatsu which was developed by Shizuto Masunaga (1925–1981), a psychologist. Masunaga emphasised the diagnostic and medical treatment aspects of shiatsu and expanded the original Chinese meridian system and the understanding of psycho-emotional relationships to disease states. He was the first to present a sound theoretical basis to shiatsu therapy.

Shiatsu has evolved over the years to become one of the most popular forms of oriental therapies in the West. In Japan, it has its own respected standing within the national health system and is widely practised.

Shiatsu is used to treat existing conditions, their symptoms and the source of these problems as well as being an effective preventative health measure. Its strength as a preventative health therapy is that well-trained therapists are able to diagnose and treat any imbalance before it develops into an illness, by realigning the body's energy flow and internal organ functions.

The shiatsu therapist believes that illness is caused by an imbalance in the Ki flow through the various meridians and internal organs of the body. The extent of this imbalance will determine the general state of the person's health. The energy flow along these meridians can be deficient, stagnant or excessive.

THE CONSULTATION PROCESS

In the initial consultation, a case history will be taken with any relevant information concerning your health. You will receive an individual diagnosis — generally derived from palpation (touching) of your hara or abdomen. This will determine the course of treatment.

To a shiatsu therapist, the condition of your hara is central to your overall health and vitality as all the meridian pathways connect into this area. From the hara, there are referral zones to all the internal organs and functions of the body.

After diagnosing your hara the shiatsu therapist may confirm the diagnosis through facial signs, back diagnostic zones or pulse diagnosis to find the essential key to your particular condition. When they have located the cause of the Ki imbalance, they will stimulate the appropriate meridians or Tsubo ("acu-points"). These are situated along the pathways and are where the Ki of the meridian focuses or accumulates, so they can be influenced by pressure. They act as gateways for an intake or release of Ki between the channels and the environment, and are transportation points as well as a means of regulating Ki within the meridian and the body.

An excess of Ki is called Jitsu and a deficiency of Ki is called Kyo. Kyo areas may look and feel slightly empty, i.e. soft and spongy to touch, lacking in tone, with some discomfort occurring below the surface and a tendency to be cold, exhibiting poor circulation.

A Jitsu area is tense and can be painful prior to touching or when touched by the therapist. It may look or feel full, i.e. raised above the normal surface of the body and tight relative to surrounding areas, with constricted circulation or a tendency to warmth.

The therapist aims to bring Jitsu points and meridians back into balance through "sedation" and improve Kyo points and meridians by "tonification" techniques. This yang/yin relationship between Jitsu and Kyo and the approach to treatment is the key to effective shiatsu. It is different from massage which tends to concentrate on the surface tension, caused by excessive functioning or blockage (Jitsu) in the body.

Stretching is also an important part of shiatsu. At the beginning or during a treatment, your shiatsu therapist may use their bodyweight to gently stretch your body. The stretching and application of bodyweight pressure is co-ordinated with the breath. This heightens one's awareness and helps release blockages in the meridian pathway or area of the body being activated by the stretch, thereby promoting the circulation of Ki.

When practitioners move on to use the pressure of thumbs, elbows or knees, they will also use their body-weight, rather than muscle power, to apply pressure.

If practitioners are working correctly they will be relaxed and steady in the application of pressure. This allows them to work for extended periods of time without becoming tired and to tune into your body as they treat you. If therapists remain centred and relaxed and apply pressure simply by shifting their bodyweight correctly, you will feel the pressure as firm but gentle. This then ensures that you remain relaxed. It is while you are in this state that therapists are able to sense any changes as they occur in the meridian system of your body and respond accordingly.

A BASIC SEQUENCE

There are quite a few shiatsu techniques, e.g. vertical pressure, kneading, tapping, rubbing and shaking, depending upon the style of shiatsu used. During a session a number of sequences are followed that cover the entire body through a system of tonification and dispersion that suits the individual diagnosis.

YOUR SHIATSU THERAPIST

To give quality shiatsu your therapist needs to have quality Ki. For this reason, a good shiatsu therapist should be fit and healthy and regularly practise some form of breathing exercises and energy-increasing exercise such as yoga, Tai Chi, Do-in or Qigong. A fully-qualified practitioner will have graduated from a recognised college with a minimum of a diploma and be registered with a natural therapy association.

Shiatsu is applied through a cotton gown (Yukatá) or cotton pyjamas supplied by the practitioner. A cotton cloth (Tenuguí) is used where contact with the bare skin is likely to occur. No oils are used. The shiatsu will be given on a futon mat, which again is made with cotton fibre. This will not interfere with the "energy body" as the cotton fibre does not have a static charge of its own like synthetic materials do.

A basic shiatsu sequence is likely to start with hara diagnosis, then stretching and applying pressure to the leg and arm meridians. From there the therapist may work, in the side position, along the meridians of the side of the head, neck, shoulders and arms, employing stretches where necessary.

TREATING COMMON CONDITIONS

Some of the common conditions and disorders which respond to shiatsu therapy include:

- Anxiety and Depression
- Arthritis
- Back pain
- Digestive Problems
- Fatigue
- Headache and Migraine
- Insomnia
- Menstrual Problems and uro-genital conditions
- Sciatica
- Sinusitis
- circulatory problems
- respiratory conditions
- conditions following strain and injury
- internal organ dysfunctioning.

Treatment of these conditions is given according to oriental diagnostic techniques and medical principles.

It is recommended in the treatment of serious or long-term illness that the experience of a senior practitioner be employed, i.e. someone with at least five years of clinical experience. Pregnancy is another situation that would require the services of an experienced practitioner.

They would generally apply palm pressure first then thumb or elbow pressure, beginning with a more general pressure to prepare the area for more specific pressure where appropriate. These techniques would also be used along either side of the spine and muscles of the back, down through the hips and legs to the feet. The usual movement of treatment is from head to feet.

After the side position, you would lie on your stomach; the practitioner would probably then work along your back. Starting from the head, neck, shoulders and arms they would work methodically down through the hips and legs to the feet.

The pressure should be smooth, unforced and gradual, although often the effect will be experienced as quite deep.

The treatment could finish with sitting position shiatsu followed by you lying on your back again as your head, face, arms and hands are worked. The practitioner would then recheck the hara for changes.

The final sequencing of the treatment is determined by the individual diagnosis which indicates the best way to access the different meridians around the body.

The average treatment time is $1^{1}/_{4}$ to $1^{1}/_{2}$ hours.

BENEFITS OF SHIATSU TREATMENT

With a good shiatsu treatment you are likely to feel immediate benefits to your health and these will build in the days that follow. Symptoms should fall away as your vitality (your Ki) flows through your system unimpeded. From your response to the initial session, the therapist would be able to suggest a suitable course of treatment, corrective exercises and dietary suggestions to help maintain your health and support the effects of the first treatment.

HOME SHIATSU THERAPY

You can learn shiatsu for self-treatment or to use on others. In this way you can do a self-diagnosis of your hara or specific Tsubo points and apply self-shiatsu or stretch the appropriate meridians of their body to create balance. This has the effect of addressing any imbalance and realigning the energy flow to maintain health on a daily basis. This is also one way shiatsu therapists ensure their own health and well-being.

THE ROLE OF DIET

Shiatsu is often combined with dietary advice in macrobiotic eating. Macrobiotics is based on the yin/yang or expansive/contractive nature of foods, and the use of foods as medicine.

From a precise and individual diagnosis, your therapist may advise you to keep a balance between the five tastes — sweet, salty, bitter, sour and pungent. These different flavours can both stimulate or support the various internal organs of the body.

You may also be advised to reduce your intake of certain strong foods and stimulants such as tea, coffee, alcohol and sugar, as well as refined foods. These are considered harmful to various energy and chemical levels within your body and can reduce the body's natural immunity.

SHIATSU—HOW TO PROPERLY APPLY PRESSURE

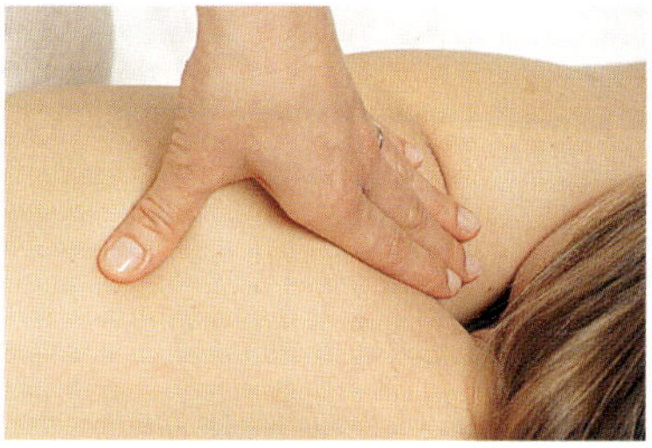

THUMB PRESSURE
Use the soft pad, or "ball", of the thumb. Do not use either the boney inside of the thumb joint or the very tip of the thumb. Lightly rest the fingers on the skin to aid control and help give a steady, even pressure.

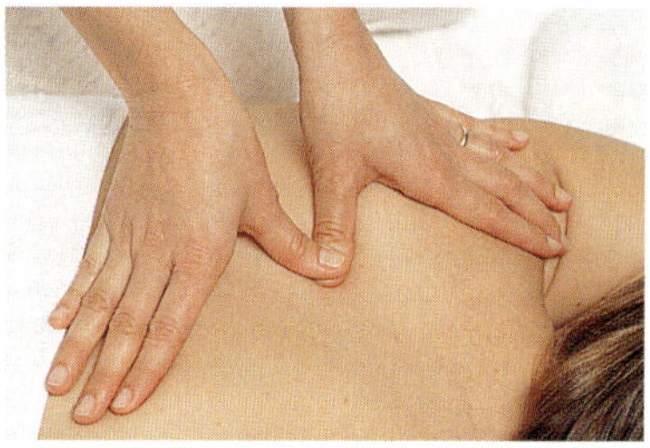

DEEP THUMB PRESSURE
Placing one thumb on top of the other will give extra depth when working on the buttocks, shoulders, back, and the soles of the feet.

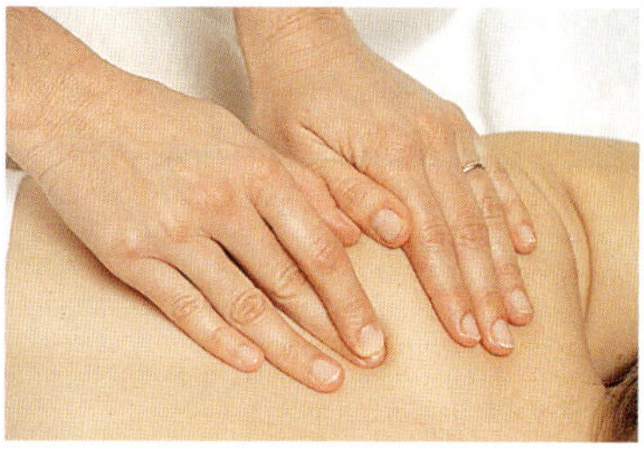

FINGER PRESSURE
When using your fingers to apply pressure, greater depth is achieved by placing the index finger on top of the middle finger. This is a good alternative to thumb pressure when thumbs are tired or the muscle area is sensitive.

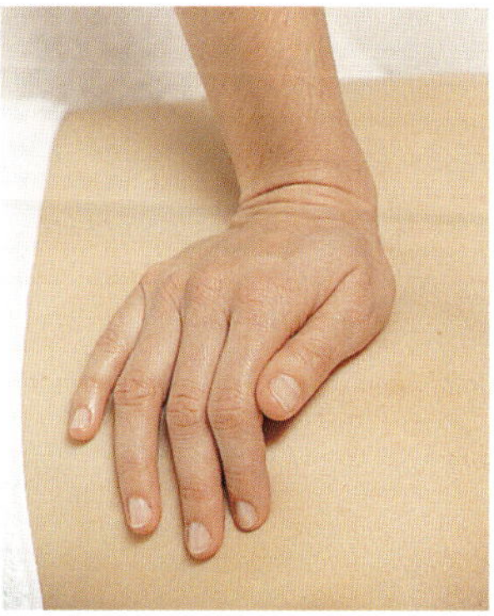

HAND PRESSURE
Using the heel of your hand provides a more general stimulation to the shiatsu point and surrounding area. This technique is most useful when working the back or the legs.

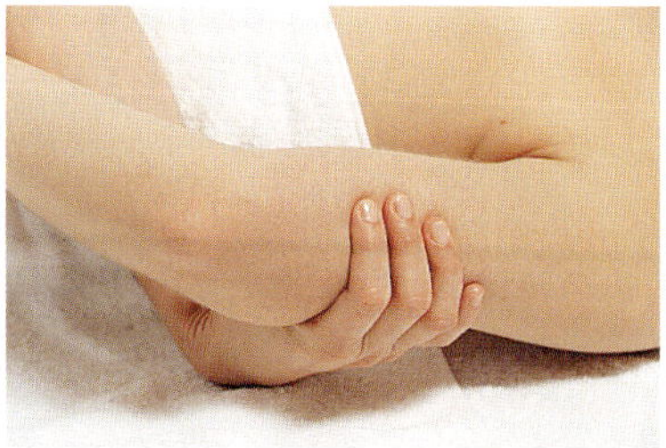

SQUEEZING
Smaller areas, such as the arms, are more easily treated by squeezing them between the thumb and fingers.

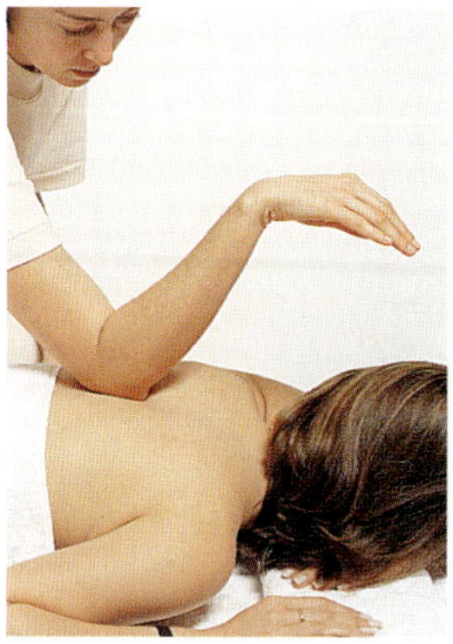

ELBOW PRESSURE
When using your elbow, keep your arm and hand loose and relaxed so that a gentle pressure is applied. This technique is useful for larger muscle areas such as the shoulders, buttocks and hamstrings.

TRADITIONAL CHINESE MEDICINE

TRADITIONAL CHINESE MEDICINE IS A TOTAL HEALTH CARE AND MAINTENANCE SYSTEM. IT INCLUDES ACUPUNCTURE, INTERNAL MEDICINE (CHINESE HERBALISM), TAI CHI CHUAN (PHYSICAL EXERCISES), QI GONG (CHINESE BREATHING EXERCISES), TUNINA (CHINESE MASSAGE), BONE SETTING AND CHINESE DIETARY THERAPY.

The various practices within this system of medicine are based on a central philosophy that owes much to the early Taoist philosophers who taught the importance of balance in life. The fundamental principle of traditional Chinese medicine is to establish and maintain, by regular review and adjustment, the body's ideal internal balance which promotes health and longevity.

THE MERIDIAN SYSTEM

Qi refers to the life force of the body. This energy flows through channels in the body in much the same way as blood flows through veins and arteries. These channels are called meridians. Each corresponds to a particular body organ and its energy flow corresponds to fluctuations in the body's electromagnetic field. Even though they are separate channels, the meridians do overlap with the circulatory and nervous systems.

YIN AND YANG

Qi energy is composed of the counter-balancing elements of yin and yang. In the poetic Chinese manner, yin is described as the shady side of the mountain, yang the sunny side. Yin is understood as passive, cold, contracting, internal, negative, and feminine. By contrast, yang is active, warm, expanding, external, positive, and masculine. The terms "positive" and "negative" are not value judgments but indicate polarity.

Both yin and yang elements are always present in the body and in constant flux. If an imbalance lasts too long or is too severe, illness will result. For instance, too much yin may cause a chill, too much yang a fever. If you are too yin, you might feel lethargic, be sensitive to cold, catch cold easily, perhaps be pale or even anaemic. If you are too yang, you might be hot-tempered, your pulse excessively fast or strong, your skin reddish or prone to rash.

THE BODY AND ITS ORGANS

The Chinese characterise the organs by observing the relationship between each organ and various emotions.

The organs are also associated with the elements: heart with fire, spleen with earth, lungs with air, kidneys with water, and liver with wood. The liver is associated with wood because the ancient Chinese realised, long before Western medical practitioners, that the liver is the only organ capable of tissue regeneration as is the wood of living trees. The poetic image of the organs as natural elements is also used to describe the ideal flow of energy throughout the body: fire from the sun energises the earth to create vegetation which in turn affects the air which compounds to metal. Air/metal condenses to water which gives life to trees/wood which burns to create fire. And so the cycle continues.

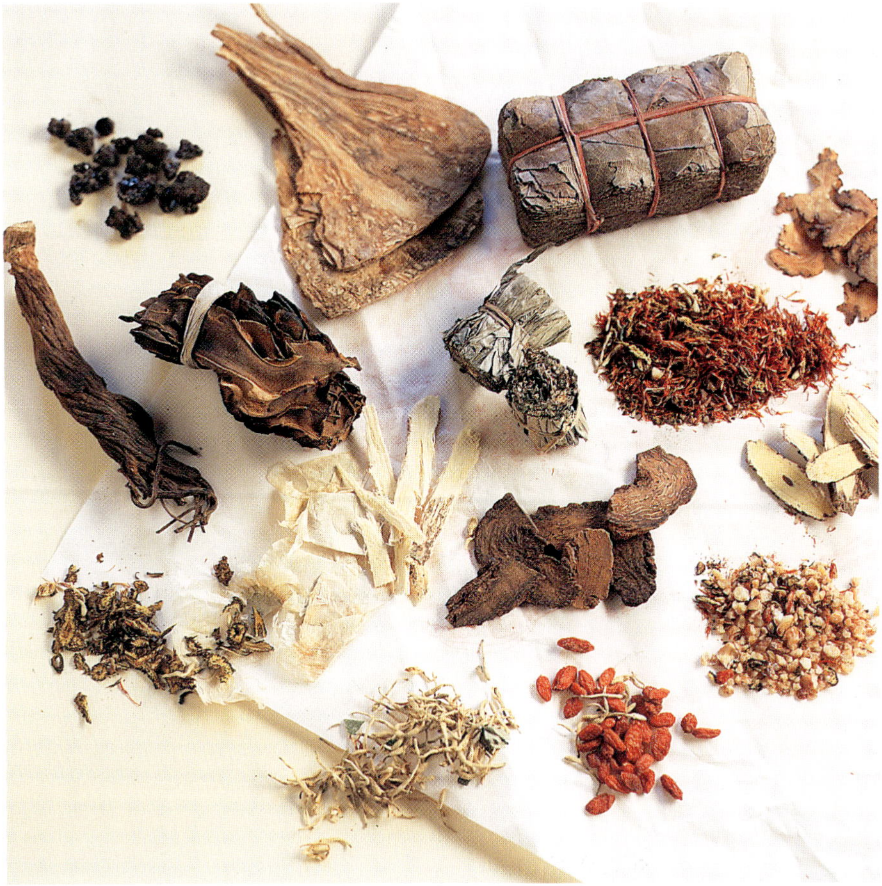

Chinese herbs may be sourced from minerals and animals as well as plants. They are available in various forms, including powders, pills and granules.

The Chinese also categorise each organ as primarily yin or yang. Yin characterises lungs, spleen, heart, pericardium, kidneys, and liver. Yang dominates the large intestine, stomach, small intestine, bladder and gall bladder.

There are many Western-educated doctors interested in the entire field of Chinese medicine, and almost all accept at least some parts of the Chinese system. Some forms, like acupuncture, have been more readily taken up than others.

DIAGNOSIS IN CHINESE MEDICINE

Traditional Chinese medicine is concerned with all aspects of your health — mental and emotional and physical. A consultation will begin with an overview of your medical history and other relevant lifestyle details, including your age and occupation.

The practitioner uses the 12 pulses to help in diagnosis (three places in each wrist, and two depths in each place). The pulses give an insight into the balance of yin and yang in the body. The tongue, skin, eyes and hair are all carefully checked as well as a person's gait and the quality of their voice.

Traditional diagnosis involves ascertaining the underlying causes behind an ailment. The same symptoms may be treated differently depending on the person and factors behind this disharmony.

The number of consultations you need, how long each will last, and for how long treatment will be required are all determined by your individual case after diagnosis.

IMPORTANT

It is essential that you prepare the herbs in the manner the herbalist has directed as some of the herbs are potentially toxic. Preparation usually involves boiling the herbs for 60–90 minutes which significantly reduces the toxicity.

Ask your herbalist for specific advice as to what effects the herbs are likely to have. You could experience an allergic reaction to some Chinese herbs. If you have an adverse reaction of any kind, discontinue the treatment and consult your herbalist for advice.

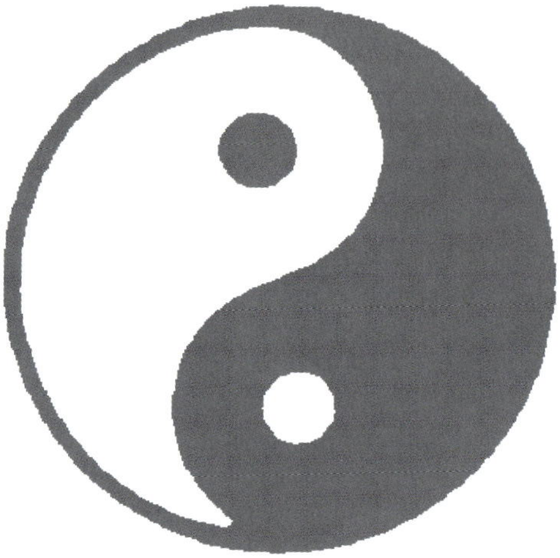

The philosophy of yin and yang is a cornerstone of traditional Chinese medicine. It is based around the idea of harmony through a balance of elements.

PROTECT YOURSELF

Chinese medicine believes that it is important to protect yourself against external factors such as heat, cold, wind and damp, which can invade your body and upset your internal yin/yang balance. Practitioners advise you keep your neck, shoulders and lower back warm and covered (wear a scarf if you are going to be in the wind, especially if you have a haircut that leaves your neck bare). Plus, if you have painful knees, ankles or other joints, keep them warm.

Too much heat can also cause problems, so in hot weather take care not to overexert yourself, dehydrate or get sunburnt.

You will be encouraged to be aware of what you eat. Chinese medicine is not overly keen on salads or cold food. Living on salads does not provide enough yang energy and it is advised that no more than a third of your diet should be raw except in very hot weather. Cold foods such as items straight from the refrigerator should be avoided as they make your stomach cold, lowering your energy levels and impairing the function of certain organs. Likewise, overly hot or spicy foods can have a detrimental effect if you already have too much energy or "heat" in your body. As in all things, balance is the key.

CHINESE HERBALISM

Chinese herbalism classifies herbs based on qualities such as their nature (warming, cooling or neutral); their shape, moisture-content and texture; their colour; their taste; and their properties — whether they are dispersing and circulating, consolidating, purging, or toning and nourishing. Each of these characteristics links the herb to a corresponding healing principle (earth, metal, wind, cold, damp etc) and thus has an expected effect on the body.

The Chinese herbs themselves are drawn from a wide range of plant, mineral and animal substances, including fungus, seeds, prickles, burrs, bark, roots, leaves, and crystallised tree sap.

After consultation, Chinese herbalists may prescribe a selection of raw herbs in various combinations. These are simmered with water in a Chinese soup pot until reduced and then drunk. The "soups" or "teas", which can be unusually powerful in taste, should be sipped, not swallowed in one gulp. Tastebuds familiar only with Western food often need time to adjust to Chinese herbs. These herbal mixtures can be stored for only a few days in the refrigerator, and are usually taken in the morning and evening, before eating. Different combinations may be prescribed for different days, or blends may be advised to enhance the effect of one herb or counteract any undesirable reactions.

Ready-made, patent medicines in the form of dried herbs and herbal teas, as well as powders and fluids are available over the counter. From the beginning of Chinese herbalism, various herbs have been used in standard formulas, many of which are aimed at chronic conditions. Those formulas which have a wide-ranging effect are being turned into granules and pills, ensuring a consistent quality and making them more suitable to our modern lifestyle. In general, pills tend to be non-concentrated at a relatively low dose, while the granulated form is a higher concentration.

But if you have a serious or obstinate condition, you will need to see a qualified Chinese herbalist for a correct diagnosis and remedy designed for your specific needs. A steady approach is intrinsic to Chinese herbalism which, like the herbalism of the West, does not pursue overnight cures. If yours is a chronic condition, a few courses of treatment are usually necessary.

Chinese herbalism can be used for health maintenance and prevention or can be used medicinally to treat specific conditions.

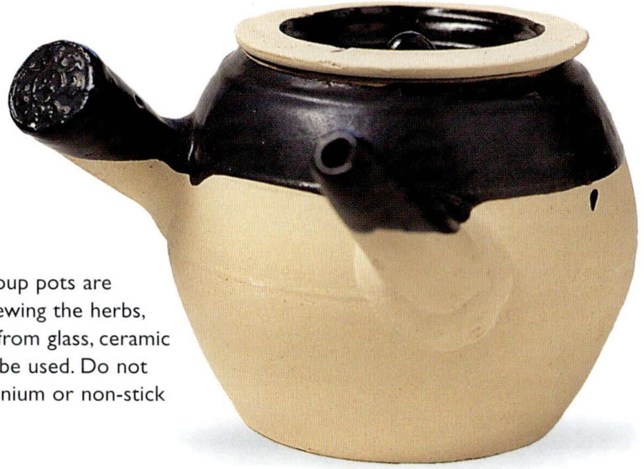

Traditional Chinese soup pots are recommended for brewing the herbs, but containers made from glass, ceramic or stainless steel can be used. Do not use plastic, iron, aluminium or non-stick cookware.

TAI CHI CHUAN

Tai Chi Chuan, meaning "supreme ultimate power", is the result of a meeting between traditional Chinese martial arts and a Taoist system of internal breathing. Today it is practised throughout China and the West as a form of moving meditation, a subtle, gentle exercise with a focus on deep breathing that also incorporates mental discipline and creative visualisation.

It is a minutely choreographed sequence of movements, with precise directions as to the placement of each part of your body, and each motion is co-ordinated with your breath. This sequence is known as the "form" and may be from five to 60 minutes in length. There are a number of different forms and, within them, different styles.

Tai Chi is aimed at slowing down the mind, refreshing the body, restoring balance, strenghtening the muscles and bringing about a reconnection of your body with your mind and your surroundings.

As an exercise system, Tai Chi has many levels and should be learnt under the guidance of an expert teacher. It may take some time for a person to learn the sequence of movements so that they can be performed without thinking. Some very proficient practitioners can learn "sets" which incorporate the use of swords or sticks. The practitioner will breathe deeply and rhythmically, activating the circulation of Qi. Then as the mind and body harmonise, a meditative aspect emerges almost without effort.

You can increase your personal Qi and ensure its smooth flow through your body by learning to breathe correctly. You are taught to breathe through your nose and into your abdomen in harmony with the movements.

Many of the movements draw inspiration from the natural world with names like "white crane spreads wings". When you perform this posture you are encouraged to visualise yourself as the white crane.

To perform Tai Chi effectively you need to incorporate these four disciplines:

1. **Relaxation** — stand easy, let go of any forcing, find strength through gentleness.

2. **Meditation** — focus your mind on each movement, visualise as you go, move slowly and evenly and feel the circular nature of all things.

3. **Harmony** — find harmony by moving all parts of your body as one.

4. **Breathing** — increase your Qi by breathing through your nose and bringing your breath down into your abdomen. Then relax your abdomen exhaling smoothly. Don't force your breath, breathe naturally and experience the tranquillity when your Qi connects you to all things.

Tai Chi will lift fitness levels and is useful in treating a range of imbalances including stress, depression, fatigue, asthma, digestive problems and back strain.

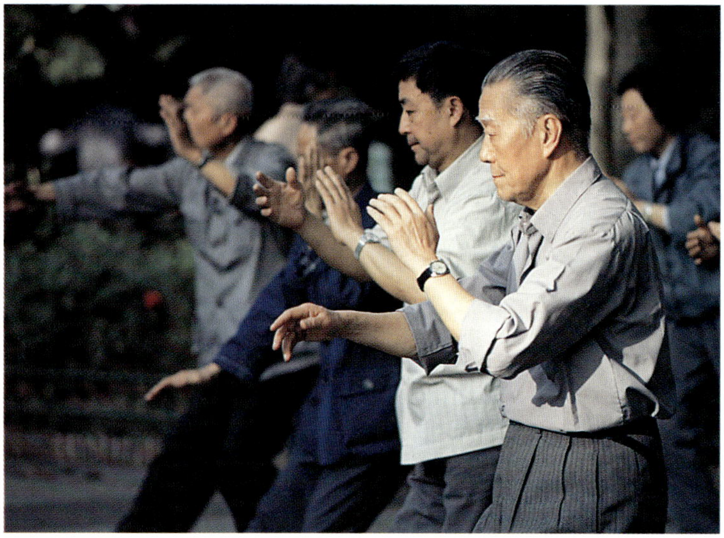

Fitness levels and age are not barriers to practising Tai Chi, and it has appeal to many due to its contrast with the "no pain, no gain" motivation of many Western exercise programs.

YOGA

THOSE UNFAMILIAR WITH YOGA MAY THINK OF IT AS AN INDIAN STYLE GET-FIT CLASS, BUT YOGA IS MUCH MORE THAN THAT. IT WORKS ON ALL ASPECTS OF HEALTH TO ENCOURAGE A STRONG BODY, A SHARP MIND, AND A REDUCTION IN THE EFFECTS OF STRESS.

The word yoga comes from the Sanskrit root word *yuj* which means to yoke or to bind. And this is the essence of yoga — to unify the physical body with the mind and with the vital energy flowing within. When these components move closer together, you experience a sense of harmony. In the modern world, life is busy and it is common to feel fragmented. Yoga helps to reconnect the fragments and bring calm to your existence.

WHAT DOES YOGA INVOLVE?

The practice of yoga involves grasping a number of basic techniques. It is the combination of breath, mind and body awareness which works together to bring about health and tranquillity.

These techniques include:

- physical postures (asanas) — the basis of yoga, these postures work gently to increase flexibility, strengthen the muscles and tone all body systems
- breathing exercises (pranayama) — help increase energy levels, calm the emotions and sharpen the mind
- meditation (dhyana) — brings a quietness to the whole being and offers refuge from internal and external stresses
- total relaxation (yoga nidra) — a deep relaxation of the body and mind which soothes and rejuvenates.

THE HISTORY OF YOGA

Yoga is thousands of years old. It was first developed in India as a philosophy of life and the practices were developed to sustain this philosophy.

Patanjali, a Hindu sage, was the first to rationalise and commit to writing the basic philosophies of yoga practice. He did this in eight concise aphorisms or small paragraphs known as the Yoga Sutras. These aphorisms, written about 200 BC, are easy to comprehend.

They offer a set of practices and principles for a healthy and contented life.

The eight limbs to yoga practice are:

1. Yama: moral codes of a universal nature
2. Niyama: personal conduct
3. Asanas: the practice of postures
4. Pranayama: breath control
5. Pratyahara: control of the senses
6. Dharana: the power of concentration
7. Dhyana: the stillness of meditation
8. Samadhi: contemplation and reflection

Yoga was first introduced to the Western world as a result of the process of colonisation of India during the 18th and 19th centuries. This interest has continued into the 20th century, with enthusiasm escalating rapidly in the "alternative" era of the 1960s and 1970s.

Today yoga is very popular in the West. In most cities and towns, yoga classes are available. The gentle exercise, the relaxation, and refuge from daily stress prove yoga to be an ideal pastime for the modern world.

IS YOGA SUITABLE FOR YOU?

With few exceptions, everyone can practise yoga. Yoga is suitable for people at all levels of fitness and all body shapes. It is equally suited to men and women, and people of all ages will benefit. It is the perfect activity to practise throughout a lifetime.

Children love yoga. As many of the poses imitate animals, children view them as fun. The calming attributes of yoga make it especially therapeutic for hyperactive children. The postures will also help the child develop a healthy body and good posture. See page 75.

For the elderly, yoga is an effective way to maintain a finely tuned body and peace of mind.

YOGA CLASSES

Although you can teach yourself yoga from books or video cassettes, these can't really be a substitute for a good yoga teacher. A teacher can guide your body into the postures ensuring no strain takes place and, most importantly, a teacher can make sure you are breathing correctly. Correct breathing techniques are essential to the practice of yoga.

There are now many yoga classes available for different types of yoga. For example:

- **hatha yoga** — this is a general term that refers to the practice of yoga postures. It teaches techniques to improve physical control of your body through postures and breathing techniques. These are designed to increase your level of energy or life force. Most beginners' hatha classes concentrate on gentle poses and include a relaxation session.
- **Iyengar yoga** — this is hatha yoga as adopted for the Western world by B.K.S. Iyengar. It is still the most popular form of yoga in these countries. The classes focus on a large spectrum of postures which strengthen and maintain the body.
- **Oki yoga** — this is a Japanese version of yoga.

Meditation and relaxation techniques are also taught in yoga classes. These are aimed at releasing physical and mental tension in order to strengthen an inner calmness of spirit.

Depending on the teacher and the style of yoga, some classes concentrate more on postures, while others emphasise breathing, meditation and relaxation techniques. The best way to find the ideal class for your own needs is to ask the teacher for a general description of the class content.

Sample a number of styles and classes, and see which you prefer.

YOGA AND WOMEN

There are many postures which are not recommended during menstruation. At this time, the temperature of the body is raised. Some women may be experiencing pain or generally feeling unwell. Concentrate on cooling and calming postures, for example, rests and gentle stretches. Avoid inverted and bending postures.

Yoga can be of great benefit physically and emotionally to the expectant and new mother. There are many postures and breathing techniques which will ease the birth process and help maintain vitality after the birth. See page 68.

However, it is essential that you consult a health practitioner and a yoga teacher before attempting any postures during pregnancy.

The best option is to attend special pre-natal yoga classes.

Always avoid any postures which constrict the abdomen.

PRACTISING YOGA

Yoga can be practised at any time during the day. First thing in the morning when the stomach is empty is a good time to do yoga as it will stretch and loosen your muscles and energise you for the day. Practising after work or before bed can be very beneficial to the body and mind, as you will release accumulated stress. Several short sessions throughout the day are ideal.

YOGA AND HEALTH

Yoga works because it balances health on three levels: the physical body, the mental sphere and the vital energy. In this way all contributing factors to ill-health are treated and harmony resides again.

Yoga practice complements all other health therapies. Whether the chosen treatment is modern medicine or one of the array of alternative health systems, yoga can be safely incorporated into the treatment routine. Yoga encourages self healing, strength of body and clarity of mind. This can only boost the healing process.

However, consult your health practitioner before beginning yoga for the first time, and discuss your health details with the yoga teacher who can give you postures suitable for your condition.

Not all postures are suitable for everyone.

There are some illnesses which should be approached with special care. See Box.

A YOGA SEQUENCE

A yoga sequence that you can easily incorporate into your daily exercise program is salute to the sun (Surya Namaskar). It can be used at any time to increase vitality, decrease stress and "massage" the internal organs. It is a set of stretches and bends formed into a flowing movement which can be performed slowly or dynamically. Traditionally there are 12 postures, each of which is associated with a sign of the zodiac. There is a different mantra which can be used with each posture.

The sequence is an effective way to get your energy flowing in the morning, but remember to start with a few warm-up exercises, especially if you are not long out of bed.

IMPORTANT

Before commencing yoga practice, it is advisable to consult a health practitioner if you have any of the following conditions:

- high blood pressure
- eye or ear problems
- ulcer
- cancer/tumor
- multiple sclerosis
- a recent operation
- heart problems
- vertigo
- hernia
- HIV/AIDS
- any long-term illness
- pregnancy.

If you do have any of the above conditions, it does not mean you are excluded from practising yoga. A carefully planned program will be both safe and therapeutic. It is important to know which postures to avoid — consult a teacher.

WARM-UP EXERCISES

1. Stand on one leg, your other leg extended in front of you. Stretch your foot and toes away from you.
2. Then, holding the same position with leg extended, stretch your foot and toes towards you.
   Do a few times and repeat with your other leg. Now, rotate your free ankle in one direction and then the other. Repeat with other ankle.
3. Reach for the sky. Stand on tip toes and reach your arms up over your head, extending the stretch through to your finger tips. Relax and repeat a few times.
4. Rotate each wrist, making the circles as big as you can.
5. Roll your shoulders forwards in large circles. Then roll your shoulders backwards.
6. With your arms and shoulders relaxed, drop your chin to your chest in a neck stretch.
7. Return your head to its normal position and tilt your head as far as possible to the right.
8. Now tilt your head as far as possible to the left.
9. With your hands and knees on the floor, hands below your shoulders, knees directly under your hips, stretch your spine like a cat does. First lift your head and buttocks so your spine lowers towards the floor.
10. Then allow your chin to move towards your chest, your buttocks to tuck under and your spine to curve upwards.

SALUTE TO THE SUN

It is important to move each step of this sequence in time with your breath. When you know the routine you can do it at a pace which best suits you. One leading yoga teacher says that three complete rounds each day is all you need to benefit from this exercise. Of course, you can do as many as you want. Some people choose to do as many as 30 rounds, using salute to the sun as a type of yoga aerobic workout. However, do not push yourself too hard — increase the number of rounds gradually.

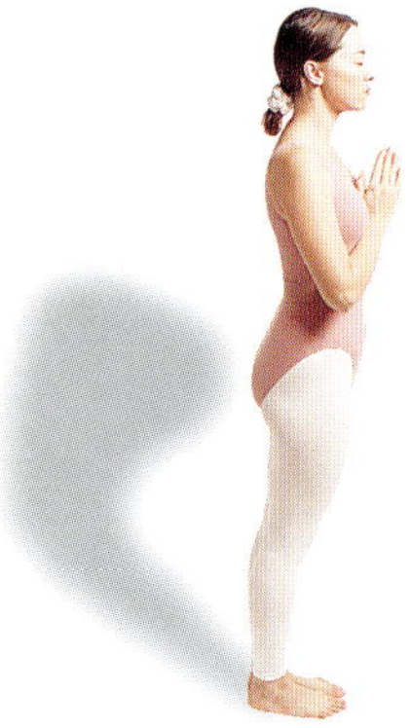

POSITION 1

1. In a standing position, bring your hands together in a prayer position at chest level. Relax your body and breathe normally.
2. Breathing in, raise your arms over your head so that your chest opens, and bend back slightly, looking towards the ceiling. Keep your head in line with your arms.
3. Breathing out, bend forward so your palms rest either side of your feet. (Bend your knees if necessary.)
4. Breathing in, take your right foot back, lower your right knee to the floor, and tuck the toes of the right foot under. Angle your head slightly and gaze towards the ceiling. Feel your hips move towards the floor. Your left leg should be bent and your arms straight.
5. Breathing out, take your left foot back to your right foot and stretch so your buttocks move toward the ceiling. Keep palms and heels pressed on the floor, and drop your head between your arms. Imagine your body forming two sides of an equilateral triangle — feel the spine lengthen from the base. Be sure to keep your arms and legs straight.
6. Holding the breath, bring your knees to the floor. Push your buttocks backwards and upwards so that you can slide along the floor. Push your upper torso forward between your arms. Try to keep your elbows close to your body.

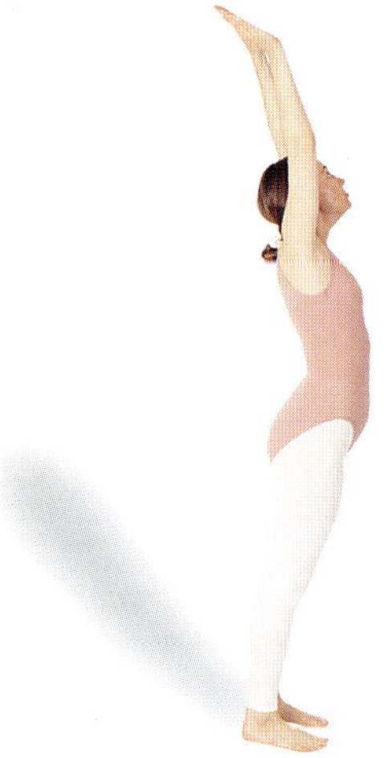

POSITION 2

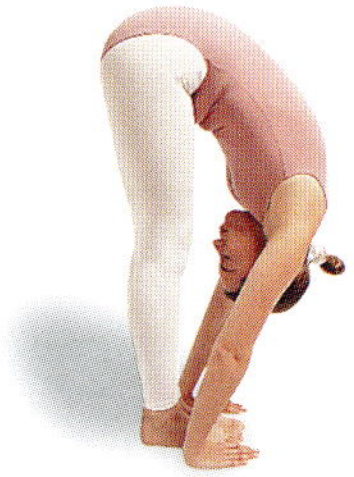

POSITION 3

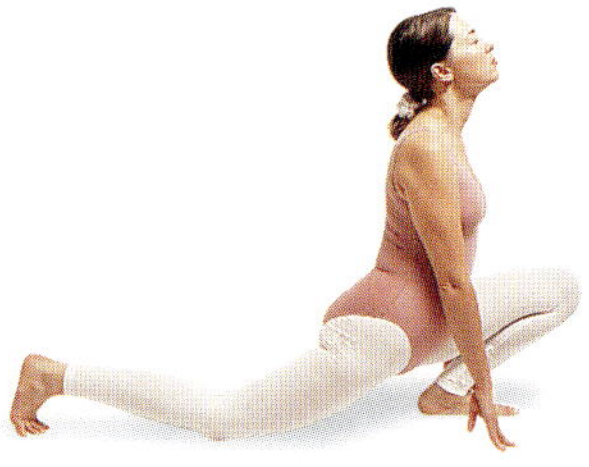

POSITION 4

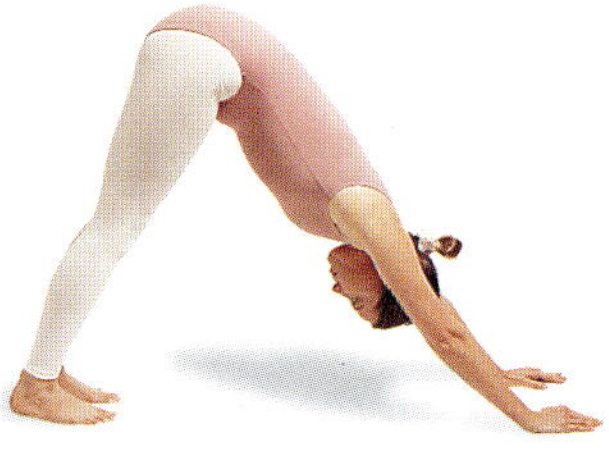

POSITION 5

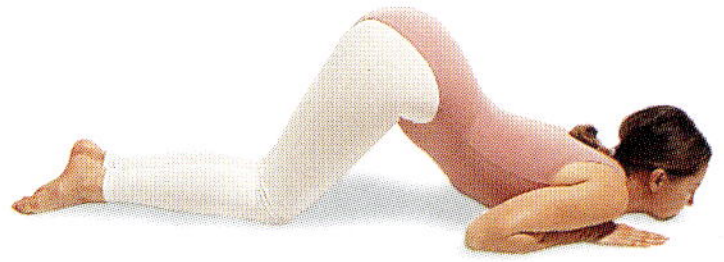

POSITION 6

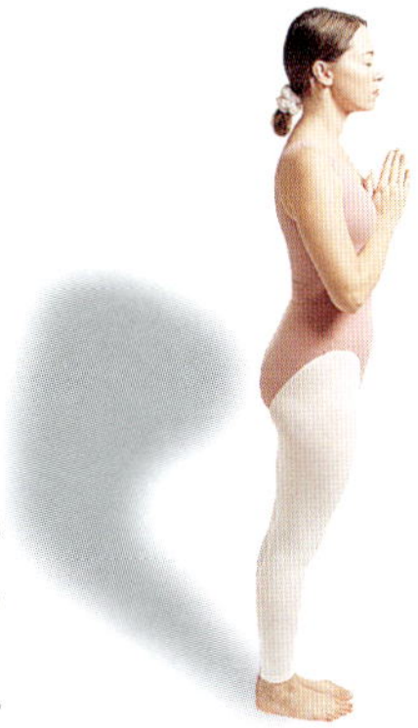

POSITION 12

7. Breathing in, continue to slide your body forwards, lowering the hips onto the floor and raising your upper torso from the waist. Stretch the spine and neck, tilting the head back.
8. Breathing out, bring your toes under again, palms flat on the floor, move your buttocks to the ceiling, press your heels into the floor and drop your head between your arms. (*See position 5.*)
9. Breathing in, step your left foot between your hands and bend your right knee to the floor, look slightly towards the ceiling and allow your hips to move downwards. (*See position 4.*)
10. Breathing out, bring your right foot to your left foot. (*See position 3.*)
11. Breathing in, straighten while lifting your arms above your head and bend back slightly. (*See position 2.*)
12. Breathing out, bring your hands together in the prayer position. (*See position 1.*)

Repeat the whole cycle but this time step back with the left leg instead of the right in positions 4 and 9.

Now you have completed one full round of salute to the sun. Once you have finished as many rounds as desired, rest on the floor in the breathing to relax position (see page 193) and allow your breath to return to normal.

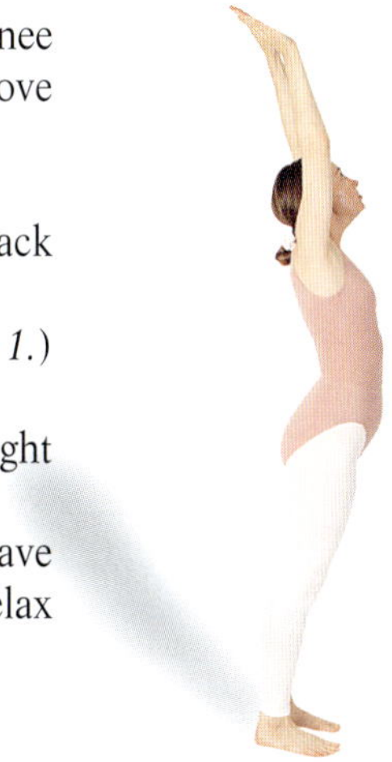

POSITION 11

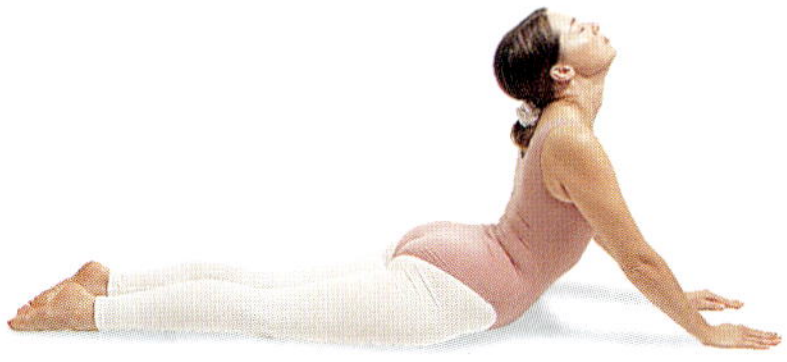

POSITION 7

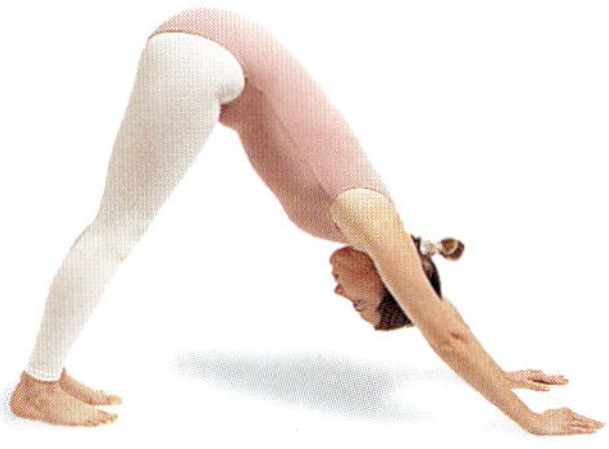

POSITION 8

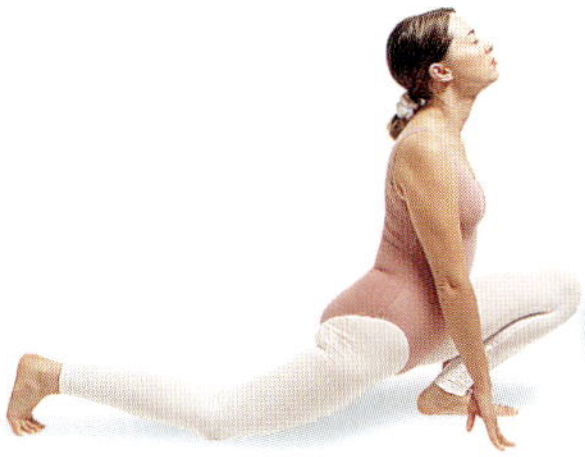

POSITION 9

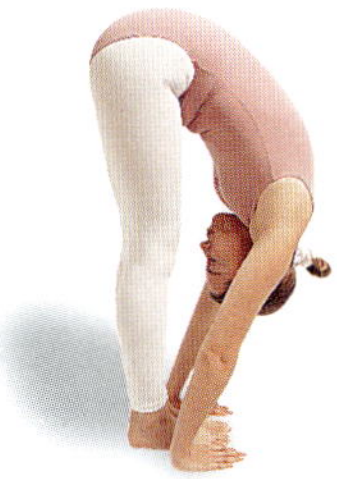

POSITION 10

BASIC ADVICE

- Unless your room is carpeted, you will need a thin mat on which to practise your exercises. It should not be soft or spongy. Yoga mats can be purchased from rubber stores and some yoga schools. Camping mats are also suitable.
- One or two light blankets or large towels are required for some postures.
- Always wear light comfortable clothing that does not restrict the abdomen.
- Ensure your bladder is empty.
- Do not practise yoga on a full stomach. Wait several hours after a heavy meal and an hour or two after a light meal.
- Pay attention to your breathing. Always breathe through your nose, not your mouth. Unless instructed, do not hold your breath.
- Always ease into a posture — do not force or push beyond your limits. Work at your own pace.
- Check your alignment — a mirror may help.
- Focus on what you are doing and be aware of your body and how you feel.
- There are many different kinds of yoga postures. Some work to loosen our bodies, others to encourage stillness in our minds. Yoga is about balance and harmony. Backward-bending postures such as the cobra can be balanced with forward-bending postures such as the butterfly.

EXAMPLES OF POSTURES

- Inverted postures included in this book are the half-shoulder stand, the inverted corpse and the plough.
- Forward-bending postures include the nerve stretch, neck tension release, right-angle stretch and yoga mudra.
- Breathing exercises include alternate nostril breathing, balloon-blowing breathing, breathing and stretching, breathing to relax, chair breathing and deep relaxation.

ALTERNATE NOSTRIL BREATHING

KNOWN AS NADI SHODAN PRANAYAMA

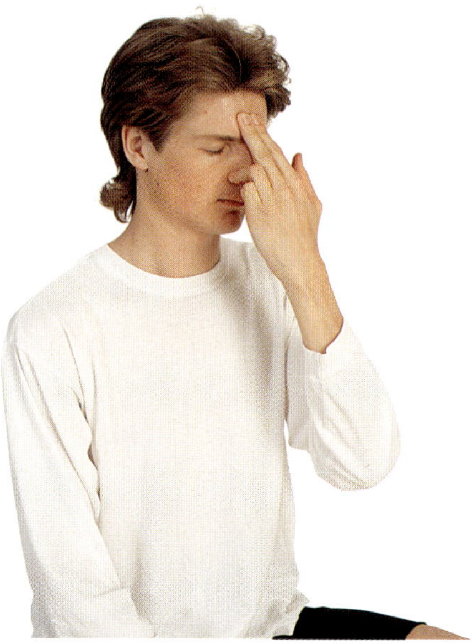

1. Using your left hand, place the index and middle fingers on your brow, centred between your eyes. Rest your thumb beside your left nostril and your ring finger beside your right nostril.

2. Block the left nostril with your thumb and slowly and evenly inhale through your right nostril.

3. Block the right nostril with your ring finger and slowly and evenly exhale through the left nostril.

4. Next, inhale through the left and exhale through the right. Keep the inhalations and exhalations the same length. Continue for a few minutes — the time of each breath will become longer as you practise.

BALLOON-BLOWING BREATHING

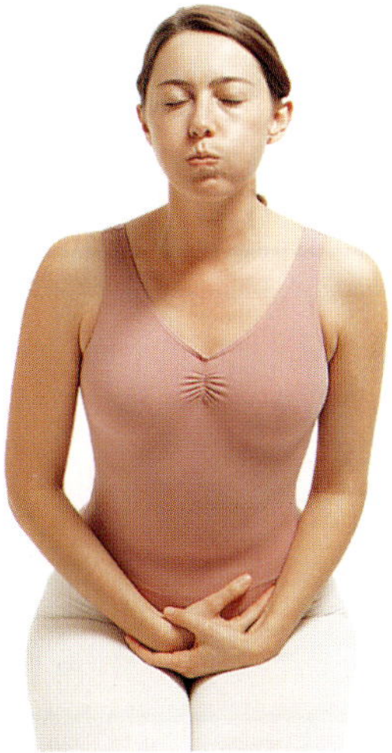

1. Imagine you are blowing up a balloon. Breathe in deeply then breathe out through pursed lips. Make sure you dispel all the air in your lungs. Do not force the air and make sure you allow yourself time to normalise your breathing by taking a couple of deep and slow breaths before "blowing up the next balloon".

BREATHING AND STRETCHING

1. Lie on your back. Breathe in and expand your rib cage, then breathe out and contract your rib cage. Make sure your abdomen is relaxed during this exercise. Repeat this breathing technique five times.

2. Breathe in and stretch your arms behind your head and push your toes down as far as they will go.

3. Breathe out and release your body from the stretch letting your hands go to your sides.

4. Repeat this exercise four times.

BREATHING TO RELAX

KNOWN AS SAVASANA OR THE CORPSE

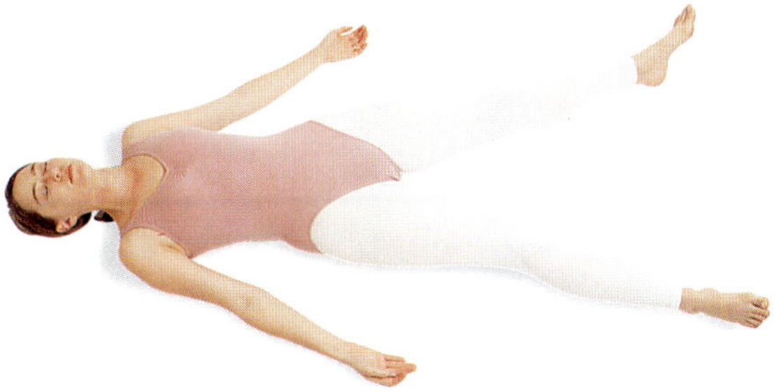

1. Lie on your back, lift your knees to your chest and slide your legs down to the floor. This will reduce the gap between your lower back and the floor.

2. Spread your legs about three feet apart and your arms about two feet from your body. Keep your palms facing upwards.

3. Be aware of your breath and your body as it breathes. Count ten of your deep and even breaths. Feel your next ten breaths going in and out of your body and expanding your abdomen. For the next ten breaths, feel the air coming into your body is energising it while the outgoing air is relaxing it.

4. When you have finished don't rush up from this exercise — give yourself time to adjust to normal pace.

BUTTERFLY

KNOWN AS BADDHA KONASANA

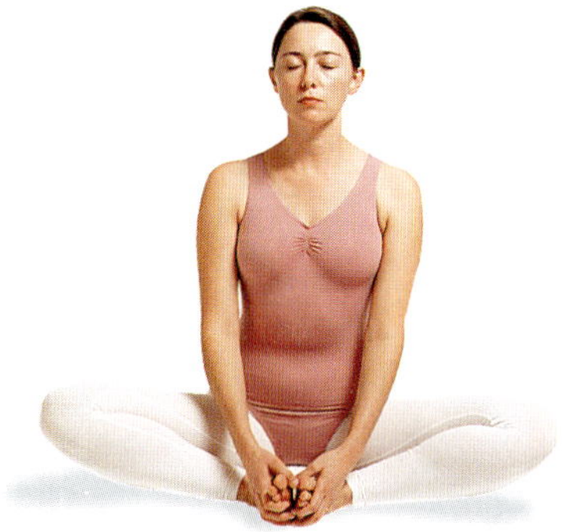

1. Sit on the floor with your knees bent. Bring the bottoms of your feet together and hold them with your hands pressing on the balls of your feet with your thumbs. Pull them in towards your body.

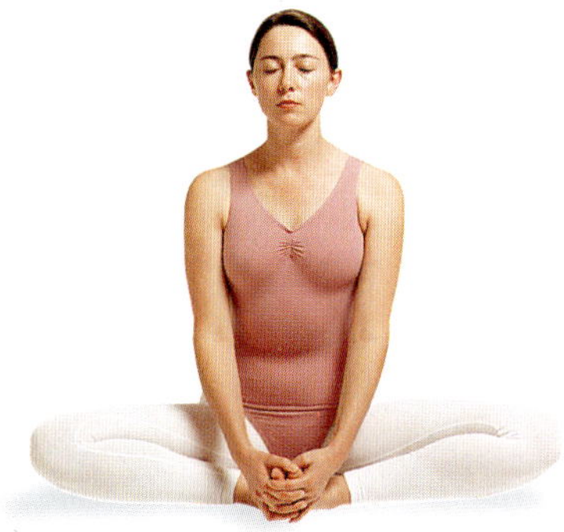

2. Widen your thighs and lower your knees as far as they will go towards the floor — don't worry if they don't touch the ground, and don't force them. Breathe evenly and deeply for a few minutes (5 to 10 minutes if possible).

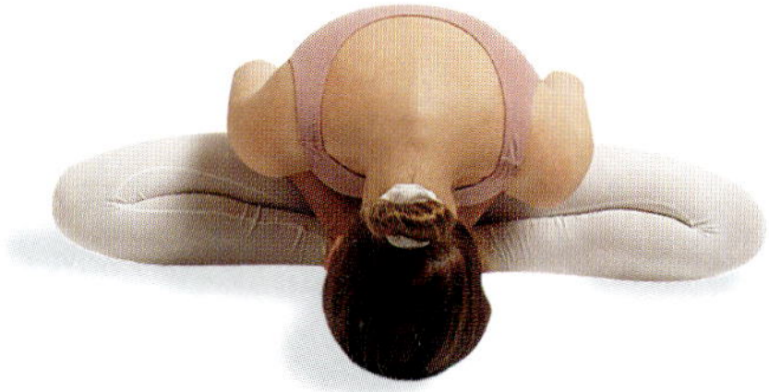

3. If you wish, incorporate a forward bend. Breathe in as you straighten your spine and breathe out as you bring your forehead towards your toes without hunching your back. Repeat this ten times but be careful not to stretch to the point where there is pain. Don't feel you have to bring your forehead to your toes, just bend as far as it is comfortable.

VARIATION

Known as supine butterfly or Supta Baddha Konasana

A soothing variation of this position can be even better, particularly for period pain.

Lie down on the floor on your back but with your knees bent and your soles together as described above. Your arms and hands can lie out at your sides. You may like to have a firm pillow or folded blanket or bolster lengthwise under your back for support. You can also position yourself so that your toes are against a wall — this can help you maintain the posture.

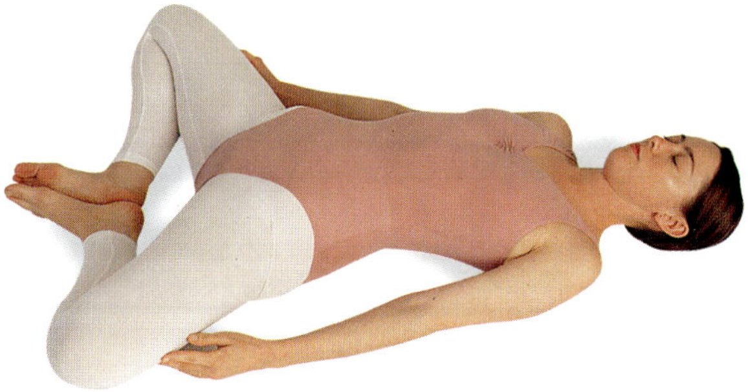

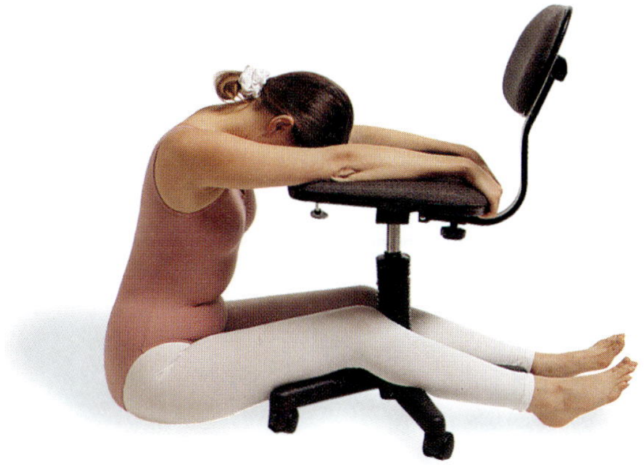

CHAIR BREATHING

1. Sit on the floor with your legs stretched out under a chair (you may need to put a cushion under your buttocks if the floor is uncomfortable). Lay your head and arms on the seat.

2. Pull your whole body tense from your head to your toes

3. Next, release each part of your body, one bit at a time.

4. Move your head back and forth slowly about five times.

5. Repeat another five times but this time breathe in as your head goes back and out as your head goes forward.

6. Continue to move your head back and forth for another five counts but this time say "Ahhh" while coming forward and synchronise the sound with the movement.

7. Finish by doing five more movements but this time with the sound "Mmmm" rather than "Ahhh".

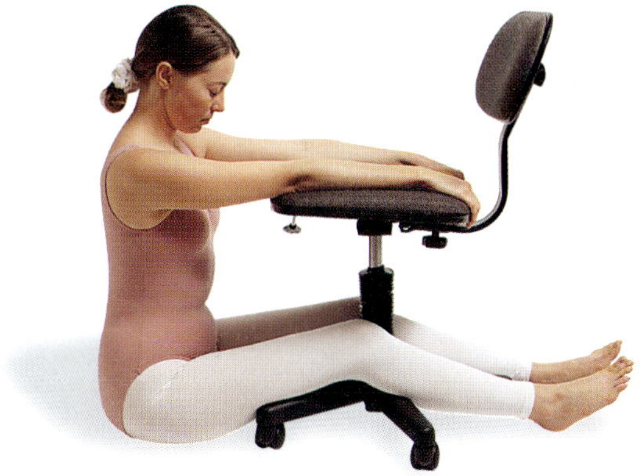

CHEST-OPENING POSITION

1. Fold or roll a light blanket or towel so that it is about 1 metre long and 15 cm wide. Place this on the floor.

1. Lie on the floor on your back with the blanket underneath the bottom part of your shoulder blades. The blanket should lie crossways — you can tuck the ends between your upper arms and your torso. Your feet should be a small distance apart, your arms resting out to your sides with the palms facing upwards.

2. Close your eyes. Let every muscle in your body soften and relax. Breathe deeply and slowly through your nose for 5 to 7 minutes.

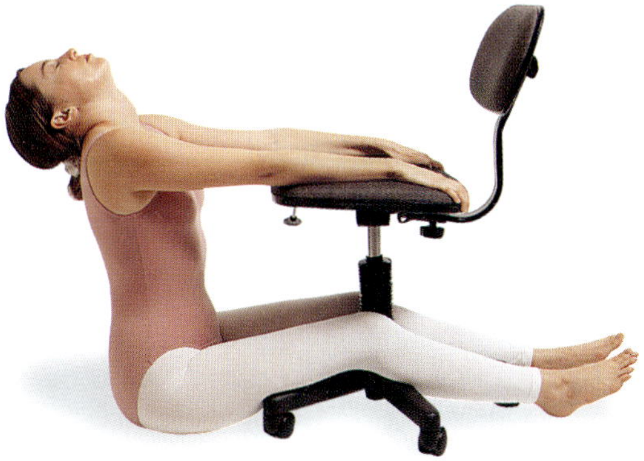

COBRA

KNOWN AS BHUJANGASANA

CAUTION: *Do not attempt this exercise if you have a peptic ulcer, hernia, hyperthyroidism, or have had recent abdominal surgery. Avoid during menstruation and take care if you have high blood pressure.*

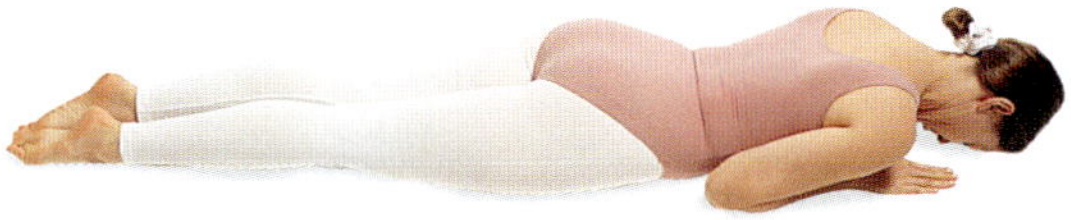

1. Lie on your stomach with the palms of your hands in line with your shoulders on the floor and your elbows close to your body. Place your forehead on the floor and keep your feet together.

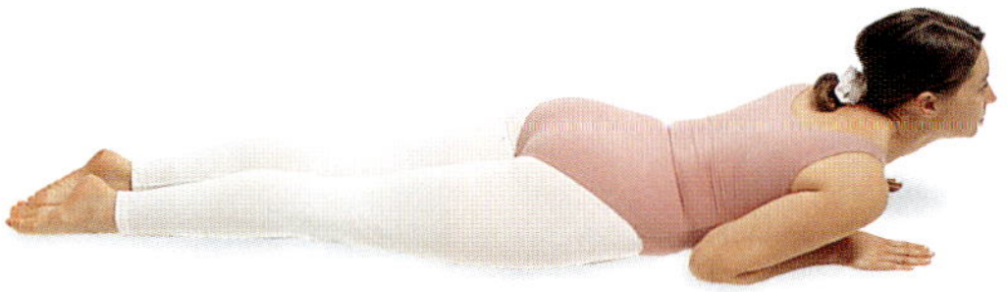

2. Inhale then exhale and slowly begin to raise your head and then shoulders off the floor while keeping your legs relaxed.

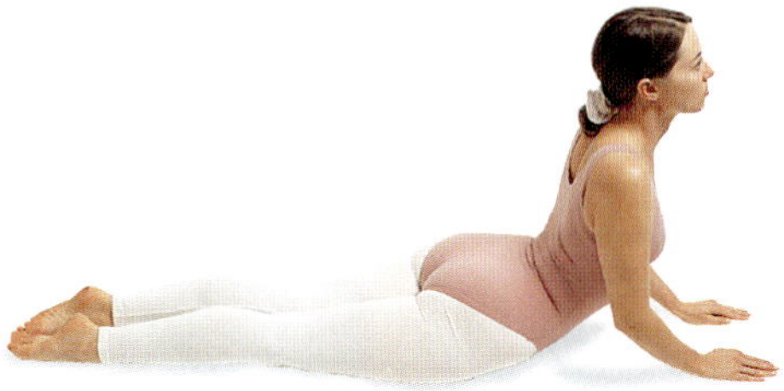

3. Continue to raise the chest and lengthen the arms, keeping the navel towards the floor. Make sure you don't straighten your elbows, keep your thighs and hips on the floor and your shoulders down.

4. Exhale then lower your upper body, in reverse order, until your forehead is once again touching the floor. Rest briefly with your head to one side.

Repeat this exercise four times then rest. Keep breathing while in the pose then come down on an exhalation.

DEEP RELAXATION

KNOWN AS YOGA NIDRA

1. Lie on the floor or in bed in the corpse position (see breathing to relax exercise). Cover yourself lightly. Close your eyes — you could cover them with an eyebag or small folded towel.

2. Inhale and squeeze every muscle in your body as tightly as possible. Then with one strong exhalation, release every muscle. Let your body become heavy—so heavy you could not even raise an arm if you tried.

3. Listen to the sounds outside the room. Observe these sounds. What can you hear? Then concentrate on the space around you. Can you hear any noises? Can you smell anything? What is the temperature like? Finally, focus on your body. Hear the breath in and out. Feel it. Follow it as it moves through your body. (You may like to incorporate the sectional breathing exercise). Your mind and body is still and quiet.

4. Now, relax each part of the body in turn. In your mind, name each part and imagine it becoming even more heavy and relaxed. Start with the fingers of your right hand: right thumb, second finger, third, fourth, little finger, palm, back of hand, forearm, elbow, upper arm, right shoulder, neck, head, right side of back, right buttock, the thigh, knee, lower leg, ankle, big toe, second toe, third, fourth, little toe. When the whole right side of your body is relaxed, move your attention to the left side. Release the muscles of the face — the forehead, eyes, nose, mouth, jaws, ears. Let go of the chest and abdomen. Your whole body is completely relaxed. Go back to quietly observing your breath.

NOTE: *You can "return to the world" after this exercise. Slowly bring your awareness back to the space around you then stretch your whole body and open your eyes. Rest for a while on your right side before getting up.*

FOOT STRETCH

1. Lie on your back on the floor or on your bed with your legs straight. Inhale and flex your feet, pulling your toes back towards you while breathing in. Release and exhale.

2. Push the outside of both feet towards the floor and inhale. Release and exhale.

3. Push the inside of your feet towards the floor and inhale. Release and exhale.

4. Repeat this whole sequence five times.

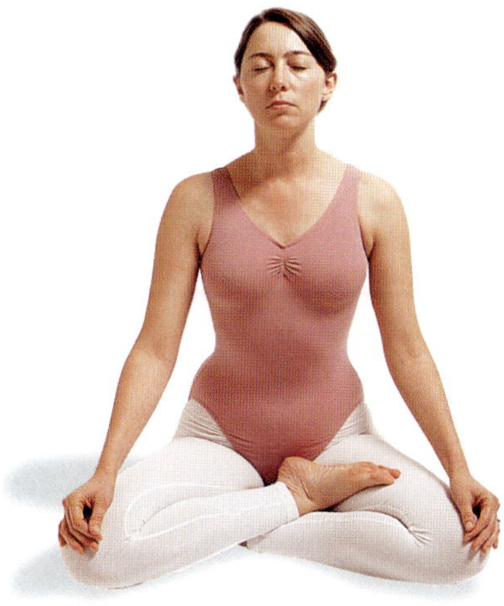

HALF-LOTUS POSE

This posture is a classic meditation posture, as is the full lotus posture. See page 152 for more information on meditation.

1. Sit on the floor with your right foot resting on your left thigh and your left foot tucked under your right thigh. A folded blanket or pillow beneath the buttocks will help keep the spine erect and aid comfort. Sit up and make sure your back is straight. Breathe deeply and rhythmically while your eyes are closed.

HALF-SHOULDER STAND

CAUTION: *Do not attempt this exercise if you have high blood pressure, fluid retention, heart problems, eye or ear problems, an enlarged thyroid or spleen. Avoid during menstruation.*

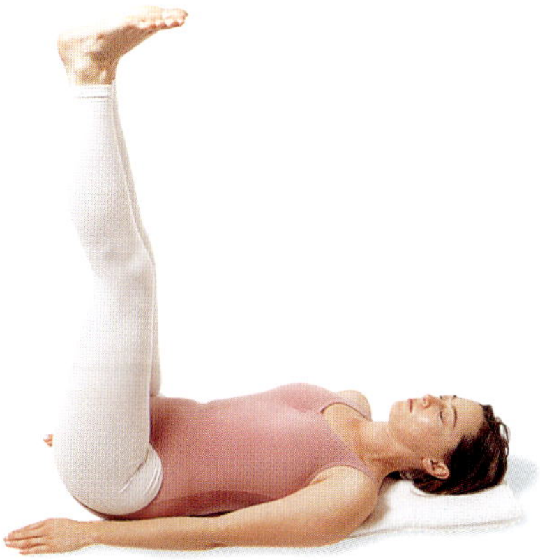

1. Place a folded towel or blanket on the floor and lie on your back with your shoulders and neck resting on the towel. While breathing in, raise your legs.

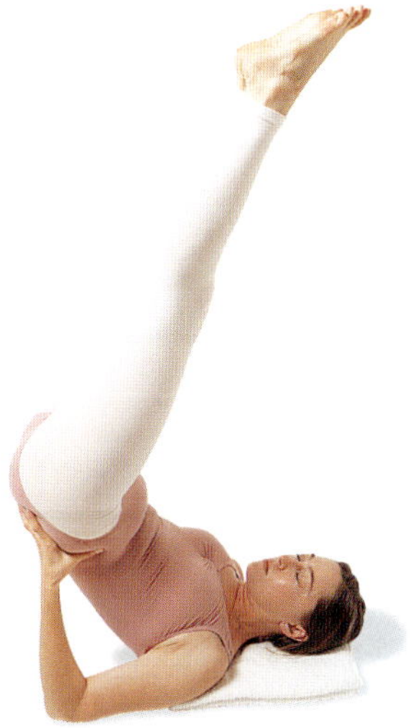

2. Breathe out and at the same time raise your legs higher by bringing your hips off the floor and supporting them with your hands (your elbows should be on the floor/towel). Hold this position for three counts while breathing normally.

3. Let your legs go with your hands and roll out of the position while exhaling.

HALF-WHEEL POSE

CAUTION: *Do not attempt this exercise if you are pregnant or if you have a fever.*

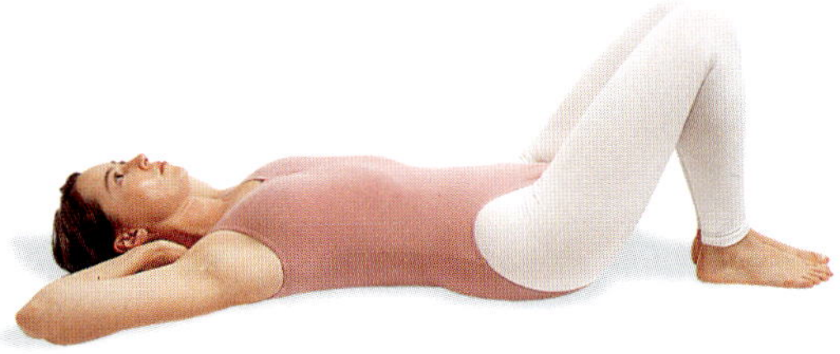

1. Lie on your back with your knees bent and your feet flat on the floor. Cup your hands and put them under your neck with your knuckles and backs of your hands together. Make sure your smallest finger knuckles are pressing on the base of your skull. Spread your index finger and thumb apart.

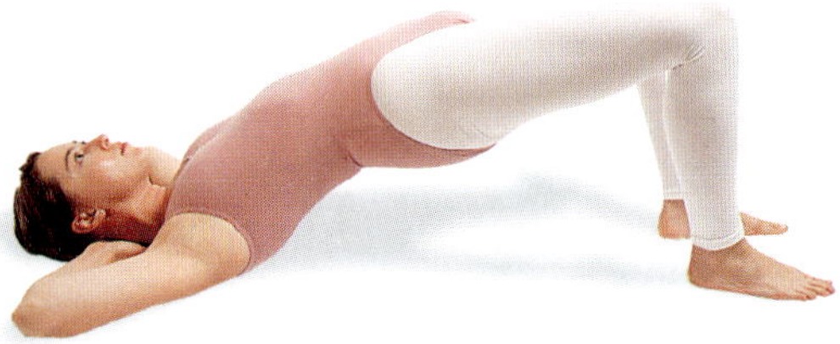

2. Breathe in and lift your hips off the ground. Keep this position for twenty counts while breathing deeply. Breathe out then gently lower your spine to the ground, vertebrae by vertebrae, from the top to the base. Lie on your back and relax.

HEAD ROTATION

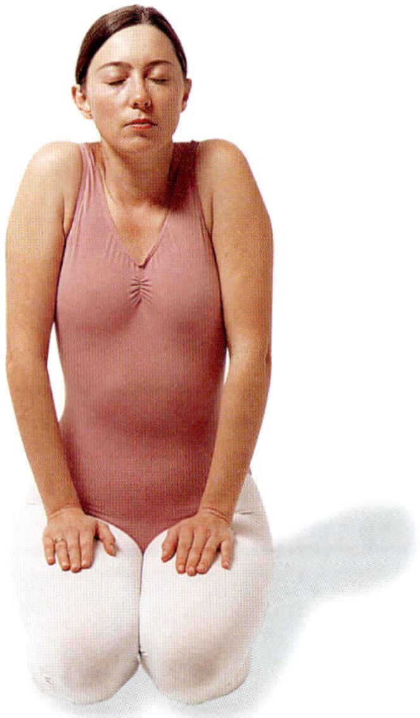

1. Bring your shoulders up to your ears, hold for three seconds then release them.

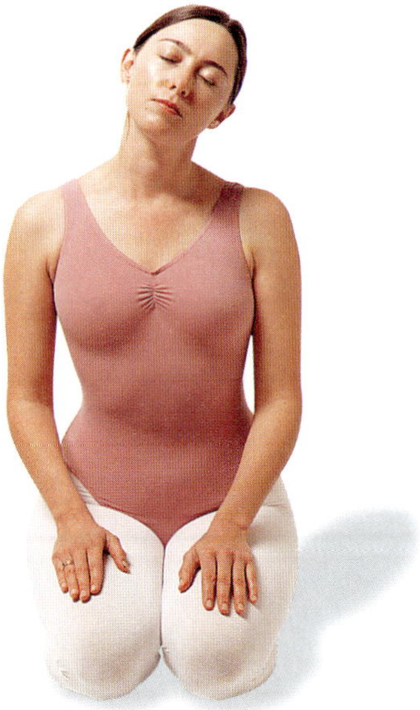

2. Gently bring your left ear towards your left shoulder.
3. Hold then release to normal position.
4. Do the same again with your right ear and shoulder.

Make sure you hold each shoulder as high as possible towards your ear and make slow, gentle movements.

HEAD-TO-KNEE EXERCISE

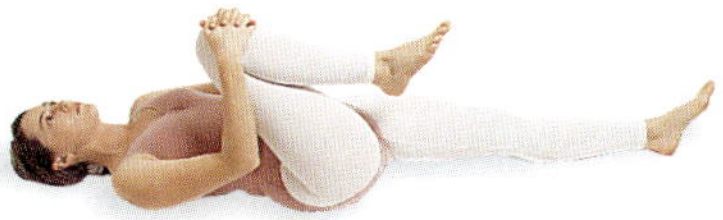

1. Lie on your back with your arms by your sides and your legs together. Breathe in and out and then bend your right leg and hug it towards your chest.

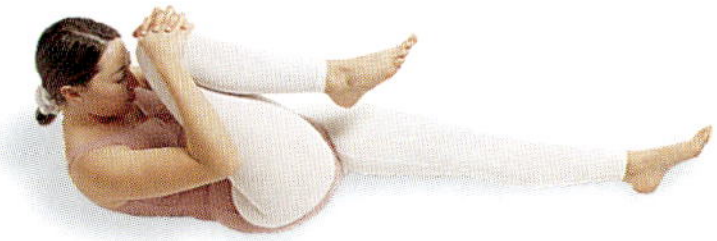

2. Breathe in slowly and as you are breathing out bring your head towards your knee, pulling your abdomen in to release all the air. Inhale and rest your head then breathe out.

3. Repeat this exercise three times with alternative legs. When you are finished rest on your back for a few minutes.

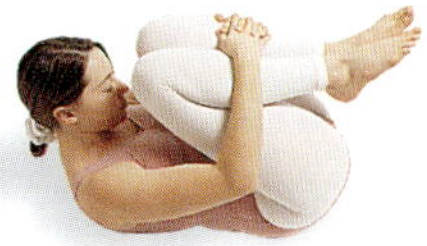

VARIATION

Try the above with both legs as well. Keep your breathing synchronised.

HEADACHE TENSION RELEASE

1. Lie on your stomach and place your forehead on the floor. Check that your feet are about 30 cm (1 ft) apart. Put your hands behind your head so that you are pressing the base of your skull with your thumbs while your elbows are touching the floor.

2. Breathe in as you lift your head, arms and feet 10 cm (4 in) off the ground. Breathe deeply for about 1 minute.

3. Relax and rest your head on one side with your arms by your side.

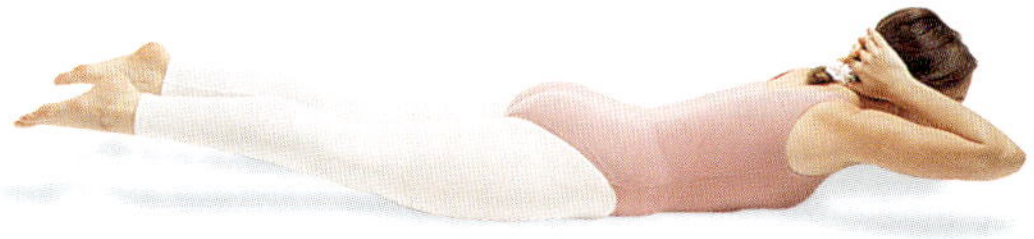

INVERTED CORPSE

ALSO KNOWN AS A WALL STAND

CAUTION: *Do not attempt this exercise if you have high blood pressure, heart problems, eye or ear problems, an enlarged thyroid or spleen. Avoid during menstruation.*

1. Lie on your back and raise your legs against a wall either vertically or at a 45 degree angle, keeping them straight — you may like to put a few folded blankets under your buttocks for added comfort. Cover your eyes with an eyebag, scarf or a folded, small towel. Relax and focus on your breathing. Stay in this position for about 5 minutes breathing deeply. You can move your legs apart so they are split.

When you have practised this exercise quite a few times you may be able to gradually build up to holding it for up to 20 minutes. Don't worry if you fall asleep in this position — the worst thing that can happen is that your legs go a bit numb.

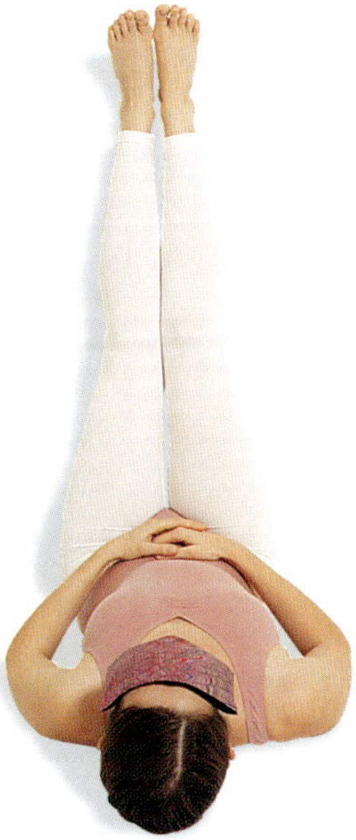

LIFTING THE HEAD

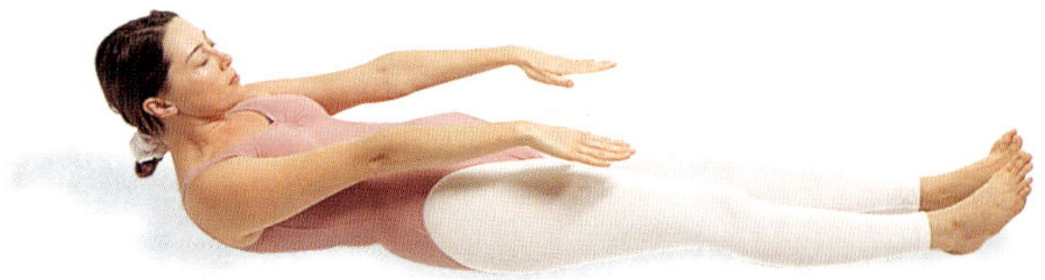

1. Lie on the floor on your back and inhale. Exhale while raising your head, shoulders and arms straight out in front of you. Hold this position for about 30 counts.

2. Inhale and relax.

Repeat this exercise 10 times then relax for a minute and do another 10.

If you feel any pain in your neck or abdomen while doing this exercise stop for a minute; when you start again only raise yourself as much as is comfortable.

NAUSEA RELIEF

KNOWN AS SUPTA VIRASANA

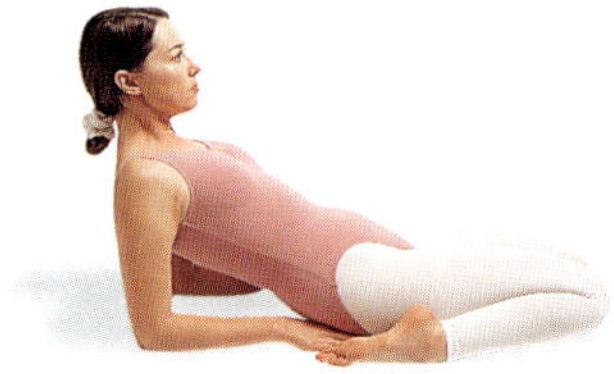

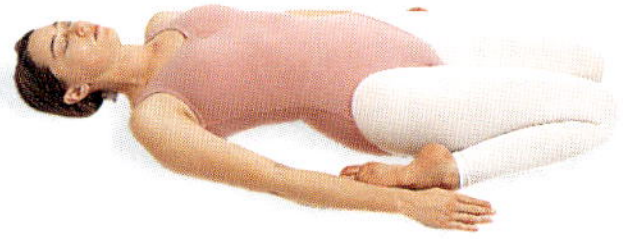

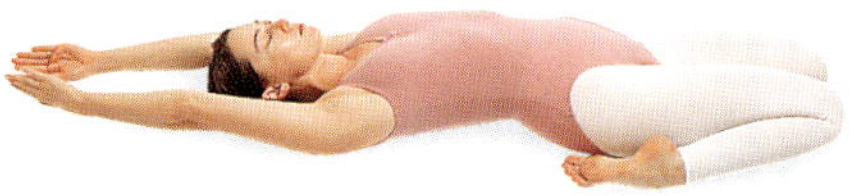

1. Sit on your heels with your knees close together and your feet positioned in a straight line near your hips — your bottom between your heels and resting on the edge of a bolster or a blanket/towel that has been folded lengthwise. Breathe out then lean back on your elbows.

2. Lean even further back until you are lying back along the floor by placing your arms down beside you and stretching them out. Your head and back should be supported along the pillow, blanket or bolster.

3. Take your arms over your head and lay them out straight. Hold this position for as long as it is comfortable — preferably 3 to 5 minutes — and breathe evenly and deeply.

To get up, place your arms once again beside you and lift yourself slowly on your elbows. You can keep your knees apart while you are doing this exercise if it makes it easier for you. Once you are well practised you will be able to do it with your knees together.

VARIATION

Known as Virasana

The simple sitting pose at the beginning of position 1 will also stretch the stomach meridian and thus help with nausea and stomach ache.

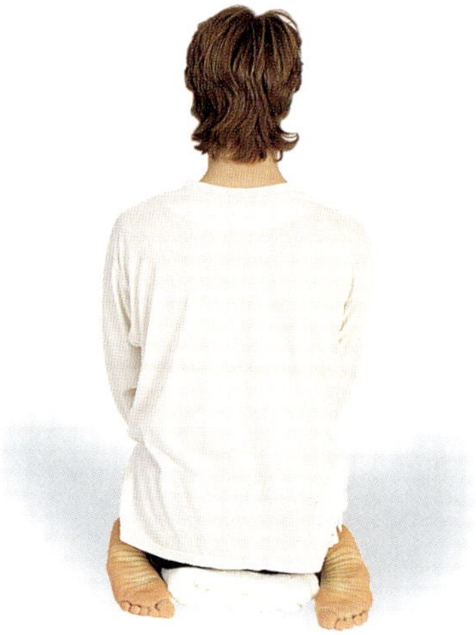

NECK TENSION RELEASE

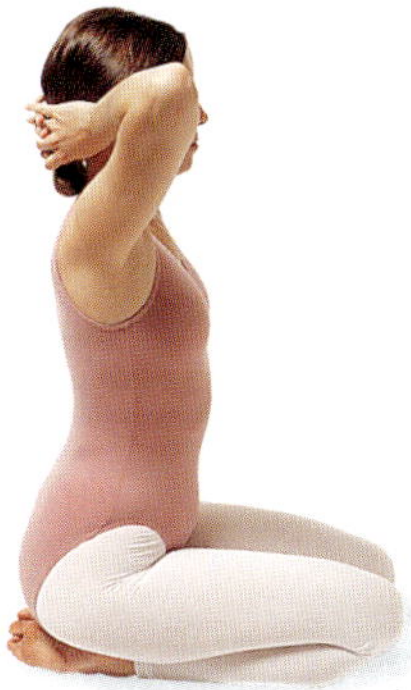

1. Kneel on the floor and sit on your heels. Breathe in then clasp your hands behind your neck.

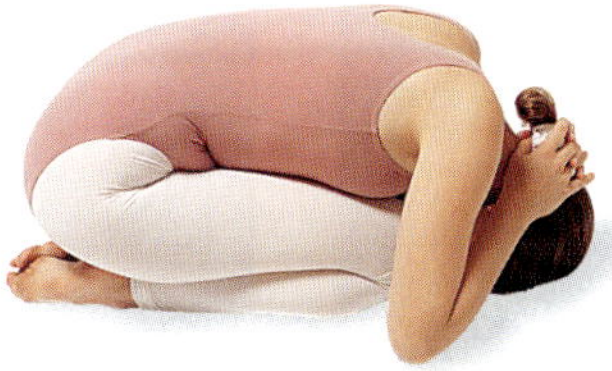

2. Lean forward as you breathe out and put your head on the floor while tucking your chin into your chest.

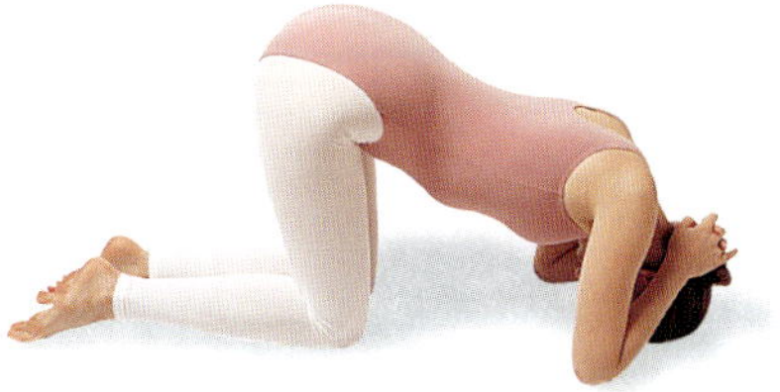

3. Lift your buttocks upwards and put a little weight onto the top of your head (not too much as you should be careful not to strain your neck muscles). Breathe deeply.

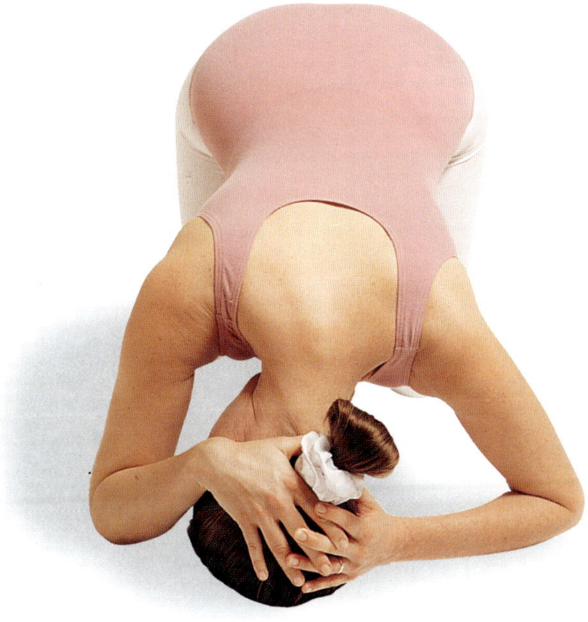

4. Gently turn your head to each side and lean forward to stretch each side of your neck.

5. Release yourself from this position and lie on your back for a few minutes breathing deeply.

VARIATION

If you can't get your head to the floor simply stretch your neck to the ceiling with your chin tucked in slightly. Do this for a few minutes while you are in an upright position on your knees. Pretend someone is pulling you up by a string which is placed on the crown of your head.

NERVE STRETCH

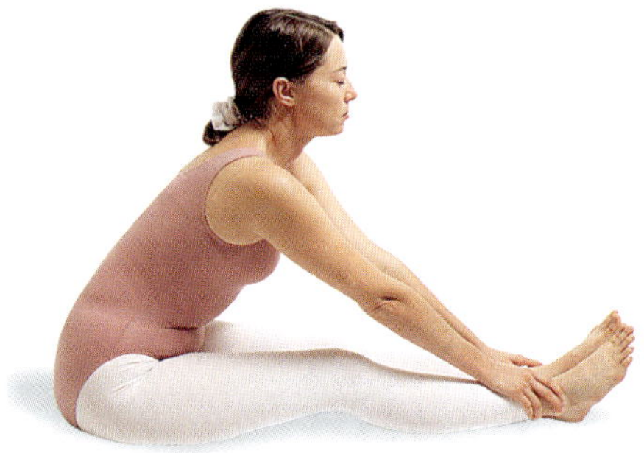

1. Sit on the floor with your legs stretched out in front of you. Breathe in and lean forward and hold your legs at the furthest point you can without causing pain.

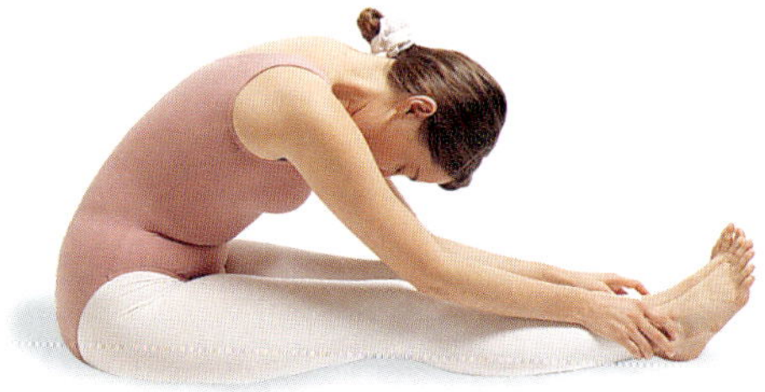

2. Breathe out while you pull your back away from your legs in an arch. Keep holding onto your legs while you do this but make sure they are on the floor.

3. Repeat this exercise five times, starting very slowly. You may find that the deeper you breathe the easier the stretch will be. Lie on your back to rest after completing the repetitions.

4. Follow this exercise with the cobra (see page 196) as this stretches your back the other way thus avoiding strain. If your back causes you problems while doing this exercise, you should consult a yoga teacher.

PELVIC FLOOR EXERCISE

1. Lie on your back (you may do this in bed) and inhale while squeezing your pelvic muscles (specifically, the perineum) for a count of five.

2. Exhale and release the squeeze.

3. Take a minute to relax, breathing in once and out once, then repeat.

THE PLOUGH

CAUTION: *If you have a bad back consult your doctor before trying this exercise. Do not practise this posture if you have high blood pressure or sciatica. Avoid during menstruation.*

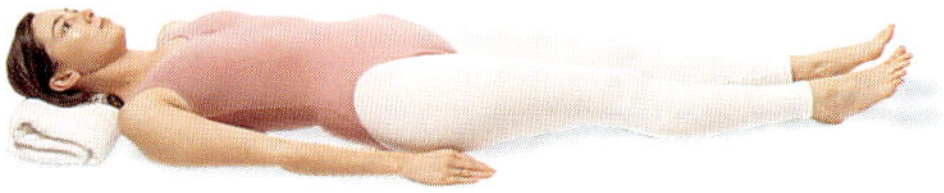

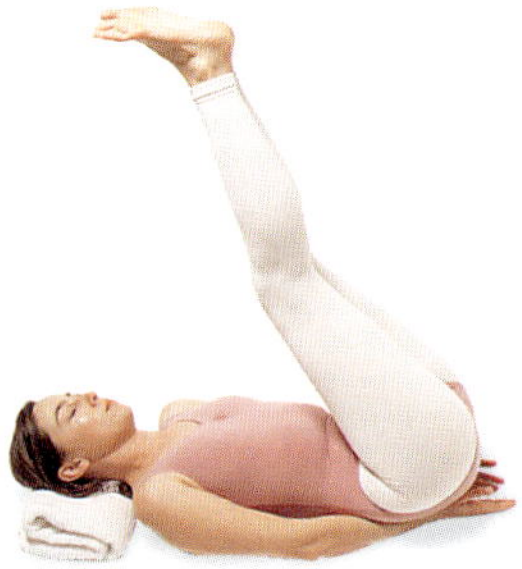

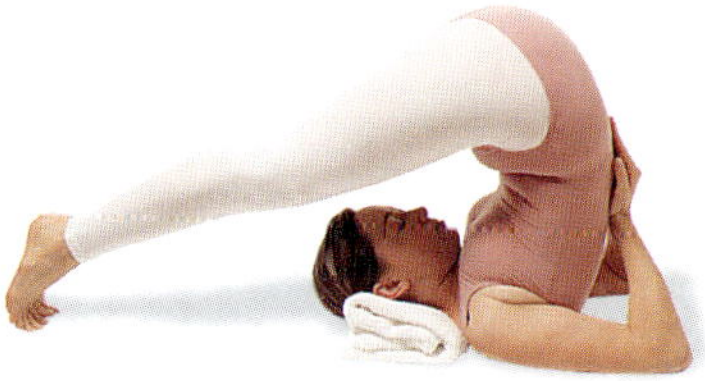

1. Lie on your back with your hands at your sides. Breathing out, raise your legs, keeping them straight and using the stomach muscles for strength.

2. As you raise the legs, begin to bend the hips upwards then the rest of your torso. Raise the buttocks toward the ceiling and gently lower the legs, toes touching the floor behind your head. If you can't reach the floor, rest your shins on a chair or your feet against a wall. Keep the head towards the chest and try to keep your legs straight. Support the back with your arms. Try to keep the elbows in (a belt tied above the elbows may prevent them slipping). Relax into the position, breathing steadily. Hold for a comfortable period only (preferably 3 to 5 minutes but you can start at 1 minute and build up).

3. Gradually uncurl the body onto the floor. Relax on your back while breathing deeply. You may like to follow this exercise with the exercise suggested for nausea relief (Supta Virasana).

A folded blanket under your shoulders for this exercise is recommended for comfort and support. Be very careful of your back and neck. If you experience any pain when you get into the position gently unroll your body and take a break lying on your back.

RIGHT-ANGLE STRETCH

1. Stand facing a wall with your feet 30 cm to 1 metre apart.

2. Bend forward from the hips until your upper torso is at right angles to your legs. Keep your back straight and your head in line with the spine so that you are looking down.

3. Reach your hands out to the wall so that your arms are straight and parallel to the floor. Your legs should still be straight and parallel to the wall. You may have to adjust your distance.

4. Push into the wall from your palms so that you can really stretch along the back. Do this for a couple of minutes, while breathing slowly and deeply through your nose.

ROCKING BACKWARDS

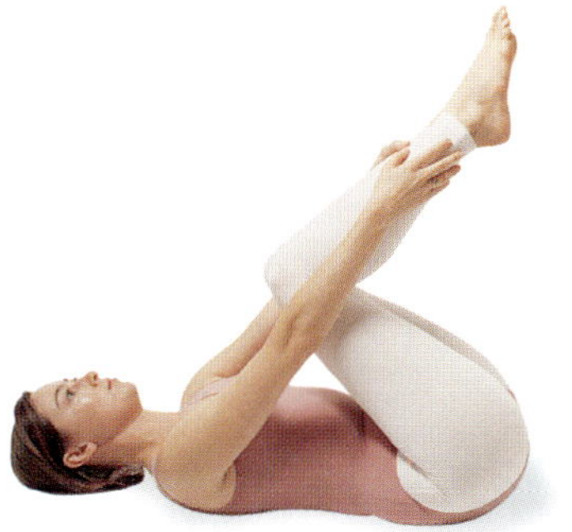

1. Lie on your back with your feet together. Breathe in and bring your knees in towards your head and hold your calves with your hands.

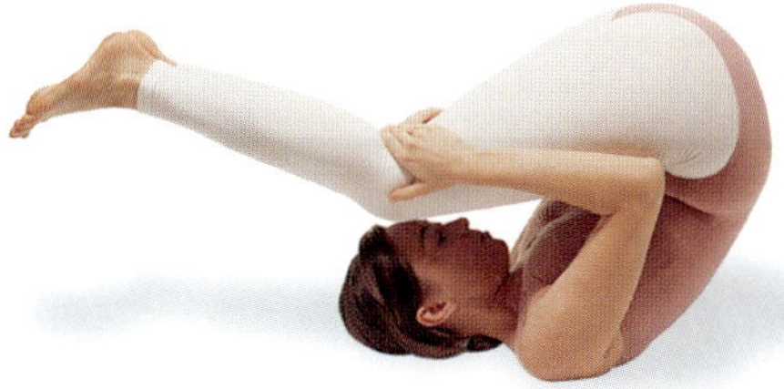

2. Rock back and forth in this posture. Relax in this posture and breathe deeply and evenly for 1 minute.

3. Release the posture, lie on your back and concentrate on deep and relaxed breathing.

4. Repeat this exercise five times. If you feel any pain in your back, stop and relax.

SECTIONAL BREATHING

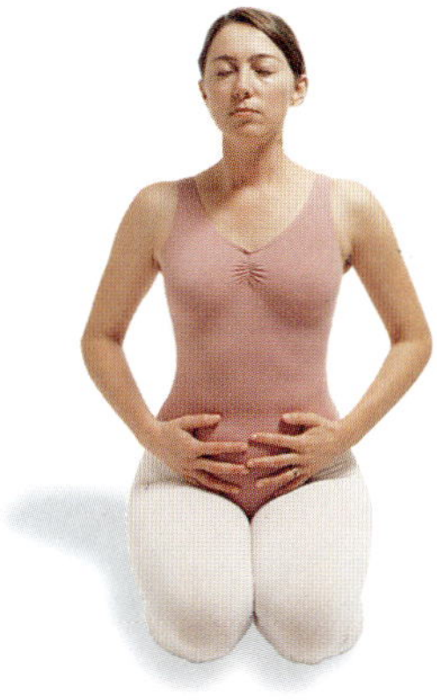

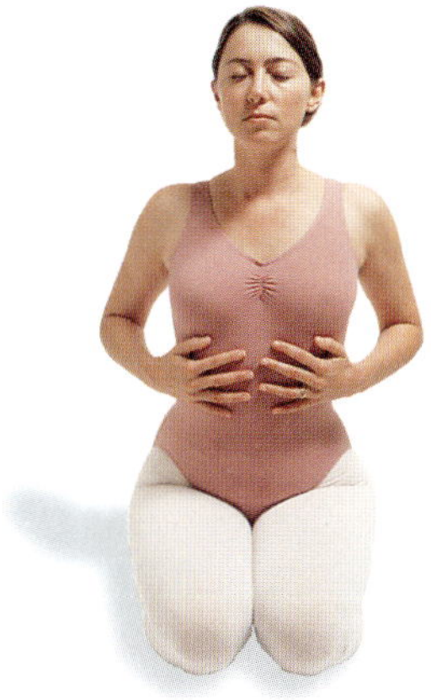

1. Inhale and let your abdomen protrude, then exhale by slowly pulling your abdomen in. You may like to put your hands on your abdomen when you begin this exercise so you can feel the movement.

2. Inhale by expanding your rib cage while keeping your shoulders and abdomen still. When you exhale release your rib cage. Again, you may like to feel your rib cage move in and out with your hands.

3. Breathe in by moving your shoulders while keeping your rib cage and abdomen still. Breathe out using the same technique.

4. Finally combine all three exercises by breathing in using your abdomen, let the air expand your rib cage and finally rise up to your shoulders. Reverse the order to breathe out.

When practising this breathing, you can sit on your knees or cross-legged on the floor or in the lotus or half-lotus position, with a folded blanket under your buttocks and your hands in your lap or on your knees. Alternatively, you can lie in the corpse position (see breathing to relax exercise). Keep your eyes closed and focus on the air moving through you.

SHOULDER STRETCHES

1. Lie on the floor or on a bed with a pillow or towel under your head. Breathe in and push your chest forward while rolling your shoulders back towards the floor or bed.

2. Breathe out then pull your shoulders towards each other and away from the ground. Keep your head on the pillow. Repeat this exercise five times.

SOLAR PLEXUS POSE

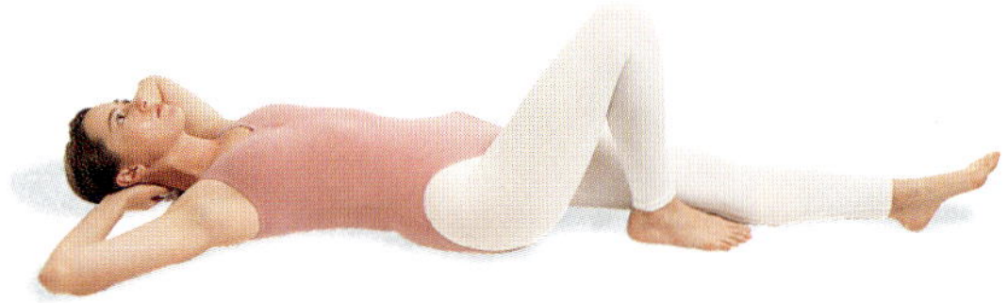

1. Lie on your back with your left leg stretched out and your right leg bent with your foot placed on the floor. Place your hands behind your head.

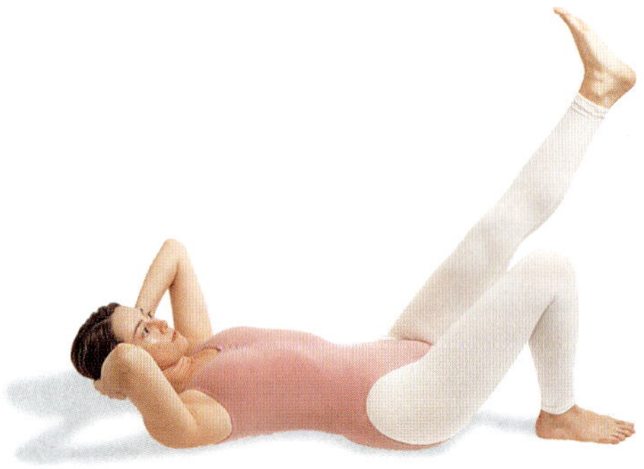

2. Inhale as you raise your head and left leg from the ground and exhale as you lower your head and leg to the ground.

Do this exercise five times with your left leg then rest. Swap legs and raise your right leg and repeat exercise five more times.

SPINAL FLEX

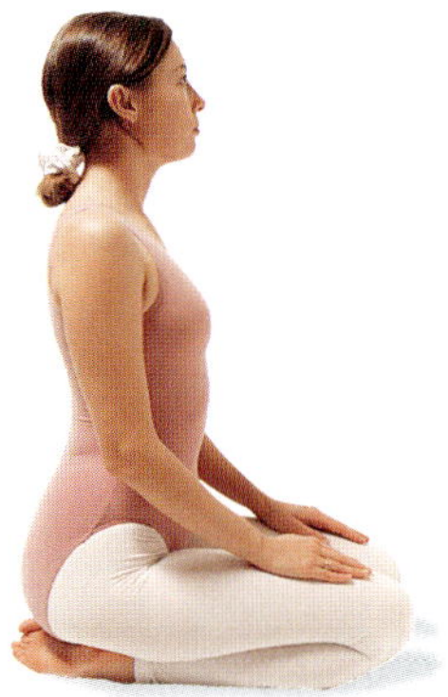

1. Sit back on your heels with toes touching, back arched and head held in line with spine. Feel length in the spine. Inhale.

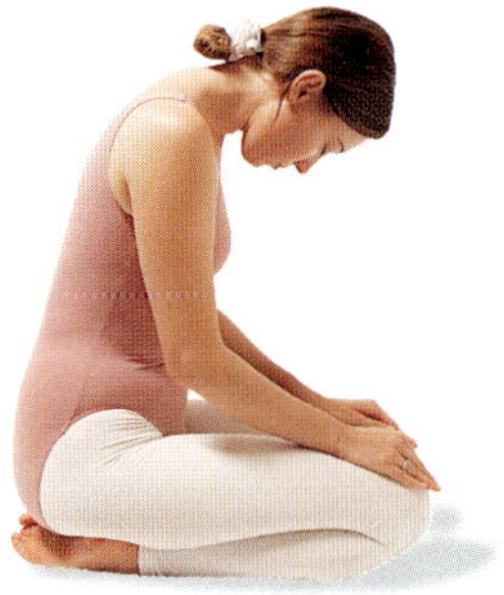

2. Exhale and relax spine, arching forward slightly, and allow the chin to drop to the chest.

Repeat five times.

STANDING

KNOWN AS TADASANA

1. Stand with your feet a few inches apart so that they are directly under your hips. The outside edges of your feet should be parallel.

2. Stretch the toes so that they are flat on the floor but not gripping (you may want to bend over and lift each one off the floor). Keep the weight evenly balanced on each foot — feel the weight at the base of the big toe down your arch through to the heel.

3. Tighten the knees and pull up the knee-caps and the thigh muscles.

4. Keep your spine and upper body straight. Your head should be aligned with the spine and you should feel it lengthening upwards. Keep your shoulders down. Let your arms fall by your sides. Stretch out through the fingertips towards the floor. Both sides of your body should be balanced.

SUPINE TWIST

KNOWN AS JATHARA PARIVARTASANA

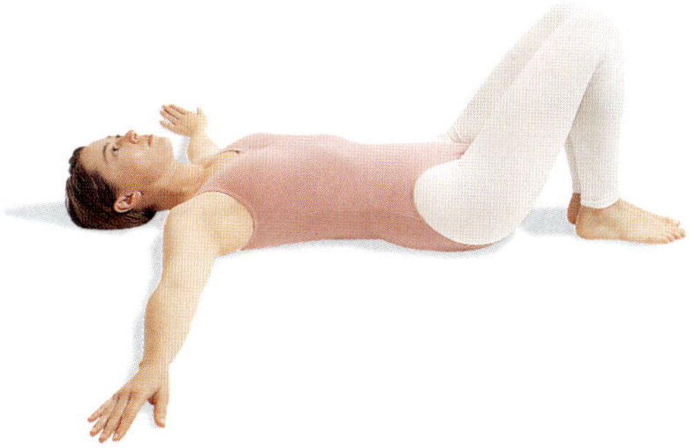

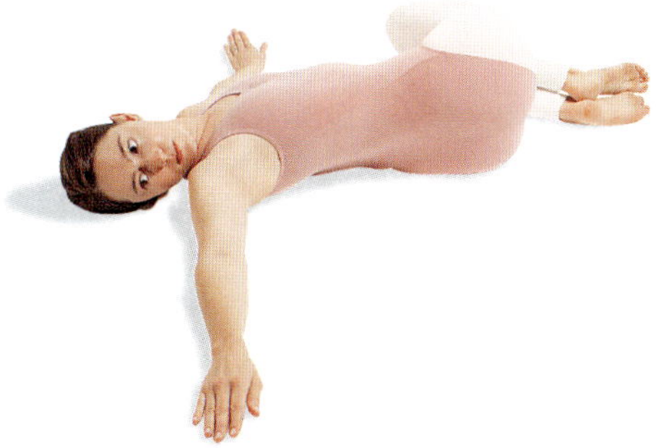

1. Lie down on your back, raise your knees, keep your feet on the floor and slide them towards your buttocks. You may like to place a small pillow under the crown of your head if you feel there is constriction in the back of your neck. Stretch out your arms so that your body forms a "T" shape. Alternatively, you may want to place your hands, palm down, under your buttocks for extra support.

2. Inhale, then as you exhale move your knees towards the floor on your left. If this feels in any way painful only lower your knees to the point that is comfortable for you. As you lower your knees to the left, turn your head to the right and look to the side.

3. Inhale again as your raise your legs back up. Repeat to the right.

Repeat this exercise five times on each side, synchronising your breathing with the movement, then rest by stretching out your legs.

OTHER THERAPIES IN BRIEF

AUTOGENIC TRAINING

The aim of this therapy is to achieve a semi-hypnotic state in order to relieve stress and help the body heal itself. This system of relaxation therapy was developed by German doctor, Johannes Schultz. Working in the late 1920s–30s, Schultz observed that patients who were able to put themselves in a light hypnotic trance responded better to treatment even without positive suggestion from a therapist. There are six specific steps in the autogenic process. These are sets of phrases that are silently repeated to induce physical sensations in different parts of the body, from heaviness in the arms through concentration on heartbeat and breathing to feeling the coolness of the forehead. The technique is widely used by a range of health practitioners from natural therapists to medical doctors and psychiatrists. Some practitioners of autogenic training have incorporated the use of affirmations (see page 48).

AYURVEDIC MEDICINE

This is the traditional health system of India. Ayurvedic medicine is not dissimilar to Traditional Chinese Medicine in that it encompasses body, mind and spirit. The term itself comes from the Sanskrit words ayur, meaning "life", and veda, meaning "knowledge" or "science".

In this system, there are five basic elements which are linked to three forces, or doshas, that control everything and everyone in the universe: vata (which is like the wind; it also governs the nervous system), pitta (which is like the sun; it also governs the digestive system) and kapha (which is like the moon; it also governs cell growth and fluid balance in the tissues). In addition, the human body is seen to be made up of seven basic constituents, or dhatus.

Balance in all these elements is seen as the key to good health. Poor health occurs when these are out of balance. Therefore, the ayurvedic practitioner aims to keep the elements in harmony; the emphasis is on prevention — maintaining stability, pre-empting problems and suggesting changes.

The approach to this is personal. Practitioners will identify the innate disposition/constitution of the individual (this is believed to be determined at the time of conception) and then continue to monitor that person's lifestyle. The whole person will be taken into account: diet, medical history, work, personal habits, choice of spouse etc. They will also undertake detailed physical examinations of urine, stools, sweat, skin, eyes, nails, tongue and even voice to assess your condition and to determine treatment.

No ailment is ever considered in isolation, but all conditions can be categorised under four principal groupings: accidental, mental, natural and physical.

Treatment plans can include dietary changes, enemas, inhalations, exercise, yoga, massage, breathing techniques and exposure to the sun. There are approximately 8000 different herbal medicines.

An ayurvedic practitioner will help create an individual health maintenance system tailored to your constitutional type.

In India, ayurvedic practitioners work closely with orthodox Western medical doctors. In the West, Deepak Chopra has been the most high profile exponent of the ayurvedic system.

BIOFEEDBACK

Biofeedback is the process of using electronic machines to monitor bodily functions such as heart rate, blood pressure, breathing and muscle tension. (A lie detector machine is one well-known example.) The information or "feedback" is usually given in the form of electronic sounds or flashing lights. The machines use receptors attached to the skin; they do not have any effect on a person's body or thought processes.

With the use of biofeedback machines, researchers discovered that with training a person can alter these "involuntary" functions (such as heartbeat and breathing). The machine enables people to recognise their body functions/responses (by following the bleeps or blinking lights) which can then be controlled through willpower or a variety of techniques such as meditation, visualisation or breathing exercises — sometimes after only a few sessions.

Western medicine still does not fully understand how it is we can alter these body functions, but if you are looking for relief from stress or stress-related conditions, biofeedback training may help. It is also used to assist in the management of epilepsy.

COLOUR THERAPY

Colour as seen by the eye is actually some of the component wavelengths of light. There are also non-visible wavelengths, like infrared rays and ultraviolet rays. Just as ultraviolet radiation has a physical impact on our bodies (enabling us to produce vitamins, but also causing sunburn), the electromagnetic components of colour can affect us physically. Research shows that exposure to red light will increase blood pressure whereas blue light will have a calming effect.

Colour therapists believe that the body absorbs some of the electromagnetic components of light and radiates them in a field known as an aura. An unhealthy body radiates an unbalanced pattern of vibrations. The application of various colours is used to correct this imbalance.

During a lengthy consultation, which may involve Kirlian photography (see page 121), a colour therapist will try to "read" your colour vibration and identify what part of the body is affected. The treatment is linked to the concept of chakras (see page 124), although there is variance

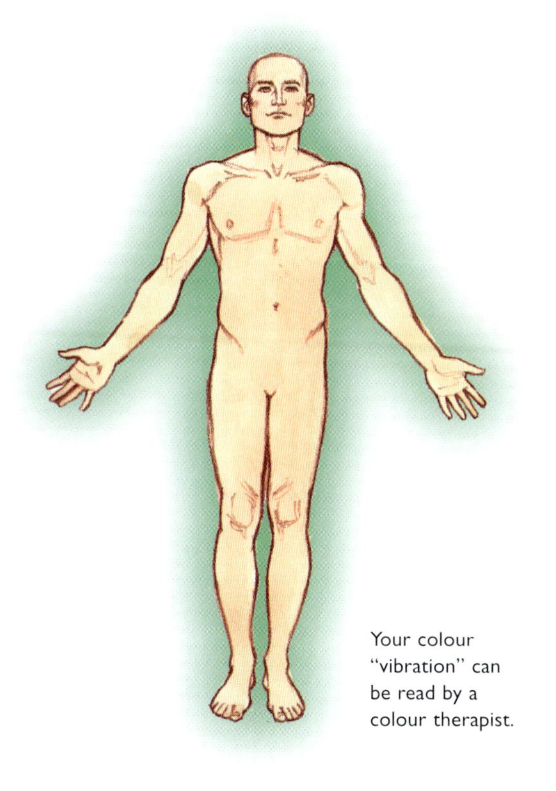

Your colour "vibration" can be read by a colour therapist.

between therapists when defining the healing qualities and uses of specific colours. The appropriate colour will be recommended by the therapist and may be applied in sessions with beams of light. Or it may be recommended that you incorporate the colour into your surroundings, clothing and food.

The use of colour in healing stretches as far back as ancient Egypt and Greece, and scientific research in modern times has supported the theory. It has been shown that coloured lights influence hormone production and, in turn, body functions. Internationally, public institutions such as hospitals and rehabilitation centres, and many private offices have utilised the theory of colour therapy in the design of their buildings to influence the behaviour of the people inside. This might be to aid relaxation, minimise stress or stimulate energy.

HYDROTHERAPY

Hydrotherapy is a broad term used to describe the use of water in treating health conditions. This may range from the application of ice packs to bathing, taking saunas and spa baths to making use of flotation tanks. A variety of health professionals use hydrotherapy in its many and varied forms. For example, physiotherapists often recommend gentle exercise taken in warm water where muscles can relax; naturopaths may prescribe hot and cold compresses or sitz baths (where water only covers the abdomen and pelvis); an aromatherapist may offer steam inhalations using essential oils.

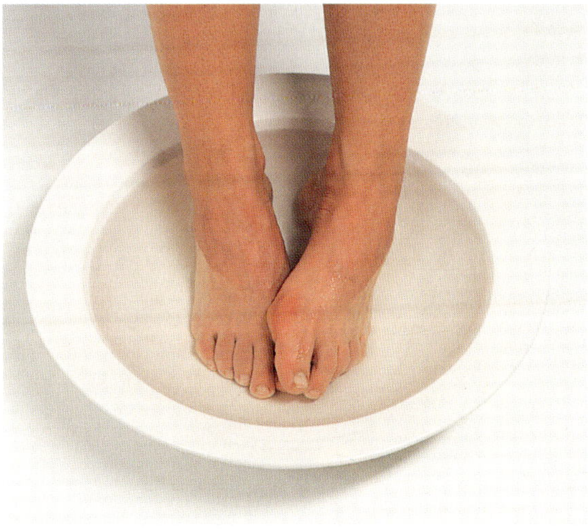

Hot and cold footbaths are a form of hydrotherapy.

The temperature of the water is of the greatest significance in many treatments. In general, heat is used for relaxation, to dilate the blood vessels and encourage sweating, while cold constricts the blood vessels, reduces surface inflammation and stimulates blood flow to the internal organs.

HYPNOTHERAPY

In recent decades, hypnotherapy has been recommended for a number of physical and psychological disorders, including addictions and stress-related problems that require behaviour modification as well as the management of chronic pain and respiratory conditions.

IMPORTANT

Hypnosis can be dangerous if administered by an unqualified or inexperienced person. It is essential you ensure the hypnotherapist is properly trained and accredited through a professional association. Psychiatrists and clinical psychologists often have training in hypnotherapy.

People suffering from severe mental disorders should not undergo hypnosis in most cases.

Not everyone can be hypnotised effectively.

Modern hypnotherapy was founded on the explorations of Austrian doctor Franz Anton Mesmer (1734–1815) who worked with magnets, music and dim lighting, which helped clients relax into a tranced state. He was eventually dismissed as a charlatan although elements of his work continued to be researched.

One of the researchers was James Braid, a Scottish surgeon. In a book he published in 1843, Braid coined the term "hypnotism" referring to the combination of relaxation and heightened awareness that could be induced in patients using some of Mesmer's techniques. Braid was able to perform some surgery using hypnotism as the only form of anaesthetic. However, quicker anaesthetics such as chloroform were being developed and hypnotic techniques fell into disfavour again.

Although its controversial history has resulted in misconceptions, hypnotherapy is now one of the most popular complementary medical techniques and is widely endorsed by Western medical practitioners.

The hypnotic state has been recognised as an altered state of consciousness somewhere between waking and sleeping. It enables a person's attention to be focused and increases their receptivity to suggestion. Thus a problem can be explored and positive input can be made to maximise the healing process (see also THE MIND BODY CONNECTION and AFFIRMATIONS AND VISUALISATIONS).

The therapist does not control the person being hypnotised but works with them to solve a problem. In addition to sessions with a therapist, self-hypnosis is often taught to tackle challenges on a daily level.

IRIDOLOGY

Iridology is a diagnostic tool used by naturopaths, herbalists and other health professionals. It is thought that internal changes in the body (such as nutritional deficiencies, the impact of injuries, the effect of stress, the state of your glandular system, even emotional conditions) are reflected in your eyes. The fine nerve filaments of the iris are linked to every organ through the body's nervous system. Any alteration in the nerve impulses affects blood flow to the iris which, in turn, alters the pigmentation. An iridologist will study the shape and colour of any flecks in your iris and their location. They will also note the texture of the iris, and any deterioration or lines, and compare this with an iridology eye map.

A form of iridology seems to date back to the ancient Greeks and Egyptians. Ignatz von Peczely (1826–1911) published the first modern treatise on the subject in 1881 and many health professionals have furthered his work since then.

Iridology charts show which areas of the eye correspond to specific parts of the body.

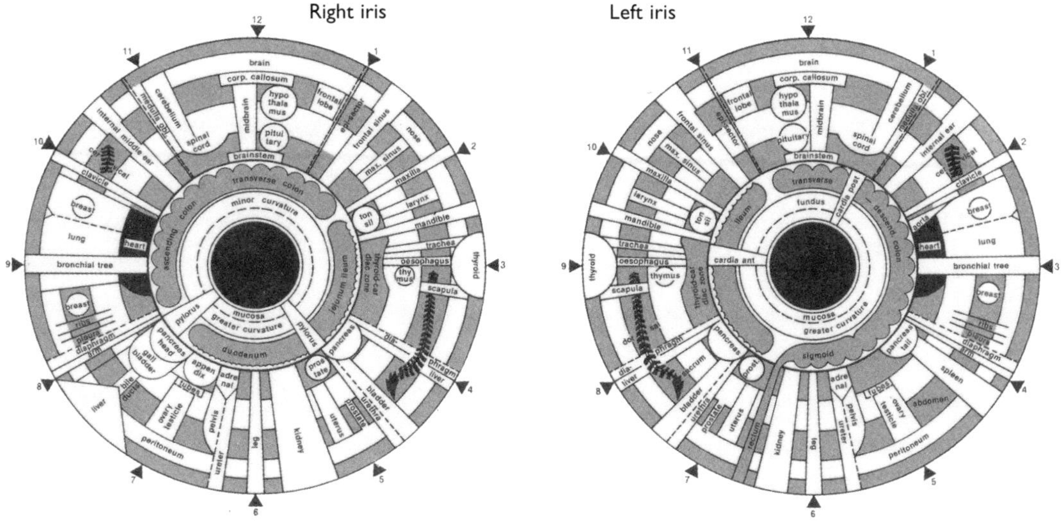

PHYSIOTHERAPY

The aim of physiotherapy is to rehabilitate people disabled by pain, injury or disease affecting their motor functions. Physiotherapists work with people who have injuries; disabilities caused by arthritis, osteoporosis etc; breathing problems; congenital abnormalities; or movement disabilities which result from multiple sclerosis or stroke. They may also work with children to promote motor development or treat their problems of co-ordination.

Your doctor can refer you to a physiotherapist who will assess your condition, looking at muscle strength, endurance and tone, posture, joint movement, muscle co-ordination and the way you walk. Physiotherapy uses a range of techniques including heat and massage to stimulate circulation and relieve pain and muscle spasm. A program of exercises will be devised to bring your muscles and movements back to normal level. The therapist may also recommend manipulative therapy which involves passive mobilisation of joints and soft tissues by the therapist, or manipulation of joints.

Electrical currents of very low strength may be applied to help train weakened muscles. Functional training teaches handicapped people how to carry out the activities of their day to day lives.

POLARITY THERAPY

The aim of this therapy is to balance the body's vital energy. It was developed by Dr Randolph Stone (1890–1983), a chiropractor, osteopath and naturopath. Dr Stone also studied herbalism, acupuncture, shiatsu, yoga and Ayurvedic medicine. He combined principles from these health systems with his interest in the electro-magnetic energy flows within the body to formulate a wide-ranging health therapy.

Stone accepted the concept of a universal energy and that the body has its own energy grid. Good health, he wrote, depended on the "polarity relationships — positive, negative and neutral, between different parts of the body and its five energy centres". These centres followed the Indian concept: air (respiratory and circulatory systems), earth (bladder, rectum), ether (throat, ears), fire (bowels, stomach) and water (glands, pelvis/reproductive system).

He believed that ill-health, especially recurring problems, is caused by imbalances and blockages in the body's energy currents. Polarity therapy tries to remove the blockages and achieve the correct balance by stimulating the flow of positive and negative energies through the body. To do this, Stone recommended manipulation and touch (with different types of pressure linked to the different polarities), diet (including fasting, colonics and a regime to "flush" the liver of toxins), stretching exercises, and modifying mental attitude. The breakdown of blockages and resultant release of toxins may manifest as urine, faeces, sweat or an emotional release.

Polarity therapy is rarely practised as a speciality of its own; more often chiropractors, osteopaths, naturopaths and massage therapists incorporate it into their work.

A-Z OF HEALTH CONDITIONS

PAGE 211

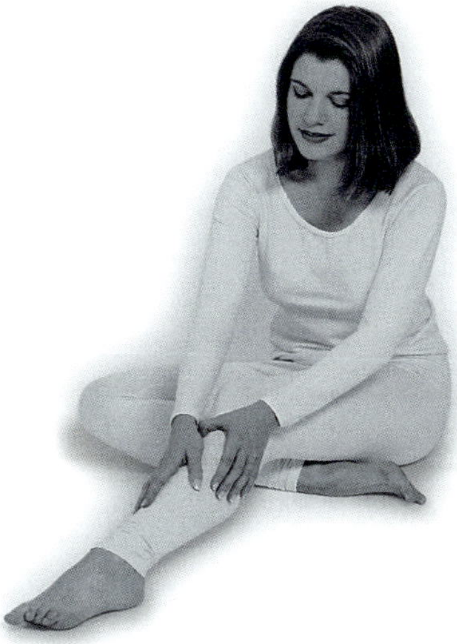

ACNE

Acne is an inflammation of the sebaceous glands in the skin, and is most likely to appear on the face, neck, upper chest and back. It can leave permanently open pores and scars on the skin.

The exact reason why acne affects some people badly and not others is not yet known, although heredity seems to play a part. Other contributing factors may include:

- changing hormone levels during puberty or due to the menstrual cycle
- an inadequate diet (high in fat or iodine, or low in nutrients)
- lack of exercise and thus poor circulation
- poor elimination of toxins from your body
- certain drugs such as iodides and bromides (found in some cough medicines), steroids or some contraceptive pills
- dirt, oil or cosmetics blocking the pores of the skin
- stress.

All these factors may cause sebum (an oily substance produced by glands in the skin) to build up, especially in the oily areas. Excess sebum can block pores, resulting in whiteheads and blackheads. These may in turn become infected, inflamed and pus-filled, resulting in pimples. When this inflammation is severe, large painful cysts may form.

Most natural therapists believe that particular skin conditions, like acne, are the body's reaction to "poisons" in the system. Therefore they will treat the cause of this imbalance rather than the acne which is only a symptom. Treatment will probably take about six weeks before improvement is noticed.

WHAT YOU CAN DO

• Discuss treatments you are using with your health professionals as some treatments used together may reduce each one's benefits.

• Ensure your diet is low in fat, high in fibre to help eliminate toxins, and high in vitamins and minerals to help your body rebuild cells, enabling your skin to repair itself.

• Drink plenty of water — at least eight glasses per day — to flush out your system.

• Get regular exercise, fresh air and sunlight.

• CHIROPRACTIC and OSTEOPATHY may help alleviate acne by assisting the healthy working of your body and its immune system and the FELDENKRAIS METHOD can help with oxygenation.

• Learn how to cope with stress (see page 40).

• In some cases, there may be underlying emotional causes for acne. In such cases, it may be useful to try to balance the emotions through exercises such as AFFIRMATIONS AND VISUALISATIONS. Therapies such as COUNSELLING may also help you deal with any distress you feel about your appearance.

• Try to regulate your hormonal system (see advice under MENSTRUAL PROBLEMS).

• Keep your skin clean and exfoliate regularly to clear away dead skin cells, but remember that excessive washing and harsh soaps may aggravate your condition.

• Rubbing the skin of your body with a loofah or towel may improve circulation, although any kind of scrubbing may aggravate the problem in some people.

• Avoid water that is too hot.

• Avoid touching your skin with your fingers or other items that may transmit grime or bacteria. Become conscious of habits like resting your chin on your hand, for example, and make sure your phone is regularly wiped clean.

• Avoid picking or squeezing which may increase inflammation.

• Shaving can irritate your skin. Keep shaving to a minimum, shave in the direction of the hair growth and consider using an electric razor.

• Try a facial steam bath, similar to a steam inhalation (see page 104), to open and cleanse the pores. A facial mask, particularly one made of clay, can also help.

• Spots can be disguised with a water-based cover-up cream — just make sure you cleanse your skin beforehand.

AROMATHERAPY

CAUTION: *Read the information on pages 102 to 105 before using these essential oils.*

Tea tree oil may be applied directly to a pimple, using a cotton bud to stop infection and assist healing.

The essential oils juniper berry and lemon can reduce the level of sebum in your skin. Add 5 drops of each to a basin of spring, distilled or bottled water. Soak cotton balls in this mixture, squeeze them out gently, then store them and the mixture in separate airtight containers in the refrigerator. When pimples occur, wipe your skin every 2 hours with the cotton balls and bathe your skin every night with the mixture.

To reduce inflammation and soothe irritation, mix 3 drops each of petitgrain, atlas cedarwood and lemon in 5 teaspoons jojoba oil (an oil that is very effective for use on oily skin). Apply 5 drops to your skin each night using a clean cotton ball. Wipe off excess with a tissue after 5 minutes.

A professional aromatherapist can give more specific advice on particular oils for your skin type.

BACH FLOWER REMEDY

Take crab apple remedy for cleansing the skin. If you are depressed about your appearance it may have an adverse effect on your skin condition, so larch is recommended for building self-confidence.

CHINESE HERBS

Chinese herbs are effective for helping all kinds of skin conditions. See a Chinese herbalist for specific advice and treatment.

HERBALISM

Dandelion root can be used to reduce acne because it helps your liver to remove toxins from your system. Try drinking 2 cups dandelion root tea per day.

Other herbs that can assist include echinacea, burdock, clivers, yellow dock, calendula and red clover. These have a purifying effect on your blood.

A herbalist will prescribe specific herbal formulas, taking into account the various possible causes such as diet or hormonal changes.

Herbal home remedies can also be applied directly to the skin. You can try dabbing fresh lemon juice or cabbage juice onto the pimple, or the juice of aloe leaves to prevent scarring and promote healing. There are commercial products available that contain herbs such as witch hazel (which has an astringent action on the skin) or soothing chamomile.

HOMOEOPATHY

There is no single homoeopathic remedy for acne. However, a homoeopath can prescribe an individual remedy which is likely to have a very successful result.

MASSAGE

Lymphatic drainage may assist in eliminating toxins, and may be even more effective if performed in association with aromatherapy massage. You can also try a facial massage at home using some of the essential oils recommended above — follow the steps for facial massage detailed in the full-body massage on page 148.

MODERN MEDICINE

Creams are available over the counter and from your doctor. The most effective active ingredient is benzoyl peroxide, although others contain salicylic acid, sulfur or other drugs. You should try a low concentrate first as the creams can dry the skin and cause irritation.

Prescription creams may contain topical antibiotics and your doctor may prescribe oral antibiotics to stop the cycle of infection. Some oral contraceptives help reduce acne by balancing hormones; they are sometimes prescribed by doctors for this purpose (note, however, that some other forms of the Pill may actually be the cause).

A synthetic form of vitamin A is applied for some cases of cystic acne. New medications are continually being developed to treat severe cases — some are effective but they can be expensive and have side effects. One of the most popular, isotretinoin, has been linked to birth defects and is not to be used in pregnancy.

Minor surgery may be required to lance large cysts. Depending on your case, you may be referred to a dermatologist (skin specialist). Dermabrasion (the removal of the top layers of skin by abrasion) is an option for the treatment of acne scars in some cases but it may cause further scarring and should be carried out by a specialist.

NATUROPATHY

CAUTION: *Read the information on page 167 before taking supplements.*

Help your body eliminate toxins, balance hormones, and get sufficient nutrients by eating plenty of fruit, vegetables, wholegrain foods, soya bean products (instead of dairy foods), free-range chicken and eggs, nuts, seeds and garlic. You can also control androgenic hormone levels, by avoiding animal products for example. Also avoid foods that contain refined carbohydrates such as white sugar and white flour and stimulants such as chocolate, spices and coffee. A naturopath may check for food allergies as an underlying cause of your acne.

Zinc, with its healing and anti-inflammatory functions, is the most important mineral for acne. Zinc tablets (25 mg elemental per day) and vitamin A (5000 iu per day) can be very effective in helping to clear the skin. Vitamin E oil straight from capsules or a vitamin E cream can be applied locally to the acne to reduce scarring, or you can take 500 iu of vitamin E tablets internally per day to help skin healing and hormone balancing.

Vitamin C will help improve your immune system — it is also anti-oxidant and will aid in collagen production and healing. Fatty acids, particularly evening primrose oil, will reduce inflammation and improve hormonal balance. If your acne is tied to menstruation or PMS, take vitamin B6 and a kelp supplement.

See a naturopath for a complete analysis of your physical and emotional condition for the best result.

REFLEXOLOGY

Work the following points: the small intestine for efficient digestion, the kidneys and colon for elimination of solid waste, the liver to aid detoxificiation, the pituitary for hormonal balance and the diaphragm for relaxation. Try this on both feet or hands for a total of 15 minutes three times a week.

SHIATSU

A shiatsu therapist would treat the liver, kidney and spleen meridians to regulate hormonal imbalances, help manage stress, boost the immune system and eliminate toxins, and the lung and large intestine meridians for cleansing the blood and skin. Shiatsu may also address any underlying emotional factors.

YOGA

To keep your skin in a healthy condition, yoga teachers recommend you do specific breathing exercises. If your breathing is impaired or shallow because of SMOKING, incorrect posture, or lack of exercise, your cells may be starved of oxygen and unable to clear away waste products properly. A good breathing exercise, like the alternative nostril breathing exercise on page 192, will help supply your cells with oxygen.

Acne can also be aggravated by stress so this yoga exercise and others recommended by a yoga teacher should have a calming effect on your whole disposition.

ALLERGIES

An allergy is a reaction in your body to a foreign substance known as an allergen. Because your body cannot tolerate this substance (which could be harmless to many other people) your immune system rejects it, producing antibodies to combat it. Whenever you are in contact with the allergen, your antibodies produce histamine, which causes disturbances in the body.

Symptoms vary depending on the allergen and your body's reaction to it. Some common ones include skin rashes and itching (including the raised red lumps that are known as *hives*), ECZEMA, HEADACHE AND MIGRAINE, DIGESTIVE PROBLEMS, vomiting, ASTHMA and ear infections (see page 80).

Rhinitis and *hay fever* are others: the mucous membranes of the nose and sinuses become inflamed causing sneezing, runny nose and eyes, and coughing (see SINUSITIS).

An allergic reaction can occur in just about any part of your body and vary greatly in severity.

Many are acute, but others develop more slowly. The range of symptoms can make the allergy difficult to diagnose and some symptoms (such as FATIGUE or a drop in mental alertness) can be subtle, thus many people continue to have undiagnosed or incorrectly diagnosed health problems that are the result of allergies.

Most symptoms disappear once exposure to the allergen is withdrawn. Consult the index on pages 408 to 413 for treatments for specific symptoms.

It is important, however, to positively identify the condition as an allergy, as it might be the symptom of a more serious illness.

There may be an hereditary link in the tendency towards allergy.

Intense emotions, such as stress, ANXIETY, fear, grief, anger and excitement, can trigger an allergy attack.

Although allergies commonly appear in childhood, the first symptoms may only become apparent in later life and sensitivity to foods can develop later on.

IMPORTANT: *In a few cases (usually involving medication, seafood or insect stings), allergic reactions can be life threatening, requiring emergency treatment of an injection, oxygen and intravenous fluids. See FIRST AID on page 386.*

COMMON ALLERGENS

It is possible to be allergic to almost anything, even the air you breathe. The most common allergens include:

- *Environmental:* pollen, dust mites, fungal spores, pollutants, animal hair, chemicals within substances such as detergents.
- *Diet:* dairy products, yeast, wheat, seafood, eggs, tomatoes, strawberries, citrus fruits and many food additives. To identify the foods that may be involved in your allergic condition, an elimination diet is recommended.
- *Medication:* all reactions to drugs should be reported to a doctor. Penicillin is one of the more common allergens.

WHAT YOU CAN DO

The primary factor in dealing with allergies is to avoid contact with the allergen. This is easier in some cases, such as a food item, than others, such as dust. There are some basic guidelines, however, for those prone to allergies:

- Try to trace a pattern in your symptoms to help pinpoint possible causes.
- Avoid processed foods and additives.
- Use low-allergenic products, and avoid chemicals where possible, or protect yourself when using such products.
- Clean your home and working environment regularly to avoid dust build-up. Don't forget hidden places like the springs of your bed or under the fridge.
- Choose domestic items that do not harbour dust (floor boards are preferable to thick carpets, for example) and that are easy to wash regularly.
- Modify your garden — stick to non-flowering plants and choose paving rather than grass.
- Good general health — particularly liver function — and learning how to cope with stress will assist in managing an allergy. See page 31 for information on strengthening your immune system.
- If you are prone to allergies, you could try a healing meditation daily (see page 155).
- Relieve the irritation of hives by bathing the area with a solution of 1 teaspoon bicarbonate of soda (baking soda) in a cup of water.

ACUPRESSURE

If you have hives or are prone to them, try massaging the acupressure point Kidney 2 in the reverse direction (towards the sole of the foot) two or three times per day for 5 minutes to ease the condition. For hayfever and rhinitis, use Liver 20. Treatment and advice from a qualified practitioner will give the best results.

ACUPUNCTURE

Acupuncture from a qualified practitioner can be extremely effective in dealing with allergic conditions.

AROMATHERAPY

To reduce the symptoms of allergic reactions such as hay fever and rhinitis, mix 1 drop of lavender oil in 1 teaspoon of base carrier oil and massage into your sinus area throughout the day. Carry this mixture around with you in a small bottle for easy access. You can also apply this mixture to skin rashes.

For hives, add 2 drops of German chamomile oil to 1/4 cup baking soda and add to your bath.

BACH FLOWER REMEDIES

Allergies are often related to emotional problems. Remedies that reduce anxiety and calm the emotions include rescue remedy, aspen, mimulus, red chestnut and impatiens. Find out which one will be most suitable for you, based on the cause of your anxiety. In its dosage form, take 4 drops four times a day.

CHINESE HERBS

A Chinese herbalist can prescribe various herbs to treat your allergies depending on your individual case. Bi Yan Pian can prove an effective first-aid patent remedy (and a preventive strategy) for respiratory allergies where symptoms include sore throat, itchy eyes and nose, sneezing, cough and headache.

CHIROPRACTIC

Dysfunctions of the bladder, bowel, and small and large intestine often contribute to allergic conditions. Any dysfunctions in these organs respond well to chiropractic adjustments.

HERBALISM

If you experience regular bouts of hives, ointment containing the herb nettle can be applied to the affected area a couple of times a day to reduce inflammation and irritation.

Garlic and horseradish tablets — often combined with vitamin C — may help reduce hay fever and rhinitis. These herbs strengthen your immune system against potential allergens. Take them according to the directions on the label.

Other herbs that may help include echinacea, elder, eyebright, fenugreek and golden seal. In their raw form, they should be prescribed by a herbalist.

HERBAL TREATMENT FOR PARENTS-TO-BE

Most parents-to-be do not realise that if they suffer from allergies they are likely to pass these allergies onto their children. The good news is their babies can be helped if the parents take herbal remedies before conceiving and also while the baby is nursing (breast-feeding helps boost the immune system). Take 10–15 drops of gentian root tincture in water three times a day before meals. This remedy will also help if taken by nursing mothers whose babies have eczema or other skin irritations.

HOMOEOPATHY

Allergic reactions such as inflammation and swelling can be effectively reduced, often through the use of the homoeopathic remedies *Urtica urens, Rhus toxicondendrona* or *Arsenicum album*. Other allergic reactions require different remedies which must be prescribed by a homoeopath.

There are also homoeopathic remedies available that boost the immune system against allergens, though these are prescribed in the context of improving overall health.

MASSAGE

Lymphatic drainage and aromatherapy massage may assist some allergies which cause inflammation of the mucous membrane.

MODERN MEDICINE

For allergic reactions, doctors may prescribe antihistamine medication and/or cortisone in the form of a nasal spray or cream. Nose drops and bronchodilators may also be prescribed. Ensure you discuss any medication in detail as some can cause side effects such as drowsiness, and others are habit forming.

Your doctor may recommend calamine lotion to relieve the itchiness of hives and other skin rashes.

Though no longer considered standard treatment, a course of injections or drops may be suggested to desensitise you to allergens. Complications may result.

NATUROPATHY

A naturopath will use an elimination diet technique to find out which foods you are allergic to. They may start you on fruit, rice and vegetables (plus non-allergenic protein substitutes) for a week and then introduce other foods. These are introduced slowly because it can take your body up to five days to react.

You can improve your immune system by taking vitamin C (try 2000 mg per day). And if your allergic reactions are linked to digestive problems, make yogurt with acidophilus part of your daily diet or take acidophilus tablets as directed on the label.

REFLEXOLOGY

For allergies of any kind, a reflexologist will work points on your feet and hands to discover and assist the organs in your body affected by the allergy.

Working the toes and fingers helps the nose, eye, ear and throat area. For hay fever, working the chest and lungs relieves tension and improves breathing. At home, you can try whichever of these is appropriate for a total of 15 minutes on both feet or hands twice a week.

SHIATSU

Shiatsu practitioners see your allergy as an inability of your liver to process protein as well as a weakness in your immune system. They will use shiatsu to "tonify" your liver and clear the meridians in your body to build up your immune system.

YOGA

If you are prone to allergic reactions such as sneezing or a runny blocked nose, yoga can help you through breathing exercises (such as those on pages 192, 193 and 195) that will increase your nasal lining's tolerance to allergic agents, aerate your lungs and soothe your nerves. Inverted postures such as the ones on pages 197, 199 and 202 are also beneficial. Some of these are quite complicated and will be more effective if you do them in a class under the direction of a yoga teacher.

ANAEMIA

Anaemia is a condition where your blood is deficient in red blood cells or the haemoglobin that transports oxygen around the body. Sufferers often feel tired because not enough oxygen is being delivered to the tissues which need it.

Other symptoms may include paleness or jaundice, easy bruising, HEADACHE, dizziness, and shortness of breath. Sometimes the tongue is slick or smooth.

There are numerous types of anaemia as there can be many causes. Anaemia can be brought on by excessive blood loss — gastro-intestinal bleeding is a common cause and may be indicated by black stool. It can be a part of a person's genetic make-up — sickle cell anaemia is one example.

Anaemia can be due to nutritional deficiency from inadequate intake or poor absorption of nutrients. Iron-deficiency anaemia is the most common. Pernicious anaemia is due to poor absorption of vitamin B12. A deficiency in folic acid can lead to megaloblastic anaemia.

Other illnesses can cause anaemia, e.g. KIDNEY PROBLEMS, DIGESTIVE PROBLEMS, an infection or an infestation of worms.

IMPORTANT: *You need to find out exactly what is causing your anaemia before you treat it. Blood tests must be taken by a doctor to determine whether you have anaemia and at what level. The condition then has to be monitored. Treatment will vary greatly depending on the type of anaemia you have, as the specific cause of the anaemia must be dealt with.*

WHAT YOU CAN DO

- Ensure your diet is well-balanced and contains folic acid and iron-rich foods such as dried peas and beans, nuts, whole grains, eggs, green leafy vegetables, and red meat (especially liver). Salmon and mackerel are good sources of B12.
- Dietary care is especially important for children, pregnant women, the elderly and those on a vegan diet who are all more likely to suffer from a diet-deficiency anaemia.

• Some chemicals such as benzene (found in petrol and paint strippers) can damage bone marrow (where red blood cells are produced) if inhaled in high concentration or over long periods. This in turn can lead to anaemia. Take care when using these products.

• If you are taking an iron supplement, it will be far more effective if it is organic iron.

ACUPUNCTURE

Acupuncture has been known to help anaemia. See a qualified acupuncturist for advice and treatment.

AROMATHERAPY

Lemon essential oil is good for circulation. Use a few drops in your bath or in a massage oil, or burn some in an oil burner throughout the day.

BACH FLOWER REMEDIES

To help reduce your exhaustion when you have anaemia, try the remedy olive. If you are lacking energy, hornbeam can also help. Take 4 drops of each of these four times a day.

CHINESE HERBALISM

Chinese herbs can be useful in treating this condition. Dang gui (also known as tong kuei or dong gui) is one commonly used example. See a Chinese herbalist for details. They may also advise you on diet changes.

HERBALISM

Herbs should be prescribed by a herbalist who can monitor your condition. The aim here is to improve the body's absorption of food. This is often done using the herb gentian root. To start, take 10–15 drops of gentian root tincture in water before meals.

A herbalist will also advise you to take herbs such as slippery elm and marshmallow to protect and soothe your internal mucous membrane. Other herbs that can improve your anaemic condition include yellow dock root, rose hip, hops, dandelion leaves, nettles, sorrel and chickweed. These contain organic iron and can be taken in herbal infusions or tinctures or the leaves may be eaten as part of a salad, as appropriate.

HOMOEOPATHY

Homoeopaths often have good results treating iron deficiency and other forms of anaemia, often with individually prescribed remedies such as *Phosphoricum acidum, Silicea* and *Ferrum metallicum.*

MODERN MEDICINE

Iron, B12 or folic acid tablets or injections may be prescribed for nutrient-deficient anaemias.

More severe types of anaemia may be treated with anabolic steroids, a hormone known as erythropoietin, even blood transfusions.

NATUROPATHY

Iron-rich foods include dark green leafy vegetables such as parsley and spinach — try eating them at the same time as vitamin C-rich food to assist iron absorption. Organic iron and vitamins B, E, C and B12 are the supplements that most commonly help anaemia, but take them only on a naturopath's advice. High levels of magnesium, calcium and zinc (and antacids which may contain them) will compete with iron for absorption so these minerals should be consumed at different times.

REFLEXOLOGY

Work the points for the liver and spleen as both these organs store iron, and the thyroid to encourage metabolic balance. Try this on both feet or hands for a total of 20 minutes twice a week. It is suitable for all types of anaemia.

SHIATSU

A shiatsu practitioner will work on your spleen meridian to support the spleen's ability to cleanse the blood of old blood cells and produce new blood cells, to increase and strengthen the flow of Ki energy throughout your body, and to ensure the proper absorption of nutrients and Ki to produce blood. Working the channels of the small intestine also assists absorption.

ANXIETY

Anxiety is a form of stress. It is an emotion you feel when you are frightened or distressed. It may be a state of apprehension, frustration with everything or fear of the unknown.

Physical symptoms may include INSOMNIA, PAIN (often in the chest, abdomen, back or head), tense muscles, trembling, dizziness, HEADACHE, a dry mouth, DIARRHOEA, frequent urinating, NAUSEA, vomiting and DIGESTIVE PROBLEMS.

Sometimes it is obvious what you are anxious about and other times it is unclear — just a strung-out feeling. You may feel some problems in your life are too difficult to address. Some obvious causes of anxiety are events such as job loss, serious illness, the death of someone close to you or a relationship breakdown. This kind of "rational" anxiety is normal and will usually lift when the problem is solved. Deep "irrational" anxiety or habitual emotional overreacting are indicative of a more serious condition which requires assistance.

Seek professional advice if your anxiety interferes with your enjoyment of life, especially if it prevents you going out or makes you avoid certain situations.

Panic attacks are sudden surges of intense anxiety which can strike at any time, sometimes without cause, sometimes triggered by an event. Symptoms differ from person to person but faintness, trouble breathing (particularly hyperventilation), trembling, dizziness, sweating, or heart palpitations are common.

Chronic anxiety of any kind can involve recurrent attacks over a period of months. Any long-term anxiety is detrimental to your physical and mental health.

WHAT YOU CAN DO

- Search for a reason. Once the cause is identified you are halfway to regaining control of your life.
- When the source of stress is identified, work to remove it from your life. For example, if your work is causing the problem, a change of job may help.
- Learn how to manage stress. See page 40.
- Talk about your fears and concerns to a supportive and understanding friend, relation or partner, or visit a counsellor or other trained therapist. Communicating your phobias can help you assess them rationally and enable you to overcome them.
- Establishing a routine and being better organised may help you cope by giving you a sense of control over your life.
- Keep active, physically and mentally, in areas that interest you.
- Try to focus your attention on the task at hand.
- Concentrate on positive solutions to a problem rather than worrying about the problem itself or imagining worst case scenarios.
- Be kind to yourself — and also to others. Don't place too high demands on yourself. Take a little time out.
- Avoid caffeine and alcohol as these give a temporary lift but make it more difficult to deal with anxieties long term.

ACUPRESSURE

Wrap the palm of one of your hands around the middle finger of the opposite hand and gently breathe for 5 minutes. This will help you relax when anxious.

ACUPUNCTURE

Acupuncture is excellent for mild anxiety through to panic attacks, and also for associated problems such as INSOMNIA.

AFFIRMATION

When you feel anxious try repeating this affirmation to yourself until peace returns. "I accept that I feel anxious. I now choose to feel at peace. I am able to deal with all challenges that life offers me. I am at peace."

AROMATHERAPY

Aromatherapy is found to be a very effective relaxing agent for stressed people. There are many oils that are sedative, and an aromatherapist may have you choose one for massage because you can often instinctively choose the oil that most corresponds to your current state of mind.

Although treatment from an aromatherapist is recommended, you can also use essential oils at home.

Essential oil baths are one way to soothe anxiety especially if the bath is taken just before you go to bed. Add 3 drops each lavender and sandalwood to the warm water, making sure the oils are well dispersed.

For a panic attack, you need treatment that is readily available to stabilise your body before the anxiety takes over and this is one of the benefits of aromatherapy. Sprinkle 2 drops of lavender on a tissue and inhale deeply and slowly. Lavender calms the mind and body, while the act of deep breathing calms the body. Keep the tissue with you all day.

There are other oils you might like to try. Frankincense, for example, is good for lengthening the breath. Marjoram, patchouli, vetivert, basil and clary sage also have useful properties. (Be careful with prolonged use of any oil, particularly marjoram as it can cause drowsiness and depression.)

BACH FLOWER REMEDIES

Aspen is suitable for all types of emotional challenges, including fear of the unknown. Mimulus is a remedy specifically for fear of a known origin. Rescue remedy can be taken for any kind of shock and is recommended for panic attacks.

CHIROPRACTIC

When your nervous system is under stress and you are feeling anxious it can be helpful to see a chiropractor for an adjustment. The adjustment will correct your nervous system and increase the flow of energy to all parts of your body, helping to reduce anxiety.

COUNSELLING

A counsellor can help you deal with any fears which may be triggering your feelings of anxiety. These fears may not be obvious to you and you may need an objective person to help identify them. Counselling can help with panic attacks as it is thought the fear you feel is related to unresolved issues.

THE FELDENKRAIS METHOD

A Feldenkrais practitioner can help you develop breathing strategies to counter anxiety or a panic attack. Anxiety can be reflected in restricted movement patterns. The Feldenkrais Method can teach people awareness of how they hold themselves and how to be more comfortable in their bodies.

HERBALISM

Herbalists can help people reduce anxiety. Herbs often prescribed include valerian, passion flower, oats, skullcap and hops because of their calming, sedating effect on the mind and body.

When you feel anxious, you can try taking 15 drops of oats tincture and 15 drops of passion flower tincture in 1 cup of water and sip it slowly. Take this herbal mixture as often as required. For a panic attack, you may wish to use 30 drops of each tincture in half a glass of water.

Chamomile tea is another mild herb favoured for home use due to its soothing qualities.

HOMOEOPATHY

One of the most common homoeopathic remedies given for anxiety is *Arsenicum album*. It is prescribed if your anxious feelings are connected to insecurity in the world and needing other people around in case something goes wrong. You may be also be treated with this remedy if you give the appearance of being capable but inside worry needlessly.

Other remedies include:

- *Phosphorus* if you are feeling too diffused or nervous
- *Aconitum napellus* if you are feeling frightened after an event
- *Argentum nitricum* if you can't face the outside world because of your highly irrational anxiety.

If one of these four remedies suits your form of anxiety, you could try taking a 6C potency three times a day. Stop taking the remedy as soon as you feel normal again.

If you feel a panic attack impending with sweating or trembling, suck one 6C potency of *Aconitum napellus* every half hour for three doses (usually in a form such as a granule or tablet).

MASSAGE

Swedish massage and aromatherapy massage from a friend or a professional are highly recommended as they relax, soothe and comfort.

MODERN MEDICINE

A good doctor will check to see if any of your symptoms have a physical cause. They will generally recommend COUNSELLING for this condition and may send you to someone who specialises in the area. Medication may be used to reduce the symptoms of anxiety (but not the cause), so for some cases doctors may prescribe tranquillisers. There are a few drugs that help panic attacks such as lorazepam and alprazolam.

Heavy medication such as tranquillisers and barbiturates is seldom prescribed for anxiety by doctors these days. They are more likely to prescribe a sedative or muscle relaxant such as diazepam or oxazepam. Caution should be exercised — see the table on page 162.

NATUROPATHY

A naturopath will need to find out the cause of your anxiety in order to treat it. If they find that the cause is stress they may prescribe magnesium supplements or B group vitamins. If it is diet-related, they will adapt your diet by reducing caffeine (tea, coffee, cola drinks and chocolate) and fatty foods and checking for food sensitivities.

Naturopaths advise taking calcium, magnesium phosphate, potassium phosphate and high potency B complex vitamins (as directed on bottle) to nourish the nervous system. These should be taken on a regular basis rather than when a panic attack is coming on. In cases of long-term anxiety, vitamin C is also important for the adrenal glands.

OSTEOPATHY

Stress and anxiety will irritate the nervous system. This may cause strain and discomfort throughout the body's joints and muscles. Long term, this can cause a disturbance in blood supply and affect overall body function. Osteopathic treatment can alleviate the immediate symptoms of stress, such as neck and shoulder discomfort, by relaxing muscles and improving joint mobility. Osteopathy will also help to improve circulation and the function of the nervous and immune systems to reduce the effects of recurring or long-term stress.

REFLEXOLOGY

To help reduce long-term anxiety or calm a panic attack, work the diaphragm reflex on both feet or hands for a total of 10 minutes once a day. This point is specifically for relaxation and stress reduction.

SHIATSU

A shiatsu practitioner will give you a full shiatsu treatment. They will start by "tonifying" and increasing the circulation around the areas of your body where the meridians are empty and then disperse any blocked energy. They will then "calm" your heart meridian. This can set your mind at rest and make you feel able to once again cope with what lies ahead.

Regular shiatsu treatment can be used as a preventive measure against panic attacks and fear by supporting kidney function and the bladder meridian to stabilise the central nervous system.

YOGA

A yoga teacher will recommend you release the muscular tension in your body using various yoga exercises. Deep breathing will also help calm your system — try the alternate nostril breathing exercise on page 192.

The hips are often affected by anxiety as they are associated with your will (consider how you may put your hands on your hips to gain control of a situation). The supine twist on page 205 will bring down your pulse rate, relax your breathing pattern and promote a sense of well-being. Try the inverted corpse position too.

ARTHRITIS

Arthritis is a general term for more than 100 conditions in which the joints are inflamed causing swelling, PAIN and restricted movement.

The most common areas of the body to be affected by arthritis are the wrists, knees, hips, ankles and fingers.

There are two main types of arthritis: osteoarthritis and rheumatoid arthritis.

Osteoarthritis starts gradually with stiffness and pain in a joint followed by the enlargement of the joint. This is caused by wear-and-tear and usually affects middle-aged and elderly people.

Rheumatoid arthritis can progress from joint to joint with chronic inflammation, pain and swelling which may eventually lead to deformity. It is sometimes accompanied by fever, and a loss of appetite and general well-being. Rheumatoid arthritis is less common than osteoarthritis although both forms are much more likely to affect women than men.

The specific cause of rheumatoid arthritis is unknown, but the immune system seems to be attacking tissues in the body. ALLERGIES and VIRAL INFECTIONS could be a trigger. It has also been linked to the bowel and bacterial balance in the intestines.

Heredity and stress may be factors in many types of arthritis.

Gout is another form of arthritis, caused by a build-up of crystals of uric acid in the joints. Symptoms include pain and swelling of the joints and tenderness and redness around these areas. The pain is usually worse at night. Gout often runs in families but can also be a symptom of KIDNEY PROBLEMS or an inadequate diet that produces too much acid. Weight and alcohol reduction is often advised as is avoiding cigarettes and drinking six to eight glasses of water per day.

IMPORTANT: *Before seeking treatment it is important your arthritis is medically diagnosed. Rheumatoid arthritis can be diagnosed through blood tests and X-rays. Most forms of arthritis can't be "cured" but many can be treated or managed.*

WHAT YOU CAN DO

- Gentle, regular stretching exercises such as Tai Chi (see page 186) will help keep limbs, tendons, joints and muscles flexible, more resilient and relaxed. They act both as a prevention and a treatment.
- Take it easy. Learn to pace your efforts, take plenty of rest breaks and don't rush or overexert yourself on days when your symptoms are minimal.
- Learn how to relax and deal with effectively with stress (see page 40).
- Avoid cigarettes as they restrict circulation which makes the condition worse.
- If applicable, you may need to reduce your weight. Obesity puts further strain on weight-bearing joints.
- Creative visualisations may help you manage your pain (see page 48). Try them for 10–20 minutes each day, twice a day if possible.
- Hydrotherapy (see page 208) is recommended for this condition. Swimming and bathing takes the weight off the joints. Soak in hot baths with bath salts or Epsom salts to relieve aching joints — try it in the morning when joints are often particularly stiff. Sea water is believed to be of assistance and spa baths should also help.
- Apply an ice pack for 15–20 minutes every four hours or so when the pain is sharp and intense and joints are stressed from overuse. At other times, a hot compress applied in the same way will provide relief. You can use a cloth that has been soaked in hot water and then squeezed out, or try a hot water bottle. Salt packs heated in a microwave oven are excellent.
- Rub a warming oil such as wintergreen into joints. Dry skin rubbing will also increase blood flow to the affected area.
- Infra-red lamps can provide soothing warmth.
- If you use an electric blanket, use it only to warm the bed and turn it off when you get in. Although warmth is good, studies have shown that the electric current may adversely affect arthritis.
- Support devices such as light splints may give rest and protection.

ACUPRESSURE AND ACUPUNCTURE

Arthritis can be effectively relieved by acupuncture. See a qualified, experienced acupuncturist for advice and treatment.

Acupressure from a qualified practitioner may also be of assistance, particularly for oestoarthritis.

THE ALEXANDER TECHNIQUE

An Alexander Technique practitioner can teach you to relieve and prevent arthritis through changing your habitual movement patterns.

AROMATHERAPY

CAUTION: *Read the information on pages 102 to 105 before using these essential oils.*

Aromatherapy administered with a massage can help relieve the pain of arthritis because it stimulates the body's own healing by improving circulation to the affected joints and can be extremely effective if used after the onset.

For those with long-term arthritis, aromatherapy can help reduce pain, improve mobility and prevent further damage.

If you have severe arthritis, it is recommended you see a professional aromatherapist for an extensive treatment. They will gently move painful joints and advise you on compresses you can use at home.

It is important that immediately after a massage or bath in essential oils the affected joint be moved as much as possible to keep the circulation going. If a joint is not moved after the application of aromatherapy, congestion can occur which makes the arthritis worse than before. Any movement which exercises the joint and long muscles is fine — just walking a little is a good example — but be careful not to overdo it.

If you suffer from arthritis, you may like to try add 3 drops lavender and 3 drops rosemary essential oils to a warm bath. The rosemary is for swelling and the lavender is for inflammation. If the joint is particularly painful, you can add 4 drops of chamomile instead as it is an effective analgesic. Diluted oil of fennel is also recommended for baths or massages.

BACH FLOWER REMEDIES

Some people believe arthritis is connected to negative emotional climates of bitterness and anger. The way the joints and muscles are constricted can be an indication of your state of mind. The remedies of holly and rockwater are good for loosening these emotions and constriction of the mind.

Impatiens and vine are remedies that can help people with gout.

CHINESE HERBS

Warming Chinese herbs that harmonise the spleen and kidney are often prescribed for people with arthritis. These are especially effective in the early stage of arthritis and are often used in conjunction with acupuncture treatment.

CHIROPRACTIC

Osteoarthritis can be greatly helped by chiropractic adjustment which releases the abnormal stress on the joints and spine. It also restores normal nerve function and increases movement in the joints. Results may vary depending on the stage of your condition. Chiropractic care can also help rheumatoid arthritis, although very gentle and subtle techniques are always recommended.

When choosing a chiropractor make sure they do peripheral adjustments (limb adjustments) as well as spinal adjustments. Some chiropractors only do spinal adjustments.

COUNSELLING

Some people believe arthritis is connected to "holding on" physically and emotionally — a counsellor can help you learn how to "let go" of any number of things from common, everyday frustrations to a traumatic past experience.

THE FELDENKRAIS METHOD

A Feldenkrais practitioner can teach you gentle, smooth, non-stressful, and efficient ways of moving, which will allow you to reach your movement potential and decrease stress on your joints which can reduce pain.

HERBALISM

The herb guaiacum is specifically for arthritis. Other useful herbs include dandelion root and greater celandine for the liver; the anti-inflammatory herbs comfrey, black cohosh and wild yam; burdock and fennel seed to combat fluid retention and to flush toxins from the body; meadowsweet and corn silk to normalise acidity; and celery with its high silica levels which will help break down calcium deposits. Look for these herbs in teas, tablets, or herbal mixtures at health food stores, and drink fresh celery juice.

You can also try rubbing the herbal ointment rue into the parts of your body which are affected by arthritis as it may ease the pain. Massage for about 30 minutes at least once a day for the best results.

In addition, you may get relief from warm or cold compresses with a chamomile infusion or a cold compress with cider vinegar.

Comfrey can also be used as either a poultice or an ointment.

HOMOEOPATHY

Specific remedies for this condition must be prescribed by a homoeopath because the prescription will vary greatly depending on numerous factors including what type of arthritis you have, what emotional state you are in, your environment, your lifestyle, and your medical history.

If you have gout and your joints are especially painful at night, consider taking one 6C potency of *Colchicum autumnale* every hour for five hours then lower the dose to 1 tablet three times a day. If the pain persists see a homoeopath who will give you a complete assessment.

MASSAGE

Swedish massage, aromatherapy massage and lymphatic drainage can assist pain relief and minor joint swelling, improve joint mobility and relax tight, hard muscles.

However, the joint itself should not be massaged when it is in a swollen, inflamed state. Be sure you are treated by a qualified practitioner.

For gout, too, very gentle massage in the area affected may give some pain relief.

MODERN MEDICINE

Depending on which type of arthritis you have, the treatment will differ accordingly. All drug treatments should be discussed fully with your doctor as many have side effects, particularly when taken long term or in combination with other medication.

You may also be prescribed analgesic and anti-inflammatory medication and/or physiotherapy may be recommended to treat the symptoms. Steroids may be used for acute flare-ups of rheumatoid arthritis. In severe cases, arthritic joints (particularly hips) may be surgically replaced with artificial ones.

For gout, medication may be prescribed to reduce the level of uric acid in the blood.

NATUROPATHY

CAUTION: *Read the information on page 167 before taking supplements.*

Due to the link with the bowel, diet is extremely important when treating all forms of arthritis. Naturopaths will suggest you avoid acid-producing foods such as meat (although fish is suitable), citrus fruits, strawberries, rhubarb, spinach and tomatoes; dairy foods (replace with soya bean products); wheat (other grains are better); food additives; and stimulants such as tea, coffee and alcohol as they lead to an increase of uric acid in the joints which causes inflammation.

They will also encourage you to eat plenty of other fruit and vegetables, and wholegrain foods as opposed to processed foods and those made from refined white flour, salt, and sugar.

Rheumatoid arthritis can be helped by fish oil (1000 mg three times a day) and evening primrose oil (1000 mg three times a day).

Osteoarthritis can be helped with prescribed doses of multi-mineral supplements and green-lipped mussel extract which is a nutritional supplement. See a naturopath for details of the exact dose you need.

For gout, a naturopath will advise you to avoid high protein foods such as meat and dairy foods; they may even tell you to change to a vegetarian diet that includes fruit, vegetables, tofu and soya bean products as well as nuts and seeds.

OSTEOPATHY

Osteopathy can assist with many forms of arthritis, both inflammatory (such as rheumatoid arthritis) and degenerative (such as osteoarthritis). Treatment is aimed at reducing inflammation, alleviating muscle contraction, and improving and restoring mobility in your joints. This is carried out gradually by relaxing the soft tissues and gently articulating the joints, thereby improving movement and circulation, reducing discomfort and enhancing the body's natural anti-inflammatory responses.

Osteopathy will not "cure" arthritis but, along with the dietary and lifestyle advice they give, an osteopath can assist with slowing the degenerative process and enable better management, both in the short and long term.

REFLEXOLOGY

A reflexologist can help your condition by working points on your feet with particular emphasis on the areas of your body which are affected by the arthritis. Treatment will also focus on the points for the adrenal glands as they help control inflammation, as well as the thyroid, kidneys and pituitary. The points for the kidneys are also worked for gout to assist in the elimination of excess uric acid.

You can try working these points at home if you are not restricted by arthritis in your hands. Also, it may be easier for you to work on your hands if you find it difficult to reach your feet. Work the suggested points for a total of 15 minutes on both feet or hands once a day.

SHIATSU

When the arthritis is not acute, shiatsu can relieve pain by increasing the mobility in your joints and improving the flow of Ki energy around your body. It can also strengthen the kidneys and disperse blockages in the gall bladder and liver meridians which are often affected in arthritis sufferers. A shiatsu practitioner will work around your joints rather than directly on them.

For gout, a shiatsu practitioner can work on your spleen and liver meridians as well as advising you on a diet more in keeping with your body's needs.

YOGA

You can ease your body into a state where your breathing slows, your muscles relax and your mind is calm, which can be helpful in alleviating the stress often associated with arthritis. Gentle yoga stretching exercises will warm up your joints.

The most important thing to remember about yoga and arthritis is that, if you are in acute pain, you should rest, relax and wait until the pain lessens before starting to exercise.

The head rotation exercise on page 198 may help ease stiffness in your neck. Problems with the wrists and ankles may be helped by rotations (see page 20). For the hips, try the variation on the butterfly exercise on page 194.

Other exercises for specific parts of your body affected by arthritis can be recommended and supervised by a yoga teacher.

ASTHMA

Asthma is a condition where the bronchial tubes spasm making it difficult to breathe. Sometimes there is excessive mucus in the lungs.

Asthma attacks may last a few hours, days or even weeks and can range from being short of breath to a life-threatening situation when you cannot breathe. There may be tightness in the chest, a rapid pulse, and coughing attacks with sweating.

Attacks may occur frequently or become prolonged. This is known as chronic asthma.

Asthma is usually the result of ALLERGIES and thus may be linked to ECZEMA and other reactions. It can also occur if your air passages are hypersensitive. Heredity may play a role.

Attacks can be triggered by allergens like dust, pollen, animal hair, certain foods, food additives, drugs, chemicals and smoke (including passive smoking). Asthma can be brought on by an infection, emotional stress or sometimes physical exertion. The incidence of pollution-related asthma appears to be rising.

The condition may begin in childhood, although adult onset is not uncommon.

IMPORTANT: *Do not replace your inhalant drug with other treatments without consulting your doctor and other health practitioners. If an asthma attack is severe, do not attempt to treat yourself — seek medical attention immediately.*

WHAT YOU CAN DO

- *First aid for an attack:* Sit up or stand up straight and breathe from your abdomen, loosen your clothing and try to get some fresh air. Drink plenty of room-temperature water. Avoid overdosing with anti-asthmatic drugs.
- Try to identify and avoid allergens (see page 214).
- Try to avoid situations where you will be exposed to tobacco smoke or high levels of air pollution. The juice of an onion sipped before exposure to irritants is said to reduce symptoms.
- Some food products may trigger an asthma attack. Products containing food additives, particularly sulphite preservatives or MSG (monosodium glutamate) should also be avoided — some wines, orange juices and potato chips fall into this category. Refined foods should be kept to a minimum.
- It is very important to avoid dairy products as they dramatically increase the mucus content in your body.
- Aspirin, drugs known as beta-blockers and some anti-arthritic medication can have an adverse effect on asthma sufferers.
- Try using a negative ioniser in the rooms where you spend a lot of time.
- Swimming is the best exercise for those who suffer from exercise-induced asthma because the nose and mouth won't dry out and cause irritation, but be careful of sensitivity to chlorinated water.
- Specific breathing control methods have had much success in drastically reducing the symptoms of asthma, even in chronic sufferers. See THE IMPORTANCE OF BREATH for details.
- Try a visualisation (see page 48) during an attack. Envisage cool blue air flowing easily into your lungs and spreading through your body, then a grey cloud of air leaving you fully as you exhale.
- Hot and cold compresses applied alternately to the upper back and chest may assist the functioning of your lungs.
- Most importantly — learn to recognise your own pattern. If you are aware of the early signs of asthma, you are able to intervene right away and prevent the symptoms turning into a severe attack. Biofeedback training and hypnotherapy (see page 207 to 208) have been very helpful in this way.

ACUPRESSURE

A qualified practitioner may be able to assist in managing this condition and provide you with information on techniques you can use at home during an attack.

ACUPUNCTURE

Acupuncture has been effective in giving relief to people with asthma that is not accompanied by complications.

AFFIRMATION

You can try to strengthen your resistance to asthma attacks with this affirmation. Repeat it to yourself as often as possible each day.

"I breathe easily knowing it is safe for me to take in life and fully express myself."

THE ALEXANDER TECHNIQUE

Originally known as "the breathing man", Alexander developed procedures for investigating, understanding and re-educating faulty breathing patterns which can both induce and intensify asthma attacks.

AROMATHERAPY

Because asthma can be caused by a variety of factors, an aromatherapist will be flexible in the treatment of this condition. If the asthma is triggered by an emotional condition, they may choose to use bergamot or chamomile essential oils which are antispasmodic and reduce depression. Lavender may be used if the asthma is linked to a chest infection. Regular aromatherapy massage from a qualified practitioner can help reduce the number of attacks and is a worthwhile support measure for chronic sufferers.

There are some first aid aromatherapy techniques you can use at home when you are having an attack. It is recommended that you inhale essential oils from a tissue rather than a steam inhalation as this can inflame the mucous membrane and increase congestion. Try 2 drops of peppermint on a tissue. Keep this with you and inhale it deeply throughout the day. It will help clear your air passages.

BACH FLOWER REMEDIES

Useful remedies include water violet (for unblocking energy, a possible psychological cause of chronic asthma) and rescue remedy (a good all-round remedy for coping with crises and useful in treating acute asthma). Rock rose is a good support measure for those with asthma.

CHINESE HERBS

Chinese herbalists can assist with this condition. There are specific anti-asthmatic herbs as well as expectorant herbs and those that clear the body of retained fluid.

CHIROPRACTIC

People with asthma respond well to chiropractic care in conjunction with important dietary changes (restricting sugar, fat and dairy). In chiropractic terms, lesions and subluxations around the neck and chest area affect breathing; releasing them allows the lungs to drain correctly and the air passages to open so the lungs can work more effectively.

COUNSELLING

You can be more prone to an asthma attack when you are feeling emotionally distressed. If you think there is an emotional component in your asthma, counselling may help.

THE FELDENKRAIS METHOD

This method, studied with a practitioner, enables people to recognise habitual breathing patterns which lead to decreased lung capacity and to learn breathing strategies that may help to reduce asthma.

HERBALISM

Grindelia is one herb used specifically for asthma. Others used for their particular affinity to the respiratory system include elderflowers, thyme, sage, plantain, passion flower and comfrey. To reduce infection in the lungs, echinacea, elecampane and wild cherry bark may be prescribed. A herbalist can put you on a complete herbal program and advise as to self-help remedies you can use during a mild attack.

HOMOEOPATHY

There are quite a few remedies that can help reduce the severity of an asthma attack by reducing the congestion of mucus in your body, "toning" your lungs, and dilating the bronchial passages. The specific remedy prescribed by a homoeopath will depend on the exact nature of your asthma and your general health.

MASSAGE

Massage should not be used during an attack of asthma; however, it can be used between attacks to relax muscles, relieve stress, and remove excessive mucus from the lungs. Although massage from a qualified practitioner will bring the most benefit, you can try massages at home, concentrating on the back, shoulders and chest.

MODERN MEDICINE

Doctors usually prescribe an inhalant drug known as a bronchodilator. Alternatively, they may recommend a form of cortisone spray. The drugs are also available in tablet form but these tend to have more side effects. This medication opens the airways by shrinking swollen tissue and reducing mucus secretion. It can be literally life saving in drastic attacks, but care must be taken against overuse which can cause tissue damage and overturn effectiveness. Long-term use may also result in an increase in the duration of the attacks. See page 163 for details on steroids.

If the asthma is related to an infection, antibiotics may be prescribed.

In severe attacks, intravenous drugs, oxygen and adrenaline may need to be administered.

NATUROPATHY

The condition can be stress related and naturopaths may suggest a change of diet combined with meditation or yoga breathing techniques. It is best to see a naturopath for a full assessment.

In addition to the all-important dairy restriction, other food sensitivities should be explored including those to gluten and sugar. You can try adding garlic and onions to your diet to counteract mucus production, as well as ginger, chilli and horseradish.

OSTEOPATHY

Osteopathy can assist in both prevention and alleviation. Treatment is aimed at enhancing the mechanics of breathing by working on the ribcage, the muscles that move the ribs that pump air in and out of the lungs, and the spine. Osteopathy also works to affect those parts of the body which control the air passages themselves, the amount of mucus secreted into them and their ability to deal with irritants.

An osteopath will work alongside drug or other therapies and assist in reducing the need for medication.

REFLEXOLOGY

Although reflexology can be used during an attack, it is primarily used for chronic conditions and as a support therapy. The points to work are the chest and lungs to assist breathing, the diaphragm and adrenal glands to help muscle tone in the chest/diaphragm area, and the ileocecal valve to reduce excess mucus which can impair breathing. Try this yourself on both feet or hands for a total of 15 minutes three times a week.

SHIATSU

In shiatsu, asthma is thought to be a weakness in the lungs and kidneys as well as an excess of wind and cold. The kidneys are responsible for "grasping" the Ki from the lungs. A shiatsu treatment will strengthen and relax your lungs and kidneys to make breathing easier and more effective. This is done by working with gentle pressure down the bladder and kidney energy channels on your back, concentrating on the upper back for the lungs and the lumbar region for the kidneys. The pressure then moves to the lung meridian in the arms and chest, finishing with the liver meridian to relax the chest muscles and diaphragm.

YOGA

Yoga is effective for people with asthma as it prepares and strengthens the body against an attack. Yoga breathing cycle exercises help with asthmatic conditions as they increase the stamina of the respiratory system, drain mucus from the lungs, and lessen tension in the chest. A yoga teacher will be able to pinpoint your strengths and weaknesses and put you on an appropriate exercise program to reduce the recurrence of attacks.

The balloon-blowing breathing exercise on page 193 is a good example of a yoga breathing cycle exercise. Another exercise that will help you avoid an impending attack is the chair breathing exercise. If you start this when you feel an attack coming on it will bring you into a calmer state. The chest-opening position is another beneficial posture.

BACK PAIN

Back pain is an extremely common problem that inspires more people to seek "alternative" therapies than any other condition. It can occur anywhere from your tail bone to the base of your skull.

It can be caused by a muscle being strained from over-exertion, lifting an object the wrong way, awkward movement, or an accident — this is often acute or sudden pain. In other cases, the cause may be ARTHRITIS, poor posture, general stress or emotional factors such as DEPRESSION. These often cause chronic (i.e. lasting or recurring) pain. Or it can be caused by physical pressure (such as a slipped disc) being placed on the nerves.

See also INFERTILITY, MENOPAUSE, NECK PAIN, PELVIC INFLAMMATORY DISEASE.

IMPORTANT: *Back pain can indicate serious problems such as a kidney infection or gynaecological complications. If the pain is not relieved after a few treatments, seek medical advice to further investigate the cause.*

WHAT YOU CAN DO

- As the abdominal muscles help support the spine, gentle exercises that strengthen these muscles will benefit your back.
- Swimming will not only strengthen the back and abdominal muscles, but will also support the body and reduce strain while exercising. However, when doing breaststroke, put your face in the water every few strokes to avoid overstretching the spinal ligaments.
- The stress on joints and muscles from jogging or running can aggravate back pain, however, the risks can be minimised by wearing shoes that are properly cushioned on the sole. You should also avoid running on hard surfaces — grass is preferable.
- Avoid high-heeled shoes as they place extra strain on your back.
- Be conscious of the position of your spine and your posture when sitting and sleeping. Avoid low soft chairs from which it is difficult to rise. Sit in a relaxed position with both feet flat on the floor, your back straight and well supported. Sleep on your back without a pillow or sleep on your side with your legs bent and a pillow between your knees to prevent hip rotation. This will help you get a good night's sleep. See also INSOMNIA.
- Give some relief to your lower back. Rest on your back with no pillow under your head — try a pillow under your knees instead. Or lie with your legs elevated, your knees and lower legs on the seat of a chair.
- Both hot and cold compresses will help relieve the pain of back ache.

ACUPRESSURE

Acupressure can help relieve moderate back pain especially in the lower part of your back. It is best to consult a qualified practitioner but you can give it a try at home.

Ask someone to apply firm pressure to the acupressure points Bladder 22 and 23 on your lower back three times daily for 10 to 15 minutes. Massage of the points Bladder 16 and 40 can also release lower back spasm.

ACUPUNCTURE

Acupuncture is known to be extremely effective on all kinds of back pain which is often due to blockages of energy in the body. It can also be used to lessen severe cases to the point where other therapies, such as massage, can be utilised.

THE ALEXANDER TECHNIQUE

The Alexander Technique can relieve and prevent back pain by re-educating you on the way you move and its effect on your body. When you observe the way you sit, walk and bend with an Alexander teacher, you will realise there are ways of moving that are more efficient and put less strain on your back.

AROMATHERAPY

CAUTION: *Read the information on pages 102 to 105 before using these essential oils.*

If your back pain is due to tension or muscular fatigue aromatherapy can be effective, especially if used in conjunction with other therapies.

A massage or bath with essential oils can be effective in relieving physical pain, reducing stress which can cause tension in your back, and relaxing your body so it can better respond to other treatments. Oils that are appropriate include lavender, chamomile, geranium and rosemary, and ginger or cinnamon if you feel cold.

You can use aromatherapy as a preventative measure if you are prone to back problems, by taking baths or having massages regularly, even when your back is not hurting. Try a warm bath containing 2 drops of rosemary and 2 drops of lavender.

BACH FLOWER REMEDIES

Rescue remedy is effective for an unexpected onset of back pain as it calms the shock of the pain. Other remedies include elm if you feel overwhelmed and oak for strength both physically and mentally.

CHIROPRACTIC

In chiropractic terms, back pain in different areas is often due to subluxations in the spine which occur when the nervous system is under stress. Chiropractic is known to be extremely effective at reducing back pain of all kinds. You may need a series of adjustments over several weeks or months, depending on your condition. X-rays may be required. A chiropractor can give you a full assessment — they are qualified to diagnose the cause of the pain, as well as offer treatment or refer you to the appropriate specialist if the pain is not of spinal origin.

COUNSELLING

A variety of emotional causes can contribute to back pain. A counsellor will focus on any stress you may be feeling which triggers the pain. They will encourage you to look at any "burdens" you are carrying in your life and to let them go. If you relate to these concepts, counselling is worthwhile pursuing.

You may also like to try an affirmation like this one: "I have all the support and strength I need. I gladly release any burdens I am carrying. I trust in the process of life." Repeat it to yourself as many times a day as possible.

THE FELDENKRAIS METHOD

Lessons in the Feldenkrais Method can be very effective in preventing and relieving back pain by identifying and eliminating possible causes. A practitioner will look at the movement patterns you use in your everyday activities and give you new movement options.

HERBALISM

Massage with a herbal ointment containing rue may bring relief.

MASSAGE

Remedial massage can assist other modalities such as CHIROPRACTIC, OSTEOPATHY and physiotherapy with back problems where the pain is caused by tight, stressed, overworked muscles or poor posture.

MODERN MEDICINE

Analgesics, anti-inflammatory medication, or muscle relaxants may be prescribed. Applying heat treatment creams or packs to the sore area of your back may also be suggested. Often physiotherapy will be recommended as well. Surgery is usually a last resort for structural problems such as a slipped disc.

OSTEOPATHY

Osteopaths specialise in treating people with back pain and are qualified to diagnose the cause of the pain as well as offer treatment. They will check for osteopathic lesions and misalignments in your body which interfere with nerve activity and blood supply. They may ask for X-rays to be taken. Osteopaths relieve the pain using a combination of gentle manipulation, massage, and techniques to improve or restore spinal joint motion. They will also suggest specific exercises to suit each individual's needs.

REFLEXOLOGY

Work the points for the whole spine as well as the throat and neck. Try this on both feet or hands for a total of 20 minutes twice a week — be careful not to overstimulate. You can also include the diaphragm and solar plexus points to encourage relaxation and thus pain reduction.

SHIATSU

Shiatsu can help if your back pain has a structural cause, or is linked to a weakness in your kidneys, or to the lack of flowing Ki energy in your hips and buttocks. Shiatsu stretching and corrective exercises will help strengthen your abdominal muscles which support your lower back and improve your posture for general back health. They are exceptionally good for relieving back pain when practised along with twisting movements. However, study them with a shiatsu therapist because the wrong exercise can do more harm than good.

Shiatsu therapy works well in combination with Chinese herbal medicine and moxibustion (see pages 182 and 95) in the treatment of chronic back pain.

YOGA

Yoga is known to be very effective on back pain but you should be careful to do the exercises very gently and slowly so that you protect your back from further damage. Stretch but don't strain. Try the supine twist, the spinal flex and the right-angle stretch exercises on pages 203 to 205.

IMPORTANT: *These exercises are best learnt under the supervision of a yoga teacher who will advise you on how to protect your back. Also make sure you take all yoga movements at your own pace.*

BLADDER PROBLEMS

The bladder forms part of the urinary tract which expels urine (formed in the kidneys) from the body.

Infections in this body system can result in difficulty or pain when urinating. In some cases blood appears in the urine. Discomfort can be considerable as the urge to urinate may be frequent with little output. There may be a stinging or burning sensation during urination. Pain in the abdomen and back can also be a symptom.

Cystitis is usually an inflammation of the inner lining of the bladder. Acute or chronic *urethritis* may accompany it. This is an inflammation of the urethra (the tube leading from the bladder).

Sometimes the urethra is bruised during sex. If symptoms occur immediately after sex, a bacterial infection may not be involved. Some of the self-help measures below should be successful in avoiding one.

Some women seem prone to inflammation of the urinary system. If the inflammation is chronic, recurrent and does not involve infection, the problem may be related to yeast in the diet. Other causes include an inappropriate diet, the Pill, antibiotics and DIABETES. Inflammation is rarely caused by bacteria, but may make you susceptible to bacterial infection.

Infectious organisms can come from the kidneys, vagina or bowel, hence THRUSH, CONSTIPATION and infections of the kidneys can also be associated with bladder infections.

Sexually transmitted diseases can be the cause of urethritis, particularly for men. Often there will be a discharge from the penis.

For women, the contraceptive diaphragm may be involved.

Stones are sometimes the cause of bladder problems. These are collections of hard salt which build up anywhere is your renal system/urinary tract (the kidneys, ureters, urethra and bladder). They can then travel to the bladder where they may cause severe abdominal pain. By blocking outflow, they can cause urinary retention which then leads to infection.

See also FLUID RETENTION, INCONTINENCE, KIDNEY PROBLEMS, PELVIC INFLAMMATORY DISEASE, PROSTATE PROBLEMS.

IMPORTANT: *Consult a doctor if you suspect an infection, particularly if you have blood or mucus in your urine as it may indicate a serious problem.*

WHAT YOU CAN DO

- At first signs of cystitis/urethritis, stay warm and relaxed, and lie or sit down if possible. An attack should pass within a few hours unless a bacterial infection is involved.
- When urinary tract symptoms occur, drink a urine alkaliser — either a commercially available preparation or a teaspoon of bicarbonate of soda (baking soda) in a glass of water (unless you have high blood pressure or heart problems).
- Apply acidophilus yogurt to the genital area.
- Avoid alcohol and coffee and other products containing caffeine which adversely affects the muscles of the bladder.
- Eat mild, non-irritating food. Avoid hot or spicy food, and animal protein (eggs, fish, meat, poultry).
- Drink plenty of water or mild herbal tea, even if you have a bladder weakness, as it will help tone your bladder and take stress from your kidneys.
- If susceptible to urinary tract inflammations, drink cranberry juice daily to balance the acidity of your urine and prevent bacterial infection.
- Highly acidic urine can make you prone to bladder infections. In such cases, avoid citrus or sour fruit, and foods containing vinegar.
- Avoid constipation and obesity.
- Do exercises to strengthen the pelvic muscles.

Try clenching and unclenching your buttock muscles, for example. Women should try stopping and starting the flow of their urine by using their pelvic muscles.

• Alternating hot and cold compresses over the lower abdomen, or taking hot and cold sitz baths, will improve circulation to the area thereby assisting bladder and bowel function.

• Go to the toilet as soon as you feel the need as retaining urine gives bacteria an opportunity to multiply.

• Wipe paper from front to back after urinating.

• Women prone to bladder infections can try splashing their genital area with cold water (preferably cooled, boiled water containing a selected herbal extract or essential oil if desired) after urinating rather than using toilet paper. The anus should be washed with unscented soap after a bowel movement.

• Choose showers over baths and avoid cosmetics such as bubble baths and talc.

• Dryness during intercourse causes irritation, so use a lubricant if necessary.

• Change your form of contraceptive; as well as the Pill, spermicidal creams may cause irritation and diaphragms may put pressure on the bladder.

• Women who experience recurring infections should try to avoid sexual positions that expose the urethral opening to excessive friction or pressure.

• Empty your bladder before and after intercourse.

• Wear cotton underwear (or none at all) and wash them in a mild, non-irritating washing powder/liquid.

• Try sanitary napkins instead of tampons.

• Avoid perfumed soaps, bubble bath, talcum powders etc and do not use vaginal deodorants.

• Avoid physical irritations such as extreme temperatures (sitting on cold ground, standing in draughts) or long bicycle rides. Chlorine in swimming pools may affect some people.

ACUPRESSURE

Treatment from a practitioner would vary depending on the cause of the problem. At home, massaging Conception Vessel 6 and 4 may be useful.

ACUPUNCTURE

Bladder problems have been known to be effectively relieved by acupuncture. A qualified acupuncturist can give you specific advice and treatment.

AROMATHERAPY

Bladder inflammation can be relieved by essential oils that are detoxifying and antiseptic. Baths are an effective way of using the oils to treat cystitis. Try 2 drops each of sandalwood, eucalyptus and cajuput in a bath; make sure the oils are well dispersed before you get in. Women should swish the water towards their urethra, like a douche, before they sit down.

BACH FLOWER REMEDIES

Bladder problems in general can be associated with "holding on" and an ability to "let go". Walnut is the all-round protector and the link breaker for letting go. Crab apple is for cleansing the mind and body.

The emotion related to the kidneys is fear. Mimulus is for known fear (it protects the kidneys) and aspen is for unknown fear. There may also be anger involved thus holly may be a suitable remedy.

CHINESE HERBS

Chinese herbs can be very effective in treating bladder problems but these should be prescribed by a herbalist based on an individual assessment.

CHIROPRACTIC

Chiropractic adjustment has been known to help with bladder problems of all kinds. A chiropractor is likely to work specifically on your tail bone, lower back, and rib cage as this area is directly connected to your bladder. Pelvic problems are often associated with bladder problems. If you display symptoms of cystitis, a chiropractor will check that your nervous system is fully functional. If it is not, this may be a recurrent cause of the infections.

COUNSELLING

Some bladder problems can be associated with "holding on" to emotions or with feelings of anxiety so counselling may be helpful in such cases.

THE FELDENKRAIS METHOD

Bladder problems are often related to weakness in the pelvic floor. A Feldenkrais practitioner can teach you awareness and control of your pelvic floor. This is then integrated into total body movement.

HERBALISM

The herbs bearberry, corn silk and marshmallow root as well as slippery elm in a powder form can help relieve the symptoms of cystitis.

Buchu tea is an antiseptic herbal remedy which cleanses the whole urinary system and helps to relieve most bladder dysfunctions, including cystitis. Try drinking 2 cups of buchu tea per day to start but you may like to see a herbalist for a complete diagnosis of your condition.

HOMOEOPATHY

If you have bladder stones or other problems associated with your bladder, professional homoeopathic treatment can be very useful.

Some of the homoeopathic remedies that are most commonly used to treat cystitis are *Sarsaparilla, Causticum* and *Cantharis.* If your urine feels hot and causes pain and you feel the need to urinate all the time but not much comes out, take one 6C potency of *Cantharis* every hour for the first day. Then take one 6C potency three times a day for the next two days. If you have any doubts or if the cystitis continues, seek professional advice.

MODERN MEDICINE

Before treatment begins, a mid-stream urine sample will be requested and analysed. There are antiseptic drugs available that change the quality of the urine so that infectious organisms do not replicate. Antibiotics may be prescribed but they can encourage THRUSH. Analgesics may bring pain relief.

NATUROPATHY

If you are suffering from cystitis, a naturopath will give you a complete diagnosis and may advise you to take 5000 iu per day of vitamin A and 2000 mg per day of vitamin C to fight the infection in your body.

Try to eat alkalising fruits and vegetables, including apples, celery, cucumber, and carrots (fresh carrot juice is especially good) because bacteria cannot live in alkaline urine. Drink pure cranberry juice. Avoid oranges or only eat them when you are sure the citric acid is not aggravating your cystitis. Avoid sugar, and instead use honey as a sweetener, because excessive sugar can contribute to cystitis.

Cystitis can also be associated with food allergies and tests may be recommended.

OSTEOPATHY

Some bladder problems can be helped by osteopathy if they are related to misalignment in your body or lack of circulation to vital organs.

REFLEXOLOGY

For bladder problems generally, work these points: the bladder, adrenal glands (for muscle tone in the bladder) and the lower spine (for the nerves in the area).

For cystitis, the points for the bladder and adrenal glands are again worked — as well as the ureter tubes — to help combat inflammation. The kidneys and lymphatic system are activated to help the immune system fight infection.

Work these points on both feet or hands for a total of 20 minutes daily until the condition clears.

SHIATSU

In shiatsu the bladder meridian runs parallel to your vertebrae and therefore has a strong effect on your nervous system up and down your spine. A shiatsu practitioner will work on getting the Ki energy flowing freely along your bladder meridian in order to calm the nervous system. They will also look at aspects of your diet to balance the energy in your body. You may be advised to add more grains, legumes and beans to your diet as well as naturally high sources of minerals, and to reduce fruits, fruit juices, sugars, saturated fats and refrigerated foods.

YOGA

The cobra exercise on page 196 is good for bladder conditions because it stimulates kidney function.

BLOOD PRESSURE PROBLEMS

The measurement of the pressure exerted on the walls of your arteries can be an indication of your heart's ability to cope with stresses. The terms "high blood pressure" and "low blood pressure" are often used inappropriately, when the actual problem may be one of many other ailments.

High blood pressure occurs when there is an increase in the force of blood against your arteries and heart. This means your heart has to work harder to pump blood around your body. Causes may vary and in many cases may not be specifically identified. Heredity may have a role.

Abnormally high blood pressure is known as *hypertension*. There may be dizziness, HEADACHE, nose bleeds, heart palpitations, shortness of breath, vision problems, FATIGUE and ANXIETY as a result of this condition but usually, during the course of daily life, there are no symptoms.

The condition is serious, however, and can lead to ANGINA, heart attack, stroke, haemorrhage or KIDNEY PROBLEMS if not successfully treated.

Low blood pressure is known as *hypotension*. Low blood pressure can be a normal state for some people and is not necessarily a problem; in very fit athletes it is a sign of the fitness of their heart function.

Conversely, it can be an abnormal state, the result of a trauma such as shock or heart failure. Low blood pressure can also be a symptom of conditions like heart valve problems, rare hormonal problems, and adrenal or glandular problems which need to be diagnosed and treated.

There can also be a temporary drop in blood pressure, particularly in elderly people, caused by a slower than normal bodily response to changing positions (such as standing up after being seated), leading to dizziness and sometimes fainting. In such cases, care should be taken to move slowly and with sufficient support.

Poor circulation is often linked to low blood pressure. FATIGUE and low blood sugar levels may also be associated. Dehydration or an allergic reaction may be other causes.

Hypotension for reasons other than these is not a condition recognised by Western orthodox medicine.

See also HEART PROBLEMS.

WHAT YOU CAN DO

- Watching your weight, even in small ways, can have a considerable effect on high blood pressure.
- Reducing salt, alcohol and saturated fat intakes will benefit those with high blood pressure.
- Regular moderate exercise is advisable for both low and high blood pressure. Forms of aerobic exercise will provide the greatest benefit if pursued carefully. Isometric exercise, such as weight lifting, is not recommended as it may cause blood pressure to temporarily skyrocket.
- Choose other forms of contraception rather than the Pill.
- Reduce stress in your life as much as possible (see page 40).

ACUPUNCTURE

Acupuncture has been used to effectively treat ideopathic hypertension. See an acupuncturist for specific treatment.

AROMATHERAPY

CAUTION: *Read the information on pages 102 to 105 before using these essential oils.*

A professional aromatherapy treatment is recommended to relieve stress which in turn can lower high blood pressure. An aromatherapist may choose oils such as clary sage or melissa to help reduce your blood pressure. Or they may use lavender, the oil that induces relaxation. For relaxation at home, add 2 drops of sweet marjoram and 2 drops of ylang ylang to your bath, making sure the oil is well dispersed. Doing this twice in one week will keep your body relaxed and able to cope with the stress you face.

For low blood pressure, particular oils can improve your circulation. Either consult an aromatherapist or try adding 4 drops of rosemary to your bath.

BACH FLOWER REMEDIES

Remedies that help calm the body and therefore reduce high blood pressure are rescue remedy and impatiens (for people who are always on the go and need to slow down).

For people with low blood pressure, the remedies that are most effective are gentian (helps to reduce depression) and larch (builds confidence).

CHINESE HERBS

Chinese herbs are very effective in treating high and low blood pressure. A Chinese herbalist can give you a herbal prescription to suit your specific symptoms.

CHIROPRACTIC

Raised or low blood pressure can occur as a direct result of nerve interference to the heart, lungs and diaphragm and can be managed by chiropractic adjustment. People with high blood pressure often have underlying back problems and a degree of pain — in these cases, a chiropractor can be of assistance.

COUNSELLING

As emotional pressures can affect blood pressure levels, counselling can be invaluable in resolving these issues.

THE FELDENKRAIS METHOD

Through teaching breathing strategies and efficient ways of moving, a Feldenkrais practitioner can help you reduce your general muscle tension which can lower blood pressure. Low blood pressure can be raised by changing the rhythm and speed of movements.

HERBALISM

A herbalist will examine your diet, stress levels and sleeping habits before prescribing specific treatment for your condition.

The herbs hawthorn berries, lime blossom, oats, nettle, motherwort and damiana are often prescribed by herbalists for high blood pressure. Also used because of their calming effect are valerian, skullcap and passion flower. Adding garlic to your meals (especially raw) can help reduce your blood pressure.

Herbs can also help improve low blood pressure but it is best to consult a herbalist for specific advice.

HOMOEOPATHY

Homoeopathy can be very effective in treating people with blood pressure problems, but it is essential that a professional diagnosis be made to get the right prescription of homoeopathic remedies.

MASSAGE

Massage may be of assistance in high blood pressure where stress or tension is an associated cause. It can encourage circulation in cases of low blood pressure.

MODERN MEDICINE

For high blood pressure, doctors will recommend lifestyle changes (see What You Can Do). Drugs known as anti-hypertensives may be prescribed as well, but these do not affect the cause of the problem and can have serious side effects. These drugs include vasodilators, ACE inhibitors and calcium channel blockers. In rare cases, surgery may be recommended.

For low blood pressure, doctors would look at your fluid and salt levels.

NATUROPATHY

CAUTION: *Read the information on page 167 before taking supplements.*

If you have high blood pressure a naturopath will recommend you reduce your intake of salt and fats and increase your intake of fibre. They will also prescribe high amounts of vitamin E tablets (500 iu per day) as well as daily intakes of fish oil (1000 mg per day) and garlic tablets (2000 mg per day).

For low blood pressure a naturopath will check your iron levels, and your liver and digestive system, and then prescribe the appropriate vitamins and minerals. Regular gentle exercise is also helpful.

In either case, consult a naturopath for advice.

REFLEXOLOGY

Using a holistic approach, a reflexologist can assist in the rebalancing of your body systems. Although there are no specific points for circulation, there are areas you can work at home which can help in the control of blood pressure, both high and low. These are the diaphragm to aid relaxation as well as the thyroid and pituitary gland.

In cases of high blood pressure, the points for the kidneys should also be worked as the condition can lead to kidney damage.

Try this on both feet or hands for a total of 15 minutes three times a week.

SHIATSU

Shiatsu treatment can help reduce high blood pressure by relaxing your constricted artery walls and generally calming your nervous system. If your high blood pressure is linked to a constriction or lack of Ki energy flowing to your kidneys, intestines, heart, liver or adrenals, a shiatsu therapist can diagnose and treat this.

For low blood pressure shiatsu offers general "tonifying" of all your essential organs (e.g. heart, liver, intestines) which will help increase your blood pressure. Correct diagnosis by a qualified practitioner is necessary for effective treatment.

VISUALISATION

If you have high blood pressure, read AFFIRMATIONS AND VISUALISATIONS and prepare yourself for visualisation.

See yourself in a stressful situation which makes your blood pressure rise. Feel the impact of that stress on your body then say to yourself, "I am at a point of choice. I choose to feel relaxed and calm under any circumstance."

Now visualise yourself in those same stressful circumstances, but this time behaving in a relaxed and calm manner, being empowered by your strength.

Visualise yourself undergoing your next blood pressure check-up. See your health professional congratulating you on an excellent blood pressure result. Take time with this part, using all your senses, imagining how relaxed you feel now your blood pressure is under control.

Do this creative visualisation daily, and practise feeling the peace and calm from your visualisation during stressful circumstances in your daily life.

YOGA

If you have high blood pressure yoga is ideal, especially the relaxation techniques. Many people have been successful in lowering their blood pressure through yoga. Join a class and inform your teacher of your condition and they will select special postures for you until your blood pressure returns to normal. You will probably have to avoid inverted postures as these can aggravate the problem, but forward stretches can be helpful because they are very sedating.

If you have low blood pressure yoga can also help, but you need an overall exercise program to suit you so it is advisable to seek a yoga teacher's advice rather than teaching yourself.

BRONCHITIS

Bronchitis is an inflammation of the bronchial tubes (air passages in the lungs). When the tubes are inflamed it is difficult to breathe; generally there is a persistent cough that brings up a lot of phlegm.

Acute bronchitis, caused by a viral or bacterial infection, comes on suddenly and usually passes within three weeks. It is often a complication of another illness such as cold or flu. Chronic bronchitis is a prolonged disorder and involves structural damage to the bronchial tubes due to repeated bouts of acute bronchitis, irritations such as air pollution or SMOKING, or a hereditary predisposition. Untreated, the symptoms may worsen over time and can develop into emphysema.

In both cases, there may be shortness of breath, coughing and thick, coloured mucus. Symptoms of acute bronchitis may include fever, wheezing and chest pain.

IMPORTANT: *Any kind of persistent coughing should be checked and treated by a doctor as it could indicate a serious problem. Mild coughs should be treated in initial stages to avoid worsening.*

WHAT YOU CAN DO

- A steam inhalation, over a basin of hot water with a towel over your head, will help to soothe, open and clear the air passages. Do this every couple of hours during a heavy bout.
- Drink plenty of fluids to help break up the mucus thus making it easier to expel. Reduce intake of alcohol and caffeine as they are diuretics.
- Keep your body warm, especially your chest area.
- A herbal pillow, filled with lavender and sage, for example, can also bring some relief at night.
- Avoid dry, overheated rooms.
- If a smoker, the best thing you can do is stop. Bronchitis sufferers should.
- Do breathing exercises (see page 25).
- Avoid smoky or polluted environments.

ACUPUNCTURE

Traditional Chinese Medicine, of which acupuncture and acupressure are part, recognises seven types of asthma but does not differentiate between asthma and bronchitis. Acupuncture is heralded for its success rate with a range of respiratory conditions.

AROMATHERAPY

CAUTION: *Read the information on pages 102 to 105 before using these essential oils.*

Aromatherapy steam inhalations can be great for clearing chest congestion. Add 3 drops each of eucalyptus and lemon into a bowl of steaming water. Sit with your head over the bowl, your eyes closed and your head covered by a towel. Inhale the steam deeply for as long as is comfortable. If the steam irritates your breathing it may be best to inhale the oil mixture from a tissue instead. You can also try an oil burner in your bedroom at night (or in your surroundings during the day) — make sure you have a deep bowl if you are burning the candle for a prolonged period.

Use these techniques at home but if you have chronic bronchitis, a professional aromatherapist can give you further advice.

BACH FLOWER REMEDIES

Remedies that are useful for bronchitis include willow as it lessens resentment and bitterness — emotions that some believe may be linked to bronchitis.

CHINESE HERBS

Chinese herbs can be used as a preventive measure against an attack of bronchitis if you know you are prone to it. Chinese herbalists will try to improve your lung energy with particular herbs and improve the flow of Qi energy in your body.

CHIROPRACTIC

Chiropractic adjustment can increase the effective functioning of your nervous system which in turn can help your immunity to illnesses like bronchitis. The direct mechanical benefit of your chest and rib cage moving better will allow the lungs and airways to function more freely and return to good health.

THE FELDENKRAIS METHOD

The breathing strategies taught by Feldenkrais practitioners may help you understand why you are experiencing bronchitis and therefore may help you to reduce its incidence.

HEALING MEDITATION

You can use the time when you are lying in bed recovering from a bout of bronchitis to visualise blue healing light flowing into your body and clearing your lungs and airways. See Healing Energies.

HERBALISM

Herbs that are useful include echinacea, elecampane, euphorbia, golden seal, grindelia, hyssop and wild cherry bark as well as chilli, ginger, garlic, thyme and cloves. Use a combination of these herbs — available from health food stores — preferably under the guidance of a herbalist.

HOMOEOPATHY

Homoeopathic remedies, when properly prescribed by a homoeopath, are excellent for helping people with bronchitis. They can improve the constitution of your body making it less prone to bronchial problems.

MASSAGE

Massage can be of benefit, by relaxing tight muscles in the back and chest and by loosening mucus. In acute cases care should be taken not to spread infection with massage. In chronic conditions, massage should only be performed between attacks.

MODERN MEDICINE

Antibiotics are often used by doctors to treat this condition. Some doctors may prescribe medication known as expectorants to ease coughing, although others feel that coughing is necessary to ensure phlegm is removed from lungs.

Also recommended are over-the-counter balsam inhalations and chest rubs such as friar's balsam, eucalyptus oil and camphor.

Regular physiotherapy may be recommended for chronic bronchitis to help drain the phlegm.

NATUROPATHY

Those who get bronchitis should avoid dairy products and chocolate due to the effect on mucous membranes. Adding garlic to your diet will be of benefit.

To reduce an acute infection, take 1000 mg or 1/4 teaspoon of powdered vitamin C every hour during the acute period, then reduce to 1/2 teaspoon twice a day — the powder form is more easily digested than tablets. In addition, take 5000 iu vitamin A per day. You can also dilute the juice of 1 lemon in 1 cup of hot water — add 1 teaspoon of honey, a clove of garlic, a pinch of chilli powder and some grated ginger for additional benefits — and drink 2 cups daily.

In chronic cases, maintain the same level of vitamin A supplement but take only 3000 mg of vitamin C daily between attacks.

OSTEOPATHY

Bronchial congestion is sometimes related to restrictions in the vertebrae and lungs, so osteopathy may be of help (see ASTHMA). Cranial osteopathy (a very gentle osteopathic approach which incorporates the treatment of the head as well as the rest of the muscle-skeleton framework) is also known to be effective.

REFLEXOLOGY

Work these points: chest/lungs and diaphragm to relax the chest area and assist breathing, the adrenal glands for muscle tone and to combat inflammation, the ileocecal valve to reduce excessive mucus, and the lymphatic system for any infection. Try these for a total of 15 minutes on both hands or feet three times a week.

SHIATSU

In shiatsu, bronchitis is seen as a weakness in your lungs and an imbalance in your water metabolism. A practitioner will strengthen your lungs by clearing phlegm from them through the application of sensitive pressure to the meridian channel and lower parts of your lungs and intercostals. This will in turn open up your chest and reduce bronchial problems.

They will also "tonify" the function of your spleen and kidneys which controls water metabolism in the body and the ability to fight infection and inflammation.

YOGA

See yoga exercises for COLDS AND INFLUENZA.

BRUISES

A bruise is a discolouration and swelling just under the surface of the skin which occurs due to a bump or strong pressure. The skin changes colour because blood capillaries break under the skin.

Age, overexposure to the sun, and some medications such as cortisone and aspirin can weaken our ability to withstand knocks or undue physical pressure without bruising.

IMPORTANT: *If you bruise very easily or without apparent cause, or a bruise lasts longer than two weeks, it is worthwhile having a medical check as it may indicate another problem such as a blood clotting disorder. Serious bruising should also get medical attention to check for further damage.*

WHAT YOU CAN DO

- Apply a cold compress or ice pack as soon as possible after injury to constrict the blood vessels and minimise bruising.
- After about 24 hours, a hot compress may help relieve the pain and promote the healing process.
- If severe bruising occurs on a leg or arm, keep the limb rested and elevated for one to two days.

ACUPUNCTURE

In traditional Chinese medicine, bruising indicates a problem of spleen Qi. Acupuncture can be used to strengthen the spleen to reduce susceptibility to bruising.

AFFIRMATION

If you are the type of person who bruises easily or seems to bump into things a lot it is worthwhile considering whether you are doing this as a form of self-punishment. If you might be, try repeating an affirmation throughout the day along the lines of "My body is precious and I release the need to punish myself."

AROMATHERAPY

Aromatherapy can help heal minor bruises as it has pain-killing and anti-swelling effects on the skin. Add 3 drops of sweet marjoram, 3 drops of geranium and 1 drop of chamomile to 2 teaspoons of base carrier oil. Apply this mixture to the bruise immediately, then keep applying it every 2 hours until the bruise clears up. Avoid contact with broken skin and if pain persists see your doctor.

BACH FLOWER REMEDIES

Rescue remedy is good for the emotional shock of bruising and walnut is for protection against any further accidents.

CHINESE HERBS

If you bruise easily a Chinese herbalist will give you herbs to protect and supplement your spleen network.

HOMOEOPATHY

One of the most well-known and effective homoeopathic remedies for bruising is *Arnica montana.* It can help a bruise to heal very quickly. In cases such as soft tissue injury, apply it to the bruise or take it internally immediately after injury. Keep applying the ointment until the bruise begins to clear. Do not use externally on open wounds.

If your bruise is on a part of your body that has a concentration of nerve endings (for example, your fingers, toes and ears) consider the use of *Hypericum perforatum.*

MODERN MEDICINE

Cold compresses are recommended. Bruise-resolving creams are available over the counter. They contain heparinoid which dissolves the clot. Analgesics may be used to relieve pain.

Doctors often advise people who bruise easily to avoid aspirin as it thins the blood.

NATUROPATHY

If you bruise easily, take 1000 mg vitamin C per day but ensure the supplement contains bioflavinoids as these strengthen the capillaries.

REFLEXOLOGY

Gently work the reflex that corresponds to the area that is bruised. Try this for a total of 10 minutes on both hands or feet once or twice a week.

If the bruise is on the foot, work the points on the hand and vice versa.

SHIATSU

Shiatsu should be avoided on areas of the skin that have been bruised but if you are prone to bruising from minor bumps, shiatsu can help. A practitioner would work on increasing Ki energy to your spleen and heart as the spleen holds the blood in the blood vessels and the heart controls the strength of the blood vessels. They would also work on bladder and small intestine deficiencies which can lead to the susceptibility to bruising in different areas.

BUNIONS AND CORNS

A *bunion* is a swollen, inflamed bulge at the side of the foot where the largest toe joins the rest of the foot. It is made worse by wearing shoes that are too narrow.

A *corn* is a hard, cone-shaped piece of skin caused by tight shoes that rub. It often occurs on the joint of the smallest toe.

The way your body distributes its weight can make you prone to this type of problem, as can carrying excess weight.

WHAT YOU CAN DO

- Resist the temptation to slice, cut or pare down your corns, bunions and calluses — this can lead to infection or possibly serious injury if the implement slips.
- Soaking feet in a solution of warm water and Epsom salts or chamomile tea will help soothe, reduce inflammation and soften hard skin. Then gently rub with a pumice stone to lightly erode the top layers of dead skin.
- Every night liberally massage each foot with moisturiser to promote blood flow, and wear cotton socks to bed to enhance the effect of the moisturiser.
- Don't wear shoes that don't fit properly. There should be a thumb width of distance from the end of the longest toe to the end of the shoes. They should also be wide enough to comfortably span the width across the ball of the foot, and have enough room to prevent pressure on the toes. Natural materials like leather are best because they "breathe". High heels are not recommended.
- Remove shoes whenever possible and wiggle and flex your toes.
- Try to lose weight if you are overweight.

THE ALEXANDER TECHNIQUE AND FELDENKRAIS METHOD

These practitioners can help you learn to distribute your weight more efficiently.

AROMATHERAPY

A therapeutic foot massage with essential oils such as German chamomile or calendula can help relieve the pain of bunions and corns. See a qualified aromatherapist who will be able to work on your feet more easily and effectively than you could at home.

BACH FLOWER REMEDIES

Walnut is a good remedy for "letting go". This is the required psychological response, according to Bach's philosophy, when you experience bunions and corns.

CHIROPRACTIC

Chiropractors can give you a full spinal check and observe your stance and gait. From this they can work out what kind of adjustments will best help you return to normal posture and balanced weight bearing, whereby the joints are not stressed and you are less prone to problems such as bunions and corns.

HERBALISM

For bunions, nettle tea may assist through its effect on calcium deposits.

Corns can easily be removed with the herb comfrey. Take a fresh comfrey leaf and crush it in your hands until it becomes moist. Before you go to bed, place the crushed leaf over the corn and put on an old sock. Do this for a few nights and the corn will disappear very quickly. Gently rubbing the area with a cut clove of garlic is another traditional remedy.

MODERN MEDICINE

Doctors will recommend corn pads to remove the corn and perhaps send you to a foot specialist known as a podiatrist or chiropodist. Some more serious bunions may require surgery.

SHIATSU

In shiatsu, the location of the bunion or corn indicates the particular meridian channels that are blocked. An experienced shiatsu practitioner can relieve the pain associated with these conditions and prevent them from getting worse or recurring by freeing the energy blocked in these channels.

YOGA

Most people do not stand correctly and this leads to foot problems. Some throw their weight onto one leg or bear their weight on only their heels or the inside or outside edges of their feet. You can see how you stand by looking at the soles of your shoes. Yoga standing poses can teach you how to distribute your body weight evenly. See a yoga teacher for guidance, but to begin practise the standing position on page 205.

BURSITIS

Bursitis — also known as housemaid's knee — is the inflammation of a bursa. A bursa is a fluid-filled cavity which lubricates the joints, helping the tendons pass over the bones. The inflammation is usually caused by misuse, overuse or trauma of the joint and its soft tissues, or by infection or ARTHRITIS. This injury is often accompanied by reduced mobility in the joint, redness and sometimes fever.

Bursitis most often occurs in the knees or shoulders.

WHAT YOU CAN DO

- Resting the joint is the best initial treatment — don't ignore or try to "work through" the pain.
- If the elbow is affected, place the arm in a sling (see page 404).
- A hot or cold compress, or alternating the two, can help relieve some of the pain.
- Once the acute pain of bursitis has subsided, gently exercise the joint by moving, swinging and stretching, gradually increasing the range of your movements and the length of time spent exercising. Begin with just a minute or two of exercise taken several times a day.
- Try to avoid the repetitive and strenuous activities that put strain on the joint in the first place.
- If you have to kneel for long periods, use a support such as a foam rubber pad.

ACUPRESSURE

Treatment from a qualified practitioner can be effective. At home, you can try massaging Liver 11 (for the elbows) and Stomach 35 plus Bladder 40 (for knee problems) a few times daily.

You can also try the Ah Shi points which are tender points over the sore area of your body. These can be found by applying deep pressure over the sore area and noting which areas are most tender. Continue to apply deep digital pressure until the pain eases. This may feel a bit uncomfortable at first but it can give you some relief.

ACUPUNCTURE

Acupuncture is also effective because the pain may be "referred", especially if it is in your elbow.

AROMATHERAPY

CAUTION: *Read the information on pages 102 to 105 before using these essential oils.*

A massage using aromatherapy can move blood around the affected joint and help reduce swelling. It is best to consult a professional for advice on specific treatment so as not to aggravate the problem. As a first aid measure, however, you could try compresses with anti-inflammatory oils such as rosemary, juniper, eucalyptus, lavender and German chamomile.

CHINESE HERBS

Lung and liver disharmony is usually the Chinese herbal explanation for bursitis so a herbalist will often prescribe herbs that harmonise these two organs.

CHIROPRACTIC

Chiropractic adjustment can help relieve the pain by increasing mobility in the joints of your knees and elbows and reducing stress on the associated nerves.

THE FELDENKRAIS METHOD

A Feldenkrais practitioner can help you understand how your total body organisation causes inflammation in your joints. You can learn new movement strategies that will be less painful.

HERBALISM

Rub rue herbal ointment into the affected joint for 30 minutes once a day for relief from pain. A herbalist may also prescribe specific dosages of anti-inflammatory herbs including celery seed and devil's claw.

MASSAGE

Massage alone can give limited relief to this condition but can assist other treatment such as CHIROPRACTIC, OSTEOPATHY and physiotherapy (see page 210).

MODERN MEDICINE

Bursitis is managed with analgesics, although antibiotics may be prescribed if there is an infection. Doctors will recommend you rest the affected area and physiotherapy may also be suggested.

In some cases, the fluid may be drained using a fine needle under local anaesthetic (although this could increase the chance of infection) and in other chronic cases, surgery to remove the bursa may be suggested.

NATUROPATHY

CAUTION: *Read the information on page 167 before taking supplements.*

Anti-inflammatory vitamins can be taken to reduce the swelling of bursitis. These include fish oil (1000 mg three times a day), evening primrose oil (1000 mg three times a day), vitamin B6 (250 mg per day) and vitamin C with bioflavinoids (1000 mg three times a day). Bromelain, an enzyme taken from pineapple, is effective in high doses (1000 mg three times a day).

OSTEOPATHY

Osteopathy will address the mechanical strains of the affected joint and also of the other joints that contribute to the movement of the limb.

Anti-inflammatory procedures such as hot and cold compresses and specific exercises may also be recommended.

REFLEXOLOGY

Work the points for the adrenal glands on both hands or feet for a total of 10 minutes twice a week to help reduce inflammation. Be careful not to overstimulate.

SHIATSU

Shiatsu practitioners can help release pain in the knees by working on the gall bladder and kidney meridians. Pain in the elbow may be eased by working the meridians of the large and small intestine in combination with the "triple heater" and gall bladder. A qualified practitioner will use the precise location of the pain to select the particular channels.

YOGA

Yoga exercises can help relieve your bursitis through gentle yet effective movement. Make sure the yoga teacher is aware of your condition.

CANCER

Cells in your body sometimes don't grow normally but build into a lump or tumour. These may be benign or they can be cancer cells. If cancer cells are not treated they can spread to other parts of your body and starve other tissue.

There are many types of cancer because there are many types of tissue in your body that can become cancerous.

Some of the more observable symptoms of possible cancer in different parts of your body can include:

- a sore that doesn't heal normally
- extreme and unexplained weight loss
- severe abdominal pain
- a lump in your breast
- extreme headaches
- the appearance of a mole that bleeds and gets larger or changes colour
- testicles that change shape
- constant hoarseness in the throat
- problems with swallowing
- bleeding between menstrual periods.

It would appear that cancer is a result of a multitude of factors — genetic, physiological, psychological and environmental. Keeping the body's immune system strong is of primary importance in both prevention and treatment (see PROTECTING YOUR IMMUNE SYSTEM).

There is substantial evidence to show that psychological factors have a strong impact in cancer treatment. Positive attitudes to yourself, your health and to healing seem to play an important part. There are a number of therapies and techniques that can offer assistance in this area: see THE MIND BODY CONNECTION, RELAXATION AND DEALING WITH STRESS, COUNSELLING, HEALING ENERGIES and MEDITATION.

SPECIAL NOTE: *By law, non-medically qualified alternative therapists may not treat cancer. However, with the cooperation of a medical doctor, they may be of assistance in treating the general health of a person with cancer. They may also be of assistance in the prevention of cancer in people of high risk.*

ACUPUNCTURE

Acupuncture is useful to boost the immune system and assist people to cope with the effects of chemotherapy.

AROMATHERAPY

CAUTION: *Essential oils should not be used at the same time as chemotherapy and massage should not be given to patients with bone cancer. Read the information on pages 102 to 105 before using oils at any other times.*

Aromatherapy can provide comfort and relaxation and also stimulate your immune system.

Rosemary has been known to stimulate hair growth after chemotherapy but this should be used only after the body has been cleared of drug residues by an extensive cleansing diet. For more details speak to your doctor, aromatherapist and naturopath for advice on how to detoxify.

Lavender oil has a beneficial effect on pressure sores caused by long periods in bed, and it can aid sleep. The gentle touch of an aromatherapist can also do a lot to improve the morale and state of mind of cancer patients.

It is recommended that you see a professional aromatherapist for specific treatment. They are found more often these days in hospitals and other places where cancer is treated.

PREVENTING BREAST CANCER

- Check your breasts once a month to detect changes in tissue. This should be a few days after the end of your period as breasts often feel lumpier during menstruation. Post-menopausal women can check at any time. Ask your doctor to guide you through a breast examination to make you familiar with the technique.
- Mammograms are special breast X-rays used to investigate breast tissue. A doctor may advise this form of examination if you are at higher risk.
- Consider the possible side effects of the contraceptive pill or using oestrogen replacement therapy.

PREVENTING CERVICAL CANCER

Abnormal cell growth in the cervix is usually identified by a cervical pap smear. This test is undertaken by a doctor or nurse, and involves sample cells being taken from the cervix in a quick and painless procedure. Early detection and treatment of abnormalities can prevent cervical cancer. It is recommended that all women have a pap smear every 1 to 2 years, especially if you:

- are sexually active (especially at a young age or with numerous partners)
- take the Pill (consider other forms of contraception)
- smoke
- have other viruses such as genital HERPES or genital WARTS (seek prompt treatment of any vaginal infections)
- have your first child during your teenage years.

The risk seems to increase with each pregnancy.

BACH FLOWER REMEDIES

Bach flower remedies known to relieve the accompanying psychological symptoms of cancer include: rescue remedy for shock, star of Bethlehem for shock and grief, holly and willow for anger, water violet for releasing blocked energy, and wild rose to combat apathy and fatalism.

> **PREVENTING TESTICULAR CANCER**
>
> Although not as well publicised, cancer of the testicles is a disturbingly common problem. It can be treated effectively if detected in the early stages.
>
> Men should give themselves regular checks, preferably after a warm bath or shower when the skin is relaxed. Use the thumb and fingers of both hands to press gently around one testicle at a time. Check that the testicles are smooth and without swelling, about matching weight (one is likely to be a little larger), and no harder or softer than usual.
>
> After a few checks, you will become familiar with what is normal for you. There will be a soft lump at the top of each testicle, towards the back; this is the tube that carries sperm.
>
> If you do notice anything unusual, consult your doctor.

CHINESE HERBS

Chinese herbs are often used to build up the immune system after a program of chemotherapy or radiation therapy for cancer.

HERBALISM

There are immune-boosting herbs, antioxidant herbs and herbs to strengthen the body for other treatments and to relieve side effects, e.g. by aiding the digestive system and liver during chemotherapy and alleviating nausea. There are also herbs that have a special affinity with specific parts of the body.

HOMOEOPATHY

Homoeopathy is currently being trialled around the world in the treatment of some forms of cancer. See a professional homoeopath for advice on how to treat your general health.

MASSAGE

In general, massage is contra-indicated for cancer, however, massage may reduce stress and give relief from pain so check with your doctor. If massage is approved, ensure you seek treatment from a qualified practitioner and cease treatment if any problems arise.

MODERN MEDICINE

The main ways that doctors treat cancer are: surgery, radiotherapy, chemotherapy and hormone treatment. All of these treatments have side effects so it is important to discuss treatments carefully with your doctor. Be sure to ask about any adverse reactions you may have.

Cancer treatment is one area where practitioners of modern medicine are usually more supportive of working with other therapies to improve the general health of the person. You may like to find a doctor who takes a holistic approach. Discuss your options with your current medical doctor.

MEDITATION

What follows is a well-known meditation to assist people with cancer. Read it through then choose images that are strongest for you.

The idea is to empower your white blood cells — the front-line troops in your immune system — to deal with the errant cancer cells. You can imagine them doing battle "Star Wars" style with the cancer cells if that image feels comfortable for you.

Some people prefer to swap the war-zone images with more peaceful visualisations, for example, the white blood cells quietly shrinking the cancer cells. It is important to choose the method with which you feel most comfortable.

Prepare for meditation (see pages 48 and 120). See a blue healing light descend into your crown chakra and spread throughout your body enlivening and invigorating every cell. When you feel yourself vibrating with healing energy focus your attention on the part of your body exhibiting the symptoms of cancer.

Imagine your white blood cells are charged with the healing energy then, using the images you have chosen, see the white blood cells grow in strength, becoming victorious over the cancer cells until the cancer cells disappear.

Take as long as you need to do this meditation. When the healing is completed see the blue light leave your body.

Do this meditation at least once a day. Meditation is particularly recommended for cancer patients. Read the chapter MEDITATION for other styles and incorporate them into your daily life. Some people who have recovered from cancer report spending several hours a day in meditation as part of their recovery process.

NATUROPATHY

You can incorporate naturopathic remedies such as improved nutrition and vitamin supplements into your recovery strategy.

Various "anti-cancer" diets share some similar principles: high fibre, low fat, mostly vegan or vegetarian with an emphasis on organic and raw foods and avoidance of salt and sugar. Fasting is often recommended, under strict supervision, to rid the system of toxins.

Antioxidants are recommended: beta carotene (found in carrots, pumpkin, green leafy vegetables), vitamins C and vitamin E, and zinc. See pages 14 to 15 and 406. Grape seed extract — available in supplement form — is another powerful antioxidant.

Abnormal cervical cells have been linked with deficiency in folic acid, which is also depleted by the Pill and smoking. If at risk, a folic acid supplement may be recommended.

OSTEOPATHY

Osteopaths will treat some patients with cancer to assist with their overall comfort and well-being. Osteopathic care may assist with rehabilitation after surgery, e.g. osteopathy may help to reduce the swelling caused by poor lymphatic drainage in an arm after a mastectomy. A consultation with an osteopath, with a very detailed case history and examination, will determine whether a patient would be suitable for osteopathic care.

REFLEXOLOGY

CAUTION: *Reflexology should not be used for lymphoma.*

To boost your general health, you could consult a reflexologist for treatment on reflexology points on your feet and hands. The points for the lymphatic system, spleen and thymus can help strengthen the immune system along with the solar plexus and diaphragm for relaxation, and the adrenal glands to reduce inflammation and stress. It is also necessary to work the reflexes that correspond to the parts of the body affected by cancer and to any specific symptoms that present themselves. You can try these at home, working both feet or hands for a total of 20 minutes three times a week. If you have any doubts, consult a professional reflexologist.

SHIATSU

An experienced practitioner can give an individual diagnosis and treatment, with emphasis on the "tonification" of the depleted internal organs and related functions, combined with specific dietary advice.

Shiatsu can also help improve your quality of life by helping you achieve a calm and relaxed state of mind and body.

YOGA

Yoga can help physically and psychologically by cultivating a positive state of mind, as well as helping you sleep and reduce stress and anxiety.

Find an experienced yoga teacher to put you on a complete yoga program that will work most effectively for your specific problems.

Yoga is especially useful for people recovering from surgery or undergoing chemotherapy.

CANDIDIASIS

This condition occurs when there is an overgrowth of the yeast-like fungus *candida albicans* on the skin and mucous membranes. Usually candida causes no problems but an overabundance produces toxins that can affect every part of the body, including tissues and organs. Diagnosis is difficult because of the possibility of a multitude of associated symptoms which include:

- vaginal and oral THRUSH
- DIGESTIVE PROBLEMS and abdominal pain with intermittent CONSTIPATION and DIARRHOEA

- Depression
- Headaches
- Insomnia or excess sleeping and fatigue
- poor concentration and memory, indifference, mental dullness
- hives, rashes, dermatitis or Eczema
- muscle aches and Pain
- inexplicable weight loss or gain
- respiratory infections, sinus problems.

The disturbance in the number of these fungi can be caused by a variety of influences including antibiotics, steroidal drugs such as the Pill, hormone shifts, a depressed immune system, a diet high in refined starch and sugars, stress and environmental factors.

WHAT YOU CAN DO

• Starve the candida fungus for at least five weeks by adopting a special yeast-free and mould-free diet containing none of the following:

— sugar or refined starches

— fruit or fruit juices (they're high in sugar)

— dairy products

— fermented foods such as vinegar and alcohol (wine and beer are particularly bad)

— wheat and yeast (including bread and extracts such as Vegemite and Marmite)

— preserved meats (such as salami, devon)

— soya bean products (such as tofu, soy sauce, miso, soy milk)

— fungal foods such as mushrooms

— mould-containing foods such as peanuts

— coffee, tea or cola.

• Adopt a high-fibre diet including plenty of vegetables and wholegrains. Foods that kill or inhibit candida include raw garlic, kale and cabbage.

• A teaspoonful of olive oil taken four to six times a day helps inhibit candida.

• Avoid anti-bacterial broad-spectrum antibiotics and steroids, including the Pill.

• Check any vitamin supplements you are taking — some contain yeast.

• Avoid yeast spores in the environment, particularly damp mouldy areas. Clean and dry out such areas in your home — your bathroom, basement and laundry, for example.

AFFIRMATION

Repeat this affirmation as many times as possible each day to strengthen your body against *candida albicans:* "My body absorbs all the nutrition it needs to make my immune system strong and powerful".

HERBALISM

The herbs wild yam, echinacea, golden seal, black haw, St John's wort, calendula and buchu are often used for treating candida. They boost your immune system and assist digestion. St Mary's thistle acts as a powerful antioxidant and can be used to "mop up" the dead cells. A herbalist is likely to combine these herbs with a yeast-free diet.

HOMOEOPATHY

Homoeopathy can help stem candida by moderating your oversensitivity and improving your immunity. See a homoeopath for a complete assessment and prescription of a homoeopathic remedy.

MODERN MEDICINE

Anti-yeast drugs may be prescribed. Vaginal candida (thrush) may be treated with pessaries and local creams. For babies with oral candida there are local drops available.

NATUROPATHY

In addition to the yeast and mould free diet, a naturopath will advise you to take acidophilus and bifidus tablets internally (according to the dosage on the label) to balance the bacteria in your body.

Garlic tablets can also help kill excessive yeast in your body. Take them according to the instructions on the bottle and separately from the acidophilus tablets for the best result. Incorporate garlic into your diet.

Use the home remedies but also seek the advice of a naturopath. This condition can be complicated and treatments vary according to the person.

REFLEXOLOGY

The main reflex point is the uterus together with the spleen and lymphatic system to combat infection and improve the body's defences. Work the points for the adrenal glands to counter inflammation and stress. Try this on both feet or hands for a total of 15 minutes three times a week.

SHIATSU

In shiatsu terms, candidiasis originates from a damp condition in the spleen and intestines leading to an imbalance in intestinal flora. These meridians are worked along with moxibustion (see page 95) and specific dietary advice.

CELLULITE

Cellulite is the build-up of "orange peel-like" fatty flesh which occurs on thighs and buttocks. It is more common on women than men, especially at menopause, and is difficult to get rid of.

The cause of cellulite has not been fully clarified. The "puckered" appearance is said to be due to strands of fibrous tissue pulling the skin inwards.

Many health practitioners associate cellulite with the build-up of toxins in the body tissues. It has been linked to poor circulation, poor lymphatic drainage, and weak kidney and liver function.

WHAT YOU CAN DO

- Gradually reducing excess weight can help.
- Eat a low-fat, low-salt diet that is well balanced with plenty of grains, fruit and vegetables.
- Do not smoke and avoid caffeine as they contribute to a sluggish system.
- Avoid CONSTIPATION — it has been linked to cellulite.
- Drink six to eight glasses of water every day to flush out toxins and enhance body functions.
- Exercise regularly to improve circulation.
- Circulation can also be stimulated by massaging the skin or just vigorous towel-drying after a shower or bath. Try a daily dry-skin rub with a natural bristle brush, loofah or friction glove, using a sweeping upward motion on the arms and legs and a clockwise circular motion on the stomach.
- Soak in a home mineral bath: add 2 cups of sea salt to a warm bath and relax for at least 20 minutes.

AFFIRMATION

Affirmations like the following can be excellent anytime you need to overcome self-consciousness: "I am beautiful just the way I am, and I love and accept myself right now."

AROMATHERAPY

Caution: Read the information on pages 102 to 105 before using these essential oils.

Massage with aromatherapy oils is recommended to reduce cellulite in conjunction with a change in diet. Mix together 2 drops of rosemary and 4 drops of juniper berry with 3 drops each of patchouli and cypress. Add this to 5 teaspoons of base carrier oil. Gently massage this blended oil into the area affected by cellulite every morning and every night.

BACH FLOWER REMEDIES

Bach's philosophy regards cellulite as a result of the emotional characteristic of not "letting go". Walnut is a remedy that helps you let go of problems. Crab apple is good for cleansing the system.

MASSAGE

Massage may be useful as it improves muscle tone and aids lymphatic drainage and the removal of waste products from body tissues.

MODERN MEDICINE

Moderating your lifestyle would be recommended. In some cases, surgery known as liposuction to reduce the fatty tissue is an option (an incision is made in the skin and then the fat is removed in a curette-like procedure); this involves pain and extensive bruising and is not always effective.

NATUROPATHY

Naturopaths can give you directions about a specific diet. They will recommend you eat plenty of fresh fruit and vegetables and whole grains and suggest you avoid fatty and processed foods, reduce your salt and dairy intake, increase your water intake, and avoid alcohol. Drink fresh celery and beetroot juices as they are good cleansers.

You may also like to try alfalfa tea or tablets, and liquid chlorophyll.

REFLEXOLOGY

Reflexology could be of some benefit if you work the points for the kidneys to improve fluid waste elimination, the liver for detoxification and circulation, and the lymphatic system for better drainage of cellular fluids. Try this on both feet or hands for a total of 20 minutes twice a week.

SHIATSU

Shiatsu can help stimulate a sluggish system and also assist with natural elimination, detoxification and lymphatic drainage by working the kidney, gall bladder, liver, large intestine and "triple heater" meridians, in conjunction with dietary changes suggested by the therapist.

CHAPPED SKIN

Chapped skin is dry and cracked, and is often found on lips, hands, and the face as well as other areas exposed to the elements.

It is caused by moisture loss in the outer layers of skin and can occur when you are out in the wind or cold for an extended period of time or in air conditioning, through overexposure to sunshine or chemicals, or due to frequent washing or contact with water.

Chapped lips may be caused by constant licking of the lips.

WHAT YOU CAN DO

- Moisture in the air helps prevent skin from drying out, so use a humidifier in your home or workplace.
- Keep your hands out of water, particularly hot water, and avoid all detergents, soaps and cleaning products. Use rubber gloves for cleaning as well as washing up.
- Even shampoo can irritate dehydrated skin. If your hands are already dry, wear plastic gloves for shampooing to give your hands a chance to heal.
- Use a non-soap cleanser for hands, face and body.
- Wear gloves or mittens outdoors in winter.
- Apply moisturising cream to your skin morning and night and any time during the day after exposure to sun, wind, cold or water. For extra effect, wear cotton gloves to bed after moisturising.
- Cold creams, petroleum jelly and lanolin are effective barrier creams, repelling liquid and preventing dehydration (some skins may be sensitive to them).
- Avoid tight clothing that rubs against your skin.
- Always use a lip balm containing sunscreen when outside or in airconditioned buildings. Continue to reapply throughout the day. If you find your lips continue to dry out, change brands.
- Drink plenty of water — six to eight glasses a day — to prevent dehydration.

AROMATHERAPY

CAUTION: *Read the information on pages 102 to 105 before using these essential oils.*

Once a week, add 2 drops of geranium essential oil to a basin of water and use this to steam your face or the part of your body that is chapped. After steaming, blend 2 drops of chamomile, 1 drop of patchouli and 1 drop of lavender to base carrier oil (4 teaspoons if using on your body or 2 teaspoons if using on your face) and massage into the skin.

HERBALISM

To reduce dryness, rub a mixture of calendula and comfrey ointment into chapped skin twice a day.

Internally you can take capsules containing evening primrose oil for its essential fatty acids. Use according to bottle instructions or a herbalist's prescription. For the same reason, linseed oil and cold-pressed oils may help.

Look for herbal cosmetic cleansing lotions, toners and moisturisers containing herbs such as chamomile, comfrey or rose.

HOMOEOPATHY

Homoeopathic remedies that are generally used to reduce the occurrence of chapped skin include *Natrum muriaticum, Graphites* and *Petroleum.* See a homoeopath for the correct prescription for your individual condition.

MODERN MEDICINE

Doctors will advise the use of urea-based or lanolin-based creams.

NATUROPATHY

CAUTION: *Read the information on page 167 before taking supplements.*

Take fish oil (1000 mg three times a day), evening primrose oil (1000 mg three times a day), vitamin A (5000 iu per day) or vitamin E tablets (500 iu per day) to help revitalise and increase the moisture in your skin.

If you are using a moisturiser, it will be more effective if it contains natural vegetable oils rather than mineral oils which can strip the skin of vitamins. For example, cold pressed oils like almond would be suggested rather than paraffin which can be found in petroleum jelly, sorbolene cream and baby oil. Try sesame oil on the body, jojoba on the face and rosehip oil around the eyes.

REFLEXOLOGY

Work the points for the thyroid for metabolic balance and the adrenal glands to help maintain cellular water balance. Try this on both feet or hands for a total of 15 minutes three times a week.

SHIATSU

A shiatsu therapist will "tonify" the functions of the spleen (which nourishes the flesh), kidney (controls fluid circulation), lung (opens the pores of the skin) and "triple heater" (for the even distribution of fluids and heat). They will also remove blockages from the gall bladder meridian, ensuring the overall distribution of Ki and oils.

CHILBLAINS

These are swollen parts of the skin that itch and burn as a result of being exposed to the cold. They most often occur on the hands and feet.

Chilblains can be a result of poor circulation, as well as cold weather, due to blood vessels shrinking and severely reducing the supply of oxygen to the skin. People with sensitive skin may be especially susceptible to chilblains.

They usually clear up in two to three weeks even without treatment.

WHAT YOU CAN DO

- To prevent chilblains, you should keep your feet and hands warm and avoid extremes of temperature.
- Avoid tight shoes as they will restrict blood flow.
- Exercise is recommended to increase circulation.
- Avoid smoking which restricts the blood vessels and impedes circulation.
- Never scratch chilblains — it will only aggravate the condition.
- Keep the affected area warm.
- Some people find relief in hot footbaths or alternating warm and cold footbaths.

AFFIRMATION

If it feels appropriate to you, repeat this affirmation throughout the day to help ease your chilblains.

"I feel my blood pulsing throughout my body, nourishing my fingers and toes."

AROMATHERAPY

CAUTION: *Read the information on pages 102 to 105 before using these essential oils.*

Add 4 drops of rosemary essential oil (or 3 drops of rosemary and 3 drops of geranium) to 2 teaspoons of base carrier oil and massage into your feet or hands to increase circulation and relieve swelling. You can also apply this mixture directly to the chilblain for immediate relief.

THE FELDENKRAIS METHOD

Peripheral circulation can be improved through Feldenkrais movement lessons and the development of body awareness, thus lessening your chances of getting chilblains.

HERBALISM

Drink a cup of ginger tea twice a day to reduce the condition. Adding garlic and chilli to your meals will help too, and is an easy way of taking a herbal medicine. You can also try prickly ash in fluid extract or tincture form. If you start taking these herbs before cool weather sets in you are less likely to get chilblains.

A hint: sprinkle a little cayenne pepper in your shoes to bring blood to the surface.

HOMOEOPATHY

If your chilblains are red, very itchy and irritated, consider taking one 6C potency tablet or liquid form of *Agaricus muscarius* homoeopathic remedy three times daily until the condition heals.

If your chilblains differ in any way to this, see a homoeopath who will prescribe a specific remedy.

MASSAGE

In some cases, massage can give relief from pain caused by this condition. It is also an excellent way to stimulate circulation, as a treatment or as a prevention.

MODERN MEDICINE

Doctors will prescribe local lanolin-based creams to ease irritation and stop the skin from swelling.

NATUROPATHY

CAUTION: *Read the information on page 167 before taking supplements.*

A supplement of bioflavinoids is recommended. Doses of vitamin E (500 iu per day) will help increase circulation as will vitamin B3. Chilblains may also indicate a lack of calcium and silica — see page 12 for good dietary sources.

REFLEXOLOGY

If your toes are affected by chilblains, it will assist if you work your fingers and vice versa. Also work the heart reflex for circulation and the spine for nerve function in the affected area. Try this on both feet or hands for a total of 20 minutes four times a week.

YOGA

Regular practise of yoga exercises will improve your circulation. Try a few rounds of salute to the sun (see page 190) each day and see a yoga teacher for other suitable exercises.

CHRONIC FATIGUE SYNDROME

Chronic Fatigue Syndrome (CFS) is also known as Myalgic Encephalomyelitis (ME) or "postviral fatigue syndrome".

The symptoms of CFS include extreme FATIGUE and lethargy, muscle PAIN and tenderness, chest pain, HEADACHE, swollen or tender glands, DEPRESSION and loss of concentration. Accompanying conditions include ringing in the ears, sight problems, lack of circulation, disturbed sleep, DIGESTIVE PROBLEMS and problems in the bladder, bowel and upper respiratory system (see separate entries for specific symptoms). People who have CFS often find they sleep a lot but rarely feel refreshed. They also find the slightest exertion requires a prolonged period of rest and recovery.

CFS is currently believed to involve both the immune system and the central nervous system. The symptoms and their severity depend on the person. Some people recover after a few months and others take years.

It is not known how CFS is caused, and is

difficult to diagnose. Some believe it is triggered by a viral or bacterial infection or immunisation. In many cases, it is first apparent as a failure to recover from some other illness such as flu or glandular fever.

It may be linked to metabolic dysfunction — if the liver and mitochondria (the energy-producing units in the cells) do not function properly, it can lead to an accumulation of toxic waste in the body and a decrease in oxygen supply to the tissues.

It is important to investigate any underlying factors such as recurrent ALLERGIES, emotional difficulties, poor nutrition or chemical exposure.

There is no proven cure for this condition. The main focus of treatment is to get plenty of rest, boost the immune system (see page 34), avoid physical and mental stress (see page 40), and detoxify the body.

Poor oxygen supply may have an effect, and improved breathing techniques can make a difference (see page 265).

The illness also seems to have strong psychological links, with stress playing a significant role. Consequently, techniques such as MEDITATION and HEALING ENERGIES can be very effective in some cases. See also THE MIND BODY CONNECTION, and AFFIRMATIONS AND VISUALISATIONS.

WHAT YOU CAN DO

- Due to the many possible factors that may contribute to both the cause of the disease and your recovery, it is recommended you keep a diary to monitor your condition: record what makes it better and worse — including foods, environment, events, treatments, etc.

- Although physical activity can leave you feeling even more drained, exercise is also an important element in your recovery. Gentle regular activities, such as yoga or Tai Chi, that concentrate on harmonising your body can be of real benefit.

ACUPUNCTURE

Acupuncture is useful for this syndrome and some practitioners specialise in this area.

AFFIRMATION

To increase your energy levels and assist you emotionally, it may be useful to repeat an affirmation, like the following, with enthusiasm even if you feel as though you will never be well: "I glow with good health and vitality."

AROMATHERAPY

CAUTION: *Read the information on pages 102 to 105 before using these essential oils.*

An aromatherapy massage can stimulate the immune system to fight against CFS and consulting an aromatherapist regularly can make a real difference to your energy levels. If you are often fatigued rosemary clears the head. Start your treatment by adding 2 drops of rosemary to a tissue and inhale it throughout the day to revive your spirits. If you put the tissue inside your shirt the warmth of your body will help further release the aroma.

BACH FLOWER REMEDIES

Olive is for exhaustion and will increase energy reserves; elm combats the feeling of being overwhelmed; and hornbeam relieves mental and physical tiredness.

CHIROPRACTIC

Chiropractic adjustment can ensure your nervous system is functional, thus increasing immunity and resistance to illness as well as decreasing the internal stresses within your body.

COUNSELLING

Counsellors have found that some people with CFS are "burnt out" as a result of pushing themselves beyond endurance. Many of those with CFS are overachievers who tend to ignore the body's warning signals. Counselling can assist in dealing with the underlying emotions which trigger your need to work so hard.

THE FELDENKRAIS METHOD

Feldenkrais practitioners can help you learn how to move more efficiently, therefore helping you conserve and make better use of your energy when you have

CFS. They generally recommend that you work to 60 or 70 percent of your capacity when undertaking physical activity while you have CFS.

HERBALISM

Every person who has CFS is treated as a special case by herbalists because people can be affected by CFS for very different reasons. The approach would usually involve draining the lymph nodes and improving liver function, digestive tone and thyroid function. A herbalist can prescribe specific herbs to boost your immune system and keep your energy levels up.

HOMOEOPATHY

There are remedies that have brought very good results for people with CFS. See a professional homoeopath for a full assessment and prescription.

MASSAGE

Lymphatic drainage can be of assistance. However, this condition should only be treated by qualified practitioners as minor, but inconvenient, complications can occur if a person is massaged incorrectly.

MODERN MEDICINE

Currently, there is no specific diagnostic test or treatment available. Counselling and rehabilitation are the approaches most commonly taken, and adequate rest will be advised along with maximising fitness under medical supervision. Occupational therapy or physiotherapy may be part of this rehabilitation process.

Antidepressant drugs may be suggested in some cases, as may vitamin B12 injections. Steps will also be taken to alleviate specific symptoms.

NATUROPATHY

CAUTION: *Read the information on page 167 before taking supplements.*

Dealing with digestive problems is perhaps the most important approach to treatment — a naturopath can recommend digestive tonics or enzymes and doses of acidophilus may help (take according to label).

Treating the liver (with sodium sulphate) and the nervous system (with B vitamins and magnesium) is also important. Vitamin A (5000 iu per day), vitamin C (1000 mg three times a day), vitamin E (500 iu per day) and zinc (25 mg elemental per day) will boost your immune system. Choline may be advised for the adrenals.

Avoid chemicals and other additives in foods and only eat organic and biodynamically grown food as they are free of chemicals and pesticides and higher in nutrients and thus more likely to be of assistance. The balance of acid and alkaline food in your diet may also be a factor.

Consult a naturopath for a diet specific to your lifestyle and condition.

OSTEOPATHY

Many osteopathic techniques are specifically designed to enhance the nervous, circulatory and lymphatic systems. The efficient function of the body's immune defence depends on a correct working relationship between all of these.

REFLEXOLOGY

The thyroid reflex is worked for this condition because this gland controls the metabolic rate of the body, influencing many different areas from tooth development to the reproductive glands. It can be adversely affected by CFS. The immune system needs special attention so the lymphatic system, spleen and thymus need to be worked.

You can work these points yourself on both feet or hands for a total of 30 minutes daily until improvement is evident. However, it may be best if the treatment comes from a reflexologist, especially if you lack the necessary energy.

SHIATSU

Shiatsu can help build up and protect your immune system when you have CFS by working on the flow of Ki energy, particularly in the liver, kidney and spleen meridians. See a shiatsu practitioner for treatment and advice on self-treatment once the individual source of the condition has been properly diagnosed.

YOGA

Yoga is good for CFS because it is gentle and concentrates on balancing the body's energy and harmonising its systems. You should be careful to do all yoga exercises at an even pace so as not to overexert yourself.

There are specific morning yoga exercises to prepare yourself for the day ahead. These are commonly referred to as restorative poses as they actually "recharge your batteries". A yoga teacher can direct you in these exercises.

If you feel tired during the day you can try the inverted corpse position on page 199 to give you more energy.

COLDS AND INFLUENZA

A *cold* is a viral infection of the upper respiratory tract which causes your nose to run or become blocked, your throat to feel sore and congested, and your head to ache; as well, you may have a dry cough.

Symptoms may last a few days to two weeks, although the runny nose may last longer.

This illness is usually developed when you are in close contact with someone who has a cold as the viruses are highly contagious and coughing, sneezing, even breathing can pass them on. This can make some environments — particularly public transport or air-conditioned buildings — particularly unhealthy.

Flu is the shortened version of the term "influenza virus". It has similar symptoms to a cold but is much more severe with muscular aches and pains, chest pain, fever, chills, sweating and weakness.

The cold and flu viruses mutate easily, which means every cold or flu you catch is different, preventing you from developing long-term immunity.

Colds and flu can develop when your immune system is low due to stress, allergies, poor diet, lack of exercise and sleep, or another illness.

WHAT YOU CAN DO

- Stay at home and avoid spreading the virus.
- Keep warm and stay out of drafts.
- Rest and relax to give your body the time and energy to get better, and to avoid the risk of complications.
- You may like to try a healing meditation to assist your recovery (see page 155).
- If you have a high fever you can try to cool the body with cool compresses to the forehead or a tepid bath. Rub an icecube at the very top centre of the head. For young children, keeping the hair damp can be an effective way of cooling down.
- Drink plenty of fluids, especially water and fruit juice, which will help flush out your system and replace fluid lost through sweating from fever.
- To relieve a blocked nose, lean over a bowl of hot water with a towel over your head. Inhale the steam to loosen mucus.
- Gargling hot, salted water can relieve a sore throat — stir a teaspoon of salt into a glass of warm water and gargle over a basin.
- DO NOT have a massage during this time as it can make the fever and infection worse.
- Gentle exercise and fresh air will help tackle a minor cold by stimulating circulation and the effective functioning of your immune system.

ACUPRESSURE

The acupressure point to help relieve a cough is Lung 7. Depress this point until the tenderness of the point subsides, hold it for 10 seconds then release the pressure for 10 seconds. Repeat the sequence.

ACUPUNCTURE

Acupuncturists have had much success treating people with severe viral infections such as influenza and with conditions in the upper respiratory tract. If you have constant colds, see an acupuncturist who will treat the condition after an extensive diagnosis to find underlying causes.

AFFIRMATION

One view of illness like flu is that it is your way of giving yourself some "time out" from the demands of your life. We can sometimes feel guilty about spending time resting; however, your body will benefit if you resist the urge to "soldier on". You may like to assist your healing with affirmations like: "I allow myself to rest knowing that it is OK for me to recharge my batteries."

AROMATHERAPY

CAUTION: *Read the information on pages 102 to 105 before using these essential oils.*

Essential oils can diminish the symptoms of a cold or flu and also reduce the risk of further infection by stimulating the body's immune system and killing bacteria. Two of the most common methods for treating these illnesses are baths and inhalations.

Inhalations soothe inflamed mucous membranes and clear the sinuses. A steam inhalation containing 2 drops of eucalyptus and 2 drops of tea tree will clear the nose of mucus.

Baths also help the sinuses as you inhale the rising steam, plus there is the added benefit of relaxing the body, giving it a chance to heal. If you are having trouble sleeping because of painful sinuses, try adding 2 drops of lavender and 2 drops of marjoram to enhance sleep.

Or put 2 drops of rosemary and 1 drop of peppermint in an oil burner with some water. Use it in the home or work place to fight the bacteria in the air and clear your sinuses. However, avoid these oils at night as they are stimulants and may keep you awake when you need your sleep.

BACH FLOWER REMEDIES

Remedies beneficial for colds and flu include rescue remedy, walnut for "letting go" and impatiens for people constantly on the go who do not allow themselves to ease up.

CHINESE HERBS

Chinese herbs build up your immune system and make your body less susceptible to these illnesses by "tonifying" the Qi in your body where it is deficient. There are also herbs that are effective from the acute onset of symptoms but they should be chosen specifically by a Chinese herbalist to suit your individual condition.

CHIROPRACTIC

If you have chiropractic adjustments on a regular basis you can keep your nervous system functioning properly which will improve your immune system. You may then find you are less susceptible to colds and flu, as well as many other common ailments. The aches and pains of joints which occur when you have the flu can be reduced with chiropractic treatment. Chiropractic care can increase the movement in sore joints and improve circulation throughout your whole body, helping you to fight the illness.

HERBALISM

Herbalists treat colds literally — this means they will keep you warm because you are "cold". They will advise you to wrap up and will prescribe herbs that heat your body including peppermint, yarrow and elderflower (taken as hot teas in the early stages of a cold). Change to ginger tea and prickly ash if the cold becomes chronic. You could try some of the ready-made herbal remedies available from health food stores that contain these herbs; take according to the directions.

Also available at health food stores are herbal flu tablets containing some of the following: echinacea and golden seal for infection, hyssop and coltsfoot for cough, eyebright and elder for sinus, golden rod to reduce mucus and boneset for aches and pains. Take according to package directions.

Drinking chamomile tea is recommended for relieving headache and fever. Good quantities of chilli in your food can also ensure a quick recovery. The key is not to fight the flu but allow your body time to heal itself.

Garlic and horseradish tablets, particularly with vitamin C, and echinacea tablets can be taken daily as a preventive measure — they strengthen your body's immune system.

HOMOEOPATHY

If you get a cold every year or two, in homoeopathic terms there is nothing to worry about. It is just your system reminding you that you need to take more care of yourself. But if you get colds on a regular basis (every month or two) then a homoeopath will give you remedies to promote the healing process in your body. These work by encouraging your body's own immune system to fight the infection.

Try the following home remedies for a cold but if in doubt see a homoeopath. If you are feeling a bit "achy" and know you are about to get a cold, take 6C potency of *Ferrum phosphoricum* three times a day.

If your eyes and nose are streaming, take 6C potency of *Allium cepa* every hour for the first day and then three times a day for two more days.

If your cold begins with sneezing and a stuffy nose then moves into your chest, take 6C potency of *Arsenicum album* remedy every hour for the first day, then take one remedy three times a day for the next two days.

If you have the flu, one of the following remedies may be suitable if your symptoms fit the ones listed. If your bones ache, take one 6C potency of *Eupatorium perfoliatum* every hour for four doses, then reduce the dose to 1 tablet three times a day. If you have a bad headache accompanied by aching limbs and tiredness, take the same dosage as above along with the homoeopathic remedy *Gelsemium sempervirens.*

MODERN MEDICINE

There is no medical "cure" for either illness. Bed rest and aspirin are recommended by most doctors for pain relief and to control a fever, but for flu and severe colds antibiotics may be administered to prevent or treat secondary bacterial infection such as BRONCHITIS or SINUSITIS — antibiotics do not counter the virus, however. Cough medicine may be recommended to suppress the irritation of a cough or as an expectorant to liquefy the mucus making it easier to shift. Antihistamines may be prescribed if the condition worsens. Otherwise colds and flu that are not serious are generally left alone to take their course.

Flu vaccinations are available at the onset of winter when epidemics are most common and are quite often recommended to the frail or elderly. However, they are temporary and only effective against specific strains of virus. Like other forms of immunisation, there may be problems attached (including a link to ARTHRITIS in some elderly people) and should be discussed fully with health practitioners.

NATUROPATHY

There are many vitamin and mineral remedies that are known to be very effective. At the first sign of a cold or flu, take 1000 mg vitamin C (1/4 teaspoon powder) with bioflavinoids and 1/2 teaspoon echinacea fluid extract every hour until you feel the symptoms have subsided. Also of benefit are cod liver oil capsules, zinc and raw garlic.

You should combine these with plenty of water, fresh fruit (rather than juiced or dried) and vegetables but as little sugar as possible. Watermelon juice and herb teas are recommended if you have a fever. Avoid dairy products as they have an adverse effect on the mucous membranes. If you have a chill, try a hot bath with Epsom salts.

OSTEOPATHY

Osteopathic treatment can assist in boosting your body's immune defences so it can help to combat these conditions by treatment of mechanical stresses along with diet and lifestyle advice.

REFLEXOLOGY

For a cold, work the points for the chest/lungs and adrenal glands to relax the chest and assist breathing and loosen mucus. Work the points for the small intestine and colon to ensure good elimination of toxic waste, and the lymphatic system to deal with any infection. All the toes and fingers can be worked as they correspond to the head area. If you have the flu, work the same points plus all the glands for endocrine balance. Try this on both feet or hands for a total of 15 minutes three times a week.

SHIATSU

Shiatsu is best as a preventive measure for colds and flu or in the very early stages but it can also be effective once the infection has set in. Shiatsu techniques can strengthen the immune system by activating your body's protecting Ki energy (Wei Chi) and enhancing the function of the lungs. Once you have a cold, shiatsu can decongest your nasal passages and sinuses. With this end in mind a shiatsu practitioner will work on the lung meridian to strengthen the lungs and eliminate wind and cold in the area, and the large intestine and stomach to reduce mucous production. The gall bladder meridian will be worked to reduce muscle aches and joint pains, and the liver and spleen to strengthen the immune system and regulate fevers.

YOGA

WARNING: *Do not attempt any yoga exercise if you have a fever.*

Yoga can help reduce the occurrence and intensity of colds and flu. It boosts your immune system making you less likely to succumb to infection. The sectional breathing exercise on page 203 increases your resistance, while the half-wheel pose releases blocked toxins thus giving your body the chance to heal. A yoga teacher can instruct you in exercises to practise while you are recuperating.

COLITIS

Colitis is inflammation of the colon (large intestine). Chronic DIARRHOEA (up to 20 times a day in severe cases), stomach pain, wind, HAEMORRHOIDS, vomiting and fever often accompany this condition. Ulcerative colitis leads to ULCERS on the large intestine. These ulcers can produce blood and mucus in your stools (faeces) and can leave you weak and anaemic.

Stress is the most common cause of ulcerative colitis, and there is a genetic link that can predispose some people to the condition.

Acute colitis is usually caused by an infection.

Chronic colitis may be caused by infection, medication, stress or food ALLERGIES, and is characterised by frequent recurrence.

"Runner's diarrhoea" is a form of colitis caused when blood is diverted from the digestive tract to your muscles, and is caused by overexercising.

Mucous colitis is more correctly known as IRRITABLE BOWEL SYNDROME.

Colitis mostly affects adults.

IMPORTANT: *The condition must be properly diagnosed by a medical practitioner as it can be mistaken for other conditions.*

WHAT YOU CAN DO

- If colitis is caused by too much exercise, cut down your training and the condition should ease.
- Try to reduce and manage the stress in your daily life. See page 40.
- A high-fibre diet rich in fruit, vegetables, cereals and whole grains can help prevent colitis. However, it is advisable to take a food sensitivity test before changing your diet. Gluten, which is found in grains like wheat, can often be a digestive irritant. In these cases, grains such as brown rice are the recommended option; gluten free breads, snacks and other products are readily available from health food stores.
- Caffeine and alchohol consumption affect colitis and should be avoided.
- Seek further medical advice for any antibiotic that causes diarrhoea as a side effect.

ACUPRESSURE AND ACUPUNCTURE

Both acute and chronic colitis have been helped by acupuncture from qualified practitioners. Acupressure is also a simple yet effective way of gently relieving colitis.

BACH FLOWER REMEDIES

Emotionally, inflammation is associated with anger, the intestine with assimilation and diarrhoea with fear. Mimulus and aspen could help with fear, and holly with anger.

CHINESE HERBS

In Chinese medicine, colitis is an indication that your liver and spleen are out of balance. Chinese herbalists are very successful in treating this condition with herbs that harmonise these organs.

CHIROPRACTIC

If you have chronic colitis, chiropractors will look for spinal problems which could be linked to your colon and will adjust your spine accordingly.

HERBALISM

Slippery elm is one of the herbs used for all infections of the bowel. Add 1 teaspoon of slippery elm powder to a few spoonfuls of hot water, mix into a paste and eat before it forms into a gel which will be harder to get down. Take this mixture twice a day and 1 tablespoon psyllium husks in 400 mls (14 fl oz) water three times a day.

Astringent herbs such as cranesbill, agrimony and wild yam may be prescribed by a herbalist along with marshmallow for protection. Fortified peppermint tea will help with bloating and cramping of the bowel.

HOMOEOPATHY

There are many remedies including *Podophyllum peltatum* and *Mercurius corrosivus* that can help reduce the pain and occurrence of colitis, but they are best prescribed by a homoeopath.

If your diarrhoea is constant, you feel sick in the stomach and distressed, you could try taking one 6C potency of *Arsenicum album* every two hours until your diarrhoea subsides.

MODERN MEDICINE

Colitis can be treated with medication to reduce inflammation, in some cases by a steroid drug or an NSAID (see page 163). Antidiarrhoeal drugs may be used with caution to provide some relief. Doctors may also study your diet to pinpoint food sensitivities and suggest vegetable roughage and raw fruits be avoided.

A bowel examination in a hospital involving a colonoscopy may be requested. In severe cases of ulcerative colitis, surgery may be advised, either a temporary colostomy to provide relief, or removal of the affected area of colon.

NATUROPATHY

CAUTION: *Read the information on page 167 before taking supplements.*

You can consult a naturopath who will help you with your diet and probably conduct an elimination test, recommending you avoid allergy-associated foods such as dairy and gluten products.

They may also prescribe doses of vitamin A (5000 iu per day), vitamin E (500 iu per day) and zinc (25 mg elemental per day) to help your system heal itself.

OSTEOPATHY

As with other problems of the digestive system, this condition may be assisted by osteopathic treatment. A thorough history and examination would need to be performed by an osteopath — perhaps along with your medical test results — to evaluate whether your problem would be suitable for this type of treatment.

REFLEXOLOGY

Work the points for the colon gently. In addition, gently activate the adrenal glands to help the inflammation, the gall bladder to release bile which acts as a lubricant on the walls of the colon, the lower spine for improved nerve function in the area, the diaphragm for relaxation and possible reduction in discomfort, and the liver. Try this on both feet or hands for a total of 15 minutes twice a week — be careful not to overstimulate.

SHIATSU

Colitis is often viewed by shiatsu practitioners as a result of eating foods too high in energy or too concentrated such as oils, fried foods, dairy sugars, spices and most refined foods, including flour products. A shiatsu practitioner will therefore advise you to cut down on these foods and increase your intake of other foods more suitable to your condition, such as cooked whole grains, sweet and root vegetables and kuzu drinks (Japanese arrowroot).

In addition, the stomach, spleen and large intestine meridians would be worked to support the digestive system overall.

YOGA

The yoga exercise known as the solar plexus pose (see page 204) can help as it stimulates the abdomen and surrounding areas.

CONJUNCTIVITIS

Conjunctivitis, or pink eye, is an inflammation of the outer eye and eye lid which may be accompanied by a yellowish discharge in the corner of the eye. There may be stinging and discomfort due to dryness, but no real pain is involved. Sight should be unaffected although the discharge may bring slight blurriness.

Allergic conjunctivitis occurs when the eye comes in contact with an irritant or allergen such as smoke. This can be a recurring problem (see ALLERGIES).

Other forms of conjunctivitis are due to viral or bacterial infection and can be highly contagious.

Consult a doctor if the condition doesn't clear up within a few days or if pain or loss of vision is involved, as in rare cases these may be symptoms of a more serious eye problem.

WHAT YOU CAN DO

- Compresses, applied four or five times daily, will provide comfort and remove the crusty discharge.
- Conjunctivitis that is the result of an allergy, to pollen for example, will often itch and burn like a mosquito bite. A cold compress instead of a hot one will relieve the itching.
- Germ-instigated conjunctivitis worsens when eyes are closed for long periods, so apply any prescribed ointment or cream at night.
- Don't use an eye patch as it may cause the infection to spread.
- Thoroughly wash any washcloths, towels or other materials that come into contact with the eyes. Ensure household members use different towels.
- Be sure to always wear well-fitting goggles when swimming if suffering a bout of conjunctivitis, or even if prone to this condition. Chlorine can be a major irritant.
- Unnecessary use of eye drops and washes can also cause irritation.
- As a preventative in babies, gently massage the eyelids to stop tear ducts becoming blocked.

ACUPUNCTURE

This therapy has had much success in clearing up cases of conjunctivitis. See an experienced acupuncturist for details regarding treatment.

CHINESE HERBS

Herbs prescribed by a Chinese herbalist are also effective in treating this condition.

CHIROPRACTIC

Chiropractors have found people with conjunctivitis may also have neck problems. By adjusting the neck and spine a chiropractor can release pressure to the nerves that supply the eyes and facial structures and create a healing environment for other illnesses in the body.

HERBALISM

WARNING: *Before you use any herbal remedies directly on your eyes you should see a herbalist who will advise you on specific dilution. This is important because your eyes are sensitive organs and you can easily damage them.*

Use a herbal wash or eyebath in the form of a weak infusion. Eyebright, as the name suggests, is effective in relieving eye infections such as conjunctivitis, as is golden seal.

HOMOEOPATHY

Remedies commonly used for conjunctivitis include *Euphrasia officinalis* and *Apis mellifica.*

If your eyes are sore and your lids are sticky with a yellowy discharge, take one 6C potency of *Pulsatilla nigricans* homoeopathic remedy four times a day for the first day and then three times a day for the next two days. If your symptoms vary from the above or the condition persists, consult a homoeopath.

MODERN MEDICINE

There are local antibiotic drops that will clear up conjunctivitis completely and safely within 12 hours. In some cases, such as allergic reactions, a form of antihistamine will be prescribed by a doctor and there are also anti-allergy eyedrops available over the counter.

NATUROPATHY

Take 1000 mg of vitamin C three times a day and 5000 iu of vitamin A once a day to help your immune system overcome the problem. A naturopath can advise you on other ways to reduce conjunctivitis.

REFLEXOLOGY

Work the reflex points for the eyes as well as the adrenal glands to deal with the inflammation and for allergies, the kidneys because they have a direct link with the eyes, the upper lymphatic system for the infection, and the cervical spine for improved nerve function in the area. Try this on both feet or hands for a total of 15 minutes twice a week.

SHIATSU

A shiatsu treatment may relieve the symptoms by working the liver meridian, which relates to the eyes, and the gall bladder meridian.

CONSTIPATION

Constipation is when you have a difficult bowel movement due to the faeces passing through your system too slowly and becoming dry and hard.

Infrequent bowel movement is another form of constipation, although there is really no definition for "normal" as the necessity varies from individual to individual. Three times a day may be normal for some while three times a week may suffice for others.

Toxic substances may build up in a constipated gut and eventually leak into the bloodstream causing a wide range of health problems including migraines and skin disorders.

Constipation may be due to inadequate diet, diuretics (e.g. drugs, caffeine in coffee, tea and cola) insufficient fluid intake, or from sluggish bowel function. Emotional stress and lack of exercise can also be factors. Bottle-fed babies are at greater risk of constipation that those who are breast fed.

If you are usually "regular" and then become chronically constipated, if you have severe abdominal pain or if there is blood in your faeces, seek the advice of a health practitioner as it may indicate a more serious problem.

See also DIGESTIVE PROBLEMS.

WHAT YOU CAN DO

- DO NOT use over-the-counter laxatives except on the advice of a health practitioner. Overuse can even cause constipation by interfering in the proper action of your body's waste disposal system.
- Diet is probably the single highest contributing factor in constipation. Be sure you are not only getting enough fibre (25–30 gms per day for adults) but also that your fluid intake is adequate (six to eight glasses of water). An increase in fibre without sufficient liquid to aid bulking and removal will actually make constipation worse.
- High-fibre foods include whole grains, bran, brown rice, dried peas and beans, dried and fresh fruits, fresh raw vegetables, jacket potatoes.
- Prunes and prune juice are traditional natural laxatives as is a daily spoonful of molasses.
- A glass of warm water with a squeeze of fresh lemon juice first thing in the morning can help.
- Daily moderate exercise will help the food move through the bowel and also strengthen the abdominal muscles — walking 20–30 minutes is ideal.
- Don't put off going to the toilet when you have the urge.
- Squatting is a better position — use a footstool and have your knees up.
- Don't strain too hard as you may become susceptible to HAEMORRHOIDS or HERNIA. Take your time too — if you are in a hurry, you can become stressed and the muscles in your bowel will become tense. Reading a book may help you relax.
- Learn how to deal with stress (see page 40).
- Question your doctor about any medication you are taking — constipation can be a side effect of some drugs, including codeine and narcotics.

ACUPRESSURE

A qualified practitioner can help your digestive problems. At home, try the acupressure points Stomach 25 and Liver 4 with your thumbs on your abdomen and hand (they ease constipation because they activate the liver and stomach) as well as Liver 2. Massage these points for about 1 minute and move the pressure in the direction of the arrows. Do this at breakfast with a warm drink.

ACUPUNCTURE

Acupuncture is good for most gastrointestinal disorders and constipation falls into this category.

AROMATHERAPY

CAUTION: *Read the information on pages 102 to 105 before using these essential oils.*

Constipation can be helped by aromatherapy massage if accompanied by a change in diet. Blend 2 drops of marjoram and 2 drops of rosemary in 2 teaspoons of base carrier oil. The abdomen should be massaged very lightly with this mixture in a clockwise direction for about 5 minutes. You may choose to massage the area yourself but it is generally more effective if someone else does it for you.

If your constipation is stress related, aromatherapy can definitely help as the oils can relieve stress and promote general well-being.

BACH FLOWER REMEDIES

Take walnut for "letting go", both physically and mentally, and water violet to release blockages.

CHINESE HERBS

Chinese herbs are known to be effective at relieving constipation. Generally, Chinese herbalists use herbs to soften the stool, regulate bowel contractions, and harmonise your liver and spleen.

CHIROPRACTIC

Many people who suffer from constipation have a history of chronic low back or pelvic problems that can be helped by chiropractic adjustment. Many report excellent response to chiropractic care with problems associated with the bowel.

COUNSELLING

Issues of trust and fear may be underlying causes of chronic constipation. If you feel these might apply to you, it could be worthwhile seeking counselling.

THE FELDENKRAIS METHOD

A Feldenkrais practitioner can teach you breathing and abdominal movement exercises that may help you reduce your constipation, depending on the cause.

HERBALISM

Slippery elm is often prescribed for constipation because it protects the bowel and softens the stools so they can be passed without damaging the rectum. Other herbs used to treat constipation include aloe, barberry, cascara sagrada, rhubarb root, senna pods and yellow dock. Try a tablespoonful of psyllium husks in 300 ml (10 fl oz) of soya milk or water before bed as a natural laxative.

Constipation can have diverse causes so the herbs that work for one person may not work for another. A visit to a herbalist is recommended for the best results.

HOMOEOPATHY

Homoeopathy can be useful in dealing with the complex causes of this condition. It will take into consideration your current emotions, the events in your life, your medical history, your diet and general lifestyle.

MASSAGE

Regular back and abdominal massage (see page 135) will greatly assist this condition. In addition, a full-body massage can relieve any stress that may be involved.

MODERN MEDICINE

Doctors will determine whether or not this condition is linked to other health problems. They may prescribe laxatives to soften the faeces and contract the bowel. An enema or colonic irrigation may be recommended by your doctor or naturopath. Colonic irrigation treatment is given at specialist clinics. It assists with impacted faeces and also improves general function of the bowel, gall bladder and liver.

NATUROPATHY

In addition to a diet high in fibre and water, a naturopath will recommend you avoid white rice, sugar and flour, and decrease your dairy and meat intake. It is also advisable to take doses of acidophilus and bifidus (according to the label) plus 2 teaspoons of psyllium in a large glass of water twice a day to work as a natural laxative. You can also try 1 to 2 tablespoons of linseed oil on your cereal each morning. Colonic cleansing may be recommended but it should be carried out by a qualified practitioner and used only occasionally.

OSTEOPATHY

The sluggish mobility of the bowel can sometimes be related to dysfunction of spinal and pelvic mechanics. Osteopathic treatment can help to alleviate these.

REFLEXOLOGY

Work the points for the liver to help detoxify the body and produce bile, the gall bladder to release bile which acts as a lubricant, and the descending and sigmoid colons as these areas are directly affected by constipation. In addition, working the points for the diaphragm can help with relaxation and stress reduction and working the lumbar spine reflex can improve nerve function in the area. Try this on both feet or hands for a total of 25 minutes daily until the condition clears.

SHIATSU

Specific points on the abdomen, stomach and hand can be activated to regulate the large intestine and liver and promote a smoother function of the colon. Also, in Oriental medicine, constipation may be seen as the result of an emotional upset and "holding on", so shiatsu treatment may clear your mind as well as your body.

YOGA

The head-to-knee exercise on page 199 benefits digestion and discourages constipation. Inverted poses are also good for constipation, such as those listed on page 197, 199 and 202.

CRAMPS

Muscular cramps are spasms that can occur in any muscle in your body. They can be quite painful and are sometimes triggered by abnormal salt balance, mineral deficiences (magnesium is important for muscle relaxation, for example) or excessive lactic acid in your muscles due to overuse (this is a by-product of muscle metabolism).

Chronic stress will deplete the body of magnesium, and dehydration will lead to salt imbalance. Poor circulation can deprive the muscles of the blood they need for proper function.

Cramps can be brought on by unaccustomed exercise or when you are overheated or fatigued. A repetitive action or an awkward position can also cause cramping.

The most common types of cramps include writer's cramp (cramp in your hand from holding a pen) and a "stitch" at the side of your abdomen. Calf cramps, commonly known as charley horses, often occur during sleep and can be intense enough to wake you — they are signs of a magnesium deficiency, which may also be indicated by minor muscle twitches.

PERIOD PAIN, however, is quite different.

See also REPETITIVE STRAIN INJURY.

WHAT YOU CAN DO

- For a calf cramp, push the foot back towards the body by applying strong pressure to the ball of the foot. Get someone to do this for you if possible while you lie down with your leg straight.
- See Shiatsu (below) for first-aid for writer's cramp.
- Make sure you stretch before and after exercising (see page 20) and don't push yourself too hard. Drink water or sport drinks to replace fluids lost through sweating.

• Do not exercise immediately after eating as blood will be shunted to muscles away from the digestive tract. Swimming has the additional impact of cold water on the body's systems.

ACUPRESSURE

If you are getting cramps in your legs the acupressure points Bladder 57 for legs and Governing Vessel 26 for general cramping may help as a preventive measure. They can be used during a cramp as well. Make sure you spend at least 1 minute massaging the point, with deep finger pressure.

THE ALEXANDER TECHNIQUE

The Alexander Technique can teach you to sit, walk, and move more efficiently and put less strain on your body in order to reduce muscular cramps.

AROMATHERAPY

Essential oil baths are good cramp prevention as they relax the body. A regular massage from an aromatherapist will increase circulation thus reducing the likelihood of cramps.

Try a combination of 2 drops of chamomile, 3 drops of sweet marjoram and 2 drops of mandarin, as these oils are soothing and release tension from the body. Add to a bath of warm water, making sure you disperse them well. Or mix with 2 teaspoons of base carrier oil and massage into the area that is cramping. Just use lavender oil if there's no time for blending.

BACH FLOWER REMEDIES

Cramping is said to be the physical reaction to fear so take mimulus and aspen to reduce fear.

CHINESE HERBS

A paeonia and licorice combination is very effective in treating cramps. See a Chinese herbalist for details.

CHIROPRACTIC

Cramps may be due to an interference in your nervous system which can be reduced through chiropractic adjustment.

THE FELDENKRAIS METHOD

Muscle lengthening positions can be explored through the Feldenkrais Method to help people reduce their muscular cramps.

Calf cramps can be helped by standing on your affected leg — make sure your heel is on the floor. Slowly move your pelvis and body forward so your weight moves over your foot. This can also be done as a preventive measure.

HERBALISM

Herbs that are often prescribed to reduce cramping include valerian, wild yam, cramp bark, prickly ash and black cohosh as they increase circulation and relax tense muscles. Different herbs work differently for cramps in various parts of the body, but as an initial treatment, drink a cup of tea each day containing combinations of these herbs. If your cramps are worse at night, it will help if you drink the tea just before you go to bed. You can also take combinations of these herbs in tablet form.

HOMOEOPATHY

There are many remedies, including *Cuprum metallicum,* that can relieve aches and muscle spasms in the body but for a specific remedy for your particular form of cramping seek professional homoeopathic treatment.

MASSAGE

Massage can be used to warm muscles for exercise. At the time of cramping, massage can give relief and it will also relieve the after-effects of severe cramps. Massage the whole region, not just the local area.

MODERN MEDICINE

A doctor may recommend you take a quinine medication which is effective in relieving most kinds of cramping where circulation is poor.

NATUROPATHY

You can help reduce cramping in your legs by taking vitamins and minerals that help relax the muscles. These may be deficient in the diet thus causing cramping.

Magnesium phosphate is a cell salt that will give quick relief to cramps in most cases; take as directed on the label. For leg muscle cramps, take calcium and magnesium. Calcium and a high potency B complex tablet taken on a long-term basis, according to label directions, will help foot cramps. If poor circulation is a factor, take vitamins E and B3.

If cramping returns when these supplements are stopped, your diet will need to be modified by a naturopath to ensure you are getting all the nutrients you need.

OSTEOPATHY

The soft tissue treatment practised by osteopaths can relieve the pain of cramps.

REFLEXOLOGY

For leg and foot cramps, work the knee, hip, lower spine and sciatic areas of each foot or hand as well as the parathyroid glands which act on the muscles of the body and the adrenal glands for muscle tone. For cramps elsewhere in the body, work the points for the thyroid and adrenal glands and the reflex relating to the area that is cramping.

Try this on both feet or hands for a total of 10 to 15 minutes daily while the cramping lasts.

SHIATSU

Shiatsu practitioners see cramping as a deficiency in blood and Ki energy flowing around your body. They will improve the flow of these by clearing the meridians associated with the area of cramping, e.g. the bladder meridian (behind the knee and calf muscle), and by dispersing the liver and gall bladder meridians as these control the functioning of muscles and tendons.

Try the following simple shiatsu remedy for writer's cramp:

Hold the hand affected by cramp with your thumb and the index finger of your other hand. Press deep into the web and near the joint between your index finger and thumb. This point is known as Large Intestine or Colon 4 (see page 88). Circle your thumb while you are holding this point for about 1 minute at a time. Repeat a few times.

YOGA

Yoga is effective in healing cramps of all types, but it is especially useful for leg cramps. You may find, however, that when you start yoga you get cramps in your legs. This is because your muscles are not used to exercise of this type.

The nerve stretch exercise on page 202 will help reduce muscular spasms, stiffness or pain in the legs and also loosen the pelvic region. It will also prevent cold feet as it increases the circulation.

CUTS AND SCRATCHES

FIRST AID

1. If there are foreign bodies in the wound, flush them out with fresh water or gently wipe surface material away. Any embedded objects should be removed by a medical attendant.
2. Stop bleeding by applying pressure with a clean cloth, piece of thick gauze or, if not available, your fingers. If bleeding continues, raise the limb above heart level. Don't use a tourniquet — they are extremely dangerous if misused.
3. Once bleeding has slowed or stopped, clean the skin around the wound using clean cotton swabs and soap and water. Gently dry the area.
4. Apply some form of antibacterial or antibiotic powder and keep the wound covered. Cells regenerate more quickly when moist whereas allowing a scab to form will slow down new cell growth.
5. Apply a sterile dressing or bandage with adhesive.

CAUTION: *Large, gaping, dirty or infected wounds require medical attention. See also* FIRST AID *section (see page 385) for advice on shock (see page 391), bleeding (see page 390), fractures (see page 396).*

AROMATHERAPY

Tea tree oil is good for healing cuts as it has antiseptic qualities to prevent infection. Apply tea tree cream or diluted essential oil to your cut every time you change the dressing. If there is no dressing, apply it twice a day.

BACH FLOWER REMEDIES

Take rescue remedy to help the healing process.

HERBALISM

Healing creams are available containing the herbs calendula, comfrey and St John's wort; the latter has antiseptic properties so is recommended for wounds with embedded dirt.

HOMOEOPATHY

Some homoeopathic remedies for cuts and scratches are similar to the herbal ointments but there are other treatments. *Ledum palustre,* for example, is used for deep cuts or punctures from a sharp, thin object. Take one 6C potency of *Ledum palustre* three times on the day you receive this kind of wound to aid the healing process and fight infection within your body.

MODERN MEDICINE

Most cuts and scratches do not require medical attention if first aid treatment is followed. However, closing a clean wound will make scarring less likely. If the cut is large, particularly if it is in an exposed area, visit a doctor for stitches. Smaller cuts can be kept closed with butterfly tapes.

In some cases if the cut is hard to clean or is infected, a tetanus injection may be advised. Note that the shot will not protect against tetanus for this injury. It is part of a routine vaccination program that aims to prevent tetanus (a relatively uncommon bacterial infection that is also known as lockjaw). The initial shot is followed by another in two months, then in five years and then every five years afterwards. If you do happen to contract tetanus, there is another form of injection available as treatment.

NATUROPATHY

CAUTION: *Read the information on page 167 before taking supplements.*

Take vitamin E (500 iu per day) and zinc (25 mg elemental per day) internally. Zinc, which promotes healing, can also be found in pumpkin and sunflower seeds, and Brazil nuts and peanuts.

SCARRING

A wound that heals well is less likely to scar than one that is picked at or allowed to become infected.

Treat new scars and newly healed wounds gently. Do not rub them with a washcloth or towel and keep them covered from the sun — apply a strong sunblock if exposed.

Most scars fade over time.

- Every night, apply vitamin E or another nourishing cream (even plain cold cream) once the wound has closed. Or use aloe vera gel and alternate with vitamin E oil. Break open a vitamin E capsule and rub the oil into the area.
- Acupuncture has had a great deal of success with healing scar tissue.
- Permanent scars may be made less visible by surgery, X-rays and freezing in some cases. A medical specialist can inject pitted scars with collagen.
- Mask red scars with green-tinged concealer make-up (available from the cosmetic section of department stores) and then foundation and matt powder.

DANDRUFF

Your skin is continually shedding layers. Dandruff, however, is an excessive amount of larger-than-normal flakes of scalp that stick to the shafts of your hair where they may accumulate a build-up of oil, dust and hair products. Irritation and itching may be associated.

Dandruff on a dry scalp may be caused by a fungal infection, poor blood circulation to the area, not enough brushing to remove the shedding skin, deficiency of essential fatty acids, vitamin A or zinc, or a disturbance in the pH balance of your scalp, perhaps through the use of shampoos or hair products that are irritating to you. It can spread to eyebrows, ears and the neck.

Dandruff on an oily scalp can indicate an overproduction of sebum which, in turn, may be linked to hormones.

Severe persistent dandruff may reflect a more

serious condition such as ECZEMA, PSORIASIS or seborrheic dermatitis and should be examined by a medical doctor.

WHAT YOU CAN DO

- Massage your scalp for a few minutes each day to stimulate circulation and loosen dead skin cells. Follow with vigorous brushing to remove flakes.
- Wash your hair regularly, rinsing well to eliminate any build-up of hair products. Clean hair is necessary and some people benefit from washing every day; other scalps are irritated by frequent washing.
- For oily hair and scalp, try rinsing with fresh lemon juice or cider vinegar diluted in water.
- For a dry scalp, try a warm oil treatment once a week. Massage olive oil, castor oil or linseed oil into your hair and scalp and wrap in a hot towel for at least ten minutes (preferably a few hours) before washing.
- Try not to blow dry hair — this will reduce the hair's condition and may irritate the scalp.
- Avoid hair products (including dyes) and change shampoos to see if these have an impact on your dandruff. Try a natural allergy-free product.
- Fresh air and sunshine can greatly improve the condition of the scalp. Ultraviolet light can have an anti-inflammatory effect on scaly skin — but avoid overexposure and keep exposed areas of skin areas covered with sunscreen.
- Stress and negative emotions can play a significant role in skin conditions such as dandruff. See RELAXATION AND DEALING WITH STRESS.

AROMATHERAPY

CAUTION: *Read the information on pages 102 to 105 before using these essential oils.*

Make up an anti-dandruff aromatherapy blend.

For a dry flaking scalp: mix 5 teaspoons of jojoba with 4 drops each of lavender, sandalwood and geranium.

For an oily, scaly scalp: mix 5 teaspoons of jojoba with 6 drops each of rosemary and lemon.

Use the suitable blend every second day until your dandruff is reduced — long-term use of any essential oil is not recommended, however. Massage it into your scalp before bed and leave overnight. In the morning, shampoo your hair. For the final rinse, add 2 drops of rosemary to the water.

HERBALISM

Chickweed can be used to prevent and treat dandruff. Rub chickweed lotion into your scalp before you go to bed. The next morning wash your hair with chickweed shampoo for the best result.

Avoid commercial shampoos with a detergent base and try those with a castile soap or herbal base. Those containing soothing herbs like chamomile, rosemary, thyme, comfrey, elderflower and nettle may help ease scalp irritation.

MODERN MEDICINE

Depending on the cause, you could use an antifungal shampoo or anti-dandruff shampoo — those containing zinc pyrithione or selenium sulfide are known to be effective, although the tar-based shampoos are the strongest (and most harsh). For most effective results, let the shampoo soak into your scalp before thoroughly rinsing it out. To avoid any irritations associated with prolonged use, alternate anti-dandruff shampoo with a regular shampoo and discontinue the anti-dandruff shampoo once the dandruff clears up.

In severe cases, a doctor may refer you to a dermatologist (skin specialist).

NATUROPATHY

CAUTION: *Read the information on page 167 before taking supplements.*

Poor diet, especially one high in fats or low in essential fatty acids, may be a factor and will be examined by a naturopath. Take doses of evening primrose oil (3000 mg per day), fish oil (3000 mg per day) and vitamin A (5000 iu per day) to help balance the essential fatty acids in your body, which will reduce the incidence of dandruff, whether dry or oily. A zinc supplement may be of benefit, if there is a deficiency.

DEPRESSION

Depression is a persistent emotional state of low mood which can last a few days or, in chronic cases, go on for years. It can involve feelings of sadness, anger, guilt, alienation, inadequacy, and loss of control, which in severe cases can plummet to prolonged hopeless despair.

Symptoms can include disturbed sleep, lack of motivation, concentration and energy, loss of libido and other enthusiasms, anxiety, bouts of crying, changes in appetite and weight, digestive problems, and aches and pains (mostly muscular and headaches). Many cases of suicide, substance abuse and other damaging behaviour have been the result of severe depression.

Causes are many and varied. Depression can be triggered by events such as losing a job or the death of a loved one; by physiological problems such as a biochemical imbalance in the brain, or emotional factors like loneliness. Depression can even be caused by diet, alcohol, drugs or illness such as flu. It can also be caused by a combination of any of the above.

Hormones may play a significant role, and be involved in PRE-MENSTRUAL SYNDROME, postnatal depression, MENOPAUSE and THYROID PROBLEMS, for example.

Seasonal affective disorder (SAD) is also a recognised syndrome, where depression is linked to the change of seasons, the body's need for sunlight and the impact of this on the pineal gland.

Depression may sometimes seem to occur without any apparent reason.

Feeling a bit "down" at times is normal. If the symptoms of depression recur regularly, are severe, or last for more than a few weeks, professional help should be sought.

WHAT YOU CAN DO

- Take note of the way you approach everyday things — walk briskly, breathe deeply, and treat yourself to something special (it can be inexpensive like a nature walk or a bunch of flowers).
- Often depression can be linked to dissatisfaction or boredom. It may be you desire a significant change such as a new job or just that you need to spend some time on yourself, doing things you enjoy.
- Talk things over with someone you can confide in, a friend or a professional — sometimes sharing a problem can relieve it. It may also help you identify reasons behind your depression. See COUNSELLING.
- Expressing your feelings can often relieve melancholia. If you feel like crying, let the tears flow. Creative pursuits such as writing, painting or playing music can be of great benefit.
- Make contact with other people to overcome a feeling of isolation and loneliness. The touch involved in a massage, for example, may help.
- Breathing deeply can be effective in overcoming feelings of sadness and despair. See THE IMPORTANCE OF BREATH.
- Learn how to deal with stress (see page 40).
- Exercise regularly to increase your energy levels and boost motivation. Exercising gives you a sense of accomplishment and control which can increase self esteem and prevent and relieve the symptoms of depression. It also releases "feel-good" chemicals, endorphins, in your body.
- Maintain a healthy, nourishing diet. Depression may lead to loss of appetite, a craving for the "comfort" of highly processed foods, or a lack of motivation to prepare meals. However, your body needs nutrients to keep it healthy and junk food will only make it feel more sluggish. Opt for wholegrain toast or muffins or even porridge or mashed potatoes rather than chips, pastries and pies. Drink warming soup or herbal tea instead of coffee, and eat fruit instead of sweets.
- Avoid alcohol as it is a depressant, and even if it seems to bring short-term relief, it will, in the end, make you feel worse. SMOKING and pain-killing drugs also have a negative effect.
- Experiencing how your posture affects your moods and learning new options may help you reduce some forms of depression. See a practitioner of the FELDENKRAIS METHOD or ALEXANDER TECHNIQUE for advice and lessons.

ACUPUNCTURE

Traditional Chinese medicine cannot be equated on a one-on-one level with Western psychological disorders. What is diagnosed as "depression" in the West may be related to lung (sadness), liver (frustration), heart (lack of joy), kidney (anxiety) or spleen (worry). Nonetheless, acupuncture is known to be effective in treating people with "depressive" conditions.

AFFIRMATION

Depression can often mask other unresolved emotions. Affirmations may help prepare you for a change for the better, even if you feel your depression may never lift.

Try repeating an affirmation like this one throughout the day, say it with feeling and smile — the simple upward movement of your cheeks can sometimes help you feel better: "I have the power to change my life. I willingly release any unresolved emotions. I welcome love and happiness into my life."

AROMATHERAPY

As depression can take several forms there are many oils that suit individual types of depression. Often you will instinctively choose the oil that is best for you at the time.

A sedative oil such as chamomile can help depression when it is accompanied by INSOMNIA and restlessness.

Oils that lift the mood without sedating, such as bergamot, geranium, clary sage, lavender, orange, neroli, rose, ylang ylang and jasmine, are good for FATIGUE and lethargy. Ask someone to give you an aromatherapy massage (see page 140) using a mixture of 2 drops each of lavender, chamomile and geranium in 2 teaspoons of base carrier oil.

BACH FLOWER REMEDIES

Bach flower remedies are particularly effective on emotions, especially when a specific remedy is linked to a specific emotion. These include gentian for those who are easily discouraged, gorse for hopelessness and despair, wild rose for apathy and mustard for depression of unknown cause.

CHINESE HERBS

Chinese herbs that create harmony and balance in your organs and disperse the stagnant Qi energy in your body will relieve your feelings of depression, which is seen by a Chinese herbalist as an imbalance of yin and yang (see page 182).

CHIROPRACTIC

If your nervous system is not fully functional your general ability to cope with the stresses in life will lessen. A chiropractor can increase the function of your nervous system in order to uplift your mind and body so you are not as likely to become depressed, and to heighten your energy levels so that you are better able to cope with day-to-day stresses.

COUNSELLING

Consider seeing a counsellor, especially if you are not able to identify the causes of your depression. You need support to make changes in your life, or to come to terms with issues. The type of counselling may vary (see page 113). It may take a psychological approach or it may involve emotional release work.

HERBALISM

Herbs generally prescribed to treat depression include balm, St John's wort, valerian, oats, skullcap and passion flower. Each day, drink 2 cups of tea or herbal infusion made with one of these herbs. Combine this with counselling and a change of diet — eliminating coffee and processed foods — for the best results.

HOMOEOPATHY

A variety of homoeopathic remedies can help with depression but the one that is right for you very much depends on your personal situation. See a homoeopath for advice and treatment.

MASSAGE

You may benefit greatly by the secure, warming touch and direct physical contact with another person as well as the relaxing and balancing effect of a massage from a qualified therapist.

MODERN MEDICINE

Counselling is often advised by doctors. In times of crisis or in cases of acute anxiety, antidepressants may be prescribed for the short term to bring relief. These are usually preferred to the physically addictive sleeping pills or tranquillisers that have been used in the past. However, although antidepressants can be effective, the expected duration of the medication and any potential side effects should be discussed with your doctor (see page 159).

In severe cases, electroconvulsive treatment (shock therapy) is still used by some doctors.

NATUROPATHY

CAUTION: *Read the information on page 167 before taking supplements.*

A naturopath will advise you to take a food sensitivity test to check whether there is a dietary link and can prescribe vitamins and minerals to increase your body's vitality and balance "brain chemicals". These could include vitamin B (take a high potency B complex tablet according to the label), zinc (25 mg elemental) and magnesium (400 mg elemental) along with kelp (as directed on the label) to increase thyroid function and the amino acids tyrosine and phenylalanine.

OSTEOPATHY

Osteopathy recognises and works with the inter-relationship between the emotions and the body's framework. A healthy, functioning physical structure will enhance your emotional state and vice versa. By working on the muscles and skeleton, osteopathy can help to improve the function of the central nervous system. If your depression is a consequence of chronic pain, you may have a strain pattern which can be corrected with cranial osteopathy.

SHIATSU

A shiatsu treatment will induce an uplifted state of mind that will help counter your depression. Depending on the reason you are depressed, shiatsu practitioners will work on your heart meridian with "tonifying" movements to bring about a peaceful state of mind and improve the flow of Ki energy and blood around your body. The spleen meridian may be treated to help internally shift the condition, as well as the liver meridian in severe cases. The large intestine and lung meridians may also be treated to allow the mind/body to open up and release past issues contributing to the depression.

VISUALISATION

It is common when depressed to lack motivation. A guided visualisation may help (see page 48). Audio cassettes are available to suit all kinds of situations and moods. It can be an advantage having another person's voice lead you through the visualisation when you lack the energy to do it for yourself.

YOGA

In yogic terms, depression is a state where excess energy is trapped inside your body leading to lethargy and negative feelings. Yoga can offer a solution to depression as the exercises act as small stimulations to bring out this suppressed energy. Back-bending poses are recommended as they open the chest and encourage better breathing and circulation. It is best to see a yoga teacher if you are depressed as they will be able to advise you on exercises most appropriate for your condition, but you may like to try salute to the sun (see page 190) to begin.

DIABETES

Diabetes mellitus or sugar diabetes is a disease where the body cannot transfer sugar (or glucose) from the blood into cells to produce energy. This is because the pancreas malfunctions and does not produce enough insulin to carry out this function. When it is not burned, glucose builds up in the bloodstream causing symptoms such as excessive thirst and hunger (especially for sweets), NAUSEA, vomiting, blurred vision, FATIGUE, slow healing of cuts and bruises, cramps in the extremities, vaginal itching, frequent skin, gum or urinary tract infections, inexplicable weight loss and frequent urination. In severe cases, it can lead to coma and even death.

People with diabetes are susceptible to a further range of ailments from HEART and KIDNEY PROBLEMS to failing eyesight.

There are two main types of diabetes mellitus: insulin-dependent diabetes, which usually begins in children and occurs when the pancreas produces little or no insulin, and non-insulin dependent diabetes, which is due to insufficient insulin production or other impairments in metabolising glucose. There are also two temporary forms: stress diabetes (following a trauma) and gestational (during pregnancy).

The cause of diabetes has not been pinpointed but it can have hereditary links. If the onset of diabetes happens in the late teens or twenties, it is often after a viral infection such as the mumps.

IMPORTANT: *By law, non-medically qualified alternative therapists may not treat diabetes. However, with the cooperation of a medical doctor, they may be of assistance in treating the general health of a person with diabetes. They may also be of assistance in the prevention of diabetes in people of high risk.*

WHAT YOU CAN DO

- Get regular exercise. Walking is one of the best forms of exercise; it strengthens the heart, helps control blood sugar levels and increases circulation to extremities.

- Diet is extremely important in managing diabetes, and should focus on high fibre and carbohydrate intake and a number of small meals. Those on medication should be consistent about when and how much they eat.

- It is advisable to maintain a reasonable body weight as there is a strong association between non-insulin dependent diabetes and obesity.

- Always carry something sweet in case of hypoglycaemia (see BOX page 270).

- Always carry or, better yet, wear diabetic identification as some diabetic emergencies can be mistaken for drunkenness.

- Diabetics are more susceptible to oral infections. Brush and floss your teeth often and visit your dentist regularly.

- The feet are particularly prone to damage and fungal infection in diabetics. However, nerve damage from diabetes can lessen the sensation of pain and, consequently, wounds can go unnoticed. Poor circulation due to diabetes can mean the wounds become gangrenous in some cases. Ensure you check your feet often and keep them clean and dry.

ACUPUNCTURE

Acupuncture can be used for both hyper and hypoglycemia.

HERBALISM

Herbalists can offer excellent supportive care and useful herbal remedies to people with diabetes that can help them avoid complications (or treat these if they occur). There is also significant research being carried out on herbs that seem to reduce blood sugar levels, including oats and wood betony.

HOMOEOPATHY

A homoeopath can prescribe holistically for this complex condition. See a qualified and experienced practitioner for advice.

MODERN MEDICINE

Diabetes requires medical management. Doctors will advise you to watch your weight and diet, and prescribe insulin or other hypoglycaemic medication, depending on the type of diabetes, to keep the sugar levels in the body balanced.

NATUROPATHY

Naturopaths are diet specialists and diet management of diabetes can be a complex process. The basic recommendations may be a diet high in fibre (to reduce the need for insulin) and low in fats (to lessen chance of accompanying heart disease). A naturopath can advise on general health, in consultation with your doctor.

DIABETIC EMERGENCIES

There are two opposite and severe reactions that may occur with diabetes.

1. Hypoglycaemic reaction (insulin reaction or low blood sugar). Results from too much insulin, often due to missed meals, too much exercise or overdose. Symptoms usually develop rapidly and include light-headedness, confused/nervous/excitable/irritable behaviour, hunger, shallow rapid breathing and pale moist skin. Can be corrected by taking 1 tablespoon of honey or jam (dissolved in 1/2 cup orange juice if possible) or 2 teaspoons sugar in 1/2 cup lukewarm water, or eating a few small candies. Severe reactions (which may lead to unconsciousness) require an intravenous glucose injection.

2. Ketoacidosis or diabetic coma. Occurs only in insulin-dependent diabetes. Can result from too little insulin or from severe physical or emotional stress or trauma. Develops slowly with early stages displaying flushed dry skin, excessive thirst and urination, stomach pains and deep rapid breathing, later drowsiness then coma. Requires immediate medical attention.

REFLEXOLOGY

If you have diabetes, reflexology should only be carried out by a qualified practitioner.

SHIATSU

If you have non-insulin dependent diabetes where your pancreas is still producing insulin, shiatsu can help to strengthen your kidneys, liver, spleen and pancreas, which contribute to many of the symptoms associated with this condition. A shiatsu practitioner will also be able to give you further advice on diet in co-operation with your doctor.

YOGA

Yoga can assist a diabetic by improving blood circulation and the function of the pancreas, reducing stress levels and strengthening the immune system. There are many helpful exercises but it is best to learn from a yoga teacher who will adapt exercises for your specific needs.

DIARRHOEA

When you have diarrhoea, your stools are runny and you need to defecate constantly. This may be accompanied by cramping in your lower stomach region.

Diarrhoea is a symptom. It can be caused by a virus, a bacterial infection, a course of antibiotics, FOOD POISONING, DIGESTIVE PROBLEMS, overeating, a reaction to alcohol, or by food you have eaten which your body is unable to process properly. Emotions can be a contributing factor, particularly stress, nervousness or a change in situation.

Most natural therapists and many doctors believe that a one-off bout of diarrhoea is your body's reaction to the toxins and impurities you have put into your system. They will advise you to keep up your fluid intake to flush out your system. Once they have determined the cause of this toxic build-up, they will apply the appropriate remedy.

Diarrhoea usually passes within two days.

IMPORTANT: *Seek medical advice immediately if:*

- *it lasts longer than 48 hours*
- *it is very severe*
- *there is any blood in your diarrhoea*
- *it is accompanied by severe abdominal pain, severe indigestion, fever, nausea, vomiting, headache or exhaustion.*

WHAT YOU CAN DO

• Drink plenty of fluids to prevent dehydration, but make sure they are not very cold as this could further irritate the intestine. A good fluid replacement drink can be made by adding 1 tablespoon of glucose powder or sugar and 1/2 teaspoon salt (preferably sea salt) to 1 litre (35 fl oz) of boiled, cooled water. This should be sipped slowly with at least half a glass taken every hour. Alternatively, electrolyte replacement preparations are available over the counter at pharmacists, health food stores and from herbalists. These replace the nutrients in solution that you will have lost: sodium, potassium, phosphorus, chloride, magnesium and calcium.

• Glucose tablets can help replace lost energy.

• Avoid food for 24 hours. Consume only clear fluids (such as water, lemonade, miso, vegetable broth) until stools form. Resume eating with simple foods such as boiled rice or potatoes, poached or hard-boiled eggs and toast, bananas, or grilled fish.

• Certain foods high in fibre, which are difficult to absorb, should be avoided at this time as they can aggravate diarrhoea. These include beans, cabbage, Brussels sprouts, fresh bread, pasta, apples, corn and bran. Also reduce fatty foods.

• If your anal region becomes sore, try rinsing with soap and water rather than wiping with toilet paper. Petroleum jelly may help by waterproofing the skin. Zinc and castor oil preparations, available at pharmacists and health food stores, are even better as they promote healing.

• Recurring diarrhoea is often caused by food ALLERGIES. Keep a food diary and consult a health practitioner to guide you through an elimination diet to pinpoint the cause. Many people have a lactose intolerance and should avoid milk and dairy products with the exception of "live" yogurt. Yogurt with acidophilus and bifidus has the ability to restore protective bacteria to the large bowel.

• Some children are fructose intolerant. In such cases, fruit juices should be avoided. Give rice milk, aloe vera juice or green barley extract instead.

ACUPRESSURE

You can try the acupressure points Stomach 25, Stomach 36, Spleen 6 and Conception Vessel 6 at home as a first aid measure — it may help, depending on the cause of your diarrhoea. Move the pressure in the direction of the arrows.

ACUPUNCTURE

As with constipation, diarrhoea can be helped by acupuncture from a qualified practitioner.

AROMATHERAPY

Oils that have a soothing effect on the intestinal lining and lessen diarrhoea include: chamomile, lavender, neroli and peppermint. These oils are antispasmodic; they also calm the nervous system and allay fears which can often bring on an attack of diarrhoea. You can add them to baths and even burn them in an oil burner in your room.

For effective relief, massage your stomach and abdomen lightly in a clockwise direction for a few minutes with 2 drops of neroli mixed in 2 teaspoons of base carrier oil. Inhaling neroli from a tissue before a stressful event can calm fears and prevent diarrhoea.

CHINESE HERBS

Diarrhoea, both acute and chronic, is one of the many ailments that can be helped by Chinese herbs although this may need to be in combination with modern medication depending on the cause.

CHIROPRACTIC

Any disturbances in your bowel are often connected to your nervous system and the state of your pelvic area. A chiropractor can help correct the function of your nervous system through chiropractic adjustment. They can also check whether your pelvis is affecting your bowel movements causing diarrhoea.

COUNSELLING

As diarrhoea can often be linked to emotional states like fear or stress, counselling may be worthwhile pursuing to help with the cause.

HERBALISM

Slippery elm is the best herb for diarrhoea because it protects the bowel. For a temporary bout of diarrhoea take one teaspoon of slippery elm powder every two hours. You can mix it with a banana and some honey to make it into a meal. Keep taking this mixture until your symptoms subside. Alternatively you can eat it like a porridge without the banana if the fruit aggravates your diarrhoea.

Barley water may also help in preventing dehydration and red raspberry leaf tea can give your bowel the necessary astringency. Golden seal can be of assistance if a bacterial infection is the cause.

HOMOEOPATHY

If your diarrhoea is accompanied by pain coming in waves in your abdomen, try taking one 6C potency tablet or liquid form of *Colocynthis* four times a day. If it is accompanied by vomiting, consider taking *Arsenicum album.* Seek professional advice if your symptoms persist.

MODERN MEDICINE

Medication is available that will stop bowel movements, but these only "plug" the bowel and don't actually affect the cause of the problem. Those containing aluminium or magnesium can actually make the condition worse. They should not be relied on except when a particular situation calls for it — when travelling on a bus or before an important meeting, for example — and they are not suitable for all types of diarrhoea.

In most cases of diarrhoea, changing your diet is all that is required. Very occasionally antibiotics are prescribed when an infection is the cause but these may aggravate the diarrhoea.

In some cases, a stool culture is required to detect parasites. This would then be treated with an antiparasitic medication.

NATUROPATHY

Activated charcoal is available over the counter and may be used to ease diarrhoea. An acidophilus supplement will help improve the condition of your bowel.

If you have regular bouts of diarrhoea a naturopath will analyse your diet to find what foods may exacerbate this condition — common irritants are dairy products and gluten. Massive doses of vitamin C can cause diarrhoea.

OSTEOPATHY

Some causes of diarrhoea, as with other problems of the digestive system, may be assisted by osteopathic treatment. Your health history needs to be discussed and an examination needs to be performed by an osteopath — perhaps along with your medical test results — to evaluate whether your problem would be suitable for osteopathic treatment.

REFLEXOLOGY

Work the points for the ascending and transverse colon as well as the liver for digestion and metabolism, the adrenal glands for any inflammation and to assist muscle tone, and the diaphragm for relaxation and stress reduction. Try this on both feet or hands for a total of 25 minutes daily until the condition clears.

SHIATSU

Diarrhoea in shiatsu terms is a lack of warming Ki energy (known as Yang Ki) in your kidneys, bladder, stomach and spleen. A practitioner will work on points in your bladder meridian to regulate the movement of water and Ki in your body and warm the spleen as well as strengthen your kidneys.

If your diarrhoea is caused by overeating a shiatsu practitioner will work on your stomach meridians, and if it is due to poor digestion a practitioner will work on your spleen and small intestines. They will also advise you on diet if your diarrhoea is not emotionally based.

YOGA

Yoga has been known to clear up regular bouts of diarrhoea. There are many exercises that are beneficial because they activate the whole abdominal area relieving the condition and other associated problems such as indigestion and wind. Try the half-shoulder stand on page 197 twice a day for about 5 minutes. If you experience any discomfort in position 2, practise position 1 only.

DIGESTIVE PROBLEMS

Indigestion, or dyspepsia as it is also known, is general discomfort after eating. Symptoms include FLATULENCE, bloating, abdominal pain and NAUSEA. It can be due to inadequate digestive juices or a disturbance in the transit of food through the bowel (stress, for example, can cause a spasm in part of the intestine). If a burning sensation in the chest (often called HEARTBURN or acid stomach) is involved, there is a problem with stomach acidity or inadequate stomach mucus.

Indigestion is usually caused by a diet that is too rich, eating too much, insufficient chewing of food, or stress. Worry ("having your stomach tied up in knots") is often the emotional cause of nervous indigestion. Heartburn can be caused by some drugs such as aspirin and anti-arthritis medication.

Consult a medical doctor in any of the following cases as the symptoms may indicate a more serious condition such as an ULCER:

- if you have indigestion after most meals
- if it is accompanied by weight loss or loss of appetite
- if the attacks are severe or involve vomiting
- if the problem lasts more than 48 hours.

Gastritis is an inflammation of the stomach lining that can cause similar symptoms to indigestion, although it is usually the result of chemical irritation (e.g. alcohol or drugs such as aspirin), ALLERGIES or FOOD POISONING.

These symptoms can also be indicative of the infectious epidemic condition known as *gastric flu,* usually accompanied by chills, fever and DIARRHOEA. It should pass within 48 hours. In *gastroenteritis,* the intestines as well as the stomach suffer from an inflammation.

See also CANDIDIASIS, COLITIS, CONSTIPATION, IRRITABLE BOWEL SYNDROME, STOMACH ACHE.

WHAT YOU CAN DO

• When you have an attack of indigestion, avoid smoking (it aggravates heartburn) and eat light mild meals such as boiled rice or toast. Sometimes a glass of milk can help.

• A warm compress over the abdomen can ease stomach pains.

• Drink 1 teaspoon of cider vinegar, fresh lemon or grapefruit juice or Swedish bitters in tepid water before meals if you have a problem digesting.

• Don't eat on the run — the blood that normally flows to your stomach and intestines for digestion has to be diverted to the muscles.

• Try to eat slowly and don't rush meals — chew your food properly (at least 20 times per mouthful) and allow at least half an hour's rest after meals so your body can concentrate on digesting.

• Don't eat late at night. Keep your evening meal light and eat it as early as possible.

• Try eating the protein part of your meal first to stimulate gastric juices.

• If you have an underactive digestive system, avoid drinking liquids with meals or immediately before a meal as this dilutes stomach acid.

• If you suffer from heartburn, do not lie down or bend down too soon after eating.

• Maintain a sensible, healthy diet (See page 9)

• Avoid rich, fatty or spicy food, and alcohol, tea and coffee. Acidic foods such as vinegar, salad dressings, citrus fruits, pineapple are more likely to cause heartburn, as are peppermint candies.

• Avoid overloading the stomach. Small frequent meals may be better.

• Don't wear constrictive clothing, especially while eating.

• Learn how to relax and deal effectively with stress (see page 40). It is best to postpone eating when emotionally upset until you feel calmer.

ACUPUNCTURE

Acupuncture is known to be useful in helping relieve recurring indigestion, usually by working on the stomach, spleen and pericardium meridians.

AROMATHERAPY

Oils that have a calming effect on the stomach include chamomile, lavender, vetiver, marjoram, peppermint and bergamot. They also help the stomach process food better.

Try a gentle massage on your stomach and abdominal area (see page 137) with a mixture of 2 drops each of chamomile and lavender in 2 teaspoons base carrier oil. Massage lightly in a clockwise direction and only for a few minutes.

BACH FLOWER REMEDIES

White chestnut and rescue remedy are likely to help if worry is the cause of your indigestion.

CHINESE MEDICINE

A wide range of digestive problems, including indigestion, can be treated with Chinese herbs. See a herbalist for details.

CHIROPRACTIC

Your nervous system has an impact on your digestive process. A chiropractor can improve the function of your nervous system through spinal adjustment which will in turn help smooth your digestion.

COUNSELLING

From a counselling point of view, digestive problems can be associated with a feeling of being "eaten up" inside. They can be found in people afraid of failure and who worry about not being perfect. If this sounds like you, counselling could help.

HERBALISM

Bitter herbs and tonics have a beneficial effect on the digestive system. There are many herbs that are most useful when dealing with indigestion. Some of these include: meadowsweet, fennel, dill, ginger, agrimony, chamomile, cinnamon, valerian, oats, skullcap and gentian.

Try 4 ml of meadowsweet tincture in a little water before each meal to help digestion and prevent indigestion. Repeat half an hour later if you feel pain.

HOMOEOPATHY

Homoeopaths only treat indigestion if it is a recurring problem or a severe case. If it happens rarely and not severely they see it as an indication the body is trying to right itself, despite overeating and drinking.

For relief of mild indigestion including heartburn and flatulence, one 6C potency of *Lycopodium clavatum* 30 minutes before each meal for one day may be appropriate. See a homoeopath if it occurs on a regular basis.

MASSAGE

Regular massage may be of assistance if the problem is caused by nervousness or stress — try a relaxing, full-body massage.

MODERN MEDICINE

Doctors prescribe more acid suppressant drugs than any other kind of medication. They are very effective in the short term but overuse can lead to other digestive problems — food is not adequately sterilised in the stomach nor is protein adequately digested, and this can lead to stomach cancer.

Antacids are often recommended for indigestion but again they are only for temporary relief. Long-term use should be avoided as they contain aluminium. Extremely dilute mixtures of hydrochloric acid or glutamic acid (available in tablet or liquid form) may help people with indigestion, particularly if

HICCUPS

Hiccups are spasms of the diaphragm and are commonly caused by eating or drinking too quickly or too much and swallowing too much air, although other digestive problems may be involved. Irritants such as tobacco or alcohol can be a trigger, as can laughter and nervousness. Hiccups in babies after feeding is normal.

Simple self-help remedies include:

- Swallow a dry spoonful of sugar (in one study this was found to help 19 out of 20 sufferers). For babies, try half a teaspoon dissolved in half a cup of water.
- Hold your breath and swallow three times in a row (not as easy as it sounds).
- Bend over and drink a glass of water from the opposite side of the glass.
- Slowly sip a cup of peppermint tea.
- Slowly eat acidophilus-rich yogurt.
- Work the diaphragm and stomach reflexology points on your feet (see page 175).
- Try massaging the acupressure point Pericardium 6 (see page 87).

If your hiccups are prolonged, severe or happen often, seek the advice of a health practitioner.

the condition is due to a natural lack of stomach acid. Digestive enzymes, from a vegetable or animal source, may be given to help breakdown food into an absorbable form if the body is unable to produce sufficient quantities itself.

Weight loss, diet modification and stress reduction are also recommended.

NATUROPATHY

Digestive enzymes and celloid sodium phosphate are often used by naturopaths to reduce indigestion and for acid stomach. Take these only if they have been prescribed by a naturopath who will determine what you need.

A naturopath would also recommend you keep your diet healthy — sometimes eating protein and carbohydrates at separate times can help. A 24-hour juice fast may be recommended if the cause of indigestion was over-eating or rich foods. "Live" acidophyllus yogurt helps to maintain a healthy digestive system, and ginger and garlic can enhance digestive energy although they can irritate some people.

Activated charcoal can be purchased over the counter and is useful for gas.

OSTEOPATHY

Digestive problems may be related to a spinal dysfunction. You could consider seeing an osteopath for a full check of your spine and advice on exercises to improve your posture and aid digestion.

REFLEXOLOGY

The stomach reflex is the main point to work as well as the liver for bile production, the gall bladder for release of bile which aids the digestive process, and the diaphragm for relaxation and stress reduction.

Work the same areas if you have gastritis but add the adrenal glands to deal with inflammation.

In either case, work the points on both feet or hands for a total of 15 minutes twice a week. You can also work the points for 15 minutes before a heavy meal.

SHIATSU

Stagnation of food in the abdomen due to overeating and drinking is one of the causes of indigestion and acid stomach. The shiatsu solution is gentle treatment of the spleen and stomach meridians to improve their function. Shiatsu practitioners can also provide specific advice on diet.

YOGA

Try the head-to-knee exercise on page 199 to relieve digestive problems.

ECZEMA

Eczema is a form of dermatitis that is red, itchy and sore. It has a crusty, weepy appearance in the worst cases and peels when it heals. It most commonly occurs in the creases of your skin. It is often associated with low levels of vitamin A and zinc linked with an irritant factor such as stress, an unhealthy diet, or ALLERGIES (particularly dairy). There seem to be hereditary links. Eczema is likely to be aggravated by extreme weather changes. The condition may develop in minutes as a reaction to contact with an irritant. Eczema may also be connected with anger or mental irritation, turned inward.

Many people who develop eczema as children develop other allergic reactions such as ASTHMA.

Eczema is likely to recur. Chronic eczema leads to a thickening of the skin which is more resistant to treatment.

WHAT YOU CAN DO

- Be patient but persistent. Any form of treatment is likely to take some time.
- As stress and anxiety can make eczema worse or bring an episode on you should learn relaxation techniques and stress control (see page 40).
- COUNSELLING may help you identify and deal with any underlying problems.
- Get checked for food sensitivity by a doctor or naturopath.
- If you have severe eczema avoid hot water, wool and soap on your skin.
- Do not use lanolin or lanolin-based creams.

• Avoid deodorants and antiperspirants that contain metallic salts known to irritate sensitive skin.

• Cotton fabrics should be worn close to the skin. Avoid synthetic materials and tight-fitting clothes.

• A compress of cold water or iced milk can relieve the itch and irritation. Avoid consuming milk and dairy products, however, as they are a common allergen.

• Cabbage leaves are said to relieve eczema. Wash and pound leaves then warm them, place directly on the affected skin and tie in place.

• A soothing bath — not too hot — can be made by adding 2 tablespoons of bicarbonate of soda (baking powder) to the water. Alternatively, try adding 2 cups of finely ground oatmeal to a warm bath.

• Prevent the skin from drying out. Drink plenty of water and avoid air-conditioning.

• Moisturise your skin with a cold-pressed oil such as sesame, wheatgerm or apricot.

• Breastfeeding, which provides essential fatty acids for the baby, protects a child from eczema.

ACUPUNCTURE

Eczema has been helped in many instances by acupuncture. Acupuncturists believe it is caused by heat, damp and wind and work to counter these and balance energy. They may suggest dietary changes if they think that the liver is involved and will also consider psychological causes.

AFFIRMATION

If anger and irritation are the cause, try repeating an affirmation like the following as many times a day as possible: "I accept that I am angry and I will find positive non-destructive ways of releasing my anger. I am at peace with myself at all times."

AROMATHERAPY

There are particular oils that not only relieve stress, they are also anti-inflammatory and reduce the irritation of the skin.

Combine 4 drops each of chamomile, juniper berry and geranium with 5 teaspoons of base carrier oil. Apply this mixture to the affected areas of your body every morning and night.

BACH FLOWER REMEDIES

Take crab apple remedy for its cleansing effect and rescue remedy if the eczema is stress related.

CHINESE HERBS

Chinese herbs are effective in reducing the occurrence of eczema. A Chinese herbalist can tell you the best ones for your particular condition.

CHIROPRACTIC

Chiropractors see many clients who have both asthma and eczema. By adjusting the spine for asthma and general spinal health, the eczema is also reduced.

HERBALISM

Chickweed is the herb that is most effective in soothing eczema. It is available in an ointment, cream and tincture and different forms of the herb should be used at different times — it is best to ask the advice of a herbalist. A wash of comfrey or chamomile infusion may also bring relief.

Chronic eczema can be treated internally with burdock and yellow dock as specific herbs in a skin remedy but see a herbalist for quantities.

HOMOEOPATHY

If you want to treat your eczema homoeopathically you should see a homoeopath who will determine which remedy you need.

MASSAGE

The area of skin affected by this condition should not be massaged as it may be further irritated. In allergic eczema, lymphatic drainage may be of benefit if performed by a qualified practitioner.

MODERN MEDICINE

In addition to identifying the source of the problem, doctors will prescribe local cortisone creams to relieve itching and reduce swollen, inflamed tissue to normal size — these should be used with caution and only for limited periods as they cause thinning of the skin which leads to stretch marks and bruising, and the steroid may be absorbed internally leading to problems with the adrenal glands. Antihistamines may also be prescribed to relieve the itching. Antibiotics may be prescribed if an infection is present. Some doctors may also suggest a desensitisation treatment to any allergens involved.

NATUROPATHY

CAUTION: *Read the information on page 167 before taking supplements.*

A naturopath will check that your digestive system is functioning properly and check for allergic reactions. Acidophilus and bifidus may be prescribed to help your digestive system process foods more efficiently.

Vitamins that could help your condition include vitamin A (5000 iu per day), vitamin C (2000 mg per day), vitamin E (500 iu per day), evening primrose oil (3000 mg per day) and zinc (25 mg elemental per day).

OSTEOPATHY

Osteopathic treatment can assist in boosting your body's immune defences, thus osteopathy can help to combat these conditions by treating mechanical stresses along with providing diet and lifestyle advice.

REFLEXOLOGY

Work the points for the diaphragm for relaxation and stress reduction, the liver for metabolism and detoxification, the kidneys and colon to ensure healthy elimination, the adrenal glands for anti-allergy and anti-inflammatory actions, the thyroid for metabolic rate, and the pituitary for hormonal balance. Try this on both feet or hands for a total of 15 minutes three times a week.

ENDOMETRIOSIS

Endometriosis is a disease where tissue from the lining of the uterus, which is normally released during menstruation, develops in other areas such as on the ovaries and Fallopian tubes — the lymph system can even carry it to other parts of the body. These pieces of tissue bleed, just as they would in the uterus, causing inflammation, cysts and scar tissue, severe PERIOD PAIN, and chronic BACK PAIN; they can also cause pain during sex or bowel movements.

This disease can cause INFERTILITY if the tissue interferes with the function of the Fallopian tubes and the ovaries.

Endometriosis can be difficult to diagnose due to the type of symptoms that are displayed. It is not always evident in ultrasounds. Confirmed diagnosis is by laparoscopy (an internal investigation). Iridology may also be used (see page 209).

The causes are unclear. However, it is definitely linked with high oestrogen levels, which may in turn be linked with exposure to chemicals and toxins. Stress, especially when linked to sex, femininity and sexuality, seems to play a significant role, and there may be links to CANDIDIASIS. Treatment is a slow process, whichever therapy you choose.

WHAT YOU CAN DO

- Heat treatment may assist in relaxing the cramps in the abdominal area. Try a hot water bottle, heating pad and warm drinks to relieve pain.
- Alternatively, a cold pack applied to the lower abdominal area may provide relief.
- Ensure you exercise regularly — this increases the production of endorphins and reduces oestrogen levels.
- Avoid caffeine completely and steer clear of alcohol and refined foods.
- On an emotional level, some believe endometriosis is connected with blocked creativity so pursuing a creative outlet could be of assistance.
- COUNSELLING may assist in uncovering and dealing with any underlying psychological issues. Also, learn how to relax and deal with stress (see page 40).

ACUPRESSURE

A qualified practitioner can give you advice on treating the causes and symptoms of this condition.

For relief of the abdominal cramps that accompany endometriosis, try acupressure at home. Move the pressure from Kidney 7 to Kidney 8 which is just above it.

ACUPUNCTURE

Acupuncture is effective in balancing hormones, reducing pain and regulating blood and Qi.

AROMATHERAPY

Oils to balance hormones, relieve stress and assist with psychological issues include rose, geranium and clary sage. They can be used in compresses, baths or in oil for a back or abdominal massage.

BACH FLOWER REMEDIES

Rescue remedy can be used for general stress and during an acute attack. Star of Bethlehem is good for prolonged stress and helps body and soul to work together for healing. Olive is recommended for physical and mental exhaustion and to give support when endurance is needed. If fear about your sexuality is a factor, mimulus and aspen can help. For lack of confidence, larch is recommended. Walnut can work as a "link breaker" to old taboos and is a good protector when going through problems.

CHINESE HERBS

This can be one of the most effective of all treatment possibilities. A Chinese herbalist will treat each case on an individual basis.

CHIROPRACTIC

Long-term chiropractic treatment can help relieve the chronic back pain associated with endometriosis and create a better environment for the body to heal.

HERBALISM

On a long-term basis a herbalist can help with herbs that balance hormones and heal and cleanse the female reproductive system. Some of these include chaste tree, false unicorn root and cramp bark. In addition, herbs can be prescribed for pain relief, such as cramp bark and black cohosh, and to alleviate stress, such as vervain. It is preferable to have a consultation with a herbalist as they can give you specific treatment.

HOMOEOPATHY

Homoeopathic remedies can help control endometriosis by regulating hormones. Due to the complicated nature of this condition you should see a homoeopath for professional advice and treatment.

MODERN MEDICINE

Medication such as the Pill can be prescribed to inhibit ovulation, reduce the symptoms of endometriosis and cause the deposits to shrivel. Pregnancy can have the same effect. Analgesics, anti-inflammatory drugs and over-the-counter antiprostaglandins can ease the pain but they don't treat the condition. Danocrine can relieve the condition but this may only be temporary; the drug is also expensive and, like the other drugs mentioned here, there are side effects. In severe cases, endometrial deposits may be lasered or cut out.

NATUROPATHY

The naturopathic way of dealing with endometriosis is through diet. A naturopath will advise you to increase your intake of fruit, vegetables, whole grains, fish, nuts and seeds and foods that contain plant oestrogens such as soya bean products and alfalfa or red clover teas. You can also take doses of evening primrose oil (3000 mg per day) and vitamin B6 (250 mg per day).

Other vitamins and minerals that can help include zinc (20–50 mg elemental per day), calcium (800 mg per day), magnesium (400 mg per day), beta carotene (6 mg per day), vitamin C (2000–4000 mg per day), vitamin B12 (400 mg per day) and potassium chloride celloids (take according to label).

OSTEOPATHY

It has been found in some cases of endometriosis that mechanical strains of the pelvic joints and muscles affect the support structures of the pelvic organs and may contribute to the condition. A consultation with an osteopath will determine if your situation may be helped by osteopathic care (this may need to be in conjunction with other treatments).

REFLEXOLOGY

Work the complete reproductive system — the uterus, ovaries and Fallopian tubes — as well as the small intestine and colon if there are adhesions in this area. Try this on both feet or hands for a total of 20 minutes twice a week.

SHIATSU

A shiatsu practitioner would treat meridians for the spleen (which "holds the blood in place"), kidneys (which nourishes the reproductive organs) and liver (which, along with the spleen and kidneys, controls hormonal balance).

FATIGUE

Fatigue is a common problem especially for people who are working hard or holding down a job and caring for a family. It can be caused by INSOMNIA and a lack of sleep or can indicate you are coming down with an illness. There may be underlying psychological or environmental causes such as low oxygen levels (from poor ventilation), oppressive heat or exposure to chemical or electromagnetic radiation (from computers, for example).

Fatigue can be a symptom of a large range of ailments — such as ALLERGIES, hormonal imbalance, parasites — which would need to be dealt with before you could expect a significant increase in your energy levels. It can also be a side effect of many drugs.

Severe fatigue can be an indicator of CHRONIC FATIGUE SYNDROME, GLANDULAR FEVER or ANAEMIA. It can also be an early sign that you are pregnant. If you are overweight, have an eating disorder or an inadequate diet, you are very likely to feel fatigued.

Ordinary fatigue from exertion can be corrected by rest and sleep, but if you have a feeling of "always being tired", you should consult a health practitioner. The practitioner should take into account your whole situation: physical, psychological, spiritual and emotional. This can take time and effort. Often a number of factors may be contributing to your fatigue.

No therapy can substitute for sensible measures such as getting sufficient sleep and exercise, eating whole foods, and reducing an excessive work load. You cannot keep "running on empty" if other parts of your life are not in order.

WHAT YOU CAN DO

- You may like to boost your diet with a good vitamin and mineral supplement.
- Avoid heavy meals at lunchtime — they can lead to a mid-afternoon slump.
- You may feel you get a "hit" from caffeine or sugar but the slump afterwards just makes thing worse — avoid them.
- Express yourself emotionally and creatively.
- Watch your breathing. Many people don't breathe properly which affects the levels of oxygen and carbon dioxide in their blood and leads to chronic tiredness. See page 25.
- Learn relaxation techniques and how to deal with stress efficiently. See page 40.
- Combat boredom — it can make you feel fatigued. Pursue an interest or a hobby.
- If you have young children, try to arrange a regular babysitter so you can have time to yourself to do things you enjoy.

ACUPUNCTURE

Acupuncture can help with all forms of fatigue once the underlying cause has been determined. See a qualified and experienced acupuncturist for diagnosis and treatment.

AFFIRMATION

If you are feeling fatigued you may also feel unsupported and wonder "what's it all for?" If this is the case, you could try repeating an appropriate affirmation as many times as possible each day. It could be something like: "I have all the energy and vitality I need to live my life to the full."

THE ALEXANDER TECHNIQUE

The Alexander Technique can teach you to increase your body awareness and efficiency of movement so that you reduce fatigue.

AROMATHERAPY

CAUTION: *Read the information on pages 102 to 105 before using these essential oils.*

Rosemary essential oil is good for mental fatigue. To uplift your mind and your body, try a bath with 2 drops each of rosemary and basil, making sure the oil is well dispersed into your bath.

BACH FLOWER REMEDIES

Olive is especially good for fatigue, supported by hornbeam if there is extreme mental fatigue, by wild rose if there is apathy and a tendency to withdraw, and by impatiens if there is impatience about recovery. Vervain can be used for perserverance and to deal with stress and tension. It is good for people who live "on their nerves".

CHINESE HERBS

Chinese herbs are renowned for helping people increase their energy levels and feel active again. Ginseng is one of the better known ones. See a Chinese herbalist for a full diagnosis of your condition and prescription of specific herbs.

CHIROPRACTIC

Chiropractic adjustment can ensure that your nervous system is functioning properly which will increase your energy and vitality.

COUNSELLING

Fatigue can be associated with DEPRESSION, grief, unexpressed anger, disillusionment, entrapment, burn-out or a feeling of "I can't go on" or lack of purpose or focus. A counsellor may help you identify these feelings and pinpoint and resolve issues underlying them. Counselling can help you to reorganise your priorities and learn to be less demanding on yourself, or increase your enthusiasm.

THE FELDENKRAIS METHOD

When you learn how to move efficiently, you can turn tiring movements into movements that are easy and invigorating.

HEALING MEDITATION

This meditation can be done whenever you feel the need for an energy boost. Read the chapter on HEALING ENERGIES and prepare yourself for meditation.

See a healing blue light entering your body through your crown chakra, revitalising every cell in your body. Focus on your breathing. With each inhalation see the blue energy moving through your body, and with every exhalation feel the heavy fatigue leave your body. You may like to visualise this as brown sludgy mud. Do this until you find yourself breathing in blue light and breathing out blue light. Follow the closing rituals to finish (see page 155).

HERBALISM

Oats and skullcap will support and nourish the nervous system. Vervain and lime blossom will ease your sleep. Lemon balm may also be recommended as a mild nerve tonic. A herbalist will prescribe a specific herbal remedy for your fatigue depending on its cause and any related symptoms.

HOMOEOPATHY

To sleep well at night if you believe your bed feels hard or lumpy, and to prevent you from feeling tired during the day, homoeopaths often prescribe *Arnica montana*. If sleeping does not leave you feeling refreshed, take one 6C potency of *Arnica montana* before you go to bed every night for a week. If this has no effect see a homoeopath for advice and treatment.

MASSAGE

If your fatigue is due to overwork or stress, a soothing full-body massage can help — either from a professional or at home. Relaxing massage may help you rest more effectively and ease tense muscles. A brisk, light massage using stimulating movements can be uplifting and energising — you can enjoy a quick, seated massage almost anywhere. See page 151.

MODERN MEDICINE

Some doctors may look at fatigue as a psychological condition and could refer you to a counsellor. A thorough examination should also involve physical investigations (perhaps blood tests etc) to determine whether allergies, hormones, nutrition or other ailments may be the cause.

NATUROPATHY

When fatigued you may crave stimulants such as sugary foods, chocolate, cola, coffee or tea. These will give you a quick energy burst but the effect will soon drop off, leaving you feeling even more tired. Complex carbohydrates, such as rice, potatoes, bread, nuts and seeds as well as proteins such as yogurt will provide a more reliable, longer-lasting energy source. Avoid fatty or refined foods as they will leave you feeling sluggish.

Naturopaths will check you don't have an iron deficiency or food allergy which may be the cause of the problem. They will also check digestive function and treat the liver. High potency B complex vitamins can help energise your body. Take them according to the label. Magnesium and potassium may help, especially if stress is involved.

OSTEOPATHY

If you are constantly tired, your body framework may be under strain. Soft tissue treatment and gentle osteopathic manipulation may be just what you need to boost your energy level.

REFLEXOLOGY

Working the points for the adrenal glands can improve muscle tone and act as a general "pick-me-up". The point corresponding to the pituitary is worked for hormonal balance, the spine for general nerve function, and the diaphragm for stress reduction and relaxation. Try this on both feet or hands for a total of 15 to 20 minutes twice a week.

SHIATSU

Fatigue in shiatsu terms is an indication of lack of flowing Ki energy around your body. Practitioners will therefore increase the flow of Ki by working on your kidney meridian and your abdomen ("hara") and lower back, both "tonifying" deficient functions and stimulating the movement of stagnant energy. After a shiatsu treatment you will find that your energy level gradually increases because the Ki is flowing more freely and your body is better able to self-regulate.

YOGA

Yoga can make a difference to your energy level because it improves the depth of your breathing, increases blood circulation and, most importantly, calms your body and spirit, especially if you attend a class regularly and practise the exercises at home. They are effective if you do them in the morning because they energise you throughout the day. The breathing to relax exercise on page 193 will give you a lift. You can try it in bed just after you wake up.

FLATULENCE

Air or gas (wind) can accumulate in the stomach or intestines, causing a bloated feeling or cramping pains. This is then released through belching or farting.

Swallowing excess air is a common cause, either through nervous action, smoking, chewing gum, gulping drink or eating food too quickly.

Some foods are not easily broken down by the digestive system so they are more likely to ferment in the bowel, causing wind.

Flatulence is often a symptom of indigestion, or may be a result of a fungal/bacterial/yeast overgrowth in the intestine.

See also DIGESTIVE PROBLEMS.

WHAT YOU CAN DO

- Consume food and drink slowly and when you are relaxed. Chew well with your mouth closed. Do not drink through a straw or out of cans or bottles.
- Avoid carbonated drinks, chewing gum and foods containing air, such as omelettes.

• Avoid sugar and refined foods as a general dietary rule as they have an adverse effect on the digestive system, as can fermented foods and those containing yeast (including bread and beer).

• Cut down on fats and oils as they tend to produce gas in your upper digestive system.

• Fibre in the diet is necessary for a healthy digestive system but sulphur can cause flatulence. People who suffer from wind should avoid foods such as cabbage, Brussels sprouts, broccoli, cauliflower, radishes and onions until their digestive systems are in better working order.

• The lectins in lentils, beans and nuts can be a problem for some. Soak beans for 12 hours before cooking to lessen their gas-producing compounds.

• Many people are lactose intolerant which means dairy foods can cause flatulence. Try eliminating them from your diet for a week or so to see if it helps — use soya bean products instead. Then, reintroduce them slowly into your diet. Notice any changes so you can identify which foods in what quantities may be causing the problems. In some cases only the richer dairy foods need be avoided.

• If your flatulence is due to nervous energy, learn how to relax and deal with stress (see page 40).

ACUPUNCTURE

Acupuncture can regulate all digestive disorders including flatulence. Moxibustion on Cu8 will give temporary relief when applied by a qualified acupuncturist.

COUNSELLING

You may be swallowing air without even realising it. This action can have emotional causes and a counsellor will help you identify and deal with these issues so you stop the physical habit.

MODERN MEDICINE

Over-the-counter preparations containing simethicone have a defoaming action which breaks down mucus-surrounded gas pockets in the stomach and intestines.

NATUROPATHY

Activated charcoal tablets are available from health food stores and some pharmacists, and work by absorbing the gas in your system. Probiotics such as acidophilus are recommended, as are bitter tonics (such as Swedish bitters) and digestive enzymes in supplement form.

REFLEXOLOGY

Work the same points that you would for Digestive Problems. Add the pancreas as it directly influences digestion. If flatulence is in the colon, work the points for the colon, in particular the sigmoid colon, in both feet or hands for a total of 15 minutes twice a week.

SHIATSU

In shiatsu terms, flatulence indicates an imbalance in the liver function and excess bacterial action in the intestines. Shiatsu is applied to the liver, stomach and intestine meridians to help regulate this condition.

FLUID RETENTION

The build-up of fluid in body cavities or tissues is known as oedema. Parts of the body swell due to water leaking from the blood supply or to interference in drainage, either from the veins or lymphatic system. It often affects the ankles, lower back, fingers, abdomen and under the eyes.

Fluid retention is a symptom of some disorder in the body, perhaps inflammation, toxicity, hormonal problems, Kidney Problems, Heart Problems, Varicose Veins, or Allergies. It may be linked to organ dysfunction in your small and large intestines, or poor lymphatic drainage.

It is common in the time leading up to menstruation (see Pre-menstrual Syndrome) and in pregnancy (see page 60). Certain drugs such as the Pill and cortisone can cause fluid retention. It may be due to a high salt intake.

Fluid retention can be eased by various treatments but it is best to treat the cause. If fluid retention is an on-going problem, ensure the cause of the condition is correctly diagnosed by a medical practitioner.

WHAT YOU CAN DO

- The blood needs to be kept circulating efficiently around your body so regular exercise is recommended as is weight loss if you are overweight.
- Avoid sodium (salt) in your diet as it holds water in the body. As well as salt, limit high-sodium foods such as prepared meats (e.g. ham, bacon, frankfurters, salami), shellfish and many brands of crackers and chips. Check the label of all packaged/canned products, including condiments.
- Drink plenty of water — six to eight glasses per day — as this actually helps flush fluids from your system. Distilled water is recommended. If drinking bottled water, check the label as many mineral waters are high in sodium.
- Ensure you are eating plenty of protein.
- Try drinking fresh cucumber juice or a mix of celery and parsley juice to reduce fluid retention.

ACUPRESSURE

You can try massaging the acupressure point Kidney 7 at home. Hold this point and then move the pressure upwards towards your heart. However, it is best to consult a qualified practitioner.

ACUPUNCTURE

Acupuncture can help. See a qualified acupuncturist as they may find your fluid retention is linked to other conditions.

AROMATHERAPY

CAUTION: *Read the information on pages 102 to 105 before using these essential oils.*

Essential oils that have diuretic qualities to help relieve fluid retention are lavender, juniper berry and rosemary. If your fluid retention is due to pre-menstrual swelling, try making a warm compress using 3 drops each of lavender and juniper berry and 2 drops of rosemary. Place the compress over your abdomen and breasts for 10 minutes for a few nights before your period.

CHINESE HERBS

Chinese herbs can help reduce fluid retention. See a Chinese herbalist for advice and treatment.

CHIROPRACTIC

A chiropractor can adjust your spine in order to improve the function of the nerves linked to the small and large intestine.

HERBALISM

Herbs that are often prescribed for fluid retention include dandelion leaf, celery, buchu, bladderwrack and barberry. These can be taken in teas or in tincture drops depending on the extent of your condition and its cause.

HOMOEOPATHY

There are many homoeopathic remedies that can be used to treat fluid retention, but a diagnosis needs to be made by a homoeopath who will take into account your emotional and physical condition.

MASSAGE

Massage can be of temporary relief for this condition. Seek a gentle massage in the direction of the heart. Regular massage, especially lymphatic drainage, can help with a sluggish system.

MODERN MEDICINE

Diuretics, usually in tablet form, are prescribed to help remove fluid from your body. Caution should be taken as long-term use can deplete the body of nutrients.

NATUROPATHY

Vitamin B6 is known to be effective in reducing fluid retention. Take 250 mg per day for the best results.

REFLEXOLOGY

At home, you can work the lymphatic system reflex to help reduce fluid in your body tissues. Working the points for the kidneys can assist the elimination of the fluid and the adrenal glands can improve muscle tone and regulate cellular water balance. Try this on both feet or hands for a total of 10 minutes twice a week. It may be advisable to see a qualified reflexologist for a full lymphatic drainage treatment.

SHIATSU

In shiatsu terms, a damp spleen and deficiency in the kidneys can be the cause of fluid retention in the body. These meridians would be treated along with the "triple heater" meridian to evenly distribute heat through the body.

YOGA

The plough pose on page 202 is beneficial for this condition but do not attempt during menstruation or if you have a back problem or high blood pressure.

FOOD POISONING

There are various forms of food poisoning, usually caused by bacteria. Symptoms can occur even 48 hours after eating contaminated food and include NAUSEA AND VOMITING, abdominal cramps, DIARRHOEA, sweating and a fever with chills.

Most cases of food poisoning pass within a couple of days. However, some forms are serious, even fatal. Seek medical advice if your symptoms are severe or if there has been no improvement within 24 hours.

WHAT YOU CAN DO

- Do not try to stop the diarrhoea and vomiting which will rid your body of the irritant.
- Drink plenty of water to flush the toxins from your system and to avoid becoming dehydrated.
- An electrolyte replacement fluid is recommended to replace nutrients lost in vomiting and diarrhoea.
- Avoid solid foods.
- Rest and remain lightly covered.
- A warm compress on the abdomen may relieve cramping.
- A cool compress on the forehead may ease the fever.

ACUPUNCTURE

Acupuncture from a qualified practitioner can be used to restore normal digestive function.

HERBALISM

Chamomile tea will have a soothing effect. Slippery elm powder may ease diarrhoea (take 2 tablespoons in 300 ml/10 fl oz water every two hours). Or take ipecac syrup as instructed on the package.

HOMOEOPATHY

There are a number of homoeopathic remedies that can be taken as first aid measures. Consider *Arsenic albicans*, especially after seafood poisoning, when there is severe diarrhoea, vomiting, chilliness, acute prostration and anxiety (worse between 12 pm and 2 am). Perhaps also *Carbo vegetabilis* for bloating, debility and flatulence.

MODERN MEDICINE

Treatment will vary depending on the type of food poisoning you have and its severity. Hospitalisation may be necessary if dehydration is severe. Antidiarrhoeal medication is usually not recommended.

PREVENTION

- Always wash hands thoroughly before handling food and cooking. Cover any cuts or scratches on hands.
- Wash kitchen surfaces, dishes and cutlery thoroughly before using.
- Proper refrigeration can avoid many problems.
- Defrost frozen food thoroughly before cooking.
- Do not leave hot, cooked food in a warm place.
- Wash hands well after handling raw meat. Cook meat, particularly chicken, thoroughly. Do not keep cooked meat near raw meat.
- If reheating food, do it thoroughly and over a relatively high temperature.
- Do not eat food you suspect may be spoiled. Never eat from a bulging can or one from which gas escapes when opened.

NATUROPATHY

To help you recover from food poisoning you can take an acidophilus and bifidus supplement as directed on the label.

SHIATSU

Shiatsu can be very good for relieving the acute symptoms of abdominal pain, nausea and diarrhoea that often result from food poisoning, once the body has naturally eliminated the irritant.

FOOT ODOUR

Foot odour occurs when you have a fungal infection on the skin of your feet, usually tinea or athlete's foot as it is also known. This fungus can be found on the skin of most people but is usually kept in check by bacteria. It flourishes in warm, humid conditions and can become chronic.

With tinea, the skin of the feet will usually appear irritated, cracked or blistered. The condition can be aggravated by wrong diet, sweat, stress, ALLERGIES and CANDIDIASIS.

Odours of the body can also be caused by food not being absorbed properly or due to the body eliminating toxins. This may be the case if your diet is inappropriate.

WHAT YOU CAN DO

- Keep feet as dry as possible.
- Keep feet immaculately clean, using warm, soapy water as often as needed. Wash in between toes but do not rub as the skin may crack. Dry thoroughly.
- Spray feet with antifungal spray or dust with talc after washing and use a foot deodorant.
- Soak your feet daily in bath salts or try foot baths with vinegar or bicarbonate of soda (baking powder). Dry thoroughly.
- Harsh chemicals such as disinfectants can irritate your feet, worsening a fungal condition. Cleaning your shower often with plenty of soap and water is effective and safe.
- Go without shoes whenever possible.
- Wear thin shoes with both uppers and soles made from natural materials such as leather and cotton as they allow your feet to "breathe".
- Change your socks often and wear cotton rather than synthetic materials.
- Always wear natural fibre socks with closed-in shoes to soak up perspiration.
- Alternate the shoes you wear and allow them to air in a well-ventilated place.
- You can insert pieces of absorbent cotton wool between your toes when wearing stockings.
- Wear thongs, sandals or clogs in public showers, at swimming pools and gyms.
- Drink six to eight glasses of water per day as this can help clear toxins.

AROMATHERAPY

Tea tree is an effective antifungal. It can be applied directly to the area (preferably diluted) or added to a footbath. Look for powders and footsprays containing this essential oil.

BACH FLOWER REMEDIES

Crab apple remedy is recommended for the cleansing effect it has on the body's systems.

HERBALISM

Gentian may help by stimulating the gut to better absorb food. Mix 10–15 drops of gentian tincture in a cup of water. Drink this mixture three times a day before meals.

Myrrh or golden seal tincture dabbed on affected parts will kill the spread of tinea and heal the lesions.

MODERN MEDICINE

If the problem is tinea, antifungal powders, creams or tablets may be prescribed. There are some available over the counter, but if the irritated skin is actually another condition such as ECZEMA, the wrong treatment could make things worse. Note that antihistamines, antiseptics and cortisone creams may exacerbate tinea.

NATUROPATHY

Naturopaths may recommend a decrease in meat intake and an increase in fresh fruit, vegetables and whole grains to clear out the system and reduce body toxins which affect body sweating and odour.

Foot odour can also be caused by a vitamin B deficiency so you may like to take a high potency B complex vitamin supplement according to the label. Acidophilus (in powder form) is also recommended.

Naturopaths will also determine whether your bowel is working properly.

For chronic tinea, a naturopath may recommend an anti-candida type diet (see page 245).

Thuja ointment can be applied to the area.

FOOT SORENESS

The most common cause of aching feet is badly fitting shoes, especially high-heeled shoes. These can give you calluses and BUNIONS AND CORNS which further your discomfort. Flat feet can cause pain due to the stretching of the arch, which means that weight has a shock effect on the tissues of the feet. VARICOSE VEINS can also contribute to aching feet.

Most people do not stand and move correctly and this leads to foot problems. Some throw their weight onto one leg or bear their weight on only their heels or the inside or outside edges of their feet. You can see how you stand by looking at the soles of your shoes.

WHAT YOU CAN DO

- Elevate aching feet to give them a complete rest. The best way to do this is by lying on the floor with your feet at a 45-degree angle up the wall. Relax like this for 20 minutes.
- Soak your feet in a tub of warm water to which bath salts have been added.
- Run your feet alternately under the hot tap and cold tap, finishing with the cold, or try an ice pack to cool away inflammation and swelling.
- Wear shoes that have thick soles to absorb shock from hard surfaces e.g. resin-soled shoes or running shoes with arch supports. Avoid wearing high heels and pointy-toed shoes.

ACUPRESSURE

Acupressure directly on the aching areas of your foot can be tried at home as a first aid treatment for this condition. A qualified practitioner can also work specific points in your feet and the rest of your body.

THE ALEXANDER TECHNIQUE

The Alexander Technique can teach you to balance the weight on your feet through lessons in movement. This can reduce any uneven strain on your feet that may be causing them to ache.

AROMATHERAPY

The skin on your feet absorbs essential oils effectively as it is often dry and hard. The use of "grounding" oils can be beneficial. Try a warm foot bath containing 4 drops of sweet marjoram to relieve pain and 2 drops of lavender to soothe. You or a friend may like to massage your feet as well to increase circulation.

CHIROPRACTIC

If one or both of your feet are aching the problem may be linked to poor distribution of weight. A chiropractor can help you with this by adjusting your spine.

THE FELDENKRAIS METHOD

Awareness of your body's movement can reduce the pounding effect on your feet. Small, dynamic movements can change the way in which your feet function so they are more flexible and supportive. A Feldenkrais practitioner can give you advice and lessons.

HEALING MEDITATION

Read the chapter on HEALING ENERGIES and prepare yourself for meditation. See blue healing light flow into your body through your crown chakra and down to your feet. See it spread throughout your body, then bring your attention to your feet and see the blue light pulsating in every cell of each foot.

You can combine this with an affirmation if you feel there may be emotional/psychological factors involved: "I release any negative thoughts and emotions and move forward in life easily and effortlessly and with peace." Do this meditation each day if you have aching feet.

MASSAGE

Massage is the best way of relieving aching feet. Seek a professional massage to your feet and legs or follow the guidelines for home massage on page 145.

MODERN MEDICINE

A doctor may advise you on the correct footwear (inserts for your shoes, for example) or refer you to a podiatrist or chiropodist, a specialist in the care of feet.

OSTEOPATHY

Aching feet may be a result of mechanical strains within your feet, legs, pelvis or back. Osteopathic treatment can alleviate these strains through gentle manipulation and help correct the discomfort in the ligaments, muscles or nerves of the feet.

REFLEXOLOGY

If you have aching feet, a reflexologist will be able to give you a full treatment to relieve pain. Feet are integral to this form of therapy.

SHIATSU

Shiatsu pressure applied to the soles of the feet helps relieve aching feet, and working the meridians in the legs helps increase circulation to the area.

YOGA

Yoga standing poses can teach you how to distribute your body weight evenly. See a yoga teacher for guidance, but to begin try the standing position on page 205.

Yoga exercises are not always done standing up so your feet get a rest while your blood flow improves — the foot stretch on page 196, for example, can be done in bed or sitting in a chair.

GALL BLADDER PROBLEMS

Your gall bladder is the pear-shaped bag on the undersurface of the liver. It concentrates and stores bile in the body.

The most common problem affecting this organ is inflammation caused by either a bacterial infection or gall stones.

Gall stones are lumps of matter (often cholesterol, bile and protein) that form in the gall bladder. The stones can exist without causing any symptoms and are usually picked up in an ultrasound examination.

If the stones block the exit from the gall bladder, they can block the flow of bile and make the gall bladder inflamed. Symptoms can include PAIN — sometimes extreme — in the upper right abdomen and sometimes pain between the shoulder blades, over the shoulder area or on the shoulder tip. There may be NAUSEA, indigestion, jaundice and fever. There can also be serious complications including liver damage, a ruptured gall bladder or an obstructed intestine.

Gall bladder problems have been linked with excess fat and sugar in the diet, some drugs (including the Pill), liver malfunction and hereditary predisposition. Those at greatest risk are "fair, fat, female, fertile and forty".

Some believe there may be an emotional connection between the gall bladder and feelings of bitterness. The common use of the term "that really galls me" is derived from this association. Problems related to gall bladder dysfunction include migraines (see page 295) and some shoulder and muscular spasms.

IMPORTANT: *If you suffer severe abdominal pain and it lasts more than a few hours, consult a medical doctor. Only follow alternative remedies under the doctor's approval. A ruptured gall bladder can be fatal.*

WHAT YOU CAN DO

• A traditional home remedy for gall bladder problems is lemon. Add fresh lemon or lemon juice to your meals (especially salads) along with olive oil.

• Eat a high-fibre diet and avoid all fats and fried foods, egg yolks, cooked cheese, oranges, coffee, full-cream milk. Keep red meat, seeds, nuts, alcohol and tobacco to a minimum.

• Weight loss is often advised for gall bladder problems. This should help control cholesterol levels.

• See LIVER PROBLEMS and HEART PROBLEMS for further ways to reduce cholesterol and to stimulate a sluggish system.

ACUPUNCTURE

Acupuncture can be used to regulate the digestive function and assist the body to assimilate fats.

AFFIRMATION

If your condition has emotional links, you may wish to repeat an affirmation like this as often as possible throughout the day: "I willingly release any negative thoughts of the past. I look for the good in all things".

AROMATHERAPY

CAUTION: *Read the information on pages 102 to 105 before using these essential oils.*

For pain relief when you have gall stones, make up a mixture of 2 drops of rosemary and 2 drops of lavender mixed with 2 teaspoons of base carrier oil. Massage this over the area of your gall bladder (below the liver and on the right hand side of the diaphragm). Be gentle when you massage and only massage lightly in a clockwise direction for a few minutes.

BACH FLOWER REMEDIES

Willow is recommended for the gall bladder because it reduces bitterness and resentment, which can be associated with the emotional side of this condition.

CHIROPRACTIC

Gall bladder dysfunction is often linked to a nervous system affected by subluxations (unnatural pressures or interferences). A chiropractor can adjust your spine to reduce these subluxations and improve the function of your nervous system.

HERBALISM

The herbs wild yam, valerian and cramp bark help relieve the pain of gall stones. Dandelion and golden seal are used if the gall bladder is inflamed. These herbs should be prescribed by a herbalist — he or she can do more for you than just relieve symptoms.

HOMOEOPATHY

Homoeopathic treatment of gall bladder problems uses preparations of plants that have a bias for the gall bladder and liver, including *Berberis vulgaris, Chelidonium majus* and *Carduus marianus.* To prepare a remedy that will dissolve gall bladder stones, a homoeopath will need to establish the composition of the stones.

MODERN MEDICINE

Surgery can be carried out to remove the gall bladder itself and some doctors will recommend this after a case of stones or once the inflammation from an attack has settled. Laser surgery and sound waves can shatter stones, enabling remnants to be passed. Strong drugs are available that can dissolve stones in some cases.

Antispasmodic drugs may be given to relieve the spasm caused by a stone passing. In some cases, a patient is hospitalised for observation to ensure there is no acute obstruction.

Colonic irrigation may be recommended by your doctor or naturopath. Treatment is given at specialist clinics. It assists in the removal of stones and also improves general function of the gall bladder and liver.

NATUROPATHY

CAUTION: *Read the information on page 167 before taking supplements.*

Diet is one way naturopaths deal with gall bladder problems. They are likely to recommend a low-fat, low-sugar, high-fibre diet with bitter greens as stimulants. You may be advised to take vitamin C (2000 mg per day) and vitamin E (500 iu per day).

Other vitamins and minerals that can help include lecithin (2 tablespoons per day), vitamin B6 (250 mg per day), zinc (25 mg elemental per day) and magnesium phosphate (taken according to the label).

OSTEOPATHY

Some gall bladder problems, as with other problems of the digestive system, may be assisted by osteopathic treatment. Your health history needs to be discussed and an examination performed by an osteopath — perhaps along with your medical test results — to evaluate whether your problem would be suitable for osteopathic treatment. If it is, then treatment would be in the form of gentle manipulation of the lower ribcage and the diaphragm as well as the liver and gall bladder themselves. This would be aimed at improving the secretion and emptying of the gall bladder. Dietary advice might also be given.

REFLEXOLOGY

Work the points for the gall bladder, of course, as well as the liver for bile formation.

If gall stones are the problem, working the points for the liver and thyroid will help your body maintain cholesterol balance.

Try this on both feet or hands for a total of 15 minutes twice a week. However, care must be taken that the stones don't become lodged in the bile duct through the overworking of these points. See a qualified reflexologist if in any doubt.

SHIATSU

Gall bladder problems often occur because of blockages in the gall bladder meridian. Problems with other organs and a lack of flowing Ki energy can also be contributing factors to gall bladder conditions. In Oriental terms the gall bladder is linked to the liver and distributes Ki around the body making it an important organ. The gall bladder usually responds well to shiatsu treatment.

YOGA

Certain yoga positions such as the half-lotus pose on page 197 can be good for gall bladder problems because they stimulate the gall bladder, promoting blood flow and triggering the immune system.

GINGIVITIS

Gingivitis is an inflammation of the gums. It can occur as the result of an infection caused by dental plaque. Plaque is a build-up of bacteria and organic matter on the tooth which can lead to decay.

Gingivitis can be linked to a vitamin C deficiency. It sometimes appears during pregnancy or at other times when you are undergoing a hormonal change.

Symptoms include bleeding gums and soreness around the base of your teeth.

If left unchecked, periodontal disease can develop which can lead to tooth loss.

WHAT YOU CAN DO

- In the early stages of gingivitis, you can treat yourself at home by rinsing with 1 teaspoon salt dissolved in a glass of water. Repeat hourly. If symptoms continue, consult a dentist.
- Even if your gums are sore, clean your teeth frequently, taking special care to clean the gum line, and use dental floss regularly.
- Alternate between two toothbrushes so they dry out between brushing.
- A homemade mouthwash you can use is a solution of half 3 percent solution of hydrogen peroxide and half water to deter bacteria.
- If you prefer not to use toothpaste containing fluoride and other chemicals, you can clean your teeth with lemon juice or a powder made from one part salt and two parts bicarbonate of soda (baking powder). Make sure you rinse your mouth thoroughly.
- Do not pick your teeth with hard, sharp or metal objects as you could injure your gums and scratch tooth enamel.
- See your dentist once a year for a clean and check up.
- Ensure your diet contains raw fruit and vegetables which clean teeth and stimulate gums. Avoid sugar and sweet foods.

ACUPUNCTURE

Acupuncture is an option if you have gingivitis. An acupuncturist will look for underlying causes for this condition, which may be stomach heat.

AROMATHERAPY

Essential oil mouthwashes are effective. Combine 250 ml (8 fl oz) cheap brandy, 3 drops each of thyme and peppermint, and 10 drops each of myrrh and fennel in a clean dry bottle and shake well. When you want to use the mouthwash shake it well again and add 3 teaspoons of the mixture to half a glass of warm water. Swish the mixture around your mouth for a minute and then spit it out. Do not swallow it. Do this twice a day.

Alternatively, you can use a solution of 5 drops of tea tree in a cup of warm saltwater.

BACH FLOWER REMEDIES

To a practitioner, gums and teeth represent decision making and the remedy scleranthus can help in making the right decision.

CHINESE HERBS

Chinese herbs are known to be effective in treating gingivitis. See a Chinese herbalist for advice and a prescription of herbs.

HERBALISM

Herbal mouthwashes can be an effective way of dealing with gingivitis because some herbs have excellent antiseptic qualities. To relieve the discomfort, try gargling twice a day with a mixture made of equal parts of thyme, sage and myrrh tinctures and glycerine in a glass of water. The glycerine is to make the mixture stick to your mouth and throat. Massaging your gums with a fresh sage leaf is a good way of keeping them healthy.

HOMOEOPATHY

Homoeopathic remedies can help reduce the symptoms of bleeding and painful gums. If your gums are bleeding and the bleeding won't stop easily take one 6C potency of *Phosphorus* homoeopathic remedy three times a day for two days. If the condition persists over a few days see a homoeopath for more specific remedies.

MODERN MEDICINE

Antibiotics are sometimes prescribed to reduce further infection, but appropriate dental hygiene should be applied on the advice of a dentist.

NATUROPATHY

CAUTION: *Read the information on page 167 before taking supplements.*

Take vitamin C with bioflavinoids (4000 mg per day), silica (as directed on the label) and calcium (800 mg per day) to help relieve gingivitis.

You can also increase your intake of protein as a lack of protein can often cause gingivitis.

REFLEXOLOGY

Work the points for the adrenal glands to deal with inflammation, the lymphatic system for the infections and all fingers or toes as they correspond to the head/mouth area. Try this on both feet or hands for a total of 15 to 20 minutes twice a week.

SHIATSU

In shiatsu terms, the gums are controlled by the small and large intestine and stomach meridians which would be treated to relieve the inflammation.

GLANDULAR FEVER

Glandular fever or mononucleosis is caused by the Epstein-Barr virus. It is most common in children, adolescents and young adults, and is transferred from person to person through the exchange of saliva.

After an incubation period that may span several weeks, symptoms include fever, swollen lymph glands, fatigue, sore throat, rash and general aches and pains. Some of these symptoms may resemble other conditions, making diagnosis difficult, but a simple blood test can confirm the condition.

The illness has a significant impact on the lymphatic system, and usually the spleen and liver as well.

Glandular fever is a difficult condition to treat because it has usually taken hold of your body by the time it is diagnosed. Symptoms can be persistent or recur. The acute illness usually lasts one to two weeks although recuperation may take months or years.

See also CHRONIC FATIGUE SYNDROME.

WHAT YOU CAN DO

- Rest is very important as the body needs a chance to become well again. Most people try to get back to their old routine too early.
- Drink plenty of fluids to combat a dehydrating fever and to flush toxins from the system.
- Gargling often with warm saltwater may alleviate a sore throat.
- Avoid alcohol during this time and for a considerable period after a bout of glandular fever as the liver is likely to be inflamed.
- Avoid fatty or rich foods. Choose high carbohydrate foods as your body will not be producing energy efficiently during this time.
- The condition can leave you debilitated. A review of your lifestyle could be of great benefit. See PROTECTING YOUR IMMUNE SYSTEM.
- If you've spent a lot of time in bed with this illness, your back may be out of alignment. A CHIROPRACTIC or OSTEOPATHY treatment may help — regular treatment will also help build your immune system.
- Once you become a little more active again, the FELDENKRAIS METHOD can help you regain movement and reduce the fatigue as can the ALEXANDER TECHNIQUE.

ACUPUNCTURE

Acupuncture can aid you in recovering from a bout of glandular fever. See a qualified, experienced acupuncturist for more details.

AFFIRMATION

It is important to allow yourself the time you need to fully recover from glandular fever. If you feel life is passing you by because of your long convalescence you could try affirmations to ease your distress.

Some believe glandular problems have a connection with feelings of apathy and poor motivation. If you feel this applies to you, try repeating an affirmation like the following as many times a day as possible: "I have all the creativity and energy I need".

HERBALISM

It is preferable to see a herbalist for specific herbal remedies as glandular fever affects people in different ways. Herbalists can rebuild your immune system with the herbs echinacea, golden seal, St John's wort, thyme and myrrh. St Mary's thistle or dandelion may be added to the formula to help rebuild liver cells — the liver becomes swollen and painful in people with glandular fever, and the health of this organ is very important in healing this condition.

HOMOEOPATHY

There are very specific homoeopathic treatments available for this condition that are known to be particularly successful. They prompt your body to fight the infection. See a homoeopath for a full assessment to suit your individual case.

MASSAGE

After this condition has subsided, lymphatic drainage massage from a qualified practitioner can help improve the lymphatic system which may prevent a recurrence of the complaint.

MODERN MEDICINE

There is no specific medical treatment. Analgesics can be given for pain or fever. Antibiotics are prescribed on some occasions for complications. Injections of vitamin C may be given to kick-start the immune system and flush out toxins.

During the acute stage of the illness, it is good to drink lemonade for energy.

NATUROPATHY

Vitamins, minerals and a healthy cleansing diet can help you recover from glandular fever. Take 1/4 teaspoon (or 1000 mg) of vitamin C powder every hour until you are feeling better. You can also take vitamin A (5000 iu per day) and zinc (25 mg elemental per day) to aid recovery. The liver needs to be looked after with sodium sulfate and liver herbs.

REFLEXOLOGY

To help speed your recovery, *gently* work these points on both feet or hands for a total of 10 minutes two or three times a week: the pituitary, for general hormone balance, and all other glands; the lymphatic system, spleen and thymus to deal with the infection and aid the immune system; the liver for detoxification; and the throat/neck reflex for any discomfort in that area. A consultation with a qualified reflexologist is recommended rather than relying on home treatment.

SHIATSU

This natural therapy can help your recovery from glandular fever as it will improve the function of your organs and strengthen your immune system. If you have had a severe case of glandular fever you could be deficient in Ki in your liver, gall bladder and kidney meridians so regular shiatsu treatment can benefit you.

YOGA

Yoga exercises can help you regain full health after a bout of glandular fever as they are gentle yet promote blood circulation and aid the immune system. You can contact a yoga teacher to give you particular exercises that suit your state of health and energy levels — there are even yoga exercises that you can do in bed.

HAEMORRHOIDS

Haemorrhoids, or piles, are swollen, painful blood vessels which build up around the anus, causing itchiness and occasional bleeding. They can restrict bowel movements and make them painful.

Haemorrhoids can be caused by a genetic weakness in the veins, CONSTIPATION or straining, LIVER PROBLEMS, pregnancy or long periods of standing, sitting or lifting. Stress and obesity can make you more susceptible.

Haemorrhoids should be medically diagnosed as similar symptoms could indicate a more serious ailment such as abscesses or cancer.

The condition should clear up by itself under the supervision of a doctor and therapist. Preparations should relieve you of the discomfort. However, consult a doctor if your haemorrhoids bleed persistently. It may indicate a more serious problem.

Haemorrhoids can be chronic or recur.

WHAT YOU CAN DO

- Rinse with soap and water then dry or use moist towelettes instead of toilet paper.
- Take hot baths or sitz baths to relieve the pain and itching.
- Apply hot and cold compresses alternately to improve circulation.
- Reduce itching with a paste of bicarbonate of soda (baking powder) and water applied to the area.
- Apply lemon juice.
- Avoid heavy lifting and other straining physical work to prevent haemorrhoids or to avoid aggravating the condition.
- Avoid sitting for long periods as circulation slows in the area. Exercise helps by promoting circulation drainage.
- Reduce straining by avoiding CONSTIPATION, ensuring good digestion (see page 272), getting regular exercise, maintaining good posture, eating a healthy diet high in dietary fibre and drinking plenty of fluids.
- Try squatting to defecate. There are platforms available commercially that fit to your toilet to make this easier.

ACUPRESSURE AND ACUPUNCTURE

These treatments from a qualified practitioner can assist in dealing with the pain of haemorrhoids.

AFFIRMATION

Some believe haemorrhoids can be associated with feelings of powerless and being rushed so affirmations may be worthwhile for this condition. Try the following if it seems appropriate: “I easily release all past hurt and angers. I have all the time I need to create the perfect life for me.”

AROMATHERAPY

To reduce pain and bowel pressure, mix together 3 drops of cypress and 2 drops of sandalwood essential oils in 5 teaspoons of calendula base carrier oil. Apply the mixture to the affected area twice a day, preferably in the morning and evening.

BACH FLOWER REMEDIES

Rescue remedy and white chestnut are effective in dealing with stress and worry, emotional reactions which can cause haemorrhoids. Walnut is also effective as it aids “letting go”, which may be another emotional factor in the condition.

CHINESE HERBS

Haemorrhoids can be reduced by Chinese herbs. Yunnan Pai Yao, for example, is one patent formula that provides an effective short-term treatment but consultation with a Chinese herbalist is usually advised.

HERBALISM

A herbalist will treat each case of haemorrhoids differently depending on the person.

The herbs that are commonly used include witch hazel, calendula, comfrey, horsechestnut, cranesbill and oak bark. These can be taken internally, dabbed on externally or used in a cream or pessary. Taking slippery elm powder will help soften your faeces.

HOMOEOPATHY

Homoeopathic remedies taken both internally and externally can help relieve the pain of haemorrhoids. See a homoeopath for a full physical and emotional assessment, but you can also try homoeopathic remedies at home. If your haemorrhoids cause shooting pain up your spine apply the homoeopathic cream *Aesculus hippocastanum* to the affected area. If your haemorrhoids bleed constantly and feel sore apply *Hamamelis virginica* cream to the affected area.

MODERN MEDICINE

Over-the-counter astringent creams, vascular tonics and rectal suppositories are available for haemorrhoids which can relieve pain to some extent. Laxatives can soften the stool to ease passing, but use with caution. In severe cases, the haemorrhoids can be injected with a chemical to make them close up. For persistent or recurring haemorrhoids, surgical removal may be suggested.

NATUROPATHY

A naturopath will advise you to take a bioflavinoid supplement (400 mg three times daily) to help reduce your haemorrhoids, and to take pressure off the blood vessels by cleansing the liver. Ensure there is a little oil in your food intake to make the faeces “slippery”.

REFLEXOLOGY

The sigmoid colon reflex is the main one for this problem. In addition, you can work the diaphragm for relaxation, the lower spine for improved nerve function, the adrenal glands for muscle tone, and the liver and heart for circulation. Try this on both feet or hands for a total of 25 minutes twice a week.

SHIATSU

Toning up your spleen and sedating your liver is one way a shiatsu practitioner can relieve haemorrhoids. A practitioner can also work on your kidney, large intestine and bladder meridians to reduce constipation and improve anal blood circulation. Toning up your heart meridian can also strengthen and clear your blood vessels to reduce the chance of haemorrhoids appearing in the first place.

YOGA

Haemorrhoids can be helped by yoga because it activates blood circulation to the anus and therefore reduces constipation.

To improve your circulation practise the half-shoulder stand exercise (on page 197) three times a day, but only if you have checked with your doctor that your condition is not linked to liver disease. While you are doing the exercise contract your anus each time you breathe out.

HANGOVER

A hangover is a self-inflicted condition which occurs after drinking alcohol, usually in excess. The body is not able to break down the alcohol before the system accumulates harmful metabolic byproducts. One of the main reasons for hangover is dehydration because alcohol robs the body of one and a half times the amount of water compared to alcohol, and with this vitamins and minerals. The resulting drop in blood pressure can lead to dizziness and disorientation.

Alcohol also irritates the stomach lining.

There may be NAUSEA AND VOMITING, DEPRESSION or HEADACHE. See separate entries for these symptoms.

WHAT YOU CAN DO

- Women should take even more care than men due to their smaller physical size. They are also more susceptible to hangovers if on the Pill, when ovulating and when pre-menstrual.

- Some drinks can make you feel worse than others due to their chemical make-up (congeners). Vodka and gin have the least of these chemicals, bourbon the most. Red wine has more than white wine.

- Activated charcoal from pharmacists and health stores absorbs congeners. Take the tablets as directed immediately after drinking alcohol, before sleeping.

- Do not drink alcohol on an empty stomach.

- Drink plenty of water before, during and after drinking alcohol. It will counter the dehydration and flush the toxins from your system.

- Have a large glass of fruit juice in the morning or eat some honey — the fructose helps the body burn alcohol faster and remove it from your system.

- Eat a light meal to replace nutrients — soups, boiled eggs and cooked cereals are recommended for an upset stomach. You may crave fatty foods because your body wants to stimulate the cleansing process of the liver thus these foods often make you feel better.

- Although you may feel like the stimulation of coffee or tea, caffeine is diuretic and will rob your body of even more water and nutrients. Choose a "sports" drink instead which contains no caffeine but will give you energy and replace electrolytes that aid rehydration.

- The traditional cure of eating raw or coddled egg may help your stomach by neutralising acid and soothing the lining.

- Try an ice pack or cold towel on the forehead, but opt for a tepid shower rather than a cold one.

- To whiten bloodshot eyes, soak cotton wool pads in cooled herb tea — chamomile, fennel, golden seal or eyebright — and place on your eyes. Or do the same with cooled wet tea bags.

- Get some fresh air and focus on your breathing (see page 25).

ACUPUNCTURE

Acupuncture is excellent for dealing with a hangover which a qualified practitioner will treat as a spleen/liver problem.

AROMATHERAPY

To revitalise you and lift your mood, use an oil burner or try a steam inhalation or bath to which one or more of the following essential oils have been added: cinnamon, aniseed, angelica, geranium, bergamot, clary sage, jasmine, juniper, lemon, orange, patchouli, rose, rosemary and vetiver. Or carry a bottle of lavender with you and massage it directly onto your temples or inhale it from the bottle.

BACH FLOWER REMEDIES

Take rescue remedy to relieve the symptoms and crab apple for cleansing the body and mind.

Bach flower remedies can also be used in dealing with why a person over-indulges in alcohol in the first place: larch may be taken for lack of self-confidence, for example, or white chestnut if they are drinking to forget their worries.

CHINESE HERBALISM

Patent formulas are available over the counter that help relieve nausea and headache. Sip a small quantity of gingseng tea often for as long as symptoms persist.

HEALING MEDITATION

See the chapter on Healing Energies for a healing meditation to restore your inner balance.

HERBALISM

Try drinking vegetable juice such as carrot and celery with 1/4 teaspoon cayenne pepper. Alternatively, peppermint tea will help settle your stomach and freshen your breath. Fresh parsley will also freshen your breath and replenish many depleted nutrients.

Take a soothing yet reviving bath by running hot water through a cloth pouch containing lemon balm, chamomile, lavender, peppermint or borage.

St Mary's thistle or dandelion before and after drinking will help protect your liver. Take it regularly if you drink often.

HOMOEOPATHY

There are many homoeopathic remedies that can help reduce the symptoms associated with a hangover. *Sulphur* is for early morning diarrhoea, *Nux vomica* is for dizziness and nausea and *Byronia* is for a severe headache which is accompanied by a huge thirst. Every hour, take one 6C potency of the remedy that matches your symptoms. Take this dose seven times.

MASSAGE

Upper back, neck and scalp massage will help alleviate symptoms as it brings fresh blood to the area.

MODERN MEDICINE

Antacids should help settle your stomach and can be taken before drinking as a preventative. Soluble aspirin should relieve your headache — paracetamol, however, could irritate your liver further.

NATUROPATHY

To avoid a hangover, you can take a high potency vitamin B supplement (according to the label), vitamin C (1000 mg per day) and zinc (25 mg elemental) before drinking, again when you finish drinking and again in the morning. You can also try magnesium, as it is severely depleted by alcohol thus producing tremors and mental confusion.

REFLEXOLOGY

Work the following on both feet or hands for a total of 30 minutes: the points for the diaphragm for relaxation and to improve breathing so that more oxygen is supplied to the brain, the points that make up the whole spine for improved muscle functioning, and all the toes/fingers because these points correspond to the head area. If you feel dizzy, also work the ear reflex for balance as well as the points for the side of the neck and the cervical spine.

SHIATSU

The stomach and liver meridians would be treated by a shiatsu practitioner to relieve hangover symptoms.

HEADACHE AND MIGRAINE

Technically your head aches when the vessels in your brain constrict, cutting off blood flow, or dilate, allowing too much blood flow.

Headaches are the most common physical complaint. Some of the usual causes are:

- muscular tension, particularly to the upper scalp and neck area
- teeth and jaw problems
- upper cervical vertebra problems
- lack of sleep (see Insomnia) and Fatigue
- excessive noise
- dehydration
- too much heat or light
- too little air
- Allergies
- low blood sugar levels

- diet
- hormones
- DEPRESSION
- fevers or infections
- toxicity
- CONSTIPATION (leading to bowel toxicity)
- LIVER PROBLEMS
- problems with congestion and drainage e.g. SINUSITIS
- other serious conditions such as meningitis, cerebral haemorrhage or cerebral tumours.

Migraines are intense, throbbing, often debilitating headaches, in many cases occurring on one side of the head and accompanied by NAUSEA AND VOMITING, blurred vision and sensitivity to light, sound and smell. They usually begin slowly and may last many hours.

Migraines are the result of a spasm followed by dilation of blood vessels. The causes are not fully understood, although they can be triggered by anxiety, shock, anger, physical stress or the release of such tension. They may be hereditary in some cases or be due to stress or diet. Common food triggers include citrus fruits, chocolate, caffeine, red wine, MSG (flavour enhancer 621), preservatives, nuts and cheese.

Cluster headaches are also intense headaches, but these tend to be continuous (rather than throbbing) and occur behind one eye. They often begin during sleep and may be associated with running eyes and nose and a swollen face (but not nausea or vomiting). The pain usually lasts 15 minutes to a few hours and several attacks may occur in one day. Such attacks may repeat over several weeks, and then disappear for months or even years. They are more common among men than women. The cause is unknown but the attacks may be triggered by stress, diet, hormonal changes or histamines, among other factors.

No matter what the therapy, treatment is prescribed for headaches according to the frequency of the headache, its position on your head, the type of pain, your emotional condition at the time of the headache and your current physical state and physical history.

For severe, prolonged or regular headaches, see a doctor who will carry out a thorough physical examination to determine the cause. Consult a doctor immediately if the headache is associated with a head injury or accompanied by confusion, loss of balance or lapses in consciousness.

WHAT YOU CAN DO

- Exercise regularly to reduce stress and the risk of tension headaches. A brisk walk and fresh air may help relieve a tension headache.

- Breathe deeply and regularly to get oxygen to your brain (see page 25).

- Eat something and drink plenty of water — dehydration and/or hunger are common causes of headache.

- Sometimes sleep can dispel a headache.

- If you have an addiction — to caffeine, tobacco or alcohol, for example — you will get headaches when you haven't had a "hit". Conversely, these substances are often the cause of headaches too. It is best to try to wean yourself off them altogether.

- If you suffer recurrent headaches, you may wish to keep a food diary to record any possible dietary trigger or try an elimination diet (see page 214).

- Bright light from the sun or the glare of a television or computer can trigger or aggravate a headache. Wear sunglasses outside and take frequent rests from the computer screen.

- Relaxation and stress-management techniques will help prevent or relieve a headache (see page 40).

- Ensure correct posture (see page 24).

- Try a 5-minute footbath at the first sign of a headache. For extra benefit, add an appropriate herbal remedy (e.g. chamomile tea, or lavender or rosemary essential oil) to water which is as hot as you can stand.

- Biofeedback, self-hypnosis and autogenic training have all had significant success in helping people manage their headaches (see page 206). At home, you can try visualisations (see 299) — focus on the blood moving away from your head.

ACUPRESSURE

There are different acupressure points for headaches occurring on different areas of your head (top of your head, on your forehead, back of your head and side of your head). Try the acupressure points that match the place the ache is occurring on your head. Make sure you hold the pressure point for at least 1 minute at a time. If you have a prolonged headache or recurring headaches, consult a qualified practitioner who may be able to bring instant relief, depending on the cause, and give you further advice to prevent the headaches and manage the pain.

ACUPUNCTURE

While in some cases acupuncture can relieve the immediate pain of a headache, this therapy is more suitable for treating recurring headaches once your doctor has determined they are not caused by a life-threatening condition. Acupuncture has had a high success rate with migraine sufferers.

Your acupuncturist will look for the underlying cause of your headaches. As headaches are often linked to what acupuncturists call 'blockages of energy' or Qi you may need a course of treatment before your headaches are relieved. Your lifestyle may also need alteration.

THE ALEXANDER TECHNIQUE

Alexander lessons can help if your headaches are related to tension in your neck, head, and shoulder areas. An Alexander Technique teacher will help you become aware of your posture, particularly the way in which you hold and move these areas of your body and show you how to avoid strain.

Consider this therapy if you find you get headaches at work, sitting at your desk, using a computer or taking notes while holding the telephone — situations where incorrect usage of your body could be the underlying cause.

AROMATHERAPY

CAUTION: *Read the information on pages 102 to 105 before using these essential oils.*

The essential oils that are most effective for headache relief are lavender and peppermint; they clear the head and relieve pain and are safer than other medications.

Make a cold compress containing 2 drops each of lavender and peppermint. Apply this to either the forehead, the temples or the back of the head, depending on where the headache is.

If your headache is due to sinusitis make up a steam inhalation containing 2 drops each of eucalyptus, rosemary and lavender. This will relieve the headache and the congestion.

If you know you are stressed and can feel a headache coming on, keep a tissue handy that has been sprinkled with 2 drops of lavender, peppermint or sweet marjoram. Inhale throughout the day as a prevention.

BACH FLOWER REMEDIES

Rescue remedy and white chestnut remedy are effective for relief of stress, migraine and tension headaches. Larch is a confidence booster and pine is for guilt, which can trigger headaches.

CHINESE HERBS

In Chinese medicine migraine headaches are an indication your organs are out of balance and the blood in your body is obstructed and not flowing freely. Cnidium and thea formula, an over-the-counter patent medicine, may provide herbal first-aid for some kinds of headache.

CHIROPRACTIC

Many people experience a reduction in the severity and occurrence of their headaches (including migraines) after they have had spinal adjustments from a chiropractor. This is because headaches and migraines can be triggered when the neck and shoulders are restricted by subluxations (unnatural pressure on the nervous system).

COUNSELLING

Recurring headaches, particularly the throbbing type, can be associated with anxiety, stress and suppressed anger. A counsellor can help you explore and resolve these issues.

FOR AN ACUTE MIGRAINE

- lie down and do not move your head
- shut out all noise and light (an eye mask may help)
- apply cold compresses to your forehead (and across your eyes if you like)
- use visualisation to counter the pain (see page 48).

THE FELDENKRAIS METHOD

The Feldenkrais Method may help reduce the occurrence of headaches if they are related to tension in your head, neck, jaw and eyes, by teaching better posture to support your head and neck and more comfortable, efficient ways of using your body.

HEALING MEDITATION

Read the chapter on Healing Energies and prepare for meditation. Visualise yourself under a waterfall of blue energy. See this energy flowing through you, particularly around your head and shoulders and along your spine. Keep this energy flowing until you feel yourself relax and the headache shift. If you feel no obvious improvement, return to what you were doing and repeat the healing meditation a short time later.

HERBALISM

The herbs that are most often used to relieve headaches are chamomile, feverfew, hops, wood betony, rosemary, fringetree, vervain, meadowsweet and Jamaican dogwood. A herbalist will ascertain the cause of the headache before prescribing specific herbs.

If your headache is related to stress the herbs that may be prescribed include valerian, skullcap and oats.

For relief from a mild headache, drink a herbal tea that contains the herbs chamomile and/or meadowsweet as often as you like throughout the day until your symptoms subside.

If your migraine eases when you put a cold compress on your head, it is known as a "cold" migraine in herbal terms. For these, try drinking an infusion containing feverfew throughout the day until the pain is relieved. Regular use of feverfew may also prevent migraine.

In addition to those used for headaches, herbs used for migraines include dandelion, ginger, valerian and cramp bark.

HOMOEOPATHY

If tension has caused your headache and the ache starts at the base of your skull and continues around to your forehead, take one 6C potency of *Gelsemium sempervirens* every hour for five doses. For other types of headache and migraine or if your headache persists longer than a day, see a homoeopath for specific diagnosis and treatment.

MASSAGE

Whole body massage or massage to the back, neck, shoulders and scalp can assist if the headaches are caused by tight muscles, overwork, poor posture, stress or tension (see page 135).

MODERN MEDICINE

For "one-off" headaches an analgesic such as aspirin or paracetamol is often recommended for quick pain relief, although effectiveness can be limited.

Antidepressants may be prescribed for people suffering recurrent headaches, depending on the cause. Muscle relaxants are available in different strengths over the counter and by prescription to ease more severe headaches and migraines.

Stronger analgesics are prescribed for migraines. Antimigraine medication is available by prescription that deals with the over-dilated arteries, but these can have side effects. As a preventive measure, there are also prescription drugs to control the hypersensitivity of blood vessels.

Drugs, including analgesics and beta-blockers, are also available to treat cluster headaches and preventive medication may be prescribed to be taken at bedtime.

If you have recurring headaches or migraines, your doctor may recommend you consult a neurologist or headache clinic for a diagnostic test known as a catscan to establish how to prevent or manage this problem. A doctor may also suggest you stop taking the Pill, if this is appropriate.

VISUALISATION

If your headache is relatively mild, read the chapter on AFFIRMATIONS AND VISUALISATIONS and try the following exercise. Though you can do it yourself, it is preferable if someone else can take you through it.

Sit in a relaxed position and take three deep breaths in and out. Bring your attention to the part of your head that is aching. What colour and shape is the ache? Picture the ache as you feel it, for example, as a red pulsing ball. Then see yourself taking that ball into your hands and squashing it until you can hardly see it.

Now picture a box or container. See yourself placing the condensed headache into your box. When you have done this think of a place you know is safe (in a cupboard, for example). Visualise yourself taking the box containing your headache and putting it there for safe keeping.

After you have done this open your eyes and look around the room. Look hard and bring your full attention to everything your eyes touch on — the arm of a chair, the lamp in the corner, the window next to you. Look at about six objects, then lightly flick your attention back to your head. Don't concentrate hard. Just do it in passing to see if your head is still aching.

If it is, repeat the visualisation. You will find your headache is usually a different shape or colour the second time. Repeat the process of putting your headache into a box and the box in a safe place. Look around the room again. Keep repeating this visualisation until your headache is lessened or completely gone.

NATUROPATHY

Naturopaths often find that migraines and headaches are related to food intolerance so they will probably recommend you avoid dairy products, wheat and other items such as oranges, chocolate, alcohol, preserved or smoked meats and tomatoes to see if your migraines lessen.

A naturopath will look at LIVER PROBLEMS or CONSTIPATION as possible causes.

You can take calcium and magnesium phosphate supplements (as instructed on the label) to regulate your nervous system.

OSTEOPATHY

Headaches and migraines can be caused by problems with the spine or cranium, affecting muscle tension, nerve pathways and circulation. An osteopath will see if there is a problem with the alignment of your muscle-skeleton framework. They will then be able to treat this with gentle manual techniques to your spinal region and cranium. They may also give advice on exercise and posture.

REFLEXOLOGY

For relief of headaches and migraines: work the diaphragm reflex for relaxation and stress reduction, the pituitary for hormonal balance and the points for the whole spine for improved nerve function. You can also work all the toes/fingers as these points correspond to the head area.

Activate other specific points depending on the origin of the headache. For example, if it came from eye strain then work the eye reflex; from neck tension, the neck and shoulder/arm points; from allergy, add the reflex for the small intestine and colon.

Try this on both feet or hands for a total of 15 to 20 minutes once a day or more frequently if necessary — be careful not to overstimulate.

As a preventative, you can encourage relaxation by regularly working the diaphragm and solar plexus.

SHIATSU

Stagnant Ki energy in your head is one of the causes of headache. Therefore a shiatsu practitioner will disperse the Ki in your head as well as applying specific pressure points to your head, feet and neck, depending on what part of your head the ache is occurring in, and work on various organs. This will clear the meridian channels and reduce headaches in general.

Shiatsu practitioners believe migraine headaches are caused by a damp heat imbalance in the liver and gall bladder meridians. They can increase the flow of Ki around your body which will bring your organs into balance and prevent blockages of Ki in your head.

A shiatsu practitioner will also advise you on diet and suggest you cut out foods that may be contributing to your headaches e.g. dairy products, saturated animal fats and oily fried food.

YOGA

If your headaches are triggered by sinus problems or you have them regularly you can see a yoga teacher who will teach you exercises to give you relief. You will need to be shown these exercises because most of them are advanced yoga breathing techniques which need the advice and supervision of a trained teacher.

Yoga can also help people who are prone to migraines because it has a soothing and calming effect on the nervous system and promotes blood flow to the head.

If your headache is related to muscle tension try the headache tension release exercise. The inverted corpse with your legs split will open up your liver meridian to relieve your headaches. See pages 190 to 205.

HEART PROBLEMS

The term "heart disease" or "cardiovascular disease" encompasses a number of different conditions of the heart and circulatory system, including:

- inflammation — various inflammatory conditions may be involved, usually a result of another illness such as diphtheria
- damage to the valves — again, an illness such as rheumatic fever may be the cause
- enlargement — due to high blood pressure (see page 234) or some types of pulmonary disease.

Pulmonary heart disease involves the obstruction of the right side of the heart due to chronic lung conditions such as ASTHMA and BRONCHITIS. It can lead to FLUID RETENTION and kidney or liver problems (see pages 326 and 329).

The most common source of heart problems is hardening of the arteries or *arteriosclerosis,* and the most common form of this is *atherosclerosis,* known in its early stages as coronary artery disease, and in its more advanced state as coronary heart disease, among other names.

In atheroscherosis, there is a build-up of fatty deposits (mainly cholesterol and triglycerides) leading to narrowing of the arteries. Eventually, this may block the flow of blood or a blood clot may form (thrombosis), resulting in a heart attack or stroke (see FIRST AID page 385).

Atherosclerosis may go undetected, although angina (see below) can be one symptom. It can begin in young people but only become apparent much later.

Blockage of the arteries (embolism) may be caused by other obstructions such as an air bubble or a ball of fungus.

In addition to heart disease, a person may be affected by congenital heart defects.

Some people suffer from irregular heart beats, either in the form of abnormally rapid or slow beating, or palpitations. These are only signs of underlying problems, and it is necessary to treat the cause.

Sometimes the pacemaker cells that control the heart rate are damaged due to heart disease.

See also DIABETES, VARICOSE VEINS.

ANGINA

Angina pecturis is a bout of tight chest pain, ranging from mild to debilitating, that can move down your arms and up your neck. There may be palpitations and dizziness. It is often accompanied by oppressive feelings of fear and anxiety.

Angina occurs when not enough oxygenated blood passes through to your heart muscle, usually as a result of atherosclerosis, which can be a serious problem.

Angina can be brought on by any activity that makes your heart work harder such as:

- sudden physical exertion
- emotional distress
- a big intake of food
- exposure to cold
- fever.

If you suffer from angina, you should avoid these potential causes and modify your lifestyle. In addition seek treatment and remain under medical supervision.

Angina sufferers may find they store tension in their neck, shoulders and back, so, in addition to the other therapies listed here, OSTEOPATHY, CHIROPRACTIC and MASSAGE may be of assistance.

Angina can be confused with other pain, such as heartburn (see page 272), and a medical diagnosis is required. See your doctor after an initial angina attack or if any subsequent attacks are worse, particularly if they occur at night.

HEART FAILURE

"Failure" in this sense does not mean the heart stops beating — that is cardiac arrest. Rather, the heart's function has been weakened and the blood flow is not enough to fulfil the body's needs. The condition is also known as cardiac insufficiency.

The main symptoms are breathlessness and FLUID RETENTION.

Underlying causes can include heart disease, high blood pressure (see page 234), a severe heart attack and lung disease — it is very important that these are diagnosed and treated.

It is important that you manage your lifestyle and get sufficient rest and gentle exercise in addition to any other form of treatment.

SIGNS OF A HEART PROBLEM

Consult a medical doctor if you display any of the following:

- chest pain
- breathlessness with even light physical activity or during sleep
- dizziness or fainting
- erratic pulse
- blue lips
- FLUID RETENTION
- extreme FATIGUE
- persistent cough
- blood in phlegm.

See also heart attack (FIRST AID, page 385).

WHAT YOU CAN DO TO HAVE A HEALTHY HEART

In addition to any other treatment, doctors and therapists agree that lifestyle and diet changes are of primary importance in both preventing heart disease and affecting the rate of its development. Most cases of heart disease can be helped by these measures, especially if caught early:

- modify your diet to keep it low in fats and salt and high in unrefined foods (grains, fruit and vegetables) and avoid rich, heavy meals
- avoid stimulants such as caffeine (in coffee, tea and cola drinks)
- reduce if you are overweight
- control your BLOOD PRESSURE PROBLEMS
- stop SMOKING
- exercise regularly
- relax and learn to deal with stress (see page 40)
- practise breathing exercises (see page 25).

OTHER FACTORS INVOLVED IN HEART PROBLEMS

Your heart is very much connected to your emotions. Think of the everyday words that reflect this link: heartache, broken heart and hardened heart. One theory about heart problems is that they can be triggered by unresolved grief.

Links have also been made between personality and heart problems with aggressive, competitive, hurried, impatient people more prone to heart attacks.

Highly stressful or life-changing situations will also put you at risk: marriage, retirement, illness, divorce, retrenchment or the death of a loved one.

Heredity seems to play a role in predisposing a person to heart problems.

To reduce the risk of congenital heart problems, pregnant women should avoid tobacco, medication and other drugs, and ensure they do not become infected with German measles (rubella).

ACUPRESSURE

If received from a qualified practitioner who will also advise on issues like diet, acupressure can be effective in reducing the symptoms of angina but alone it is not a solution or cure. At home, you can try the acupressure points Conception Vessel 17, Pericardium 6 and Heart 7 when you feel the pain in your chest and along your arm as a first aid treatment and daily as a preventive measure when you are feeling well.

ACUPUNCTURE

Acupuncture can be of assistance if you suffer from angina. Acupuncturists view the initial problem as excess yang, often from the kidneys and liver. Subsequently, when the heart is weak, it is a deficiency problem.

Technically, it is a problem with the pericardium rather than the heart, which is responsible for emotional balance in Chinese medicine.

AFFIRMATION

If you suffer from heart problems and feel this affirmation is appropriate try repeating it to yourself as many times a day as possible.

"I am willing to accept and release my grief. I feel secure in the knowledge that every ending makes way for a wonderful new beginning."

AROMATHERAPY

There are particular essential oils that have strengthening effects on the heart, including lavender, neroli and ylang ylang, but be cautious when using any oils when you have a heart condition. Consult your doctor and only see a qualified aromatherapist for treatment.

BACH FLOWER REMEDIES

Bach flower remedies for long-term maintainance of the heart include holly and willow. Dilute 2 drops each of holly and willow remedies in a 25 ml (1 fl oz) bottle of spring water, then take 4 drops of this mixture four times daily.

For acute conditions, try rescue remedy.

CHIROPRACTIC

Chiropractic adjustments may be beneficial if you have a heart problem because they can increase circulation by improving the function of your nervous system. Chiropractors employ specific adjustments when you have concerns with your heart, so be sure to inform them of your full medical history.

COUNSELLING

A counsellor can help you release grief or deal with any other underlying emotional cause of heart disease.

HERBALISM

In most cases heart problems, including angina, are treated medically but herbalists often supplement medical treatment with hawthorn berries, motherwort, lime blossom and oats, which are all effective in strengthening the heart. Herbs should be prescribed by a qualified herbalist who will assess your condition before deciding on what you need.

HEALING MEDITATION

Read the chapter on HEALING ENERGIES to learn how you can channel healing energy to yourself. Once you have the blue light flowing to you concentrate it in your heart area to strengthen and balance your heart.

HOMOEOPATHY

For attacks of angina that are accompanied by fear and panic the best homoeopathic remedy to take is *Aconitum napellus.* Take one 6C potency every 30 minutes until your chest feels less constricted. This remedy will help calm your system but if your attacks of angina are frequent, you should see a homoeopath who will be able to fully assess your condition.

MASSAGE

Massage can assist with stress reduction and relaxation but it is advisable to check with your doctor before having a massage.

MODERN MEDICINE

No drug can reverse atherosclerosis. There are hypolipidaemics which lower the level of excess cholesterol and triglycerides in the blood.

Angina and heart failure can be managed with regular medication (vasodilators) that promote coronary blood flow. For angina, the first line of treatment is nitroglycerine which is given as a tablet under the tongue when the pain starts. It is also available as patches, which have fewer side effects.

Digitalis is usually prescribed for heart failure, and diuretics to relieve the symptoms.

Coronary artery by-pass surgery (known as angioplasty) may be carried out to circumvent a blockage in an artery. Defective heart valves can also be corrected by surgery, as can many other congenital heart disorders. Heart transplant operations are now an option.

If pacemaker cells are not functioning properly, an artificial electrical pacemaker may be fitted in a surgical procedure.

After a heart attack, anticoagulants may be used to prevent blood clotting. There are also injections available for the immediate treatment of blood clots in arteries and to prevent the further formation of blood clots, thereby preventing imminent heart attacks.

Anti-arrhythmic medication can keep the heart beating regularly.

NATUROPATHY

CAUTION: *Read the information on page 167 before taking supplements.*

Vitamins and minerals that help the heart include coenzyme Q10 (30 mg three times a day), vitamin E (500 iu per day), calcium (800 mg per day), magnesium phosphate, and potassium aspartate (as directed on the label). Fish oil (which is anti-arrhythmic) and garlic are also recommended in capsule form.

Don't rely on vitamins and minerals in an attack of angina; only use them as a preventive action.

It is important to modify your diet and a naturopath would advise that antioxidants (especially vitamins E, A and C) are the most important aspect — cholesterol is only a problem when oxidation occurs. A naturopath would also check liver function as a high cholesterol problem is often due to the liver not being able to break down cholesterol effectively. A general diet guideline would be to keep fats to a minimum and avoid meat, chicken and dairy products (use soya bean products instead) but to eat lots of seafood, especially cold water fish.

REFLEXOLOGY

Gently work the point for the heart as well as the shoulder/arm for circulation, the chest/lungs and diaphragm to improve breathing and aid stress reduction, the sigmoid colon to relieve pressure on the heart, the points for the whole spine and the adrenal glands for heart function and muscle tone, the kidneys for fluid elimination, and the pituitary to stimulate endocrine glands which affect blood pressure, respiration and heart rate. Work these points on both feet or hands for a total of 15 minutes twice a week. Be sure to tell your doctor you are trying this natural therapy especially if it involves a consultation with a reflexologist.

SHIATSU

Shiatsu can be very good in the case of angina and heart problems generally as it will relax your blood vessels and increase circulation which will ease the stress on your heart. In order to achieve this a shiatsu practitioner would disperse and tone up the Ki in your heart meridian.

YOGA

Most yoga postures are quite safe for people with heart troubles but you should avoid the inverted postures and seek your doctor's advice.

Yoga can be beneficial for heart complaints because it can strengthen your heart. Yoga can also act to slow down your heart beat, which may benefit your condition.

Forward stretches (see page 192) can be quite beneficial to you, as can relaxing and breathing yoga exercises if you need to reduce your stress levels. The easy breathing to relax exercise on page 193 is one that aids your heart.

HEPATITIS

Hepatitis is an inflammation that affects the liver. The acute form may have symptoms of NAUSEA AND VOMITING, fever and FATIGUE. You may also get jaundice (yellowing of eyes and skin).

There are different types, related to different viruses: hepatitis A, transmitted by contaminated food and drink and associated with poor sanitation. Symptoms are usually mild, occur within two to six weeks and last up to six weeks.

The body will subsequently be immune to type A infection.

Hepatitis B is passed on through contact with blood and other body fluids. Symptoms may be mild or severe, occurring from six to 26 weeks after contact. There can be complete recovery (albeit slow) with future immunity, or the virus can remain active, making the person a carrier. The body's autoimmune system can react in such a way as to continue the inflammation, thus chronic relapses occur. Later this can lead to cirrhosis and cancer of the liver.

Hepatitis C is transmitted in the same ways to type B, and behaves similarly in that it is a chronic, active form of hepatitis.

Hepatitis may also be symptomless, depending on your body's reaction to the virus. Many carriers of the disease do not know they have it.

A toxic hepatitis-like condition can be caused by alcohol and other drugs (including paracetamol and the acid suppressant medication, cimethidine). It involves toxic damage to the liver, and the condition begins to heal when the abuse stops. The treatment is similar to hepatitis.

Hepatitis is a disease of the liver that is believed by some to be linked to feelings of anger and frustration (see page 6).

See also LIVER PROBLEMS.

IMPORTANT: *Hepatitis should be diagnosed by a doctor and always monitored under medical supervision, although there is no specific medical treatment. Any other treatment should only be used with this stipulation.*

WHAT YOU CAN DO

- Rest is recommended.
- Drink no alcohol for six months.
- Drink plenty of fluids, preferably distilled water and freshly squeezed vegetable juices, to flush the liver of toxins.
- Avoid fats and fatty foods.
- Get adequate protein. Choose brown rice, fish or a protein supplement drink if the appetite is weak.
- Do not take any medication without first checking with your doctor.
- Maintain strict personal hygiene.
- Make no unprotected sexual contact, depending on the type of hepatitis you have. This is an important rule of health, anyway.
- Do not share personal items like needles, toothbrushes and razor blades. An infected person should keep separate linen, eating utensils and soap.
- Be stringent in hygiene and food consumption and avoid water, seafood, and food washed in water in high-risk regions.
- Ensure any needle that pierces your skin has been properly cleaned and sterilised or is brand new. There are pre-sterilised, disposable, single-use acupuncture needles and hypodermic syringes available.
- Vaccinations are available for hepatitis A and B.

ACUPUNCTURE

Acupuncture may be used to rectify some of the debilitating effects of hepatitis A, B, C and other forms.

AFFIRMATION

Some believe there is an emotional link between hepatitis and extreme anger or rage. If you are feeling hurt or powerless about an event or person try using an affirmation like this one as many times a day as possible: "I find appropriate ways of expressing my rage. I forgive and release the past and open myself to peace".

BACH FLOWER REMEDIES

Impatiens and beech remedy combat the irritability you may feel with this condition and holly and willow will dispel anger.

CHINESE HERBS

There are a number of patent Chinese herbs available that are commonly used for hepatitis, but a practitioner will treat the condition on an individual basis.

HEALING MEDITATION

See the chapter on HEALING ENERGIES and channel the

blue healing light to yourself. Focus it on your abdomen and liver. At the same time, you may like to use an affirmation like the one above as a mantra.

HERBALISM

The best herb for this condition is silymarin. Others include dandelion root and greater celandine which support the liver and St Mary's thistle which actually acts to repair and protect the liver. See a herbalist and your doctor for advice and treatment.

HOMOEOPATHY

Homoeopaths can assist orthodox doctors with the treatment of hepatitis as they prescribe holistically. The liver-toning action of the remedies will help the liver function properly while the body is fighting the disease. These remedies are also useful because orthodox drugs can be harmful to a weak liver whereas appropriate homoeopathic remedies act gently to assist the healing of the liver. See a homoeopath and your doctor for specific advice and treatment.

MODERN MEDICINE

There is some medication available to deal with chronic active forms of hepatitis but, in general, most of the advice from doctors will be in terms of lifestyle and diet.

NATUROPATHY

High doses of vitamin C (1/4 teaspoon of powder every hour in acute cases, otherwise 1000 mg three times a day) will often help this condition as well as beta carotene (20 mg per day).

REFLEXOLOGY

Work the points for the liver and adrenal glands on each foot or hand for a total of 15 minutes twice a week. If you consult a reflexologist for this condition, make sure your doctor is aware that this is the course of action you are choosing.

SHIATSU

Regular treatment of the spleen and liver meridians from an experienced shiatsu practitioner, along with dietary support, will assist the body in recovering from this condition.

VISUALISATION

If you wish to deal with the anger that may be linked to this condition, you could try reading the chapter on AFFIRMATIONS AND VISUALISATIONS to prepare yourself for visualisation. In your mind's eye see any person or events that have caused you anger or rage. You may like to see the events as if you were watching a movie. As you watch, experience the feelings of anger in much the same way as you would allow laughter to flow through you. Anger or rage, like laughter, is simply energy in motion. You do not need to act on it.

Give the angry energy a colour and see it drain out of you as it moves through your body. Visualise the green energy of peace cover you like a waterfall. See the green energy push out the angry energy. Keep visualising this until your feelings of anger are replaced by feelings of peace and your body is full of green light.

Return your visualisation to the events that angered you and see yourself now reacting to those people or circumstances in a peaceful, forgiving manner. You may not feel these emotions but direct yourself like you would an actor. It will take practice until you can truly view these events with balance but in time this will come.

HERNIA

A hernia is the abnormal protrusion of an organ through a rupture in a weak section in the surrounding tissue. This may occur in various parts of the body including the upper thigh, the navel or the intestine protruding into the groin. In the latter case, the intestine may become strangulated, cutting off blood supply, and emergency surgery is required.

In the case of a hiatus hernia it is the protrusion of the stomach into the chest through the diaphragm. Symptoms of this kind of hernia can include heartburn (see page 272), difficulty swallowing (but not in all cases) and chest pain.

Causes are varied, although the underlying muscle weakness is thought to be a birth defect.

Hiatus hernias can be brought on by intra-abdominal pressure from heavy lifting, poor posture, pregnancy, severe CONSTIPATION, or obesity, and can be aggravated by other stresses such as severe persistent coughing. These conditions have to be dealt with to ease the hernia and prevent recurrence.

WHAT YOU CAN DO

- Lose weight if you are OVERWEIGHT.
- Take care with lifting and carrying. Lessons in THE FELDENKRAIS METHOD or ALEXANDER TECHNIQUE can show you ways to avoid strain and further damage.
- For a hiatus hernia: avoid bending forward and maintain a straight posture (particularly when sitting), eat frequent small meals and avoid spicy, acidic or fatty foods, coffee, tea or alcohol as these cause reflux.

ACUPUNCTURE

Acupuncture is used for treating hiatus hernia as well as other digestive disorders.

AFFIRMATION

As hernias are ruptures, you may benefit from repeating an affirmation such as this one as many times a day as possible: "I mend ruptures in my life and allow healing energy to flow through me."

HERBALISM

For people prone to hernias the herbs you can take as a preventive measure include: meadowsweet, fennel, peppermint, agrimony, dill and ginger. Drink tea with any one of the above herbs in it as many times a day as you like. This will help to relieve the gas that can cause indigestion and eventually hernias.

HOMOEOPATHY

Homoeopathy can improve the function of the muscles' connective tissue. If your hernia is towards the right side of your body, take one 6C potency of *Lycopodium clavatum* three times a day for a few days. If the hernia is towards the left side, take one 6C tablet or liquid form of *Nux vomica* three times a day for a few days. For hernias in general, take one 6C tablet or liquid form of *Calcarea fluorata* three times a day for a few days. If the hernia does not improve in a few days consult a homoeopath.

MODERN MEDICINE

Depending on the severity of the hernia doctors sometimes recommend surgery or supply a supportive garment (truss) to hold the hernia in place. Antacids are sometimes given for pain relief for a hiatus hernia or drugs that assist in the emptying of the stomach and thus reduce reflux.

NATUROPATHY

Naturopathic cell salts that can help are silica and calcium fluoride as they strengthen the tissues. These have to be taken long term and under the supervision of a naturopath to be effective.

REFLEXOLOGY

For an abdominal hernia of any kind, work the points that correspond to the groin area as the main reflex as well as the colon, and the adrenal glands for muscle tone. For hiatus hernia, work the diaphragm points for stress reduction along with the stomach and adrenal glands. In either case, work the points on both feet or hands for a total of 20 minutes two or three times a week.

SHIATSU

In shiatsu the spleen is the organ that "holds things up" in the body, preventing prolapse, so this meridian will most likely be treated for all kinds of hernias. Other organs that are often worked on in the case of hernias are the large and small intestines and liver, depending on the location of the hernia. A hiatus hernia would be treated by supporting the stomach meridian.

YOGA

Yoga cannot heal a hernia but it can help you avoid a recurrence of a hiatus hernia by reducing body fat through exercise, promoting body awareness and, most importantly, by strengthening your abdominal muscles.

If you have recently undergone hernia surgery consult your doctor and wait a few weeks before starting a yoga program.

The lifting the head exercise on page 200 will strengthen your abdominal muscles, but only practise it with your doctor's advice.

HERPES AND COLD SORES

Herpes simplex is a virus that causes both cold sores and genital herpes. The main symptom is clusters of infected blisters which most commonly form around the mouth or nose, or on the vulva, vagina and cervix in women and on the penis in men, although other areas of the body can be affected.

The herpes simplex virus can be passed on from person to person through physical contact with the blisters. The virus also seems to shed between attacks.

Once there, the virus remains in the nervous system but does not develop into blisters unless you are ill, undernourished, under stress or suffer extremes of temperature. Localised stress such as sunburn or friction can trigger an outbreak.

An initial outbreak usually occurs a couple of days to a few weeks after the actual infection. Recurrent infections can occur after the first outbreak without re-exposure to the virus, but these symptoms are usually milder and confined to the same physical area on the body. Attacks tend to become less severe and less frequent over time. Eventually the virus seems to burn itself out.

Although the first attack is usually the most severe, in other cases it may be so mild that it passes without notice; a second attack may not occur until perhaps years later — this is important to remember if trying to pinpoint the source of the infection.

An outbreak of blisters may be preceded by a tingling or burning sensation in the nerve endings. The blisters themselves can be itchy and painful, especially on the genitals. The attack may be accompanied by flu-like symptoms.

The virus on the cervix may not cause any noticeable symptoms, thus a woman can be a "silent carrier".

WHAT YOU CAN DO

- Treat the condition as soon as possible, even before blisters appear if you feel the warning signs.
- Apply ice to blisters to relieve pain and aid healing.
- Bathe the blisters with salt water or diluted bicarbonate of soda (baking powder) — a small handful in a sitz bath is good for genital herpes. Keep blisters dry between bathing, exposing them to air as much as possible.
- If not too painful, dab sores with witch hazel, alcohol or equal parts of lemon juice and water to accelerate drying.
- Apply a cold wet tea bag to the area. The tannin in black tea is an anaesthetic.
- Do not touch the blisters unnecessarily or they may spread. Wash hands thoroughly after treating them.
- When blisters are in evidence, avoid direct contact to prevent contagion. Depending on location of blisters, condoms may provide protection. Also avoid sharing towels, pillow cases etc. with which a blister has had recent contact.
- If you have genital herpes, wear cotton rather than synthetic underwear and clothing and do not use scented talcum powder, soaps, bubble baths or feminine hygiene products.
- Maintain good general health to avoid outbreaks. See PROTECTING YOUR IMMUNE SYSTEM.
- Practise relaxation techniques so that stress does not trigger the condition (see page 40).
- Women with genital herpes should take particular care to have regular Pap smears as the virus is associated with an increased risk of cervical cancer (see page 243).
- Pregnant women can pass the virus to their child during labour if blisters are present, causing the risk of encephalitis to the child. The condition should be discussed with your doctor.

AFFIRMATION

Outbreaks of herpes often occur when you are stressed and they can make you feel unattractive. Affirmations like the following may help: "I forgive myself for not being perfect. I love and accept myself exactly the way I am now".

AROMATHERAPY

Essential oils such as eucalyptus, tea tree and bergamot are highly effective when treating herpes blisters, especially if applied early. Add 2 drops each of tea tree and bergamot to 2 teaspoons of isopropyl alcohol (available from pharmacies) or vodka. Dab the mixture on the blisters every few hours.

BACH FLOWER REMEDIES

Take crab apple for its cleansing effect.

CHINESE HERBALISM

The Chinese herb Yin Qiao San is particularly effective for dealing with this condition. See a herbalist for details.

HERBALISM

The herb bittersweet will help prevent the growth of a blister if it is applied early and used often during the day. It is available in ointment form. If the blister becomes a wet sore, apply bittersweet in oil form instead. Distilled witch hazel can later be applied to help it dry followed by the oil from a vitamin E capsule.

Infusions or dilute tinctures of the following herbs can be applied directly to the area or added to a sitz bath: echinacea, golden seal, St John's wort, comfrey, calendula. Oils that contain these herbs may also be available commercially.

Immune-enhancing herbs such as astragalus, echinacea and garlic can also be taken internally, as can burdock, dandelion root and yellow dock to aid elimination of toxins, and calendula and poke root to stimulate the lymphatic system.

For genital herpes, herbalists prescribe a mixture of these herbs with the addition of herbs that are specific to the reproductive system.

HOMOEOPATHY

Homoeopathic remedies can be of help as they will prompt the body to provide a defence against the infection thus promoting rapid healing. If you have a dry cold sore that gives you a burning sensation on your lips, take one 6C potency of *Natrum muriaticum* four times a day for three days or until the cold sore starts to heal. For other treatments, see a homoeopath.

MODERN MEDICINE

Accurate diagnosis of herpes can only come from a swab of an active sore. Idoxuridine ointment may be applied directly to the sore. L-lysine is a commonly-used natural antiviral medication, taken in tablet form for both genital herpes and cold sores, as a prevention and treatment. Both of these are available over the counter. For genital herpes, acyclovar may be prescribed to reduce the frequency and severity of an outbreak.

NATUROPATHY

Naturopaths will examine your diet and lifestyle if you are prone to outbreaks to determine how great an impact these may be having. You may be advised to avoid foods that contain arginine which the virus needs to thrive such as chocolate, red wine, peanuts, cola, coffee, tea, sugar, most nuts, gelatine, beer, peas, carob, chick peas, soya beans, wheat, coconut, tomatoes, mushrooms, eggplants, sesame and sunflower seeds, brown rice, oatmeal and popcorn. Avoid these foods if you have a severe recurring problem with herpes, otherwise don't eat them during an outbreak.

Lysine-containing foods are recommended. These include brewer's yeast, beans, bean sprouts, meat, chicken, fish, prawns, eggs, cheese, milk, yogurt, and most fruit and vegetables, particularly potatoes.

In addition, naturopaths will prescribe vitamins and minerals to relieve your symptoms and then work on the root cause of the problem. A practical way of dealing with a cold sore is to take 6000 mg of L-lysine on the first day you feel the cold sore coming on and then 3000 mg per day until it clears up. You can also take vitamin A (5000 iu per day), vitamin C (1000 mg three times a day) and zinc (25 mg elemental per day) to boost your immune system to prevent another attack.

REFLEXOLOGY

Work the points for all the glands for hormonal balance, and the lymphatic system and spleen to boost the immune system. Try this on both feet or hands for a total of 25 minutes three times a week. If this does not make a difference, consider seeing a professional reflexologist.

SHIATSU

Regular shiatsu treatment can help you keep your immune system up and lower your stress level. It will do this by improving the flow of Ki energy around your body, in particular around the areas of the liver, spleen and kidney meridians.

HIV/AIDS

AIDS (Acquired Immune Deficiency Syndrome) is a condition that so severely weakens your immune system that it is vulnerable to infections of all kinds, which can then devastate the body, often fatally. AIDS develops in people who have HIV (Human Immunodeficiency Virus) although not everyone who has HIV will develop AIDS.

Different symptoms of HIV/AIDs are developed by different people depending on how their bodies reacts to the virus. Some people do not show any symptoms at all for many months, even years.

Some of the symptoms of HIV/AIDs that can develop include fever, persistent swollen glands, unexplained, significant weight loss, and persistent diarrhoea.

Opportunistic infections may affect the lungs, skin, nervous and digestive systems and may include COLITIS, CANDIDIASIS, HERPES, pneumonia, Kaposi's sarcoma (a type of skin cancer) and other cancers (see page 242).

Treatment can be sought for symptoms and infections, although there is no cure for HIV/AIDS itself.

HIV can be contracted through infected blood, semen and vaginal fluids. Transmission is most common through unprotected sex, shared needles, or blood transfusion.

The presence of HIV antibodies, which develop three to six months after contact, can be ascertained through a blood test. This does not necessarily indicate that there is active virus in the body but that there has been contact.

WHAT YOU CAN DO

• The most important thing you can do if you have HIV/AIDS is to build up your immune system. If your immune system can be strengthened, there is evidence that full-blown AIDS is less likely to develop. See PROTECTING YOUR IMMUNE SYSTEM.

• Mental attitude seems to be of primary importance in managing the condition. See THE MIND BODY CONNECTION and RELAXATION AND DEALING WITH STRESS for some background information.

• There are many specialist clinics and support groups for those with HIV/AIDS and their families and friends. They can be located through a hospital, health practitioner or the telephone directory.

• Alternative therapies should be used under medical supervision, with a collaborative treatment recommended to nourish mind, body and spirit. By law, non-medically qualified alternative therapists may not treat HIV/AIDS. However, with the cooperation of a medical doctor, they may be of assistance in treating the general health of a person with HIV/AIDS. They may also be of assistance in the prevention of HIV/AIDS in people of high risk.

• To safeguard against contracting the virus, the following preventive measures are recommended:

— Safe sex practices — avoiding direct contact with semen, vaginal fluids and blood and the use of condoms and other latex barriers.

— Ensure any needle that pierces your skin (e.g. injections, ear piercing, tattooing) has been properly cleaned and sterilised, that is with hydrogen peroxide and alcohol and by boiling. Or, better still, is brand new. There are pre-sterilised, disposable, single-use acupuncture needles and hypodermic syringes available.

— Do not share personal items such as needles, toothbrushes or razors that could have been in contact with blood and other fluids.

ACUPUNCTURE

Acupuncture is used extensively to alleviate symptoms and strengthen the immune system.

AROMATHERAPY

Aromatherapy can provide relaxation through massage and, most importantly, strengthen your immune system. It can help you improve the quality of your life by offering relaxing massage and mood-enhancing oils. Aromatherapy can also relieve the symptoms of some related infections such as skin, bowel, and lung infections.

BACH FLOWER REMEDIES

These can be useful for HIV positive people, their friends and families in supporting the emotional upheaval that may be involved in dealing with the condition. Remedies range from mimulus for fear of illness or death and sweet chestnut for despair to pine for guilt and willow for resentment.

CHINESE HERBS

Many of the symptoms brought on by HIV/AIDS and the side effects of the prescribed drugs can be treated with Chinese herbs.

CHIROPRACTIC

Your immune system is affected by the condition of your nervous system. A chiropractor can free up your nervous system with spinal adjustments that can help improve your immune system. See a chiropractor and give them a detailed history of your health condition so they can decide on the appropriate techniques.

HEALING MEDITATION

Read the chapter on HEALING ENERGIES and prepare yourself for meditation.

Open your crown chakra and allow healing blue light to flow from the divine life force into your crown chakra and down through your entire body. Feel the light open every cell, ready to receive the strengthening energy it needs. As you feel the energy see yourself connected with all life through this beam of blue light which links you back to all creation. Feel your heart expand with love for yourself. Acknowledge that the path you are on offers special opportunities for growth. Know you have the courage to deal with what life offers you. Continue visualising the blue energy filling you and repeat this affirmation to yourself like a mantra: "I am a brave and courageous spirit. I attract to me all the help I need. I am love, all is love."

HERBALISM

Herbalists can work with your doctor to improve your general health. Herbs have been found to be especially useful in strengthening particular organs and keeping the immune system strong in people who have HIV/AIDS. Herbs that are often used for this purpose include astragalus, echinacea, golden seal, St John's wort and thyme. Detoxifying herbs that can also help are burdock, yellow dock and blue flag. In addition to antimicrobial herbs and antioxidants, herbal prescriptions can also include herbs to nourish your nervous system, to counter depression, to restore energy and aid digestion.

HOMOEOPATHY

Homoeopathic treatment from a qualified practitioner can be very beneficial to your general health and in alleviating associated problems.

MASSAGE

The process of touch can be extraordinarily soothing in itself. Massage can also be used for pain and stress relief and relaxation. It can benefit the lymphatic system and aid circulation and digestion.

MODERN MEDICINE

In addition to treating associated conditions and symptoms, there are experimental (and expensive) medications available for people with HIV/AIDS such as the antiviral drug AZT which is said to reduce the replication of the retrovirus.

NATUROPATHY

The course of the condition appears to be significantly modified by good nutrition. A naturopath can help keep your immune system strong with dietary advice and vitamin and mineral supplements such as beta carotene, vitamin B complex, vitamin C with bioflavinoids, vitamin E, magnesium, selenium and zinc.

REFLEXOLOGY

Work the points for the lymphatic system, spleen and thymus to assist the immune system, the liver for detoxification, the diaphragm for relaxation and stress reduction, and the pituitary for hormonal balance. Try this on both feet or hands for a total of 25 minutes every second day. You could ask a friend to work these points for you but to make a real difference see a reflexologist first who will massage your feet and hands and advise on other reflexes, depending on your specific symptoms.

SHIATSU

Shiatsu from an experienced practitioner is a good supportive therapy. Practitioners can help build up the low Ki energy in your immune system through the kidney, spleen and liver meridians of your body. Shiatsu "tonification" techniques will bring up your energy level and keep you relaxed. An immune system-boosting diet would also be recommended.

YOGA

The harmonising practice of yoga can help you face the challenges ahead more positively, assist your body's immune system and build up your strength gently. Consult a yoga teacher who will put you on an exercise program that will suit your particular needs.

IMPETIGO

Impetigo is a highly contagious skin infection caused by staphylococcus or streptococcus bacteria. When the skin is affected by impetigo it develops red, pus-filled, swollen blisters which form yellow scabs. It usually occurs around the nose and mouth, or on the arms and legs.

The infection is contagious and may be introduced by poor diet and hygiene, swimming in polluted water, insect bites, and infected cuts. It is most common in children.

WHAT YOU CAN DO

- Hygiene is important as prevention and treatment.
- Wash the hands and face of the affected person with alcohol several times a day to prevent the spread of infection.
- Avoid scratching.
- Soak off scabs with warm water, gently rub with a soft washcloth.
- An affected person should not share items such as towels or washcloths.
- Children with this condition should be isolated from other children until the infection runs its course.

AROMATHERAPY

You can clean the sores using clean cotton wool dipped into about 1/2 cup cooled boiled water to which 6 to 8 drops of lavender or tea tree essential oil has been added. Tea tree has been scientifically proven to be even better than antibiotics in the treatment of this condition.

BACH FLOWER REMEDIES

Take crab apple for its cleansing effect.

HERBALISM

Cleansing herbs are useful in dealing with impetigo. You can administer St John's wort and calendula externally in herbal creams and you can take echinacea, myrrh and golden seal internally in tablets, teas or tinctures.

HOMOEOPATHY

Homoeopathy can reduce an attack of impetigo when it appears. If your skin is cracked and scabs appear around your nose and mouth take one 6C potency of *Antimonium crudum* three times a day for two days. If the irritation lasts longer, consult a homoeopath.

MODERN MEDICINE

Antibiotics in tablet, liquid or ointment form are usually prescribed. They are very effective in clearing the infection and must be used if the infection continues to spread despite other treatment measures.

NATUROPATHY

To strengthen your immune system naturopaths will advise you to take vitamin C (3000 mg per day), vitamin A (5000 iu per day) and zinc (25 mg elemental per day). You should not use soap but rather wash with a concentrated whey extract which has been diluted. Vitamin E ointment can be used externally for healing.

REFLEXOLOGY

Reflexologists do not treat impetigo due to its contagious nature. However, you may be able to work on your own hands. Try the following points on both hands for a total of 15 minutes twice a week: the lymphatic system and spleen to boost the immune system, the liver for detoxification, and the diaphragm for relaxation and stress reduction.

IMPOTENCE

Impotence is the inability to attain or maintain an erection during intercourse. Repeated or prolonged problems can be due to different factors:

- stress
- poor physical condition due to excess weight or lack of fitness
- chronic illness such as DIABETES and, in particular, blocked arteries (see page 235)
- hormonal imbalance (too much oestrogen and not enough testosterone)
- excessive drug or alcohol use
- physical abnormality.

Psychological factors play a significant role and are by far the most common cause. Problems include DEPRESSION, unrealistic expectations which can lead to trying too hard, feelings of inadequacy or unconsciously contradictory attitudes to sex.

The occasional difficulty with erections is completely normal. See your doctor if the difficulties continue or get worse.

See also INFERTILITY.

WHAT YOU CAN DO

- Relax and learn how to deal with stress (see page 40) — often the primary factor.
- Avoid alcohol which can block an erection even as it loosens inhibition.
- Watch what you eat — after a heavy meal the blood supply is involved in the digestive process.
- Look after your heart and circulatory system with a healthy diet and lifestyle. Blocked arteries to the genitals are a major cause of impotence.
- Exercise will help increase your libido, by improving circulation and thus lifting testosterone levels.

ACUPUNCTURE

Acupuncture can help impotence if it is related to stress. See a qualified acupuncturist for further information.

AROMATHERAPY

CAUTION: *Read the information on pages 102 to 105 before using these essential oils.*

If impotence is due to a psychological cause, aromatherapy can help. There are many essential oils that act as aphrodisiacs; some are quite powerful, including sandalwood, jasmine, ylang ylang and clary sage.

Ask your partner to give you a full-body massage (see page 143) with a mixture of 2 drops each of sandalwood, jasmine and clary sage in 5 teaspoons of base carrier oil. A relaxing aromabath to which this mixture has been added may also help sooth tension.

BACH FLOWER REMEDIES

Rescue remedy and white chestnut will help to calm your mind of the worry and stress that accompanies this condition. Mimulus and aspen can also be taken for the fear you may experience.

CHIROPRACTIC

Impotence can be linked to chronic problems in the mid to low area of the back as this affects the nerve flow which in turn reduces vascular supply. See a chiropractor for advice and treatment.

COUNSELLING

Impotence can often have psychological causes which counselling can assist in pinpointing and resolving.

FELDENKRAIS METHOD

The Feldenkrais Method can improve pelvic movement which can improve sexual function in some cases.

HERBALISM

Ginseng, damiana and saw palmetto berries are herbs used for impotence as is gingko which will assist with blood supply and peripheral circulation. It is most important that you see a herbal practitioner to identify and treat any underlying causes rather than attempting self-treatment.

HYPNOTHERAPY

A doctor or a naturopath may refer you to a hypnotherapist if it seems impotence is due to a psychological or emotional block.

MODERN MEDICINE

Because impotence is such a complex condition, it is critical to have a proper assessment from a doctor or a specialist in the area. Some drugs, including tranquillisers, antidepressants, amphetamines and those used to treat high blood pressure and prostate disease, may inhibit erection and should be discussed with your doctor. Splints can be used as can surgical implants to rectify some impotence problems and there are also medications that can be taken. Prostaglandins can be injected into the penis before intercourse to maintain an erection. Doctors may also prescribe drugs that relax muscles and encourage blood flow.

NATUROPATHY

Impotence is sometimes caused by zinc and vitamin B6 deficiency so a prescription of these from a naturopath could make all the difference. To begin, try 25 mg of elemental zinc per day and 250 mg of vitamin B6 per day. Lecithin is also good if blocked blood vessels are involved and vitamin E can help improve circulation to the area. See a naturopath for more specific advice.

OSTEOPATHY

It has been found in some cases that mechanical strains of the pelvic joints and musculature affect the support structures of the pelvic organs and may contribute to impotence. A consultation with an osteopath will determine if your situation may be helped by osteopathic care (this may need to be in conjunction with other treatments).

REFLEXOLOGY

The reproductive system is the main reflex point for this condition, but you can also work all the glands for hormonal balance, the lower spine for nerve function, and the diaphragm for relaxation and stress reduction. Try this for a total of 15 to 20 minutes on both hands or feet three times a week until the condition improves and then weekly thereafter.

SHIATSU

If your impotence is causing you to feel depressed shiatsu can help lift your spirits and reduce feelings of stress and pressure; the heart protector meridian would be treated to harmonise emotions.

Sex drive can be increased by shiatsu. Working on the spleen and stomach meridians, in Oriental terms, enhances the desire for sex. The kidney meridian also controls sexual drive, while the liver controls physical function of the reproductive organs. Dispersing the liver meridian may help reduce your impotence by increasing blood and Ki circulation in your body.

Hormonal imbalances can also be helped with shiatsu treatment that tones up your bladder and kidney meridians.

VISUALISATION

Read the chapter on AFFIRMATIONS AND VISUALISATIONS and prepare for visualisation. In your mind's eye visualise a recent difficult sexual encounter. Even if this is painful to recall, persevere and accept any feelings of inadequacy. If you wish, you can incorporate an affirmation such as: "I forgive myself and release my feelings of powerlessness". Repeat this until you are able to accept the negative feelings.

Then recall that same sexual encounter and

visualise yourself performing as you and your partner would desire. Allow the sexual feelings to flow through you. You could repeat an affirmation such as: "I rejoice in my sexuality."

Once you have accepted your negative feelings in the first part of this step in the visualisation, you do not have to repeat that step of the visualisation again. Just concentrate on how you want to be and practise that part of the visualisation at least once a day.

Be gentle with yourself. It may take some time for your body to catch up with your visualisation.

YOGA

Regular yoga practice can help with stress control and with meditation techniques as well as improve the circulatory system.

INCONTINENCE

Incontinence is the loss of control of urination or bowel movement, although the latter is more commonly known as soiling. Stress incontinence occurs with the involuntary release of urine with a sudden movement such as a sneeze. With urge incontinence, the need to urinate is caused by ANXIETY and is extremely urgent when it arises. Stress incontinence is commonly caused by weak muscles due to multiple and long births, poor pelvic tone and obesity. For men it can be an indication of a PROSTATE PROBLEM. ALLERGIES, an infection or inflammation may be the cause (see also BLADDER PROBLEMS). Some medication such as diuretics may contribute to the problem.

Loss of control of bowel movements can be a result of childbirth, paralysis or damage to anal muscles during a surgical operation or anal sex.

Both kinds of incontinence are more common in older people.

Many people find that they have to get up during the night to urinate. This is known as nocturia and is usually due to an accumulation of liquid during the day, and the inability of the kidney to concentrate the urine at night as it should. This may be a sign of kidney disease but can be caused by anything that irritates or places increased pressure on the bladder such as stress, infections, DIABETES, CONSTIPATION or pregnancy. The cause of the problem should be identified and treated by a health practitioner.

ACUPRESSURE AND ACUPUNCTURE

Acupuncture and acupressure are used for this condition to strengthen the kidney and bladder functions. Similarly, they are used to treat bedwetting in children.

BACH FLOWER REMEDIES

Bach flower remedies that can help reduce the emotional pain of incontinence include cherry plum to help those who feel they have a loss of control, and crab apple for cleansing.

CHIROPRACTIC

Adjustment from a chiropractor can help you reduce the incidence of incontinence too. Subluxations along the spine (especially around the pelvic area) can significantly affect the performance of your bowel and bladder — these are unnatural pressures on the nervous system or interferences within it.

THE FELDENKRAIS METHOD

Bladder problems are often related to weakness in the pelvic floor area. A Feldenkrais practitioner can teach you awareness and control of your pelvic floor. This is then integrated into total body movement.

HERBALISM

Buchu tea is an antiseptic herbal remedy that cleanses the whole urinary system and helps to relieve most bladder dysfunctions, including incontinence. Try drinking 2 cups of buchu tea per day to start with but you may like to see a herbalist for a full diagnosis of your condition. Cornsilk tea, bearberry, damiana and epilobium may also form part of the treatment.

HOMOEOPATHY

Homoeopathic remedies that could help reduce incontinence include *Causticum, Aloe socotrina*, and *Pulsatilla nigricans*. The remedy varies depending on the type of incontinence you have. If your incontinence occurs when you cough or sneeze take one 6C potency of *Causticum* three times a day for three days. If your incontinence is a regular occurrence, see a homoeopath for advice and specific remedies.

MODERN MEDICINE

For incontinence, medication may be prescribed — some are hormone-based and work on stress incontinence by tightening the bladder sphincter; antibiotics may be used to treat an infection linked to urge incontinence. Pelvic floor exercises such as the Kegel's (see page 69) may be of assistance; 100 contractions each day are recommended. Physiotherapy may also be suggested. A doctor may recommend surgery for either recurring cystitis, incontinence or bladder stones.

NATUROPATHY

Silica and calcium fluoride, taken as directed on the label, strengthen the tissues and can therefore help reduce incontinence. For more advice see a naturopath who will also check your diet and general health.

OSTEOPATHY

It has been found in some cases of incontinence that mechanical strains of the pelvic joints and musculature affect the support structures of the pelvic organs and may contribute to the condition. A consultation with an osteopath will determine if your situation may be helped by osteopathic care (this may need to be in conjunction with other treatments you undertake).

REFLEXOLOGY

Try reflexology points for the kidneys, ureter tubes and bladder to help tone the whole urinary system. In addition, work the adrenal glands for muscle tone, the lower spine for nerve function in the area and the diaphragm for relaxation. Work both feet or hands for a total of 15 to 20 minutes twice a week.

SHIATSU

If you have incontinence caused by weakness in your pelvic muscle, shiatsu exercises called sotai can help. Specific exercises can be provided by a shiatsu practitioner to suit your exact condition. Other ways practitioners deal with incontinence is through toning up your bladder and kidneys (as it is these organs that open and close the urethra) as well as toning up the spleen and liver meridians in your legs. Shiatsu and moxibustion heat may also be applied to the lower abdomen, lower back and sacrum areas.

YOGA

Incontinence generally happens in later life or just after childbirth. Yoga is ideal for older people and new mothers because it is a gentle form of exercise. There are specific yogic pelvic floor exercises to tone this area. Try the one on page 202 — you can aim to do three of these squeezes sequences three times a day.

INFERTILITY

Infertility is the inability to conceive. It may be a problem with the woman's fertility or the man's, or a combination of factors.

In either partner, infertility — or subfertility — may be due to chronic illness, disturbances in hormones (especially in women), poor diet, excess weight, physical or emotional stress, or exposure to radiation or heavy metals.

Among other causes, subfertility in women may be due to blocked tubes, failure to ovulate, too little progesterone, problems with cervical mucus, abnormalities of the womb or ENDOMETRIOSIS. A woman may develop antibodies to her partner's sperm and so become "immune" to conception. Previous forms of contraception such as the Pill or IUDs may have an impact. It may also be the result of PELVIC INFLAMMATORY DISEASE.

For men it may be due to low production of sperm, weak or slow-moving sperm, an obstruction in the seminal tract, inability to ejaculate, premature ejeculation, testicular trauma, atrophy of the testes, undescended testes, or other congenital problems within the reproductive system. Inadequate sperm production can be a side effect of illness such as chronic infection of the prostate or mumps, or drugs (particularly chronic marijuana use).

Men should not confuse sperm with semen, or infertility with virility (sexual performance). See also IMPOTENCE.

Finding the exact cause of infertility (there is often a combination of factors) can be a long and complicated process, so patience and perseverance is necessary, as well as expert guidance. Treatment for subfertility is also a long process in any healing field. It is recommended you seek medical advice as well as trying other therapies.

WHAT YOU CAN DO

- If you have been trying to conceive for over 12 months without success, consult your doctor. If you are a woman over the age of 35, see a doctor after six months of trying.
- Both partners should endeavour to maintain a healthy, nutritious diet, exercise regularly and get plenty of rest and rejuvenating sleep, as good general health aids conception.
- Be aware of the time of ovulation — for fertilisation to occur, sexual intercourse must take place shortly before or after ovulation. Kits that test urine samples to detect ovulation times are available from pharmacies, or your health practitioner can instruct you on determining ovulation through graphing your body temperature.
- If you are a woman having trouble conceiving and you have a heavy exercise regime, ease up on your training schedule.
- Stress can cause problems with conceiving, so learn how to relax (see page 40). Have a holiday with your partner and spend time together.
- Worrying about not conceiving can cause more stress and prolong the problem. Try not to get anxious. Enjoy passionate, joyous sex rather than strictly scheduled sex.
- To retain mature sperm and vital energies, it may be worthwhile abstaining from sex in the week before ovulation, and in the week of ovulation have sex perhaps every second day.
- The "missionary" or other "male-superior" positions for intercourse that allow deep penetration can be helpful in that it delivers sperm high in the vagina (unless the uterus is severely tilted). If, in addition, a woman remains lying down with her knees raised after intercourse, there is less semen lost.
- Some women can conceive after having problems if they increase their body weight, as research as found that body fat can produce and store oestrogen which prepares the body for pregnancy.
- Bad colds and viruses accompanied by fever can have an effect on sperm production. It generally takes 78 days to produce a sperm and 12 days for it to mature. So give yourself some time if you have been ill.
- Avoid steroids, tobacco, alcohol, caffeine and other drugs, including certain antibiotics, that can affect sperm count and ovulation.
- Sperm production occurs at a lower temperature than body temperature so keep the testicles cool by avoiding excessive physical activities, hot baths and close-fitting underwear. Cold hip baths will assist circulation and may increase a low sperm count.

ACUPUNCTURE

Acupuncturists have been known to successfully treat subfertility by unblocking the channels of Qi or energy in the body. Consult a qualified acupuncturist for more details of the treatment.

AROMATHERAPY

To alleviate stress, try rose essential oil, which has links to femininity and women's reproductive system. Lavender, rosemary and geranium also work on tension. To increase circulation and boost a weak reproductive system in both men and women, try the warming tonic oils of cinnamon, ginger and peppermint. Sage and clary have also been effective. You may like to use these oils in a bath (warm or cold depending on your situation) or a massage.

BACH FLOWER REMEDIES

White chestnut will help if you have recurring worrying thoughts concerning your infertility. Other remedies that can help include larch or gentian to help boost your confidence so you will feel likely to succeed, crab apple to help you feel positive about your body, impatiens to give you the patience to do what is necessary, and willow if you feel resentful.

CHINESE HERBS

Chinese herbalists have successfully treated people to improve their fertility for centuries. See a Chinese herbalist for advice and specific herbal treatment.

CHIROPRACTIC

Women who have problems with the balance of their pelvic floor and cannot conceive have had results with chiropractic adjustment. The alignment of the pelvis can have a significant effect on your chances of conception. Men may also be helped with specific adjustments to the spine to return normal nerve function to the reproductive organs.

COUNSELLING

There is an emotional connection with conception. Some counsellors see this as a need to relax and "let go" into parenthood. If this could be the case, it is worthwhile consulting a counsellor. Counselling will also assist you to come to terms with some of the complex issues surrounding difficulties with fertility. The ideal situation is for both partners to participate.

HERBALISM

Herbs that are useful for balancing female hormones include false unicorn root, true unicorn root and chaste tree. Additionally, the herb liquorice will support your adrenals when you have a hormonal imbalance. All these herbs help to tone a woman's system. It is best to see a herbalist for treatment rather than treat yourself.

HOMOEOPATHY

Homoeopathic remedies are known to be quite effective in helping reduce subfertility but the process of diagnosis can be complicated due to the many factors involved. See a homoeopath for specific advice and treatment.

MODERN MEDICINE

Causes of infertility can be complicated so it is crucial there is a proper medical assessment of both partners. Counselling or other psychotherapy may be recommended.

For women, hormonal drugs may be prescribed to stimulate ovulation. Various surgical techniques can unblock tubes. Artificial insemination with the partner's sperm for some cases of inadequate sperm production or hostile cervical mucus may be successful. In vitro fertilisation (IVF) is another option if there is no success with other methods.

NATUROPATHY

CAUTION: *Read the information on page 167 before taking supplements.*

For women, there are many ways a naturopath can help boost fertility. For example, take evening primrose oil (3000 mg per day), vitamin B6 (250 mg per day) and high potency B complex vitamins (take according to directions on label).

Zinc (60 mg elemental) is also particularly good for fertility, as is vitamin A (10,000 iu per day), vitamin C (2.5 g + 300 mg bioflavinoids per day), vitamin E (400–500 iu per day), calcium (600 mg per day) and magnesium (300 mg per day). Selenium (100–200 mcg per day) can help but it is not available commercially in some countries.

Diet is also a big factor in subfertility. A naturopath can advise you on changes you can make to your diet to increase your chances of pregnancy. It is best to see a naturopath rather than try home remedies because it is a complex issue that will benefit from the expertise of a professional.

For men, antioxidants are important as sperm damage can be caused by oxidation. Doses of vitamin C (3000 mg per day), vitamin E (500 iu per day), selenium (100–200 mg per day), evening primrose oil (3000 mg per day), B complex (take according to directions), vitamin A (10,000 iu per day) and zinc (25–50 mg elemental per day) can increase your sperm count and the quality of your sperm.

A naturopath may also advise you about a natural fertility program. This involves three techniques — checking mucus, taking body temperature and following the lunar cycle — which are known to be effective in achieving or avoiding pregnancy, as well as giving useful information about hormone balance and reproductive health.

OSTEOPATHY

It has been found in some cases of male and female infertility that mechanical strains of the pelvic joints and musculature affect the support structures of the pelvic organs and may contribute to the condition. A consultation with an osteopath will determine if your situation may be helped by osteopathic care (this may need to be in conjunction with other treatments you undertake).

REFLEXOLOGY

Women and men can try the following reflexology points — ask your partner to work both your feet or hands for a total of 25 minutes daily during the period of ovulation and for two days before and after, and weekly between times.

Work the entire reproductive system: the uterus/prostate for improved blood supply to the area, the ovaries/testes for improved sex hormone secretion, and the Fallopian tubes/seminal vesicles to stimulate the area and ensure a free flow of energy. In addition, work the pituitary for improved hormonal balance; the adrenal glands for improved energy, muscle tone and secretion of sex hormones; the thyroid for a balanced metabolic rate; the whole spine (particularly the lumbar spine) for improved nerve function to the pelvic area; and the diaphragm for relaxation and stress reduction.

SHIATSU

If your infertility is due to a hormonal imbalance or your inability to produce sufficient or healthy ova or sperm, or is stress-related, then shiatsu can help. A weakness of constitutional Ki in your body can cause the lack of sperm or ova so your kidneys will need toning as well as the liver to help move the blood to your reproductive organs. The spleen meridian would be worked to encourage the production of blood and Ki.

VISUALISATION

Before trying this visualisation for women, read the chapter on AFFIRMATIONS AND VISUALISATIONS and prepare yourself for visualisation. In your mind's eye see yourself pregnant. Imagine what it feels like to have a baby growing inside you. Notice the emotions this triggers. Especially notice any fears or anxiety which surface. Be careful not to judge yourself for these fears. Having a child is a life-changing experience and most women feel some fear.

See these emotions as a form of energy — perhaps as a colour. Feel and see them leaving your body, being pushed out by waves of trust, peace and love, which you can visualise as baby pink, entering your body through your crown chakra.

To aid this process repeat the following affirmation to yourself: "I lovingly accept all my feelings about motherhood and pregnancy. I acknowledge the power and beauty of being a woman. I feel whole and complete." Use this affirmation even if you feel far from perfect, whole and complete. Say the words with feeling and allow the rest of your mind, body and emotions time to believe it. They will. Feeling perfect, whole and complete without a baby will not stop you from conceiving. One theory is that it can improve your chances because it relieves the emotional pressure. Do this visualisation at least once a day for as long as you feel necessary.

Men can adapt this visualisation and affirmation to suit their needs.

If you are feeling angry with yourself or another, repeat affirmations where you forgive yourself and the other person.

INSECT BITES AND STINGS

Bites from mosquitoes and ants can be itchy and sometimes painful. If scratched, and the skin is broken, an infection can develop. Stings from bees, wasps etv can be extremely painful.

Mosquitoes can also spread diseases such as encephalitis, yellow fever and malaria in infested areas. Ticks can be poisonous.

Allergic reactions, common to bee and wasp stings, may involve intense pain, abnormal swelling, puffy eyelids and breathing difficulties.

IMPORTANT: *If you are allergic to stings, have a severe reaction to a sting or are stung in the mouth, nose or throat, seek medical attention immediately. Before any treatment is applied, the bite or sting should be identified and first aid applied. See page 392 for first aid instructions, including information on spiders and snakes.*

WHAT YOU CAN DO

- Apply an ice cube directly to the sting.
- For a bee sting, make up a solution of ice cold water and a little bicarbonate of soda (baking powder) in a bowl. Depending on position of the sting, apply a compress soaked in this or immerse the affected part.
- Apply diluted lemon juice to a wasp sting.
- Vinegar will relieve the stinging, especially of sea creatures like sea lice.
- Try a thick paste of water and a powdered meat tenderiser that contains papain or bromelain (these break down protein — the basis of most bites/stings).
- The pulp of raw onion or garlic is said to be effective in relieving pain and swelling, preventing infection and promoting healing for both bites and stings.

AROMATHERAPY

Some essential oils can be effective on stings and bites because of their analgesic and antiseptic qualities. Mix together 3 drops of tea tree and 4 drops of lavender with 2 teaspoons of base carrier oil. Apply a little of this mixture to the sting or bite. Keep applying every hour until the pain is relieved. If you don't want to use oil you can apply tea tree cream to your bite; this is readily available commercially. Lavender or tea tree oils can also be applied undiluted if necessary.

BACH FLOWER REMEDIES

Rescue remedy also comes in a cream and this can be effective in relieving the pain of insect bites and stings.

PREVENTION

- When you are outdoors, avoid attracting insects by wearing white or khaki clothing that cover the arms and legs, and by not wearing sweet smelling fragrance.
- Insect repellent is the best way to deter insects, and there are a number of natural insect repellents available. Try adding 7 drops of citronella essential oil to 15 mls of a lanolin-free cream (use a vegetable oil-based cream) and apply this to the places on your body that are easily bitten. Remember your ankles and feet. Burning pennyroyal oil in an oil burner will also keep insects at bay.
- If you are going to be in a mosquito-infested area, you can try the homoeopathic approach of taking one 6C potency of *Ledum palustre* three times a day for a few days beforehand to prevent bites.
- If you are susceptible to insect bites, try a vitamin B1 supplement.

HERBALISM

The herb chickweed can relieve itching and calendula is effective in healing. You can buy them in cream form, sometimes mixed together.

If you dab distilled witch hazel tincture on a bee sting or insect bite it will relieve the pain and swelling.

Alternately you can put a freshly peeled aloe leaf on the affected area or apply a gel with aloe in it. Crushed basil leaves can be applied to mosquito bites.

HOMOEOPATHY

Homoeopathy is good for treating insect bites and stings that swell up or bruise as long as you are not having an allergic reaction. If the bite stings and is surrounded by red swelling skin take one 6C potency of *Apis mellifica* every hour for four doses. If the sting feels bruised use *Arnica montana* ointment to relieve the pain.

MODERN MEDICINE

Locally applied creams and lotions such as calamine lotion or topical anaesthetic gels can help relieve itchiness and pain, and sometimes antihistamines are used to reduce allergic reactions.

INSOMNIA

Insomnia is the inability to fall asleep or remain asleep, either through the night or by waking too early. It affects almost everyone at some stage but can become a chronic problem. In such cases, it is best to seek professional advice.

Insomnia can be caused by stress, ANXIETY, excitement, PAIN, overeating just before bed, caffeine, poor diet, lack of exercise, or conditions that are not conducive to sleep, for example, an uncomfortable mattress or bedding that is too hot or heavy.

In the condition known as sleep apnoea, a person's air passages are blocked and they wake up continually when they find they can't breathe. As a result, they often fall asleep during the day. The cause is usually obesity or alcohol.

WHAT YOU CAN DO

- Learn how to deal with stress during your waking hours (see page 40).
- Make sure you get plenty of exercise during the day so you feel like you have used up your excess energy by night time.
- Avoid B group vitamins at night, coffee, tea, soft drinks (particularly cola), chocolate and cigarettes as they are stimulants. Alcohol may make you sleepy as it depresses your system but it also has an extremely disruptive effect on sleep.
- Avoid big meals late at night as they will activate your digestive system, and drink sparingly so you do not have to wake to empty your bladder.
- Keep regular sleeping hours. Record your sleep pattern and anything that disturbs it in a sleep journal.
- Adjust your sleep habits—including the time you go to bed and get up—so that you fall asleep easily and awake refreshed. How much sleep you need varies from person to person.
- Allow yourself time to relax and unwind before bed. Create a bedtime ritual — perhaps take a bath or listen to soothing, down-tempo music. MEDITATION, breathing techniques and visualisations (see pages 25 and 48) are effective ways to wind down physically and mentally.
- Use soft colours and lighting in your bedroom to create a restful atmosphere. Choose soft blues and purples, even green, but avoid red, yellow and orange. If possible, keep your bedroom for sleeping and not for working or thinking.
- Ensure your bed and pillows are comfortable and your bedroom is sufficiently ventilated but warm and dark. Try a quilt if you find your bedding wraps around you in your sleep. Many people in temperate climates also sleep with too-warm bedding — a common but unrecognised cause of unsettled sleep.
- A mug of warm milk with a teaspoon of honey and sprinkled with nutmeg or a cup of chamomile tea before bed can put you in the mood for sleep.
- Many people find listening to a tape of calming music or even a reading on headphones in the dark can help them drift off. Make your own or buy a talking book or pre-recorded relaxation tape.
- Finally, if you really can't sleep, don't fight it. Get up and do something useful.
- If you wake from sleep because you find it difficult to breathe, or you can only sleep propped up, it may be a sign of a heart problem so consult your doctor.

ACUPUNCTURE

Treatments of acupuncture from a qualified practitioner can be very effective on insomnia.

AFFIRMATION

If your insomnia is linked to being stressed or worried try an affirmation such as this and repeat it as many times as possible each day. "I sleep soundly knowing my life is growing and unfolding in the best possible way for me".

THE ALEXANDER TECHNIQUE

The position in which you sleep could be affecting the quality of your sleep. The Alexander Technique can teach you to use posture and movement, both in and out of bed, to help you rest better.

Before going to sleep, try resting in the semi-supine position for a few minutes. Lie on your back with your knees bent and your feet flat on the mattress, a little apart and turned out slightly. Rest your hands on top of your hips. You can place a thin pillow, folded blanket or book under your head.

AROMATHERAPY

Particular essential oils have sedating, soothing effects on the nervous system which can help reduce stress-related insomnia. Some of these include lavender, marjoram, chamomile, ylang ylang and true melissa.

Try taking an aromabath just before you go to bed, but make sure the water is not too hot as heat is stimulating. Add 3 drops each of lavender and ylang ylang, making sure it is well dispersed. You can also sprinkle a few drops of these oils on your sheets.

BACH FLOWER REMEDIES

If persistent worrying thoughts are the cause of your insomnia, try white chestnut.

CHINESE HERBS

Chinese herbalists can help this condition. Suan Zao Rentang (Zizyphus combination) is often helpful for simple insomnia, for example.

CHIROPRACTIC

If your insomnia is due to neck or back problems or general aches and pains then you may need chiropractic adjustment to realign your spine. Many people report a better night's rest after adjustment because their nervous system has been balanced.

COUNSELLING

If you suspect your insomnia is caused by emotional worries or unresolved issues a counsellor may help you deal with these.

THE FELDENKRAIS METHOD

Practitioners of the Feldenkrais Method can teach you strategies for releasing your muscle tension through gentle movements. Less tension in your muscles may mean sounder sleep.

HERBALISM

Before you go to bed take 10 drops each of Jamaican dogwood, valerian and passion flower tincture in half a cup of water. If you wake during the night take the same amount again. The herbs skullcap and hops also have a sedative effect on the body. Ready-made herbal sleep preparations containing these herbs are available at most health food stores.

You can also try sleeping with a hops pillow under your sleeping pillow.

HOMOEOPATHY

Two of the more common homoeopathic remedies used to treat insomnia are *Coffea cruda* and *Arnica montana* but there are many other constitutional homoeopathic remedies. They should be prescribed by a homoeopath to suit the complex symptoms you may be experiencing.

MASSAGE

A regular full-body massage or massage to the back, shoulders and neck should encourage relaxation and release pain and tension thus helping this condition (see page 135).

MODERN MEDICINE

Use caution if considering over-the-counter sleep medication as it usually contains antihistamines which can have pronounced side effects (including dizziness, dehydration and nausea) if used in this manner. Sleeping tablets or tranquillisers may be prescribed by your doctor. Ideally, these should only be used for a short time as they are highly addictive. Sleeping pills can also bring sleep without the important REM sleep when you dream; this is essential for health and the release of stress. When using sleeping pills, it is likely that your body won't move during the night, and this is necessary for draining the lymphatic system. Antidepressants may be administered but only if the condition is linked to depression. Doctors usually recommend relaxation classes or anti-stress programs before prescribing a course of medication.

Treatment for sleep apnoea may involve the wearing of a mask which forces the person to breathe.

NATUROPATHY

You could try taking doses of magnesium phosphate and calcium (as directed on the bottle) to help relax the nervous system.

REFLEXOLOGY

Work the points for the diaphragm and head area for relaxation and stress reduction, and the pituitary for hormonal balance. In addition, work any reflex that relates to tension in a particular part of the body e.g. the eyes, the neck/shoulders, the spine. Try this on both feet or hands for a total of 20 minutes daily until your sleep pattern improves and then once or twice weekly thereafter.

SHIATSU

In shiatsu insomnia is seen to be caused by a congested or inflamed liver, a deficiency of Ki in the heart meridian, a disturbance in the spirit due to emotional shock or trauma, or a lack of flowing Ki in the body in general. In the case of a problem liver, a shiatsu practitioner will disperse your liver channel. For the heart meridian a practitioner will "tonify" the Ki in this meridian bringing a peaceful state of mind that induces sleep.

Insomnia may also be caused by an excess of Ki in the kidneys leading to a restless body and mind. A practitioner would work on your back to sedate and the kidney meridian to balance.

YOGA

Try the deep relaxation exercise on page 196 in bed.

IRRITABLE BOWEL SYNDROME

Irritable bowel syndrome (IBS) is also known as spastic colon or mucous COLITIS. Although there is no inflammation present, the muscles in the colon fail to function properly and cause abdominal pain, DIARRHOEA alternating with CONSTIPATION, bloating, FLATULENCE, NAUSEA, and even ANXIETY and DEPRESSION.

Those who have the condition may find their digestive systems always seem to give some kind of trouble. The symptoms may persist over years, even with treatment, or come and go.

The cause of IBS has not fully been determined, but stress and emotional disturbances are thought to be the major contributing factors. Emotionally, this illness may be connected to "irritability" and low-level anger. Food intolerance (see ALLERGIES) or an unbalanced diet may also be involved.

To deal successfully with this condition, you may need to combine other treatments with a change in diet and lifestyle.

IMPORTANT: *Be cautious when dealing with these symptoms as the condition can be serious. Ensure other causes such as chronic infection or bowel cancer are investigated, particularly if you have blood or mucus in your stools, or if you experience severe abdominal pain or rapid weight loss.*

WHAT YOU CAN DO

- Take steps to reduce stress and anxiety in your everyday routine (see page 40).
- Keep a diary to record what events bring on irritable bowel symptoms and which foods and drinks you should avoid.
- Find out if you are lactose intolerant. Your health practitioner can test for this or you can give up dairy foods for a few days — this may clear up the problem.
- Maintain a healthy, balanced diet high in fibre — especially bran, grains, fruit and vegetables.
- Drink plenty of water — six to eight glasses a day.
- Steer clear of chewing gum containing sorbitol which is difficult to digest.
- Avoid stimulating laxatives and choose bulky laxatives such as linseed.
- Avoid alcohol, coffee, sweets, greasy and spicy foods and too much meat as they can cause further irritation or may be difficult to digest.

ACUPRESSURE

It is best to see a qualified practitioner for advice and treatment but you could also try the acupressure point Liver 3. Hold the point until you find the tender spot; continue to hold it for 10 seconds then release it.

ACUPUNCTURE

Acupuncture can help if you have IBS. Seek an acupuncturist for advice and treatment.

AFFIRMATION

Affirmations may help if there is an emotional side to your condition. If it seems appropriate, try repeating the following as often as possible: "I love and accept myself exactly as I am right now. I trust I fully express my emotions in a positive way. I am at peace."

AROMATHERAPY

Essential oils such as lavender and chamomile can soothe the mind and body. Try a few drops in a bath or mixed with base carrier oil for massage.

BACH FLOWER REMEDIES

Remedies that relieve stress include rescue remedy, white chestnut and walnut.

CHINESE HERBS

Irritable bowel syndrome indicates to a Chinese herbalist that your lung and liver are out of balance. They would prescribe herbs that harmonise these two organs to reduce your IBS.

CHIROPRACTIC

IBS can be helped by chiropractic adjustment because the function of the bowels improves when the spine is free of subluxations (unnatural pressure on the nervous system or interference within it). Chiropractic adjustment also helps the nervous system which in turn helps strengthen the immune system.

COUNSELLING

If you have IBS and are feeling irritable or believe life is not flowing as it should, counselling can help.

HEALING MEDITATION

See the chapter on HEALING ENERGIES for the self-healing technique on page 123. When you have the blue light flowing throughout your body focus it on your bowel and digestive system.

HERBALISM

The herb slippery elm will help regulate your bowel and protect it. Mix 1–2 teaspoons of slippery elm powder in half a glass of hot water. Mix this into a paste and take as often as you like until the pain subsides. Try to eat it before it turns into a gel because it can be difficult to digest once this happens. You should also avoid harsh fibre such as bran and take the softer fibres such as oats — try 1 tablespoon of psyllium husks with one glass of water.

Echinacea, wild yam, yarrow, St John's wort and golden seal will help heal your body from the effects of IBS. The astringent herb fringetree is also effective.

HOMOEOPATHY

There are many homoeopathic remedies that can help if you have IBS. Your prescription will depend on the exact nature of your condition at the time. If your anus feels like it is burning and you have profuse diarrhoea, you can try taking one 6C potency of *Aloe socotrina* every half hour for five doses. If you constantly feel like going to the toilet for no reason and experience spasms in your rectum, you can try one 6C potency tablet or liquid form of *Nux vomica* every half an hour for five doses. If your condition does not improve after two days with these remedies, see a homoeopath.

MASSAGE

A gentle abdominal massage can bring relief from pain and will nourish the intestine. See page 137 for self-massage, remembering to only massage in a clockwise direction.

MODERN MEDICINE

A doctor will thoroughly investigate this condition, testing your faeces and X-raying the bowel or carrying out a rectal examination, to rule out other problems. Drugs such as antispasmodic medications can be given to help reduce abdominal pain, and antidiarrhoeal drugs can be used to reduce bowel activity.

NATUROPATHY

As food intolerance may be involved, a naturopath will tell you to avoid all possible allergens which may include dairy products and gluten-containing grains such as wheat, rye, barley and oats. See a naturopath for a specific elimination diet which concentrates on easy-to-digest foods such as rice, bananas, sweet potatoes and steamed green and yellow vegetables, and slowly reintroduces foods that may be causing the problem.

OSTEOPATHY

As with other problems of the digestive system, this condition may be assisted by osteopathic treatment. A detailed interview and examination would need to be performed by an osteopath — perhaps along with your medical test results — to evaluate whether your problem would be suitable for osteopathic treatment.

REFLEXOLOGY

Work these points gently: the colon and small intestine plus the adrenal glands for muscle tone and the diaphragm for relaxation and stress reduction. Try this on both feet or hands for a total of 15 minutes twice a week.

SHIATSU

If your IBS is linked to emotional factors shiatsu can help balance these and make you feel more sure of yourself. If it is more a physical condition, shiatsu can help balance your colon and strengthen the flow of Ki around your body. Depending on the cause of your condition, a practitioner may also tone and disperse the Ki in your bladder meridian to relieve the pain in your abdomen.

YOGA

Yoga can improve IBS in a short period of time and it has been known to cure this condition within a few months. In yogic terms IBS is described as a disturbance in the flow of "life energy". The life energy is said to be moving downwards too much which causes diarrhoea. Or the life energy is also moving around the navel too much which causes constipation. The yoga way of dealing with this is to practise the inverted yoga postures to slow down the release of the down-flowing life energy which will improve the diarrhoea (see pages 197 and 203).

You can also practise deep relaxation yoga techniques to stabilise the life energy around your navel which will help decrease constipation.

JET LAG

Jet lag occurs when you travel from one time zone to another and your body's "clock" or circadian rhythm — which works on a cycle that is very close to 24 hours — is disturbed. The effect is worse on long flights east-west or west-east rather than north or south. As a rule, it takes one day to adjust for each time zone that is crossed.

The production of toxic chemicals known as "free radicals" are also thought to be a factor, caused by cabin pressurisation and exposure to radiation.

When you are "jet lagged" you feel very tired, both physically and emotionally, moody and disorientated.

See also Insomnia and Fatigue.

WHAT YOU CAN DO

- Maintain good general health — the effects of jet lag are worse among older people and those with poor levels of fitness.
- Try adjusting your eating habits for four days before departing. Alternate between a day of eating as much as you want then eating very lightly: feast then fast then feast then fast on the day of the flight.
- Make some time adjustment in the period leading up to your journey — gradually going to bed earlier or later depending on your destination.
- Do not get less sleep before flying thinking it will make you tired — it can make jet lag worse. Catch up on sleep as soon as you can after arrival.

• Try to book flights that cause minimal disruption to routine. For example, if you are taking a nine-hour flight to a destination that is five hours ahead, schedule a late night flight — a plane departing at 10:00 pm will arrive at noon local time, but your body clock will think that it is 9:00 am; you will have the day ahead in any case. This is better than a noon flight that arrives at 2:00 am local time when your body thinks it is only 9:00 pm — you won't be feeling like sleep although your new environment says it's the middle of the night.

• Avoid caffeine and alcohol and drink plenty of water before, during and after the flight to avoid dehydration which makes jet lag worse.

• Do not eat meals on board the plane if you are not hungry as a sluggish digestive system will also make your jet lag worse. Choose light foods such as salads, if possible; order vegetarian.

• Try to sleep on board the plane. Eye masks and ear plugs can help shut out disturbances, and neck pillows can prevent the head from dropping. Wear loose comfortable clothing, and socks rather than shoes when on board. Ask the flight attendant not to wake you for a meal.

• If you can't sleep on board, don't get anxious but do shut your eyes and try to relax. You could daydream or meditate. Think of the flight as "time-out" from demands and routine, time for solitude and thought. This will reduce the stress on arrival.

• Vigorous exercise at your new destination can help rid the body of toxins produced during flying.

• Some experts suggest that time spent in the sunshine at your new destination can help the body adjust by keeping the biological clock stimulated.

• If you feel tired at your destination, but it isn't time to sleep yet, socialise. It will distract you and help alter your perception of time.

• Avoid working or important decision-making for at least a day after arrival, if possible, as you won't be at your best.

• If your stay is a short one, try to keep as close as possible to your regular eating and sleeping schedule.

ACUPUNCTURE

Acupuncture is known to be effective in relieving jet lag. See an acupuncturist before you travel for treatments that will last you till your return.

AFFIRMATION

As jet lag relates to your linear concept of time, an affirmation such as the following may help your mind and body adjust. Repeat it as often as required. "My body clock adjusts well to change and is perfectly in tune to where I am right now."

THE ALEXANDER TECHNIQUE

During your flight, experiment a little to find a comfortable position that you can remain in for a while. Constantly wriggling, stretching and moving, while it may seem beneficial at the time, can actually cause more aches and fatigue.

AROMATHERAPY

Lavender essential oil relaxes and soothes and can help with nervous anxiety during the flight — try sprinkling a few drops on a handkerchief and inhaling regularly, or rub a little onto your temples. Once you have arrived, geranium added to a bath will stimulate your adrenal system. You can also inhale rosemary from a handkerchief whenever you need an energy boost.

BACH FLOWER REMEDIES

Bach flower remedies are beneficial for long journeys because they are compact, easy to take and give quick relief. White chestnut is good for jet lag as it reduces the worry and stress of travelling. Honeysuckle is also effective because it is for homesickness and nostalgia. Olive can be taken for complete mental and physical exhaustion, and clematis for grounding. Rescue remedy is helpful for adjusting to a different environment and temperature.

CHINESE MEDICINE

The over-the-counter patent medicine Gui Pi Tang (ginseng and longan combination) is recommended to the traveller to ward off the effects of jet lag.

THE FELDENKRAIS METHOD

Simple movement strategies can be used to overcome fatigue from jet lag and counteract the effect of sitting in a cramped area for long periods of time. For example, small pelvic movements that mobilise your entire spine can be useful during the flight. See a Feldenkrais practitioner for advice and lessons.

HOMOEOPATHY

Take one 6C potency of *Arnica montana* every two hours while you are flying and then three times a day after you arrive at your destination for perhaps three to four days until you feel recovered.

MODERN MEDICINE

Sleeping tablets may be prescribed for use during the flight and to conquer disrupted sleep patterns on arrival, but they are to be used with appropriate caution as they are highly addictive. Melatonin, which is taken orally, can be used to reset the sleep cycle. It is effective when used short term but the side effects of long-term use are unknown.

REFLEXOLOGY

To help relieve jet lag, work the points that correspond to all the glands and the eye/ear reflex as well as all the fingers or toes as they correspond to the head area. Try this on both hands or feet for a total of 30 minutes for a couple of days.

SHIATSU

Try pressing on the shiatsu point called Gall Bladder 20 when you need relief from a headache that may occur from travelling on a plane. Press for a minute then give it a rest for a minute and press again.

You can also try the shiatsu pressure points called Bladder 57, Gall Bladder 34 and Stomach 36 to release the tension in your legs that could occur from the pressure inside the aircraft and lack of activity. Press for a minute then give it a rest and press again.

Use these points whenever you think about it.

Once you have arrived at your destination, a shiatsu practitioner can work on the triple heater and spleen meridians to help adjust your internal body clock.

YOGA

You can reduce the effect of jet lag with yoga. If you practise yoga before bed on arrival at your destination it can help your body adjust to your new conditions and to sleep (see the deep relaxation exercise on page 196). You can also use yoga to bring your energy levels up when you are feeling tired — see the breathing to relax exercise on page 193 for one example.

KIDNEY PROBLEMS

The kidneys filter waste material from the blood to the urine and are vital in controlling the fluid levels in your body. Many disorders can affect the proper functioning of the kidneys, including obstructions and blockages or bacterial infections and inflammation, brought on by another condition such as cystitis. Children may be affected by nephritis (an inflammation) or nephrosis (a protein leak that causes severe swelling.)

The restricted blood supply associated with high blood pressure (see page 234) can cause kidney problems, and kidney problems can also cause high blood pressure as retained fluids put an extra burden on the heart.

DIABETES, gout (see page 222) and some forms of medication (particularly analgesics) can cause kidney dysfunction, as can accidents and poisoning.

Some believe there is an emotional link between kidney problems and fear.

Kidney stones are one common problem. The stones form in the kidney from calcium and salt deposits and then pass through the urinary system, or sometimes block it. The blockage can lead to infection which can, in turn, lead eventually to kidney failure.

Stones may dissolve or remain in the body indefinitely without any symptoms being displayed. Small stones may pass without notice or you may suffer dragging pains in your lower back or abdomen. When the stone enters the ureter it can cause sudden sharp, even agonising pain in the back or side, radiating to the abdomen, groin and inner thigh. This can last for a few days. There may be sweating and chills and you may want to urinate frequently, feel nauseous and vomit.

Excessive sweating or poor diet with not enough fluid may contribute to kidney stones as it concentrates the calcium/salt deposits in the urine. Other factors in stone formation may be an increased dairy intake (this is an alkaline form of calcium) or too little magnesium (which causes calcium to leach out into the system).

Some people seem more susceptible to developing stones, which has a higher incidence in men from middle age.

Consult a doctor if you experience any of the following symptoms:

- back pain, below the ribs
- burning sensation on urination
- more frequent urination
- bloody, cloudy or dark urine
- swelling of hands and feet
- eye puffiness (especially in children)
- unexplained fever
- continual fatigue.

Kidney problems can go undetected. Untreated, they may contribute to the progressive damage of the kidneys, resulting eventually in kidney failure. It is recommended you have any kidney problem properly diagnosed and use alternative therapies in conjunction with medical care.

See also BLADDER PROBLEMS.

WHAT YOU CAN DO

- Drink plenty of water every day. At least six to eight glasses a day is recommended to effectively flush toxins from the system. When the body is dehydrated urine becomes concentrated and increases the risk of kidney problems.

- Regular exercise will also aid circulation and the removal of toxins from your system.

- Empty the bladder as soon as the need to urinate is felt as bacteria can breed and minerals held are more likely to crystallise.

- If you suffer from kidney stones drink low calcium mineral water and limit your intake of dairy foods (they are high in alkaline calcium) and those rich in oxalic acid (e.g. celery, grapes, green peppers, parsley, strawberries, spinach and chocolate).

- There is a link between excessive protein consumption and kidney stones so ensure your intake is moderate. You should also watch your intake of salt and vitamin D. Vitamin C in certain forms, especially ascorbic acid, can irritate a kidney inflammation — seek advice as how to best meet your needs for this important vitamin.

- If you use an antacid, check it is not calcium-based.

- Avoid diuretic medication. If essential, ensure the drug is one that does not increase the uric acid levels in the blood.

ACUPUNCTURE

Acupuncture is useful in dealing with kidney disorders. See a qualified acupuncturist for details.

AFFIRMATION

To help the fear that may be linked with kidney problems, try an affirmation such as: "I am safe and secure at all times".

AROMATHERAPY

Essential oils can have a positive effect on the kidneys as they circulate in the blood stream. The oils that have this tonic effect include cedarwood, chamomile and juniper berry. Try a bath containing 2 drops each of cedarwood and juniper berry, making sure the oils are fully dispersed in the water. Seek the advice of a qualified aromatherapist for other treatments.

BACH FLOWER REMEDIES

Mimulus and aspen are remedies that help the emotional side of kidney conditions.

CHIROPRACTIC

If nerves directly linked to the kidneys are distorted or pinched, their function may be reduced or altered, creating disease. Chiropractic adjustment can help organs such as the kidneys to function better as it improves the nervous system.

HERBALISM

In the early stages kidney stones can be dissolved with the herbs gravel root and hydrangea. Buchu and corn silk have an antiseptic effect on the urinary system; try drinking buchu tea twice a day to help.

For nephritis, buchu and corn silk are again used as well as echinacea and golden seal.

HOMOEOPATHY

The homoeopathic remedy *Berberis vulgaris* is known for its ability to dissolve kidney stones and reduce associated pain and discomfort. See a homoeopath for specific advice and treatment for your particular kidney problem.

MODERN MEDICINE

The doctor will test a urine sample for evidence of blood, protein and cells. They will also examine the abdomen for swelling or tenderness.

If kidney function is good and stones are not large, they will be left to pass out. In cases of blockage, surgery may be required. Larger kidney stones can be broken up by sound or shock waves so they can be passed with greater ease. This procedure is known as lithotripsy. Some stones can be dissolved using medication. Calcium stones, for example, may be dissolved with injections of magnesium sulphate.

Drugs can be used to control conditions involving infection and inflammation of the kidneys. In cases of nephritis, children need to be hospitalised where they can receive steroid treatment and fluid management.

Many kidney problems will need to be monitored after initial treatment. Chronic kidney disease may require regular treatment on a hemodialysis machine or a kidney transplant.

NATUROPATHY

Diet management under a naturopath's guidance as well as vitamin and minerals can help relieve kidney problems. For example, doses of lecithin (2 tablespoons per day), magnesium phosphate (400 mg per day) and vitamin B6 (250 mg per day) may help dissolve kidney stones. For nephritis, increase your intake of vitamin C in the form of sodium bicarbonate as well as bioflavinoids and vitamin A.

Cranberry juice has an antiseptic effect on the urinary system.

OSTEOPATHY

By treating the supporting tissues, blood supply and nerve supply of the kidneys and bladder through manual techniques on the spine, abdomen and pelvis, osteopathy can help with many forms of urinary disturbance. Consult an osteopath to see if your problem is suitable for treatment.

REFLEXOLOGY

Gently work the main reflex point — the kidneys — as well as those for the ureter tubes and bladder to encourage the healthy functioning of the whole urinary system. Work the diaphragm for relaxation and stress reduction which may help with the pain of kidney stones. The parathyroid should be worked to assist with the metabolism of calcium and the lower spine for healthy nerve function. Try this on both feet or hands for a total of 15 minutes twice a week.

SHIATSU

In Oriental terms the kidneys are very important organs because they are responsible for many functions including storing Ki and transforming fluid into urine. The kidneys not only govern a lot of the water in our bodies but also the Ki which is responsible for reproduction and growth. They are often referred to as the root of all Ki in the body and are responsible for our longevity. Because of the kidney's importance it is crucial that any infection or disease in this organ be healed. A shiatsu therapist can give advice and treatment.

YOGA

In yogic philosophy, if your kidneys are strong you should have an abundance of energy and strength. Yoga aims to build this strength when there are problems. Try the butterfly posture on page 194 as an example.

LARYNGITIS

Laryngitis is a "dis-ease" that is telling your body to rest and stop talking — and that is exactly what you should do.

Laryngitis is a condition where the larynx (voice box) is inflamed and therefore causes a loss of voice or hoarseness. There is usually no soreness. If there is soreness, the condition is known as pharyngitis.

In severe cases, there may be breathing difficulties. It can be caused by strain and overuse, a virus or a bacterial infection. In such cases, it may be accompanied by a cough, fever, fatigue or difficulty swallowing.

Chronic laryngitis lasting weeks or months is often due to an irritant such as smoking or air pollution. Some prescription drugs such as blood pressure medication, antihistamines and the inhaled steroids used in the treatment of asthma can cause throat dryness.

Some believe there is an emotional link between laryngitis and not expressing yourself truthfully.

You should consult a medical practitioner if your voice does not return to normal within five days or if you have severe pain when you swallow.

See SORE THROAT *for more information.*

LIVER PROBLEMS

The liver has about 200 metabolic functions: it works to detoxify the blood and process nutrients, including the manufacture of bile to digest fat, and is involved in energy production and immunity. Disorders of this organ can manifest in all parts of the body.

Signs of liver dysfunction include:

- blurred vision
- NAUSEA
- fat intolerance
- alcohol and caffeine intolerance
- ACNE
- FATIGUE
- reduced muscle tone.

Jaundice — the yellowing of skin and the whites of the eyes — is not a disease, but rather a symptom that may be caused by a number of liver disorders.

Problems can include liver "sluggishness" or underfunctioning as well as more serious conditions such as HEPATITIS and tumours.

Alcohol can cause serious damage to the liver, as can other chemicals and pharmaceutical drugs.

Cirrhosis of the liver is a chronic disease caused by the death of liver cells that are replaced with scar tissue. It may result from alcoholism, poor nutrition, heart failure or chronic hepatitis, and although irreversible, it can be halted.

A damaged liver does have significant powers of regeneration but it is important to stop the destructive processes. If you suspect a liver disorder, seek medical advice before beginning any other treatment.

See also GALL BLADDER PROBLEMS.

WHAT YOU CAN DO

- Restricting your consumption of alcohol will help your liver stay healthy. It may be worthwhile seeing a counsellor if this poses a problem.
- Avoid all non-essential drugs and chemicals. Paracetamol, cimethidine (widely prescribed for ULCERS) and antidepressants are common examples of medication that can cause liver damage. Other drugs such as the Pill can impair liver function.

ACUPRESSURE AND ACUPUNCTURE

More than in Western medicine, the liver is seen as an extremely important organ in traditional Chinese medicine. Acupuncture and acupressure are very useful for treating liver dysfunction. See a qualified practitioner for details.

AROMATHERAPY

CAUTION: *Read the information on pages 102 to 105 before using these essential oils.*

The essential oil that has the most powerful effect on the liver is rosemary. It stimulates the production and flow of bile and is a general liver tonic. Also helpful to the liver are peppermint, chamomile and lemon essential oils. If any of these are massaged into the body they will enter the bloodstream and reach the liver quickly. Another way of absorbing the oils is through alternate hot and cold compresses over the liver area.

Try making two hot compresses with 2 drops each of rosemary and chamomile together and a cold compress with 2 drops of peppermint. Place them one at a time over your liver area. Alternate them every 5 minutes and make sure you finish off with a cold one. Do this for about 15 minutes once a day, preferably at night before you go to bed.

BACH FLOWER REMEDIES

Some believe the liver is associated with anger and the remedies that reduce the feeling of anger are impatiens and holly.

HERBALISM

In herbal terms the liver is known as "the swamp of the body" because most ailments have an impact on the liver. Herbs that are specifically for the liver include celandine, St Mary's thistle and dandelion. You should seek the advice of a herbalist before you take herbs for your liver because your diet and physical state will determine which herbs will be most beneficial.

HOMOEOPATHY

There are many homoeopathic remedies that have a toning effect on the liver. See a homoeopath for the correct prescription based holistically on your mental and physical condition.

MODERN MEDICINE

Most general practitioners would not consider the liver's role in many of the symptoms of dysfunction listed above.

If a patient had jaundice, vomiting and liver pain, a liver function test would be undertaken to pinpoint a disease e.g. hepatitis or toxic damage. There is no specific treatment for such conditions, although steroids may be given for chronic active hepatitis.

NATUROPATHY

A naturopath will recommend eating plenty of salads and vegetables, drinking fresh juices and avoiding fatty foods to keep your liver healthy. In addition, take vitamin C (4000 mg per day), beta carotene (60 mg per day) and zinc (20 mg elemental per day).

OSTEOPATHY

By treating the supporting tissues, blood supply and nerve supply of the liver through manual techniques on the spine, abdomen and pelvis, osteopathy can help with many forms of liver disturbance. Consult an osteopath to see if your problem is suitable for this kind of treatment.

REFLEXOLOGY

Work these points: the liver as the main reflex, the gall bladder to aid its healthy function, the thoracic spine for nerve function in the area, and the diaphragm for relaxation and reduced stress. Try this on both feet or hands for a total of 15 to 20 minutes twice a week.

SHIATSU

In shiatsu the liver is more important than many other organs, including the heart and brain, because it ensures the smooth, unrestricted flow of Ki energy to retain your health. A shiatsu practitioner will therefore work to ensure the flow of energy through your liver meridian, supporting the gall bladder meridian to evenly distribute the liver's energy. You would also be advised to avoid fried foods and saturated fats.

YOGA

Yoga won't heal liver disease, but certain exercises such as the rocking backwards exercise and the inverted corpse on pages 199 and 203 can strengthen your liver and your immune system in general.

MENOPAUSE

Menopause refers to the period of time when a woman's menstruation becomes irregular and finally ceases. It usually begins around the age of

45 to 50 as a result of the ovaries no longer producing oestrogen and progesterone, and may last from six months to three years.

Symptoms triggered by these changes in hormone levels include:

- hot flushes (which usually begin two to five years before actual menopause and may continue for years afterwards)
- irregular menstrual bleeding
- FATIGUE
- night sweats
- INSOMNIA
- HEADACHES
- vertigo
- dramatic changes in blood pressure and heart palpitations
- muscle and joint pain
- VARICOSE VEINS
- brown patches on the skin or recurrent skin allergies
- weight gain or redistribution
- ANXIETY, irritability and mood swings
- DEPRESSION and loss of confidence.

In the later stages, OSTEOPOROSIS can be brought on as can drying of the vagina and loss of vaginal elasticity (causing pain during sex), urinary frequency, and dry skin.

Many women find menopause emotionally difficult. It can undermine their feelings of femininity and spark concerns about aging. It may come at a time when there are other upheavals and stresses such as retirement or children leaving home.

WHAT YOU CAN DO

• Don't assume all your symptoms are due to menopause. There may be other problems: this is an age where there is an increased likelihood of developing other conditions such as DIABETES or high blood pressure (see page 234) and there may be increased stress. It is important to regularly discuss all symptoms with your medical practitioner, especially heavy bleeding between periods or bleeding after your period has ceased for six months or longer.

• Maintain a healthy, balanced diet and get regular exercise and sufficient rest to minimise symptoms.

• Drink plenty of fluids to help keep your body temperature regulated. Hot flushes occur until your body learns how to cope with the missing oestrogen. Limit alcohol and caffeine and eat smaller meals to assist in maintaining an even temperature.

• Dress in natural fibres and wear layers of clothing that you can peel off during a hot flush. Try using separate sheets and blankets to those of your bed partner so you can alter the temperature to suit you.

• Consider taking your partner to a discussion with your health practitioner so he can also get a better understanding of the changes associated with this time.

• Regular sex seems to moderate hormone levels and can be of emotional benefit too. Talk with your partner to try to overcome any difficulties associated with menopausal symptoms. The sensuality and closeness that comes from touching can be very important at this time, especially when there may be discomfort associated with intercourse. Try the full-body massage on page 143.

• As menstruation can be irregular, continue to use contraception for a year after the cessation of periods.

• Continue to have yearly pelvic examinations after menopause.

• Physically and psychologically you will benefit from learning relaxation techniques (see page 40).

• After menopause, some women feel fit and vigorous as they never had before. Stay positive and live this part of your life to the full, unencumbered by the need for contraception and by menstruation, and with a new zest for living.

ACUPUNCTURE

Acupuncture is known to be effective in relieving the emotional and physical symptoms of menopause. Seek the advice of a qualified acupuncturist for specific treatment.

AFFIRMATION

Try this affirmation to give you strength during this

time of transition. Repeat it as many times a day as possible: "I am greater than my body. I acknowledge my beauty and my power as a woman is enriched by the experience of life."

AROMATHERAPY

Aromatherapy can calm menopausal symptoms because it reduces stress and stress often triggers the symptoms. The essential oil of geranium has this balancing effect on the hormones and rose tones and cleanses the uterus and helps regulate the menstrual cycle. The femininity of rose can be an added boon. Peppermint will help because it "cools" the effects of hot flushes.

Try a relaxing bath (not too hot if you are experiencing hot flushes) with 2 drops each of geranium and rose fully dispersed in the water.

If you are experiencing a hot flush sprinkle 2 drops of peppermint on a tissue and inhale it till you feel cooler.

BACH FLOWER REMEDIES

Rescue remedy, white chestnut, aspen and mimulus are all effective in calming anxiety. Or you can take cherry plum or gorse for depression.

CHINESE HERBS

Chinese herbs are effective in reducing many of the symptoms of menopause including hot flushes, night sweats and restless fatigue. Chinese herbalists use herbs to tone moisture in your body and supplement and protect your kidney network so the hormonal changes you experience are smooth and natural.

CHIROPRACTIC

Menopausal symptoms can be reduced if the spine is free from subluxations (unnatural pressures) and the nervous system is not stressed. See a chiropractor for advice and chiropractic care.

THE FELDENKRAIS METHOD

Attending lessons in the Feldenkrais method of movement can re-establish a sense of well-being when you are menopausal.

HERBALISM

Herbs that can help relieve the symptoms of menopause include motherwort for hot flushes and black cohosh for balancing your hormone levels as well as chaste tree, false unicorn root and dong quai. St John's wort is also helpful for the anxiety often felt at this time.

A herbalist can do a lot to help so a consultation is recommended rather than self-treatment. However, you may like to try drinking cold sage herbal tea twice daily to ease hot flushes.

HOMOEOPATHY

There are homoeopathic drops that are specifically for hot flushes. These are made to the individual's requirement and so are only available on prescription from a homoeopath.

MODERN MEDICINE

Hormone replacement therapy (HRT), in the form of pills, cream and skin implants, is the mainstay of modern medical treatment of menopausal problems. The side effects of hormonal drugs should be discussed and other conditions such as heart or liver problems need to be taken into account.

Counselling may also be recommended. A water-based lubricant such as KY jelly will be suggested for use during intercourse and an oestrogen vaginal cream may be prescribed. Drugs such as clonidine may also be prescribed to alleviate hot flushes.

NATUROPATHY

Naturopathy can help to relieve the symptoms of menopause. See a naturopath for more details but doses of evening primrose oil (3000 mg per day) and vitamin B6 (250 mg per day) can be beneficial. Vitamin E (1000 iu daily) can help control hot flushes over time.

Diet is also an influencing factor in a smooth transition through menopause. Try to stay away from stimulants such as sugar, white flour and coffee. Foods such as soya bean products, parsley, cucumber and alfalfa contain plant oestrogens which will help reduce your symptoms.

OSTEOPATHY

Structural strains can affect the hormone balance by disturbing the nerve supply and blood supply to the endocrine glands, and the ovaries and uterus as supporting structures. By addressing various regions of the body and cranium with gentle manual techniques, osteopathy can reduce the difficulties of menopause.

REFLEXOLOGY

Work the following points: the reproductive system — including the Fallopian tubes — as the main reflex, the pituitary for hormonal balance, the diaphragm for relaxation, and the thyroid and parathyroid for calcium balance. You can also work any point that relates to a specific symptom, e.g. kidneys and bladder for urinary problems. Try this on both feet or hands for a total of 25 minutes twice a week.

SHIATSU

Oriental medicine explains the symptoms associated with menopause as an imbalance of Ki energy and blood in your spleen, heart and liver from a lack of cooling energy (yin) in your kidneys. By toning the kidney meridian which produces cooling yin energy and moving the blood in your organs, a shiatsu practitioner can reduce hot flushes, night sweats and general irritation.

YOGA

Relaxing yoga exercises can bring your body temperature down when you have hot flushes and keep your mind in a calm state so you can cope with the changes you are experiencing. Try the breathing to relax exercise, the inverted corpse position and the plough posture on pages 193 to 202 to make yourself calmer and prevent insomnia.

MENSTRUAL PROBLEMS

See also INFERTILITY, MENOPAUSE, PELVIC INFLAMMATORY DISEASE, PERIOD PAIN, PRE-MENSTRUAL SYNDROME and THYROID PROBLEMS.

Discomforts associated with the menstrual cycle can be alleviated — consult specific entries such as HEADACHE or FATIGUE in this book.

WHAT YOU CAN DO

To avoid or treat period problems it is important to maintain good general health:

- Eat a balanced, wholefood diet (see page 9).
- Keep your weight within a normal range.
- Avoid caffeine, alcohol and smoking as they can all interfere with hormone balance and efficient circulation.
- Get enough rest and regular exercise.
- Learn how to relax and deal effectively with stress (see page 40).

(1) DISTURBANCES IN THE CYCLE

Disturbances in the cycle are usually related to hormone balance. For example, the temporary or permanent absence of periods (known as amenorrhea) is often caused by deficiencies of ovarian or pituitary hormones with oestrogen levels falling too low. Underlying the hormone imbalance may be a number of triggers, including:

- cysts on the ovaries
- extreme or sudden changes in body weight
- stress, shock or physical disruption such as travel or moving house
- ALLERGIES, sudden or chronic illness
- LIVER and KIDNEY PROBLEMS
- poor circulation
- some drug treatments, chemotherapy or radiotherapy
- some forms of the contraceptive pill
- coming off the Pill
- the onset of MENOPAUSE
- iron-deficiency ANAEMIA or other nutritional deficiencies
- childbirth and breastfeeding.

It is normal for a period to be missed or delayed due to stress or excitement. However, if periods are absent for six to nine months (and the woman is not pregnant), the cause should be investigated medically.

Medical examination is recommended for any continuing disturbances in the menstrual cycle such as irregular periods, spotting or minimal bleeding.

IMPORTANT: *Disturbances in the cycle, even the absence of periods, do not indicate infertility. If you wish to avoid pregnancy, full contraceptive precautions should still be taken.*

ACUPUNCTURE

Hormone regulation and treating the absence of periods is one of the areas where a course of acupuncture treatment has proved extremely effective.

BACH FLOWER REMEDIES

Elm, mimulus, walnut, white chestnut and vervain may be of assistance. Rescue remedy may help if a period is delayed by shock or sudden trauma.

COUNSELLING

Your emotions can have a significant effect on your hormonal system. This is not only the case for emotional stress and any kind of upheaval but also for how you feel about yourself and issues of femininity and sexuality. A counsellor may be able to help identify and work through any such problems.

HERBALISM

Blue cohosh, chaste tree, false unicorn root, lovage, mugwort and pennyroyal are herbs that have strong effects on the female reproductive system. A herbalist may prescribe a tonic that incorporates these along with other herbs to treat other causes such as stress.

MODERN MEDICINE

The cause may be investigated through a blood test and perhaps an ultrasound. Dilation and Curettage (also known as a D and C) may be recommended, particularly in cases of bleeding after menopause which are investigated to assess for endometrial cancer.

The oral contraceptive pill is commonly prescribed to regulate disturbances caused by hormone dysfunction, but this does not actually fix the problem.

NATUROPATHY

Vitamin B6, found in tuna, salmon, egg yolk, legumes, oats, walnuts can help with hormone dysfunction — this is particularly likely to be depleted if you are coming off the Pill. A naturopath will also check that you are getting enough protein — animal and soya bean products being the highest source. Vitamin E and essential fatty acids, present in tofu, fish oils, cold-pressed olive oil, egg yolk, nuts and seeds, will also assist in the production of hormones.

REFLEXOLOGY

Work these points: the uterus as the main reflex, the pituitary and ovaries for hormonal balance, the thyroid to promote the function of the reproductive glands, the adrenal glands to supplement the sex hormones secreted by the ovaries, and the diaphragm for relaxation. Try this on both feet or hands for a total of 15 minutes daily during menstruation and in the week before.

SHIATSU

Shiatsu treatment is very effective in relieving PMT and disturbances of the menstrual cycle. Hormonal imbalance can be regulated with regular sessions.

YOGA

Yoga can be very helpful in normalising periods. Try the butterfly exercise as well as forward stretches such as the nerve stretch (see pages 194 to 202).

(2) EXCESSIVE BLEEDING

What is commonly termed "flooding" is medically known as menorrhagia. Menstrual bleeding would be considered excessive if you had to change sanitary protection every couple of hours or through the night, or if large clots formed.

It may be a sign of:

- hormone imbalance
- stress
- genetic predisposition
- blood clotting disorder
- problem with your uterus such as fibroids
- pelvic infection
- ectopic pregnancy
- miscarriage
- IUD.

It is important to get an accurate diagnosis from your health practitioner as the problem may be serious. Treatment, of course, will depend on the cause.

BACH FLOWER REMEDIES

Remedies that may be useful include rescue remedy plus willow for resentment of the body, and hornbeam and mustard for lack of energy, especially if ANAEMIA is involved. Walnut is good for protecting the self and it will enhance the other remedies.

HERBALISM

There are many herbs that have an astringent action on the uterus including golden seal and shepherds purse. A herbalist can prescribe suitable ones for your individual condition.

HOMOEOPATHY

Sepia is probably the most commonly prescribed remedy but see a homoeopath for a holistic treatment to suit your physical and mental state.

MODERN MEDICINE

The treatment varies considerably depending on the cause, from hormone therapy to hysterectomy (relatively few cases nowadays). The general practitioner may refer you to a specialist such as a gynaecologist. Diagnostic testing may include a Dilation and Curettage (also known as a D and C), which is an exploratory operation under anaesthetic, or a hysteroscopy, where a tiny "telescope" is inserted through the cervix under local or general anaesthetic.

NATUROPATHY

Deficiencies of vitamins K and C (take it with bioflavinoids) can affect your body's control of bleeding. Your iron levels should be maintained (through food or supplements) to prevent anaemic conditions from blood loss. B vitamins and zinc can also assist by regulating your hormones.

Although essential fatty acids, such as evening primrose oil, can assist with some causes of menorrhagia, excessive intake can interfere with blood clotting.

Try obtaining protein from a vegetarian diet rather than meat, as high levels of animal proteins in a diet have been linked with heavier menstrual flow.

REFLEXOLOGY

You can follow the same course of action as outlined for *Disturbances in the cycle,* page 333.

SHIATSU

In shiatsu terms, this condition is generally a result of a weak spleen not "holding" blood or heat in the blood, usually from a liver imbalance. A practitioner would work on these meridians.

YOGA

You can follow the same course of action as outlined for *Disturbances in the cycle,* page 333. Most yoga schools have a special soothing program you are advised to follow while you are menstruating — you should avoid inverted postures during this time.

MULTIPLE SCLEROSIS

Multiple Sclerosis (MS) is a disease that affects the central nervous system, causing permanent loss of function in the nerve fibres. It begins in young adulthood and early symptoms include muscular weakness, tremors and clumsiness, pins and needles in the limbs, blurry vision and disturbed speech. In more severe cases, INCONTINENCE may develop.

Symptoms may develop over hours or days but can then disappear and reappear in different forms. In some cases, only mild symptoms ever occur but the condition can progress over years, in spurts or as a slow decline, to loss of sensation, paralysis and loss of vision.

Its causes are not quite understood. Doctors think it could be connected to a weakness in the immune system or a virus, but it is not contagious. It appears to be aggravated by stress, infections, allergies and injuries.

There is no "cure" although the progress of the disease can be slowed.

WHAT YOU CAN DO

- In a condition such as this it is important to minimise the stress in your life and increase your ability to relax (see page 40).
- Ensure you maintain a healthy diet low in fats and high in fibre. Do not take stimulants such as coffee, tea, chocolate and cola and avoid cigarette smoke, sugar and alcohol as they hamper the healthy function of the body.
- Regular moderate exercise will help maintain muscles in optimum condition.
- Do not allow yourself to become overweight as this can put extra strain on muscles.
- Avoid extremes of hot and cold.

ACUPUNCTURE

Acupuncture can relieve some of the symptoms of MS and can strengthen muscle function.

AFFIRMATION

Some people believe this condition may be linked to deep feelings of insecurity so an affirmation such as the following may be beneficial: "I move freely in the world and trust that I am loved and supported at all times."

THE FELDENKRAIS METHOD

Awareness of the function of pelvic and spiral movements can help if you have limited mobility or insecure balance. The Feldenkrais Method can assist by stimulating the function of your nervous system.

HERBALISM

Herbalists don't usually treat people with MS unless they are under the direction of a doctor. Seek your doctor's advice if you would like to include herbal remedies in your treatment.

HOMOEOPATHY

Homoeopathic treatment of people with MS is known to be fairly successful. See a homoeopath for further advice and treatment.

MASSAGE

Massage is of great benefit to MS as it relaxes the whole body and helps reduce muscle spasms. Massage can also reduce numbness in the limbs if used regularly. Ensure you are treated by a qualified practitioner.

MODERN MEDICINE

Physiotherapy is the main orthodox treatment for MS but there are medications you can be prescribed, for example, short courses of steroid injections can help reduce the severity of acute attacks of muscular spasm. An eye patch may assist with double vision and speech instruction can help those affected by speech difficulties.

NATUROPATHY

CAUTION: *Read the information on page 167 before taking supplements.*

To help your nervous system when you have MS, naturopaths often advise taking plenty of essential fatty acids such as evening primrose oil (3000 mg per day) and fish oil (3000 mg per day) as well as lecithin (2 tablespoons per day), high potency B complex vitamins (take as directed on label), calcium (800 mg per day) and magnesium phosphate (400 mg per day). Also cut out saturated animal fats and ask your naturopath to prescribe a specific allergy-free diet.

OSTEOPATHY

Osteopathy can help you maintain the mobility in your body if you have MS by reducing muscle contracture and keeping joints moving.

REFLEXOLOGY

Work these points: the whole spine as the main reflex, all the glands for hormonal balance, and the diaphragm for relaxation and stress reduction. Try this on both feet or hands for a total of 20 minutes two or three times a week.

SHIATSU

If your MS is in remission, shiatsu can help boost your immune system and increase your feeling of well-being. If you are currently experiencing the symptoms of MS, shiatsu can help balance the kidney, bladder and gall bladder meridians in your body to increase your mobility and general vitality. Oriental sotai exercises are also good for strengthening your muscles. These are corrective and resistive exercises that can be performed with a practitioner or alone. A shiatsu practitioner will advise you on the best exercises for your condition.

YOGA

If you have MS you can use yoga to build up your remaining muscular capacity. Yoga relaxation and meditation techniques can also help you accept the changes happening to you while making the most of what you do have.

NAUSEA AND VOMITING

Nausea is the feeling of sickness in your stomach. It can sometimes be accompanied by vomiting.

Nausea is a symptom only and may have a variety of causes, including:

- ANXIETY and stress
- shock or distress
- side effect of a drug
- low blood sugar
- dehydration
- too much alcohol or a HANGOVER
- ALLERGIES
- DIGESTIVE PROBLEMS
- LIVER and GALL BLADDER PROBLEMS
- HEADACHE (especially in children) AND MIGRAINE
- PAIN
- virus
- FOOD POISONING
- poisoning (see page 399).

It is a symptom of a large number of illnesses such as HEPATITIS.

Some women feel nausea during pregnancy — this is known as morning sickness (see page 338).

IMPORTANT: *Seek medical advice if nausea or vomiting persists or is severe, if the nausea is accompanied by sudden severe pain in the chest or abdomen, or if there is blood in the vomit.*

WHAT YOU CAN DO

- Eat small meals without drinking and sip moderate amounts of fluid between meals.
- Try eating a dry cracker or toast to settle the stomach. A good rule of thumb when feeling nauseous is to eat small amounts of light carbohydrates first, then add some light protein when your stomach has settled. Fatty foods should be avoided.
- A few spoonfuls of concentrated syrup of sugar in water may also help as can flat, lukewarm soft drinks such as lemonade or ginger beer. All drinks should be room-temperature or just warm, but not cold.
- Antacids are not designed for nausea and will only assist if your nausea is mild and associated with indigestion. They are useless if you are vomiting.
- MEDITATION and visualisation (see page 48) can bring relief from nausea in some cases, as can channelling HEALING ENERGIES to yourself.
- Allowing yourself to vomit can bring instant relief to the relentless queasiness. Often your body needs to rid itself of that which is causing you nausea.
- Vomiting causes you to lose fluid and nutrients that need to be replaced. Sip clear light liquids, or an electrolyte-replacement fluid.

ACUPRESSURE

When you are feeling nauseous one of the best ways to deal with it is through acupressure — try Conception Vessel 24 especially in women or Stomach 12 in men.

For motion sickness and in pregnancy, the point is Pericardium 6. It can be found in the middle of your forearm, between the tendons, two thumb widths above the crease on your wrist when your arm is turned palm up. Hold it firmly then move the pressure downwards towards your hand for about a minute at a time, breathing freely.

ACUPUNCTURE

As with acupressure, needles may be used for relieving nausea and its associated stomach pains, including an acute condition. Practitioners will often advise patients on the use of acupressure points.

AFFIRMATION

If you are feeling nauseous because you are feeling afraid or anxious, you could try an affirmation such as: "I accept fear and move forward knowing courage is my guide".

AROMATHERAPY

If your nausea is associated with emotional concerns the best essential oils to use are sandalwood and lavender. If it is food that is upsetting your stomach or you have motion sickness, peppermint will provide the greatest relief.

Inhalations are the most effective and convenient ways of treating nausea: sprinkle a few drops of the appropriate oil on a tissue or handkerchief and inhale as necessary — you can keep doing this throughout the day.

You can also have a gentle abdominal massage or soothing bath to relieve symptoms, it just depends how your body best absorbs the oils.

BACH FLOWER REMEDIES

Holly and willow remedies will help your liver which may be a cause of your nausea. They are also used to soothe deep anger and bitterness — emotions associated with the liver and gall bladder. Strong emotions such as these may also be a factor in making you feel sick.

CHINESE HERBS

In Chinese medicine nausea is said to be caused by stagnant Qi energy in your body, obstructed moisture, an imbalance of your liver network and disharmony in your organs. Chinese herbs can be used to clear up these imbalances and reduce your nausea. See a Chinese herbalist for advice and treatment. The over-the-counter patent medicine Er Chen Tang (citrus and pinellia combination) is an effective first aid treatment.

CHIROPRACTIC

Chiropractors find that unexplained bouts of nausea can often be relieved by regular chiropractic care which normalises nerve function.

COUNSELLING

Recurring or unexplained feelings of nausea can present as a symptom when something is making you "feel" ill. Consult a counsellor if there could be an emotional component to your nausea.

MORNING SICKNESS

Morning sickness is a common problem in the first few months of pregnancy. Symptoms include vomiting and nausea which is caused by the change in the levels of hormones and does not always occur in the morning despite the name.

Doctors usually avoid prescribing drugs for morning sickness but in severe cases, some medication may be given. You do have other options.

Herbal teas of black horehound or ginger or peppermint can bring relief — try a cup before you get out of bed. Vitamin B6 (100 mg twice a day with food) can also help to reduce morning sickness. There are a number of homoeopathic remedies that can be used to great effect under the direction of a homeopath.

Treatment from an acupressure practitioner, shiatsu therapist or a reflexologist may also relieve your nausea but make sure you consult a qualified and experienced practitioner as incorrect treatment can cause problems (see pages 87, 170, 178).

Morning sickness is much less likely to occur if your nutrition is adequate for several months *before* you conceive.

During your pregnancy, eat small amounts of complex carbohydrates and proteins, often, to help combat fatigue by keeping your blood sugar levels stable. Almonds and other nuts, seeds and wholegrain breads are good for this. A protein food eaten last thing at night can help to prevent low blood sugar levels and nausea the following morning, as protein takes longer to digest than other foods.

MOTION SICKNESS

Seasickness, airsickness, carsickness are all likely to be caused by motion and a difficulty in communicating what your eye sees to the inner ear mechanism that makes the necessary balance adjustments. As well as nausea and sometimes vomiting, dizziness, sweating and pale clammy skin are all part of motion sickness.

- Over the counter medication is available which works as a preventative for some people. They are usually antihistamines or scopolamine — the latter is also available as a patch to be absorbed through the skin. These medications may cause drowsiness and can't be taken while controlling a vehicle. Some have constipation and dry mouth as side effects.

- There are homoeopathic remedies to prevent motion sickness. Some are available in health food stores although it is best to get a prescription from a homoeopath.

- Try chewing on candied ginger to prevent and relieve nausea. Sucking on a lemon may also stop you producing excess saliva, an early part of the problem.

- Try the acupressure points listed on page 337.

- Eat lightly before and during travel. Get sufficient rest before travelling (fatigue makes you more susceptible) and avoid alcohol if you are sensitive to motion sickness.

- Avoid cigarette smoke, exhaust fumes and unpleasant odours. Give yourself access to plenty of fresh air if possible — open a window or go onto the boat deck.

- Visual sensitivity to rapid eye movements and watching things in motion, especially when trying to focus, may be the cause of motion sickness for many people, including those who feel ill when reading in a car, baiting hooks while on a boat, or even when watching a fast-moving sport.

- Keep your head as still as possible. Sit in the front seat of a vehicle and look ahead so you can see where you are going. This will help you balance yourself — taking the driver's seat and control of the vehicle is even better. However, if you can't handle a moving environment, such as a bobbing horizon from a boat, you may be better off focusing your attention on a fixed point inside the vehicle. On a large boat, take up a position midship where the least movement occurs. Travelling at night, when you can't see details as clearly, may help.

- You can learn how to desensitise yourself to this visual problem — see an optometrist, opthamologist or natural vision specialist for details.

- Motion sickness can be largely psychological. Do not assume you are going to feel sick, and try to distract your thoughts, occupying your mind and attention with pleasant things. Stay away from any other people who are feeling sick.

HERBALISM

The herbs that are most commonly used to treat nausea include chamomile, cinnamon, fennel, marshmallow, dill, meadowsweet, peppermint and black horehound.

Black horehound can be used fresh from your garden. Pick a two-inch stem and make it into a herbal infusion in a cup of hot water. Or you can take ginger tablets or drink ginger tea. This will help relieve feelings of nausea but only if you haven't vomited.

If you have vomited, drink peppermint tea until your stomach settles down.

HOMOEOPATHY

Homoeopaths believe that nausea has constructive purposes so you should only take homoeopathic remedies if your nausea does not go away in a day.

But if you are not coping well and you feel the need to vomit but nothing comes out and you have recently eaten too much, take one 6C potency of *Nux vomica* every hour for four doses.

MASSAGE

You may like to try a gentle abdominal massage in a clockwise direction following the large intestine. See page 137.

MODERN MEDICINE

Antiemetic medication is prescribed to help relieve nausea and vomiting. It is also used as a preventative e.g. with treatments such as chemotherapy.

NATUROPATHY

Nausea is often associated with liver dysfunction. For this reason high potency B complex vitamins may help long term with your liver function but don't take them on an empty stomach.

In terms of your diet you should stick with bland foods that are easy to digest such as steamed vegetables, stewed fruit, dry biscuits or toast. You should avoid fatty, greasy foods and any foods that contain sugar.

OSTEOPATHY

Nausea can be due to disturbances in the systems that control balance and co-ordination — these are in the central nervous system, the ears and the spinal muscles. It can also be due to digestive problems and biochemical changes in the body (such as those that occur in pregnancy). Osteopathy can help to minimise these disturbances through treatment of the whole body structure and thus may help to reduce your nausea in these circumstances.

REFLEXOLOGY

To help relieve symptoms of nausea work these points or ask a friend to: the stomach as a possible main reflex, the liver and gall bladder for digestion, and the diaphragm for relaxation.

For motion sickness, work the ear reflex for balance, the neck for muscular tension, and the cervical spine for the upper nervous system.

Regularly work the appropriate points on both feet or hands for a total of 10–15 minutes.

SHIATSU

A shiatsu practitioner can help relieve feelings of nausea by settling the stomach and liver meridians. See the Acupressure entry on page 337 for advice on self-help.

YOGA

Yoga exercises are effective in relieving nausea. Try the nausea relief exercise on page 200 if the problem is mild. It stretches the abdominal organs and pelvis.

NECK PAIN

Straining the muscles in your neck can cause neck pain as a result of poor posture, awkward movement, accident or general stress. If the muscles spasm, there may be stiffness and restricted movement.

Neck pain can cause HEADACHE and vice versa. It may also cause NAUSEA. The pain may extend to the back, shoulder or arm due to trapped nerves.

Neck pain may be a sign of a more serious condition and should be examined by a health practitioner if it persists.

See also ARTHRITIS, BACK PAIN.

WHAT YOU CAN DO

- Maintain flexibility in the neck by doing daily neck exercises designed to release tension and stiffness (see page 20).
- Neck muscles can tighten when you are physically tense or under mental stress so learn relaxation techniques (see page 40).
- Try hot and/or cold compresses. You can use towels wrung out in water, or hot water bottles filled with boiling water and iced water. Use one or the other, or alternate the two. The spray from a shower can have a similar effect.
- Over-the-counter heat rubs may provide relief.
- Practise good posture especially while sitting at a desk or computer (see page 56).
- Check your bedding — too many pillows or not using a pillow may give you a stiff neck, as can a bad mattress or sleeping on your stomach (the foetal position is recommended).
- If you are susceptible to neck pain, keep your neck warm and protected from cold, damp and draughts.

ACUPUNCTURE

Acupuncture can be effective in relieving acute and chronic neck pain. See an acupuncturist for treatment.

AFFIRMATION

A lack of connection between your mind and your body or feelings of stress and worry about your ability to deal with future events may result in neck pain. If this is the case, you may wish to repeat an affirmation like the following as many times a day as possible: "I am in harmony with my body. I am confident that I can rise to every occasion. I effortlessly release all unnecessary tension right now."

THE ALEXANDER TECHNIQUE

Through lessons in posture and movement, an Alexander Technique teacher can help you discover easier and more efficient ways of moving that don't put strain on your neck.

AROMATHERAPY

CAUTION: *Read the information on pages 102 to 105 before using these essential oils.*

There is nothing better than a good neck massage when you have a stiff or sore neck. This massage can be even more effective when you use essential oils because they work on the body's nervous system to release the tension and free up the muscles.

Get a friend (or even better, a professional aromatherapist) to give you a neck massage with the following oil combination: 2 drops each of lemon, sweet marjoram and cajuput oil mixed with 2 teaspoons of base carrier oil. These oils will lessen inflammation, relax the muscles in the neck and reduce pain.

BACH FLOWER REMEDIES

Rescue remedy can help if the pain is a result of shock (e.g. whiplash) or stress (e.g. muscle tension). Physical stiffness may also indicate inflexibility in mental attitudes or emotions so willow could be a useful treatment.

CHIROPRACTIC

Returning the nerves and spinal joints to their correct positioning is extremely beneficial in overcoming neck pain and problems. See a chiropractor for advice and adjustment.

THE FELDENKRAIS METHOD

Neck pain can be reduced by finding more comfortable ways of moving and understanding how to organise your skeleton to support your head. A consultation with a Feldenkrais practitioner can be of great benefit as it will provide you with a diagnosis of the cause of your pain if it comes from behaviour patterns (as is common) as well as providing effective treatment and techniques to avoid further problems.

HEALING MEDITATION

Read the chapter on HEALING ENERGIES and prepare yourself for meditation. See the blue healing energy entering your body through your crown chakra. When your body is vibrating with the blue light, bring your attention to your neck. Breathe the blue energy into your neck, particularly the sore areas. See every muscle in your neck relax with the blue healing light.

MASSAGE

If the pain is muscular, massage can be of great benefit and in most cases can bring speedy and often permanent relief. For best results, visit a professional massage therapist. You can also consult page 135 for advice and instructions on using massage at home.

You can massage yourself: use your palm and fingers to stroke from the base of your scalp to your collarbone, working both sides. Next, bring one hand across your body to the other shoulder and knead the area by squeezing and releasing — continue this movement all the way down the arm to the wrist and then back up again. Then, work your shoulder area more deeply using fingertip frictions. Repeat on the other side of your body.

Better yet, ask someone else to massage you. With the quick, do-anywhere massage on page 151, you are seated and can remain fully-clothed.

MODERN MEDICINE

Painkillers such as aspirin and paracetamol can be quite effective on neck pain as can anti-inflammatory medications but these are only used in severe cases. Diazepam may be prescribed for severe muscle spasms. Physiotherapy, traction or a cervical collar may also be recommended in such situations. For immediate relief of moderate neck pain, doctors usually suggest heat packs and deep heat creams.

OSTEOPATHY

As with other areas of spinal strain, osteopathy has an important role to play in alleviating neck pain. An osteopath will check for alterations in the position and movement of your neck joints and relax muscle tension, gently encouraging a return of the normal function and mobility of your neck. Each patient is individually assessed to determine their own structural capabilities and needs.

REFLEXOLOGY

To help relieve neck pain have a friend activate these points or work them yourself: the throat/neck area as the main reflex point, the cervical spine for nerve function in the area, the shoulder/arm for muscular tension, and the diaphragm for relaxation. You can also work points for associated symptoms (e.g. HEADACHE) or affected parts (e.g. ears). Try this on both feet or hands for a total of 15 minutes twice a week.

SHIATSU

Shiatsu is effective in relieving any kind of muscular tension or spasm. The Ki energy which is blocked in your neck and shoulders will be released through shiatsu applied to the meridians in this area, usually the gall bladder and large intestine. The liver will also be balanced so that blood and Ki flow freely around your body. You will find your general vitality increases after a full treatment.

YOGA

IMPORTANT: *Only do movements that are comfortable for you — if you strain too far you may do damage to your neck.*

In yogic philosophy the neck is the seat of self-will or control. When there is neck pain it can reflect mental inflexibility or an inability to "bend the will". The neck tension release exercise on page 201 and its variation create more flexibility.

NOSEBLEEDS

Medically known as epistaxis, nosebleeds are usually caused by the rupture of a small blood vessel in the nose and occur when you experience a knock to the nose, blow your nose too hard or cause it irritation when the mucous membranes are dry. Some people have nose bleeds quite frequently if their nasal blood vessels are weak, and it may be associated with allergic rhinitis (hayfever), see pages 214 and 364. In children, nosebleeds may be spontaneous and are quite common. In adults, however, they may be a sign of a serious problem such as high blood pressure (see page 234).

A medical practitioner should be consulted if:

- you are bleeding from the back of the nose
- you are elderly, have high blood pressure and the nosebleed lasts longer than 10 minutes
- the episodes of bleeding are regular
- blood loss is severe
- the nosebleed follows a hit to the head that also causes concussion
- if it follows surgery such as a tonsillectomy
- if the blood is combined with a clear fluid.

FIRST AID FOR NOSEBLEEDS

1. Sit down with head slightly forward — this prevents you swallowing blood which can leave you nauseous. Loosen clothing around the upper body.
2. Pinch nostrils together with thumb and index finger and breathe through your mouth for about 10 minutes. Alternatively, you can plug the bleeding nostril with cotton or gauze until the bleeding stops.

NOTE: *There is disagreement about whether you should blow your nose before applying pressure. Doing so may release a blood clot that could otherwise keep a blood vessel from closing. However, it may also cause further irritation and rupture.*

Cold, wet towels or an ice-pack can be applied to the back of neck and face during this time to narrow blood vessels and restrict blood flow. If bleeding lasts longer than 30 minutes, seek medical advice. After bleeding has stopped, treat your nose gently for a few days and avoid blowing.

WHAT YOU CAN DO

- Stress can play a factor so if you are susceptible to nosebleeds you may wish to try relaxation techniques (see page 40).
- If you are prone to nosebleeds avoid aspirin and foods containing salicylates (see page 407 for a list).
- The nasal cavity needs to be kept moist. Avoid smoking or smoke-filled environments, humidify the air using a humidifier filled with pure water and apply a lubricant such as petroleum jelly to the inside of your nose if necessary.
- Oestrogen levels also affect mucous membranes so the menstrual cycle and the Pill can have an impact.

AROMATHERAPY

CAUTION: *Read the information on pages 102 to 105 before using these essential oils.*

Lemon essential oil is effective in stopping bleeding by speeding up blood clotting. Soak a piece of absorbant cotton or a cotton wool ball in cold water that contains 2 drops of lemon. Insert this into your bleeding nostril while you are lying down and leave in until the bleeding slows.

CHINESE HERBS

If you experience nosebleeds regularly Chinese herbs can help consolidate the blood in your body to reduce the occurrence of bleeding, and may also recommend diet and lifestyle changes.

CHIROPRACTIC

Chiropractors find people prone to nosebleeds often have accompanying symptoms of neck and head pain. This can be relieved with chiropractic adjustment and will also reduce your nosebleeds.

HERBALISM

The herb yarrow is good for reducing and stopping nosebleeds. Yarrow will easily grow in your garden or you can buy it dried from your health food shop. Apply a cold compress containing yarrow to your nose.

HOMOEOPATHY

For nosebleeds that will not stop on their own accord, take one 6C potency of *Phosphorus* every hour for three doses. Replace this homoeopathic remedy with *Arnica montana* if the nose bleed is the result of a blow to the nose.

MODERN MEDICINE

For recurring nosebleeds it is possible to get the blood vessels in the nose cauterised i.e. burnt with a hot wire to seal the vessel.

NATUROPATHY

You can strengthen the mucous membrane and capillary walls with doses of vitamin C (2000 mg per day), bioflavinoids (1200 mg per day) and beta carotene (40 mg per day).

SHIATSU

In shiatsu terms, nosebleeds are diagnosed as heat in the blood and excess energy in the liver, heart or lungs which would be sedated through shiatsu pressure applied to these meridians.

OSTEOPOROSIS

Also known as "brittle bones", osteoporosis is the gradual loss of bone density and strength. The bones become weak and may break easily.

Throughout life, bone tissues are constantly building up and breaking down. A range of minerals (including calcium and magnesium) and exercise are necessary for this bone regeneration. The reproductive hormones also play a part in maintaining this balance. As hormone production decreases in later life, the breakdown exceeds the build-up and the process of osteoporosis begins. Menopausal women are most susceptible to osteoporosis because of the drastic reduction of oestrogen and progesterone in their body. It can, however, affect people in their mid-twenties.

Osteoporosis can also be caused by anorexia nervosa or overuse of steroids and diuretic drugs which increase calcium excretion.

Osteoporosis usually begins in the spine. The body's weight compresses the weak bones, resulting in a rounded back and loss of height.

The weakened bones are neither tender nor painful. The problem is that osteoporosis makes a person susceptible to fractures and the complications these can cause. Common sites of fracture are the hip, wrist and upper arm.

Osteoporosis can be prevented and its progress halted.

See also MENOPAUSE.

WHAT YOU CAN DO

- Exercising regularly will prevent the onset of osteoporosis and help slow down the effects of the condition. Exercising strengthens bones by increasing their mineral content. Walking is one form of exercise that is effective as a preventative; the heel striking the ground stimulates bone production.
- Ensure your diet includes calcium-rich and magnesium-rich foods such as dairy products, soya bean products, nuts, seeds, fish with edible bones (such as sardines and canned salmon) and green leaf vegetables. Vitamin D should be consumed at the same time (see page 15) as this assists the absorption of calcium. Be aware, however, that excess alkaline sources of calcium can be linked to kidney stones (see page 326).
- Don't eat excessive animal protein — it increases the excretion of calcium from the body. And avoid salt because the more sodium you excrete, the more calcium you excrete.
- Cut down on alcohol and caffeine which can put you at higher risk.
- If applicable, stop smoking as this affects hormone levels and the circulation of nutrients in your body.

CHIROPRACTIC

If chiropractic adjustment is in your health regime you are less likely to be prone to osteoporosis. If you have osteoporosis, chiropractic care can help and is safe as long as your chiropractor has full knowledge of your condition. They may need to take X-rays.

THE FELDENKRAIS METHOD

The gentle movement exploration exercises that Feldenkrais offers may help you reduce the chance of getting osteoporosis by refining your body's ability to bear weight to strengthen your skeleton. By recruiting your entire spine to reduce excess load in parts of your skeleton, the general function of your body can be improved.

HERBALISM

Herbs that keep your oestrogen levels high to prevent osteoporosis include true unicorn root, chaste tree and black cohosh. The other herbs that are often prescribed for this condition include herbs that are used for ARTHRITIS. A professional diagnosis is necessary for this condition, so see a herbalist for a specific prescription.

HOMOEOPATHY

Homoeopaths often prescribe holistically so that endocrine tone can occur thus balancing your glands to prevent further osteoporosis.

MODERN MEDICINE

In addition to advice on diet, exercise and smoking, hormone replacement therapy (HRT) may be used for menopausal women with this condition but it does have side effects and is not always protective against bone loss without exercise. It is advisable to fully discuss your options with a range of practitioners.

NATUROPATHY

Vitamin C and B complex vitamins (take according to the label) can help prevent osteoporosis. Also a calcium supplement (800 mg per day) and doses of magnesium phosphate (400 mg per day) are useful. If you already have this condition you can take calcium orotate, the best form of calcium to be absorbed into your bones. Vitamin D is also important.

A naturopath will give you specific dietary advice, including details of phyto-oestrogens (found in soya bean products, linseeds, sprouts and some herbs and vegetables) which are good for preventing menopausal bone loss.

OSTEOPATHY

Osteopathy may assist in the prevention and treatment of osteoporosis. Through treatment, diet and exercise, osteopathy can help you to maintain more mobility throughout your skeletal frame. An osteopath will use very gentle techniques, relaxing soft tissue and encouraging better blood circulation to your bones. They will not use manipulative procedures on the delicate bony structures.

REFLEXOLOGY

Work these points: the thyroid for its effect on the ovaries, the parathyroid to balance calcium levels, and the pituitary to stimulate all endocrine glands. Work the adrenal glands to produce oestrogen, reduce inflammation and regulate water balance, and work the ovaries for oestrogen release. The knees, legs and hips are commonly affected and these points can be worked to stimulate blood circulation in the area. Try this on both feet or hands for a total of 15 minutes twice a week.

SHIATSU

Shiatsu can help prevent osteoporosis in menopausal women by toning the bladder and kidney meridians which will, in effect, balance the hormones.

YOGA

If started early, regular yoga practice can help prevent osteoporosis. The condition can also be alleviated to some degree by yoga. This will make the most of the movement that is in your body and stretch the back, giving blood the chance to circulate, aiding regeneration. Yoga is gentle enough not to jar your body and yet active enough to have a positive effect on the calcium content in bones and bone density.

OVERWEIGHT

People become overweight when they consume more food energy than is required by the body — the excess is then stored as fat. Reasons for this disproportion include lack of exercise, a slow metabolism, an unbalanced diet or underlying emotional issues leading to overeating. In a limited number of cases, THYROID PROBLEMS may be the cause.

Obesity exists when a person is substantially (more than 20–30 percent) above their healthy weight range.

Being overweight is a threat to health as it requires the circulatory system to work harder. Breathlessness, FATIGUE and VARICOSE VEINS may be associated symptoms as can aching feet and joints caused by the greater weight they are supporting. Very overweight people are also more susceptible to HEART PROBLEMS, LIVER PROBLEMS, KIDNEY PROBLEMS, ARTHRITIS, CANCER and DIABETES. Even being 10 percent overweight can affect your health. (Remember, however, that being underweight, exercising excessively and having an inadequate diet can all adversely affect your health as well.)

WHAT YOU CAN DO

• Aim at long-term weight loss rather than quick-fix diets and set realistic goals for weekly weight loss. A 0.5 to 1 kilogram loss per week over a number of weeks is ideal.

• See THE IMPORTANCE OF DIET, EXERCISE AND POSTURE. You need to balance what you eat with what you burn up, either by increasing your exercise, reducing your food energy intake or both.

• Eat regular balanced meals, choosing from a wide range of foods that are high in fibre (this will help fill you up) and low in fat. High fibre foods include fruit and vegetables, breads, cereals and whole grains. Avoid refined carbohydrates and saturated fats.

• Healthy, low-fat and low-kilojoule food does not have to be boring. Look for recipes and food products that will bring interest to your meals and you will find it easier to maintain a good eating pattern. Steam, grill, bake and boil rather than fry and use spices, fresh herbs, lemon juice and vinegars to add flavour instead of butter, dairy products and oils.

• Drink plenty of water and sugar-free drinks which will fill you up and flush the body of toxins — a build-up of toxins will lead to the additional problem of

Fluid Retention. Avoid alcohol and soft drinks that are high in kilojoules and low in nutrients. Drink fruit juices only in moderation.

• Exercise at least three times a week to burn up kilojoules and increase metabolic rate. A fitness expert will be able to advise you as to your optimum heart rate for burning fat. Be as active as you can — take the stairs instead of the lift and walk to work if you can instead of taking the bus.

• Avoid fad diets but keep your eye out for useful hints that can help enhance your willpower and alter your attitude to food, such as focusing on your meals rather than watching TV, and learning to recognise hunger so that you only eat when you are hungry, stopping before you are overly full.

• Do not confuse temporary water loss with fat loss. Diuretics will only flush fluid from your system, as will steam baths and saunas. Even when dieting, initial weight loss is often water.

• Stress and other emotional issues may be a factor in your weight situation. Relaxation techniques can help. They may also shift your focus from food and help you feel better about yourself (see page 40).

ACUPUNCTURE

Acupuncture can be used to suppress appetite and excessive thirst using ear "hunger" and "thirst" points. However, feelings of hunger and thirst are often not the reason behind excess weight.

AROMATHERAPY

An aromatherapist will encourage you to treat your body with respect and create a nurturing environment to help you open up to an improved self image. Massage with aromatherapy oils may help with these things as well as improving your skin and muscle tone and boosting your self confidence.

COUNSELLING

As an addiction to food can be associated with many and varied issues, counselling can assist in finding underlying emotional reasons for your overeating. Some therapists believe obesity may be an unconscious way of "protecting yourself". For example, excess weight can be used to avoid sexual attention.

HERBALISM

Spirulina and psyllium husks can help regulate your appetite, and there are other herbs such as gymnema that can curb sugar cravings.

HOMOEOPATHY

Specific homoeopathic remedies are good for regulating your appetite when you are trying to lose weight and also for regulating your thyroid when your weight gain is linked to thyroid problems.

MODERN MEDICINE

Exercise and diet management under medical supervision is the recommended course of action in most cases. In rare cases, surgery may be carried out — to remove fat (see Cellulite) or to "staple" the stomach. Appetite-suppressing drugs are available but can have a serious impact on health (including addiction) and should only be taken under strict supervision. Do not use over-the-counter aids without advice. Laxatives should never be used for weight control.

NATUROPATHY

A naturopath will put you on a whole food, junk food-free diet and advise you on regular exercise. Eating small meals often is important to keep up your metabolism. Focus on fruit and vegetables but not too many nuts and seeds. Drink plenty of water (eight glasses a day) and eat absolutely no white sugar, white flour or white rice. Avoid dairy foods and meat and replace them with soya bean products, tofu, whole grains and beans.

Taking kelp can help speed up your metabolism and a good multi and B-complex vitamin can help regenerate your body. The amino acid carnitine is also an excellent fat metaboliser, especially in conjunction with exercise.

REFLEXOLOGY

To help balance your body's metabolism when you are trying to reduce your weight, work the point for the thyroid. Try this on both feet or hands for a total of 15 minutes two or three times a week.

SHIATSU

Shiatsu treatment is effective in supporting the body's elimination systems, balancing the digestive system, and regulating the appetite and thyroid function.

VISUALISATION

Read the chapter AFFIRMATIONS AND VISUALISATION and prepare yourself for creative visualisation.

Imagine yourself in a special room where you feel completely safe and secure. There is a beautiful ornate full-length mirror. In your mind's eye see yourself as you are now, standing naked before the mirror. Take in all parts of yourself and allow any feelings that surface to come naturally without judging them. If you feel emotions such as self-loathing or anger say the following affirmation to yourself several times: "I accept my feelings of powerlessness. I am safe and secure at all times. I am at ease with all my feelings. I love and accept myself exactly as I am right now. I rejoice in my strength and beauty". Say these words even though you may not mean them. If the negative feelings keep arising just allow them to be. Be gentle with yourself. Resist judging yourself for feeling negative. The first step towards change is accepting yourself exactly as you are now.

This part of the exercise can be difficult but it is worth persevering. Each time you do it you may discover a different set of negative emotions. Just keep accepting what comes up and realise what a multi-faceted human being you are.

When you have finished this part of the visualisation take another look into the mirror. See that you are holding a large crystal that is glowing with gold light. See yourself surrounded by this light and as it clears look in the mirror and picture yourself as you can be — a strong powerful person, at your perfect weight, skin clear, eyes shining, hair lustrous, energy and vitality vibrating from your every cell. Hold this vision for as long as you can and truly revel in the physical enjoyment of it.

If you are unable to visualise yourself naked then visualise yourself clothed, wearing a new outfit that makes you feel fabulous. Spend as long as you like on this part of the visualisation and when you complete it try and bring some of those positive feelings about yourself and your body back into your daily life.

You can assist this process by using your affirmation to replace any negative thoughts you have about yourself. This takes constant vigilance but it is well worth the effort.

Do this visualisation daily. However, after you have done it a few times and have exhausted the negative emotions you feel about yourself, drop the first part of the exercise where you picture yourself as you are now. Instead focus on the image of how you want to be and repeat the affirmation to that visualisation.

YOGA

Yoga is a good way of helping you control your eating habits as it can promote mastery over the mind which helps reduce cravings for food.

Yoga is also a gentle non-competitive exercise that can assist you to reduce weight; it is easy on your heart which will be burdened if you are overweight.

PAIN

Pain can affect all parts of your body and for many different reasons. It is the body's way of telling you that you need to make a change to improve your health. It may range from a slight twinge to chronic debilitating waves of pain.

Each person differs in their tolerance of pain, and the details of pain are hard to describe. Nevertheless, it is an important part of diagnosis and you should try to convey to your health practitioner the kind of pain you are experiencing: a dull ache, sharp and sudden, burning, throbbing etc.

No matter how mild, pain can be a signal of a serious condition. Seek medical advice for any persistent or chronic pain.

Pain is a symptom of a vast number of conditions. Consult the index and see also BACK PAIN, CRAMPS, FOOT SORENESS, HEADACHE AND MIGRAINE, NECK PAIN and STOMACH ACHE.

Emotional and psychological factors can play a significant role — see THE MIND BODY CONNECTION. Relaxation techniques and MEDITATION can also help you manage pain (see pages 40 and 152).

ACUPRESSURE

One of the quickest and easiest ways to relieve pain of all types — especially muscular — is through acupressure. Different pains require pressure in different areas. Consult individual entries in this book for self-help information but in all cases it is best to seek advice and treatment from a qualified practitioner.

ACUPUNCTURE

Acupuncture is widely known for its pain-relieving effect on all kinds of conditions. An acupuncturist will give you a thorough diagnosis and look for the underlying causes of the pain you are experiencing.

AFFIRMATION

It is said that we sometimes feel pain — emotional and physical — when we resist change. If you relate to this concept try repeating this affirmation to yourself as many times as possible each day: "I am willing to release the past and make any changes in my life which are for my highest good. I am at peace".

THE ALEXANDER TECHNIQUE

Muscular pain in various parts of the body can be prevented by learning the Alexander Technique as it will help you discover more efficient ways of sitting, standing and moving.

AROMATHERAPY

CAUTION: *Read the information on pages 102 to 105 before using these essential oils.*

There are many essential oils that help reduce pain whether it is muscular or internal. These include rosemary, bergamot, chamomile, lavender and marjoram. Your skin can absorb them from a bath, body massage, steam inhalation, tissue inhalation or oil burner. You may like to start by taking a bath containing four drops of any of the above oils. If you benefit from this, it may be worth consulting an aromatherapist for further treatment.

BACH FLOWER REMEDIES

Rescue remedy may reduce pain of any kind.

CHINESE HERBS

The over-the-counter patent medicine Yunnan Pai Yao is known to be effective in providing first-aid relief for various kinds of pain, including that associated with bruising, swelling and wounds. Among the many pain-relieving herbs that may be prescribed by a Chinese herbalist, paeonia and licorice combination is recommended for muscle pain and spasm.

CHIROPRACTIC

Pain that has a mechanical cause, like a sports injury or a car accident, can be helped with chiropractic adjustment. Headache and migraine pain is also reduced with chiropractic care. The adjustments reduce the subluxations along the spine which often cause pain by interfering with the nervous system.

COUNSELLING

Physical pain can mirror emotional pain, bringing up feelings of vulnerability and fragility. A counsellor can help you deal with these emotions.

THE FELDENKRAIS METHOD

Learning the Feldenkrais Method from a practitioner may help you reorganise your movement patterns or habits so that you can recognise the relationship between pain and movement.

HEALING ENERGY

Healing energy is known to be a very powerful tool to help people work through their pain (both physical and emotional). Read the chapter on HEALING ENERGIES and ask someone to channel energy to you or channel it to yourself. In particular, focus the blue light on the painful area of your body and breathe into it — try to relax your body as much as possible.

HERBALISM

The herb or herbs that can be used depend on what type of pain you are experiencing. Herbs that help relieve pain in general include black cohosh, hops and cramp bark. White willow bark tablets, available from your health food store, are the herbal equivalent of aspirin. Other herbs that can be used for pain relief because of their calming effects include valerian, skullcap and oats. Rue is very good for muscular pain — rub a rue ointment into the affected area for about half an hour to let it sink in.

HOMOEOPATHY

If experiencing nerve pain, rub *Hypericum* cream on the painful area three times a day. If the pain is worse when you sleep, make sure one of the applications is just before going to bed. *Arnica montana* cream can be used for bruises, strains, aches and pains. You can also take either *Arnica* or *Hypericum* internally for greater effect.

MASSAGE

It is automatic for a person to rub a sore spot because touch, in itself, can soothe and comfort both the mind and the body. Massage encourages the release of the body's own natural painkillers, endorphins. It stretches tight muscles and relieves spasms as well as easing the physical and mental stress that is associated with pain. Techniques will vary depending on the cause of the pain — for example, massage at home (see page 135) can ease a tension headache but remedial massage from a trained professional is recommended for more serious problems.

MODERN MEDICINE

No drug or combination of drugs will relieve all pain. Effectiveness depends on the individual and the condition. There are numerous groups of drugs available (see page 162). Some are available over the counter as well as by prescription, depending on the kind of pain that is experienced. Over-the-counter medication should be limited to temporary, minor ailments only.

Among the drugs available are analgesics (pain relievers) which include aspirin and paracetamol. Aspirin has an anti-inflammatory effect but can irritate the gastro-intestinal tract which can lead to bleeding and, therefore, ANAEMIA, with regular use. Paracetamol does not have this side effect but it will not relieve inflammation and an overdose can cause liver damage. Other anti-inflammatories include steroids and NSAIDs with the active ingredient ibuprofen which is available without prescription. Narcotics, muscle relaxants, and sometimes local anaesthetics can be used for pain control.

Liniments may be applied topically — rubbed into sprained muscles, for example — to create warmth in the local area.

For more details on medications, see the chapter on MODERN MEDICINE.

NATUROPATHY

CAUTION: *Read the information on page 167 before taking supplements.*

Take doses of phenylalanine (DLPA) (500 mg per day), calcium (800 mg per day), magnesium (400 mg per day) and high potency B complex vitamins (take as directed) to help reduce your pain. Phenylalanine has an analgesic effect and is used to build pain-killing hormones such as endorphins. This amino acid cannot be synthesised by the body but is found naturally in cheese, nuts, bananas, avocados, sesame seeds and other foods. The other vitamins and minerals help to relax the nervous system which is often overexcited by painful stimuli.

OSTEOPATHY

If your pain is related to joints, muscles and other soft tissues, an osteopath will be able to help you. They will treat your body framework to improve blood and fluid circulation and encourage normal nerve activity thus lessening the pain. They will also give you exercises for posture and mobility to keep your body in good structural order.

REFLEXOLOGY

To relax and reduce stress in the body when it is in pain, work the points for the diaphragm and solar plexus. Also gently work the reflex that corresponds to the area of pain e.g. shoulder, stomach. Try this on both feet or hands for a total of 15 minutes three times a week. If pain persists, consider seeing a qualified reflexologist.

SHIATSU

Shiatsu is effective in relieving all kinds of pain. In shiatsu, pain is an indication that too much energy is present in a particular part of the body so a practitioner will work to disperse the painful areas to improve the flow of Ki energy.

YOGA

As well as encouraging your body to function more efficiently, the meditation and relaxation side of yoga helps you control your mind to reduce stress and pain. Relaxation also releases stress-reducing endorphins in your body which naturally reduce pain. If you attend a yoga class regularly and practise the exercises at home you will find that pain will be reduced and your state of mind will be more in tune with your body.

PELVIC INFLAMMATORY DISEASE

Pelvic Inflammatory Disease (PID) is an infection that affects the female reproductive system. The symptoms include:

- pelvic discomfort and/or lower back pain
- vaginal discharge
- bleeding after sex or between periods
- DIARRHOEA
- bloating
- pain during urination
- FATIGUE
- sometimes fever.

It can be caused by a variety of organisms, which can be the result of a sexually transmitted disease (STD), an abortion, miscarriage or childbirth, surgery or appendicitis.

Some of these require treatment with specific antibiotics, which will quickly clear up the problem. In other cases, where the organism is no longer present, there is still residual inflammation and congestion which requires a more prolonged treatment program.

If left untreated the danger is that PID could cause scarring and reduced fertility. For this reason, medical diagnosis is advised. Other therapies can be used as an adjunct or to treat the illness when bacteria are not detected.

The onset of the condition may be insidious or acute, depending on the organism involved. In many cases (such as those involving chlamydia), the symptoms of PID are so mild that it goes undiagnosed and untreated. It can then develop into a chronic condition, creating problems which may not be detected until an investigation into fertility is carried out.

The organisms involved in PID may be sexually transmitted (such as in the case of chlamydia and gonorrhoea). Protected sex should reduce the risk of infection but if you have PID your sexual partner should also be examined and treated to prevent reinfection. In men, these organisms can cause non-specific urethritis (NSU).

See also BLADDER PROBLEMS, PROTECTING YOUR IMMUNE SYSTEM.

WHAT YOU CAN DO

- Practise safe sex by using condoms.
- For many women with PID, non-orgasmic sex may be painful due to the rush of blood it causes in the congested area.
- Therapies that involve working the lower back and pelvic region (e.g. chiropractic, yoga) can drain stagnant circulation.
- Any exercise that involves rhythmic blood flow to the area will help — belly dancing is ideal but swimming, walking and cycling are also good.

ACUPUNCTURE

As with other infections, acupuncture can assist the person's system to fight the disorder and heal itself. It may be used in conjunction with orthodox medicine but should be applied by a qualified practitioner.

AFFIRMATION

Repeat the following affirmation as many times a day as possible to assist your healing and counter any negativity you might be feeling about your femininity: "I enjoy being a woman. I rejoice in my sexuality."

HERBALISM

An anti-inflammatory herb that can be used to assist with this condition is meadowsweet. Herbs that fight the infection include echinacea, golden seal, St John's wort and poke root (with caution). It is recommended you see a herbalist for treatment rather than attempt self-treatment.

HOMOEOPATHY

Homoeopathic treatment from a qualified homoeopath can be effective in reducing the occurrence of the infections.

MODERN MEDICINE

Diagnosis involves a pelvic examination in which swabs are taken and analysed. There are analgesics that can reduce the pain and antibiotics or anti-inflammatory medication are prescribed if appropriate.

NATUROPATHY

CAUTION: *Read the information on page 167 before taking supplements.*

Vitamins and minerals that help the body fight PID include vitamin A (5000 iu per day), high potency B complex (take as directed), vitamin C (1/4 teaspoon of powder or 1000 mg every hour), vitamin E (500 iu per day), zinc (25 mg elemental per day) and beta carotene (20 mg per day).

OSTEOPATHY

It has been found in some cases that mechanical strains of the pelvic joints and musculature affect the support structures of the pelvic organs and may contribute to the condition. A consultation with an osteopath will determine if your situation may be helped by osteopathic care (this may need to be in conjunction with other treatments you undertake).

REFLEXOLOGY

As the main reflex, work the point for the pelvis as well as the area surrounding it. Also work the adrenal glands to deal with the inflammation, the lymphatic system and spleen to boost the immune system, and the diaphragm for relaxation. Try this on both feet or hands for a total of 15 to 20 minutes twice a week — be careful not to overstimulate.

SHIATSU

In Oriental terms, dampness in the spleen, deficiency in the kidneys and damp heat in the liver can all contribute to PID. See an experienced shiatsu therapist for diagnosis and appropriate treatment.

PERIOD PAIN

It is common to experience pain with a period but it can also be a sign of complications. Therefore, it is important to observe the pain closely.

Period pain either starts at the beginning of your period or immediately before, ceasing when the flow starts, or during the period when a clot or piece of tissue is being passed.

It is caused by the contraction of the uterus (which may be linked to hormone imbalance) or, in more severe cases, is connected to other gynaecological problems such as ENDOMETRIOSIS.

If the pain starts in the days leading up to your period you should also check with a doctor or naturopath for secondary causes such as ovarian cysts or PELVIC INFLAMMATORY DISEASE.

Some women feel pain at the time of ovulation and generally this is no cause for concern.

Women with lower back problems often experience pain during periods as the uterus places pressure on the nerve endings; the sciatic nerve (running from below the waist down the back of the leg) can be affected. CHIROPRACTIC, OSTEOPATHY, physiotherapy and remedial MASSAGE in regular treatment may, in particular, bring relief in these cases.

See also MENSTRUAL PROBLEMS, PRE-MENSTRUAL SYNDROME.

WHAT YOU CAN DO

- Keep your lower back and abdomen warm.
- Sit or lie with your legs elevated.
- Heat applied to the abdomen using a heat pad or hot water bottle can reduce pain as can a hot bath.
- Period pain may also be associated with muscle spasm in the lumbar area. Applying heat to the back, rather than the abdomen, can bring relief.
- Ginger helps relieve cramping — use it in your cooking and drink ginger tea.
- Although some women choose to avoid sex during this time, others have found that orgasm can relieve congestion.
- Rest is advised to relieve pain. Relaxation techniques such as MEDITATION will help relax muscles and focus your mind away from the pain.
- Good circulation is important in bringing oxygen to cramping muscles. Regular exercise (such as yoga or belly dancing) and bodywork (such as massage) can achieve this and also help tone internal muscles.
- Ensure you maintain a well-balanced diet that includes calcium, plenty of iron and B vitamins. During your period, cut down on salty and sweet junk foods and don't give in to cravings or you'll feel even more bloated and sluggish — the same applies to alcohol (although a glass or two may help some women by relaxing cramping muscles).
- Avoid CONSTIPATION during your period as bowel congestion can intensify the pain.
- Keep fluid intake high, especially if you suffer FLUID RETENTION, to stimulate kidney function.

ACUPUNCTURE

Acupuncture can be extremely effective in helping to relieve period pain as it unblocks the energy channels of the body and allows blood to circulate more easily and with less resistance. It regulates contractions, is stress relieving and can also be invaluable for alleviating pain from the sciatic nerve. Moxibustion may be used by the acupuncturist.

AFFIRMATION

Some period pain is believed to be emotionally linked to feelings of unease about your femininity. If you think this may be the case, try repeating this affirmation as many times as possible throughout the day: "I enjoy being a woman and accept the cycles of my body."

AROMATHERAPY

CAUTION: *Read the information on pages 102 to 105 before using these essential oils.*

Essential oils of cypress, clary sage, chamomile, marjoram and juniper berry are all known to be antispasmodic. They relieve menstrual pain by reducing cramping of the uterus.

It is best to start using any of the above oils ten days before your period to give them time to work. They can be absorbed into your body from baths or in massage oil.

As a first aid measure when you have period pain to reduce its severity, apply a warm compress containing 2 drops each of marjoram, chamomile and clary sage to your back and lower abdomen.

BACH FLOWER REMEDIES

Rescue remedy is the best remedy for period pain, although others may include hornbeam, mustard, willow and sweet chestnut. A qualified therapist can tailor treatment to your individual needs.

CHINESE HERBS

Chinese herbs are known to be effective in reducing period pain. See a Chinese herbalist for specific advice and a herbal prescription.

For home use, the patent medicine Wu Chi Pai Feng (which comes in pill form) has been known to assist menstrual problems including fatigue, fluid retention, anaemia, irregularity, cramps and moodiness. Yunnan Pai Yao can be an effective first aid for menstrual cramps.

THE FELDENKRAIS METHOD

You can learn strategies from a Feldenkrais practitioner to release muscle tension in your pelvic region to get relief from period pain.

HEALING MEDITATION

To help you restore internal balance and prevent period pain read the chapter on HEALING ENERGIES and practise the self-healing techniques. Channel healing light to yourself each day during the week before your period is due.

HERBALISM

Herbs that regulate the hormones and thereby reduce period pain include chaste tree, calendula, wild yam, false unicorn root and cramp bark. The liver herbs such as dandelion, barberry and St Mary's thistle are also important in this process. Black cohosh is another herb that can help reduce period pain and general mental distress.

Try mixing 24 drops of chaste tree tincture with 6 drops of calendula tincture in a glass of water. Drink this mixture three times a day for five days before your period starts. This can reduce the pain and tension in your abdomen but if your pain persists see a herbalist for herbs specific to your condition and accompanying symptoms.

HOMOEOPATHY

Some of the homoeopathic remedies that are most commonly used to treat period pain are *Colocynthis, Sabina* and *Sepia officinalis*. It depends on the type of pain you are experiencing as to which remedy you should take. If you suffer severe period pains on a regular basis, you should see a homoeopath for a full assessment of your condition. However, if your periods are painful only every once in a while, try one of the following remedies. If your period pain feels like a cramp in your abdomen and improves if you hold the affected area, take one 6C potency of *Colocynthis* every two hours for four doses. If your period pain feels like it is bearing down and is accompanied by fatigue and moodiness, take one 6C of *Sepia officinalis* every two hours for four doses.

MASSAGE

You can find relief in gently massaging the abdomen and lower back at the time of pain. At home, you can massage in circles in a clockwise direction for about 5 minutes. To massage your abdomen, lie down with your knees bent and use your fingertips to massage the area. To massage your lower back, lie on your side with a pillow under your neck and one between your knees and use your palm to massage the area.

Lymphatic drainage performed by a professional on a regular basis will generally give some relief from this problem.

MODERN MEDICINE

There are a number of treatments for period pain that relieve the symptom but not the cause: a variety of analgesics and anti-inflammatories is available both by prescription and over the counter. NSAIDs block prostaglandins and thus slow down contractions. The Pill prevents ovulation and can therefore be effective in reducing symptoms. Your doctor may refer you to a gynaecologist (a specialist in the female reproductive system) if a more serious condition is suspected.

Ultrasound or laparoscopy may be used to investigate the cause of pain, and surgery may be recommended if there are abnormal growths.

NATUROPATHY

Vitamins and minerals that help relieve the cramps associated with periods are magnesium phosphate, potassium phosphate, calcium (take these three as directed on the pack), vitamin B6 (250 mg per day in the second half of your cycle) and evening primrose oil (1000 mg three times a day through the whole of your cycle). The evening primrose oil will help regulate your hormones.

Other practical naturopathic advice is to eat no saturated fats as they can cause an imbalance in prostaglandins.

REFLEXOLOGY

The uterus, ovaries and Fallopian tubes are the main reflex points for this problem. Also work all points for the lower spine for nerve function in the area, all the glands for hormonal balance, and the diaphragm for relaxation and stress reduction. Try this on both feet or hands for a total of 20 minutes daily while the pain persists and then once or twice a week.

SHIATSU

In Oriental terms period pain is a result of imbalances in your blood circulation and hormonal system. These can be caused by the weakness and interrupted flow of Ki in your body. A shiatsu practitioner will work on your liver and your spleen because your liver stores blood and keeps the Ki flowing and your spleen controls the blood in your blood vessels.

If you are experiencing lower back pain as well as period pain, a shiatsu practitioner will tone your bladder meridian to reduce the pressure in your lower back area.

Shiatsu can also help regulate your periods and reduce their heaviness.

YOGA

Period pain can be more severe if you are feeling tense. Regular yoga practice can relieve stress. Most yoga schools have a special soothing program you are advised to follow while you are menstruating — you should avoid inverted postures during this time. The butterfly pose on page 194 is particularly good as it not only releases stress but frees up the pelvic area.

PRE-MENSTRUAL SYNDROME

Pre-menstrual syndrome (PMS) is a description of the symptoms a lot of women experience, on average, one to two weeks before their period. Some of these symptoms include mood swings, irrationality, irritability, aggression, tearfulness, DEPRESSION, difficulty concentrating, abdominal bloating, FLUID RETENTION, CONSTIPATION, food cravings, HEADACHES, FATIGUE, INSOMNIA, altered libido, outbreak of ACNE, breast soreness and BACK PAIN. Emotional symptoms are also known as pre-menstrual tension (PMT). Symptoms may vary in kind and intensity from month to month. For a few women, the symptoms are so severe they affect the course of their daily life.

There are a wide range of reasons for these symptoms caused by the altering hormonal levels in your body during this time, particularly an increase in prolactin hormone. However, many of the specific factors responsible for the symptoms have yet to be precisely identified.

WHAT YOU CAN DO

- Stress seems to make PMS even worse. Relax and try to stay positive and confident during these times. Don't set yourself unrealistic goals. Listen to soft music, have a warm bath and pamper yourself. Relaxation techniques can really help (see page 40).
- Avoid drinking tea and coffee as caffeine can aggravate skin problems and contribute to anxiety and irritability. Alcohol also seems to have a negative effect, as does smoking and the chemicals contained in cola and cocoa/chocolate.
- Try eating smaller meals more often during the day to keep energy levels in your body balanced.
- Eat foods high in fibre to help with bloating and constipation and to clear excess oestrogens.
- Cut down on salt to reduce fluid retention.
- Keep sugar in food and drink low even if you are craving it — sugar can have a significant influence on your symptoms, through fluctuating blood sugar levels.
- Limit your intake of dairy products to one portion a day as these can inhibit the absorption of magnesium which helps control oestrogen levels.
- Cut down on saturated fats such as meat and dairy as they cause an imbalance in prostaglandin production, necessary for correct hormonal balance. Increase oily fish (cod, tuna, salmon) and seeds (sunflower, sesame, pumpkin) in your diet, and use cold-pressed linseed or walnut oil in salad dressing.
- Take regular exercise to relax muscles and increase blood flow — half an hour each day is ideal. Exercise increases the production of endorphins which are "feel good" chemicals.
- Sex with orgasm may help relieve sluggishness and aching muscles and improve your mood.
- Talk about your PMS. It is now a widely known problem and people can be supportive and accommodating. There are even PMS support groups for chronic sufferers.

ACUPUNCTURE

The symptoms, and often the cause, of PMS can be relieved by acupuncture. See an acupuncturist for treatment and advice.

AROMATHERAPY

Some of the essentials oils that can balance the emotions include geranium, sandalwood, chamomile and lavender. You can start using them in baths and massage in one to two weeks (10 days is about average) before you start your period for the best results.

Try a bath with 2 drops of lavender and 3 drops of sandalwood, or mix these oils with 5 teaspoons base carrier oil for massage.

BACH FLOWER REMEDIES

To help stem irritability take impatiens, willow, beech or rescue remedy. If you feel depressed when you are pre-menstrual, gentian, hornbeam or mustard remedy can be of help. If you have trouble concentrating take scleranthus.

CHINESE HERBS

Chinese herbs are effective in relieving the symptoms of pre-menstrual syndrome. Bupleurum and paeonia formula, an over-the-counter preparation, gives good results in most cases. See a Chinese herbalist for a specific prescription.

CHIROPRACTIC

PMS can be reduced through regular chiropractic adjustment of the pelvis and surrounding areas.

THE FELDENKRAIS METHOD

Feldenkrais lessons provide an understanding of the tension that habitual movement builds up in your body. Awareness of this may help reduce pre-menstrual problems.

HEALING ENGERGIES

Read the chapter HEALING ENERGIES and prepare yourself for meditation. This may seem an effort when you are feeling the effects of PMS but it's worth it.

See blue light entering your crown chakra filling your entire body but especially your lower abdomen. In this area the blue light pulsates with a deeper colour and energy. Feel it revitalise all the cells of your body and release the tension from any areas that might be stressed.

Feel your spirit lift as the blue light pushes out any negativity you are feeling. To assist this process repeat the following affirmation to yourself like a mantra: "I revel in my femininity and I rejoice in my womanhood. I release all negative emotions and allow my body, mind and spirit to vibrate with peace and love."

Do this for as long as it takes for your mood to alter. Then see the blue healing light leave your body. before you close your chakra centres.

Use this meditation as often as you like.

HERBALISM

See PERIOD PAIN for advice on herbs that regulate hormones. These herbs and the liver herbs are useful for PMS. In particular, vitex is recommended to decrease prolactin levels.

HOMOEOPATHY

The homoeopathic remedy *Folliculinum* is sometimes used as a specific treatment for PMS but the correct dosage will need professional advice. There are many other remedies such as *Pulsatilla nigricans, Sepia officinalis* and *Nux vomica,* which are chosen depending on your emotional and physical condition. It is recommended you see a homoeopath for a reduction in the symptoms.

MASSAGE

Massage or lymphatic drainage to the lower back, abdomen and chest before the problematic part of your menstrual cycle will often prevent the onset of symptoms.

MODERN MEDICINE

As well as lifestyle advice, doctors may suggest vitamin supplements and diuretics to relieve some of the symptoms of PMS. Counselling may also be recommended to deal with emotional upheavals associated with PMT. Progesterone in various forms may be prescribed for the second half of the cycle to restore hormone levels.

NATUROPATHY

In addition to diet and exercise, naturopaths suggest evening primrose oil (1000 mg three times a day) taken a few days before the onset of PMS to help relieve symptoms. An increase in your intake of vitamin B6 can provide relief for mood swings and fatigue (250 mg per day). Magnesium can also help. You may like to try a daily mineral and vitamin pill especially formulated for PMS, available from pharmacies and health food stores.

OSTEOPATHY

PMS can sometimes be affected by problems in the spine, cranium and pelvis. Osteopathic treatment of your neuro-musculo-skeletal framework may assist.

REFLEXOLOGY

Work the reproductive system as the main reflex area for the problem as well as the pituitary for hormonal balance plus points that correspond to any other painful areas, such as tender breasts, or the bladder and kidney for fluid retention. The diaphragm reflex can also be worked for relaxation. Try this on both feet or hands for a total of 15 to 20 minutes daily during menstruation and for a week leading up to it.

SHIATSU

By smoothing the flow of Ki in your body a shiatsu practitioner will be able to reduce your irritability and depression before your period. With PMS, the Ki in your body is most likely to be blocked in your liver, spleen and heart meridians. The shiatsu practitioner will work on these areas as well as the hips and lower back.

YOGA

You can use yoga to help control your mood swings. Regular yoga exercise will relax your body and mind and make you less highly strung. Any poses that are good for liver conditions such the rocking backwards exercise and the inverted corpse on page 199 can help with irritability before your period. When your period is coming on you may like to increase your yoga exercise to keep up your blood circulation and calm your state of mind. A special menstruation sequence is taught by all Iyengar-trained yoga teachers and many women feel better after practising it.

PROSTATE PROBLEMS

The prostate gland is a small organ at the base of a man's bladder which produces the fluid that forms part of semen. It is wrapped around the urethra (the tube through which urine passes).

The most common prostate problem is *prostatitis,* an inflammation of the gland, often caused by bacteria — which can be sexually transmitted — or congestion. Symptoms include frequent or painful urination and aching around the groin and lower back. The urine may be smelly or discoloured. Sex may be painful.

After the age of 50, benign enlargement of the prostate is a common problem. The gland presses on the urethra making it difficult to urinate and empty the bladder. The flow of urine may be weak. Over time, the extra stress put on the muscles in the area can lead to complications such as urinary tract infection. Zinc deficiency may be a factor in this condition.

See also BLADDER PROBLEMS.

IMPORTANT: *All prostate problems should be diagnosed by a doctor to make sure there is no cancer present.*

WHAT YOU CAN DO

- Relieve the discomfort of prostate problems with hot sitz baths — soak for 20 minutes twice a day if possible. Or try alternating hot and cold compresses, applied to the lower back or lower abdomen.
- Drink at least eight glasses of water each day.
- Avoid food and drink that seem to aggravate the symptoms: all forms of coffee, tea, chocolate, alcohol, cola, nuts and spicy foods. Yeast, animal fats and refined white sugar should also be avoided.

• Avoid prolonged sitting and any bouncing movement such as cycling, riding motorbikes or driving trucks.

• If prostatitis is caused by bacteria, it may be advisable to avoid sexual activity until the infection is controlled. If there is no bacteria involved, ejaculation may be recommended.

• For a benign enlargment, avoid or reduce chemicals in the diet, epecially pesticides.

ACUPUNCTURE

Acupuncture from a qualified practitioner is effective in treating prostatitis.

CHINESE HERBS

Chinese herbs are exceptionally effective in treating prostate problems. See a herbalist for details.

HERBALISM

Herbs specific for prostate problems include saw palmetto, damiana and epilobium. These have proved very successful in many cases and may be part of a comprehensive treatment prescribed by a herbalist. Couch grass may be recommended if the urinary tract is infected.

MASSAGE

Prostate massage can be helpful in the early stages of enlargement as it relieves prostate congestion and inflammation.

MODERN MEDICINE

If prostatitis involves bacterial infection, a full course of antibiotics will be prescribed.

Until recently, prostate enlargement could not be managed with medication; new drugs are now available. The overgrown tissue may be removed in a surgical operation — infertility is a side effect but there is not necessarily a loss of sexual function.

NATUROPATHY

Zinc will help to reduce swelling. Take zinc (25 mg elemental twice a day), vitamin E (500 iu twice a day) and evening primrose oil (3000 mg per day). You can also increase your intake of zinc and phyto-oestrogens (plant oestrogens) through your diet by eating soya bean products, sprouts, linseeds and pumpkin and sunflower seeds.

REFLEXOLOGY

Work these points: the prostate as the main reflex, the bladder for the elimination of waste, the pituitary for hormonal balance and normal cellular growth, the adrenal glands to supplement the sex hormones secreted by the reproductive glands, and the lower spine for nerve function in the area. Try this on both feet or hands for a total of 15 minutes two or three times a week.

SHIATSU

Shiatsu can help reduce inflammation and pain by treating the liver and kidney meridians.

PSORIASIS

Psoriasis is a condition of the skin where the cells grow too quickly for them to be shed easily. It is characterised by itchy red patches covered by silvery scales which may become raw with open lesions. This can be psychologically and socially disturbing due to the skin's appearance.

Psoriasis is found mostly on the knees, elbows, trunk and scalp but it can appear anywhere on the nails and skin, including the penis or vulva.

It may be triggered by minor infections and ANXIETY in many cases and may also be hereditary. ARTHRITIS seems to be linked to psoriasis as both a trigger and a consequence. The causes are not known but it is not infectious. It should be diagnosed medically to prevent it being confused with other scaly skin conditions such as ECZEMA.

Psoriasis is a chronic, recurring condition that may disappear for more than a year between bouts. It can often be difficult to heal completely, although it can be improved. There is no specific cure. Each individual case varies in how it reacts to triggers and treatments.

WHAT YOU CAN DO

- Spending time in the sun, with care, often improves psoriasis. Use a sunscreen on skin that doesn't have psoriasis but expose red patches to the sun without protection for short periods.
- Keep skin from flaking and itching by applying moisturisers which help the skin retain water.
- Warms baths can soothe but hot water can make itching worse.
- Cold baths, ice cubes or a cold pack can help relieve itching, although some cases are aggravated by cold, becoming worse in winter, and humidity.
- Remove scales daily with alkaline-free soap and water and the gentle dermabrasion of a pumice stone.
- Tar products such as shampoos and bath oils are available over the counter and by prescription and bring relief to some sufferers.
- Covering a small, coin-sized area of psoriasis with tape or plastic for several days can be of assistance, but care should be taken the skin does not become too moist or infection may follow.
- Stress and tension can aggravate this condition and trigger an outbreak. Practise relaxation techniques (see page 40).
- Maintain a healthy immune system to keep up your defences against infections which will then reduce the likelihood of attacks (see page 31).
- Being overweight seems to make the condition worse.
- Avoid alcohol as it can trigger flare-ups.
- Lesions often appear on skin that has been damaged. Avoid injuries such as scrapes from blunt razors or chafing from watchbands. Avoid irritants, including cosmetics and chemicals, and wear loose clothing made of natural fibres.

AROMATHERAPY

Aromatherapy is excellent for reducing stress especially through full-body massage. The essential oils and a non-irritant base carrier oil will also help reduce the scaly appearance of the skin as they increase moisture content. It is best to consult a professional aromatherapist for an aromatherapy massage. They will test your skin for allergic reactions to any oils and choose the safest oils.

BACH FLOWER REMEDIES

Crab apple is the best remedy for psoriasis because it has a cleansing effect on the body. If the psoriasis is stress-related, take rescue remedy as well.

CHINESE HERBS

Chinese herbs are effective in reducing psoriasis. See a Chinese herbalist for advice and herbal prescription.

CHIROPRACTIC

Chiropractic treatment can reduce psoriasis because it helps normalise the function of the nervous system which contributes to the occurrence of this condition.

HERBALISM

Herbs that help cleanse the skin include yellow dock, burdock, dandelion, gentian, celandine, calendula and echinacea. A herbalist may prescribe a mixture of these along with a cream containing either evening primrose oil, chickweed, cleavers or aloe vera to relieve dryness and irritation. Apply the cream once or twice a day.

HOMOEOPATHY

Homoeopathy is known to be successful in treating psoriasis. See a professional homoeopath for advice and treatment.

MODERN MEDICINE

Ultraviolet therapy can be used on the skin as well as local creams to reduce inflammation and relieve itching. These may be steroid-based; however, systematic steroids are not used as the size of dosage required would have serious side effects. Other drugs are sometimes used for disabling cases, but again the side effects are severe. Keratolytics — skin preparations that remove the outermost layer of skin — can be used with care.

NATUROPATHY

CAUTION: *Read the information on page 167 before taking supplements.*

A naturopath would explore a number of possible causes and treat the symptoms and the causes. They may examine the possibility of the condition being stress-related or connected to liver dysfunction or CONSTIPATION. They may recommend you try a wholefood/allergy-free diet.

Most common naturopathic treatments include doses of evening primrose oil (3000 mg per day), linseed oil (2 tablespoons per day), beta carotene (20 mg per day), bioflavinoids (1000 mg per day), vitamin E (500 iu per day), zinc (25 mg elemental per day) and fish oil (3000 mg per day). Vitamin A may also be recommended. Psoralens, either applied topically or taken orally, can make the skin more light-sensitive which seems to impact on psoriasis. They are available in synthetic form or can be found naturally in celery, parsley, lettuce, limes and lemons. Fumaric acid taken internally as a supplement or applied topically is also good.

REFLEXOLOGY

Work all points that correspond to glands to aid hormonal balance; in particular, the thyroid for the skin and the adrenals for inflammation. Also work the kidneys, bladder, the small intestine and colon for elimination, the liver for detoxification, and the diaphragm for relaxation and stress reduction. Try this on both feet or hands for a total of 15 minutes three times a week.

SHIATSU

If your psoriasis is inflamed and covers a fair amount of your body it is not recommended you undergo shiatsu treatment as touching your skin will irritate it. However, if the inflammation disappears then shiatsu can be used as a preventive measure against further outbreaks.

All the organs in your body that eliminate waste products will be treated, particularly your liver, bladder and kidney. In Oriental medicine, the skin is considered an organ of elimination as well and the shiatsu treatment will ensure that Ki flows freely through your body to reduce the inflammation of your skin. The lung and large intestine meridians will also be treated to assist elimination and the nourishment of the skin.

REPETITIVE STRAIN INJURY

Repetitive strain injury (RSI) usually occurs from misuse, overuse or trauma of a muscle or the joint it controls. It is also known as overuse injury and is often a form of tendonitis (inflammation of the tendon) or tenosynovitis (inflammation of the tendon's sheath). Tennis elbow is one form of RSI; the most common is carpal tunnel syndrome which affects the nerve that passes through the wrist.

Symptoms of RSI include pain and stiffness in the affected part and often tingling or numbness. Sufferers may find it difficult to pick up objects. It is a chronic condition that can be difficult to treat while people continue with the repetitive activity. There may also be a psychological factor to some cases and stress may predispose a person to RSI.

The wrist, forearms and hands are often affected, with the pain spreading to the neck and shoulders. The complaint is most commonly experienced by those who spend long hours on computer keyboards or by people who work on assembly lines.

WHAT YOU CAN DO

• The main advice in all forms of treatment is rest the affected part. You must try to stop the repetitive activity for a while if possible.

• Hot compresses and warm baths should ease the pain, so should a heat pad or hot-water bottle. Keep the affected area warm (with clothing) and supported (a bandage or splint may help).

• After use, the muscle may gain relief from an ice pack. Some people feel improvement with daily ice water compresses or soaks, rather than warm water treatments. *These however are not recommended for those with heart problems or diabetes.*

• Elevating the affected area will counter swelling.

• Strengthen your muscles with exercises and ensure they are warmed up before exerting them.

• Take frequent rests from your activity and stretch and move your muscles in the opposite direction to the repetitive action.

• Regularly practise progressive relaxation of all the parts of your body to rid yourself of tension (see page 196). Before sleep is a good time for this.

• If a sports injury, consider taking private lessons to correct your performance.

• Take a close look at your working conditions and get professional advice from specialists in the field. If you are working at a desk and keyboard ensure you are seated at the right height and that your arms are at an angle of 70° to 90° to your abdomen. Your feet should be fully on the floor with your back straight and supported by your chair.

ACUPUNCTURE

Any kind of overuse of the muscles or joints can be helped by acupuncture. See a qualified acupuncturist for treatment and advice.

AFFIRMATION

It can be important to find fulfilment in the work you do. A work-related health problem may be your body's way of telling you that you are not happy, especially if you are the type of person who "pushes yourself" to fulfil expectations. If you relate to this concept try repeating the following affirmation as many times a day as possible: "I willingly release unnecessary strain in my life".

THE ALEXANDER TECHNIQUE

The Alexander Technique is highly successful in identifying and dealing with the cause of RSI. It helps prevent and relieve problems through re-education of movement and posture for more efficient and less painful ways of moving.

AROMATHERAPY

See ARTHRITIS; the same technique can be used.

CHIROPRACTIC

When your muscles are working under abnormal stresses they often lack correct connection in the central nervous system. This can be improved by chiropractic assessment and adjustment. Chiropractic care can also help you get additional movement in stiff, sore joints through suggested exercises.

COUNSELLING

You may be susceptible to RSI if you do not like the work you are doing. If you think this could be the case, counselling may be beneficial to help you discover the type of work that would satisfy you.

THE FELDENKRAIS METHOD

The Feldenkrais Method is highly successful in identifying and dealing with the cause of RSI. For example, learning to sit in different ways and monitor movement patterns is a useful skill for various occupations. The Method offers you the chance to learn to sit in a way which engages your large muscles for stability and involves minimal muscle activity. This can improve the efficiency of your upper trunk muscles for fine light work and enables you to increase your postural stamina.

HEALING ENERGY

Some people with RSI report they feel as if energy is trapped in the affected part of their body. This energy imbalance can be assisted by energy healing. Either seek healing from a therapist or someone you know or read the HEALING ENERGIES section and learn to channel healing energy to yourself. When you are practising self-healing you can visualise the blue healing light pushing the excess energy from your body and the injured area returning to natural balance.

HERBALISM

Herbs with muscle relaxant and nervine properties may be prescribed by a herbalist. The herbs used for ARTHRITIS are often used to help RSI.

HOMOEOPATHY

Homoeopathic remedies such as *Ruta graveolens* are useful in reducing the pain of RSI but they should be prescribed by a homoeopath who will fully assess your condition.

MASSAGE

Temporary relief may be obtained from massage of the area, increasing circulation and bringing warmth

MODERN MEDICINE

Analgesics or anti-inflammatory drugs may be prescribed; aspirin can bring relief. Severe cases may be injected with a local anaesthetic or steroid. However, repeated steroid injections will weaken the tendons and lead to an increased risk of rupture under pressure. Doctors will generally refer you to a physiotherapist. The physiotherapist will advise you on what exercises you can do to reduce the strain on your tendons and give you postural advice. In severe cases, surgery may be recommended to relieve the compression.

NATUROPATHY

Try taking 3000 mg evening primrose oil and 250 mg of vitamin B6 each day to help reduce swelling and inflammation.

You should also make sure you are eating a wholesome diet. A naturopath can give advice about foods that will assist your condition.

OSTEOPATHY

RSI can be effectively reduced by osteopathic treatment. Osteopaths will address the mechanical strains of the affected region and also the other joints which contribute to the movements of the limb. They will use soft tissue massage and gentle articulation of the joints involved. Anti-inflammatory procedures such as hot and cold compresses, specific exercises or rest and strapping may also be recommended.

REFLEXOLOGY

To help relax the body and reduce stress when you have RSI, work the diaphragm reflex for 10 to 15 minutes twice a week. If the pain is in your hands and arms, ask a friend to work on your feet for you.

SHIATSU

Shiatsu can help relieve the pain and occurrence of RSI wherever it is in your body. By gently balancing your meridians and promoting smooth-flowing Ki energy, shiatsu reduces the general stress on your body. A practitioner can target strained body areas and give you specific exercises to prevent overstress in the future.

YOGA

Yoga is an exercise that is gentle on your joints and muscles, yet strengthening. If your body is fit from regular exercise, it is less likely to suffer strain.

The gentle exercise of yoga is also suitable for people recovering from RSI. If you have RSI ask a yoga teacher which exercises they would recommend for the strained part of your body.

SCIATICA

Sciatica is due to irritation of the sciatic nerve which passes from the lower end of the spinal cord into the back of the leg down to the foot. This irritation can be due to pressure on the nerve anywhere along its path. There are many possible causes ranging from a minor muscular strain in the lower back or pelvis causing swelling around the nerve, to a disc protrusion ("slipped disc') trapping the nerve root, or perhaps the position of a foetus during pregnancy.

It is a symptom, not a diagnosis. You need to treat the aggravation causing your sciatica. Your sciatica may be a one-off occurrence or it can flare up at times depending on the underlying condition. See also Back Pain.

WHAT YOU CAN DO

- Get lots of bed rest on a firm, supportive mattress. A board under your mattress can provide extra support.
- Try this resting posture: lie on your back with your legs lifted on a pile of pillows. Your knees should be

bent, your thighs positioned at 90° to your back and the pillows placed under your calves — like you are sitting on a chair but rather you are on your back.

• Soaking in a warm bath for 20 minutes may bring temporary relief from pain, as will long hot showers.

ACUPRESSURE

Most cases of sciatica will improve after consistent acupressure treatment from a qualified practitioner, who may also advise on how you can use acupressure at home.

ACUPUNCTURE

Acupuncture is known to be effective on sciatica and is being used by a significant number of medical practitioners, as well as qualified acupuncturists, to treat this condition.

AFFIRMATION

It is possible that, along with the physical numbness of sciatica, there may be numbness on an emotional level. If so, an affirmation like the following may help: "I open myself to experiencing my feelings because it is safe and I am supported at all times".

AROMATHERAPY

Aromatherapy massage is not recommended for treating sciatica but cold compresses may help reduce the irritation and relieve pain.

Apply a cold compress sprinkled with 2 drops each of chamomile and lavender to the affected area. Leave for 15 minutes and repeat this three times a day.

CHIROPRACTIC

Pelvic problems and chronic lower back pain can be contributing factors to sciatica. Both of these can be reduced by gentle chiropractic adjustment.

THE FELDENKRAIS METHOD

If your sciatica is a result of strained spinal movement the Feldenkrais Method can help you by teaching you new and more efficient ways of moving that don't injure your spine.

HERBALISM

Herbs that help relieve sciatica include St John's wort, black cohosh, Jamaican dogwood, calendula and yarrow. They are analgesic herbs that can dramatically relieve pain.

Ointment containing rue will give you relief from severe, deep-seated pain. Apply to your skin three times a day, massaging for about half an hour to allow the herb to do its work. Massaging the lower back with oil containing St John's wort is very effective.

MASSAGE

Massage from a professional therapist may give relief to both the back and legs and can also relax the rest of the body which may be stressed because of the pain associated with this condition.

MODERN MEDICINE

Doctors may refer you to a physiotherapist or recommend exercises. They may prescribe analgesics, anti-inflammatories or muscle relaxants. In severe cases, surgery is an option to relieve the pressure.

NATUROPATHY

Taking bioflavinoids (2000 mg per day), evening primrose oil (3000 mg per day), calcium phosphate and magnesium phosphate (take the latter two as directed on the packet) may help relieve your sciatica because they work as anti-inflammatories. Bromelain is also excellent (800 to 1000 mg three times a day).

OSTEOPATHY

By taking a thorough case history and performing a physical examination (which may also require X-rays or scans in some cases), an osteopath will be able to diagnose the cause of sciatica and formulate an appropriate treatment plan. This may include gentle manipulation, soft tissue stretching, exercise, rest or postural advice.

REFLEXOLOGY

Work the sciatic area as the main reflex point as well as the points corresponding to the hip/knee area which may also be affected. Work all the points for the lower spine for nerve function as well as the shoulders and diaphragm for relaxation. Try this on both feet or hands for a total of 10 minutes twice a week — be careful not to overstimulate.

SHIATSU

Gentle shiatsu stretching techniques can be used to decompress your lumbar vertebrae and release any pressure on the sciatic nerve. When working on your sciatica a shiatsu practitioner will also balance your kidney and bladder meridians and your large and small intestine meridians — these are near your sciatic nerve and may be the source of tension in the back which can cause pressure.

YOGA

Remedial yoga poses can be of great assistance in treating sciatica but should be done under the supervision of a yoga teacher.

SHINGLES

Shingles, or herpes zoster, appears as clusters of small blisters, mainly on the buttock/thigh region, chest, neck and forehead and on one side of the body. After the blisters break, scabs and redness may last two to three weeks, and there may be some scarring.

The blisters are preceded or accompanied by severe pain which may remain after the rash disappears (sometimes for months).

Shingles is actually an inflammation of the nerve cells thought to be caused by the chickenpox virus. The virus lies dormant in the body after the person has had chickenpox in their youth but reappears later in life when the immune system is weak. It may also be contracted as an adult. Shingles usually occurs only once.

You cannot catch shingles from contact with the shingles rash, but you can contract chickenpox if you haven't had it before (see page 78).

There are health risks involved if the blisters appear on the face or if shingles appears in early pregnancy. Medical advice should be sought.

See also HERPES AND COLD SORES.

WHAT YOU CAN DO

- Rest is necessary to give your body a chance to heal.
- Wear loose, light clothing to avoid causing further irritation to the blisters.
- Take a cool bath a few times a day to help relieve pain. Lukewarm, wet compresses may also help.
- Keep your immune system protected (see page 31).

ACUPUNCTURE

Acupuncture can help. A qualified practitioner will seek to treat the cause of shingles as well as the symptoms.

AFFIRMATION

If you believe tension or stress may have triggered your shingles, you could try repeating an affirmation like the following as many times a day as possible: "I am totally relaxed and at ease in the world. My sensitivity is a strength".

AROMATHERAPY

Essential oils can be helpful in easing the pain of shingles. The oil that does this most effectively is bergamot because it is not only an analgesic but also an antidepressant. Add 3 drops of bergamot to your bath three times a week, making sure it is well dispersed in the water. This bath should relax you as well as lessen the pain. Be careful to only use this oil for two weeks then change your oil to a gentler one, for example, lavender.

HERBALISM

The herbs St John's wort, golden seal, oats, vervain and echinacea are all effective, not only for healing the rash you get with shingles, but for strengthening your immune system against the disease.

Herbalists have excellent results from the following herbal remedy. Mix 5 drops of St John's wort tincture and 5 drops of vervain tincture in a glass of water. Drink this mixture every hour.

You can also apply the following herbal mixture directly onto your rash as often as required: equal parts of St John's wort tincture, plantain tincture and water.

St John's wort ointment can be applied to your rash when you feel you can cope with this.

HOMOEOPATHY

Homoeopathic remedies are known to be successful in eliminating the pain of shingles. Those that work on the herpes virus are often used to heal shingles. See a homoeopath for a full assessment to determine what remedies will benefit you most.

MODERN MEDICINE

There is no specific "cure". Medication such as antiviral drugs can shorten the length of this condition if treated early. Analgesics can give pain relief during an attack. Other drugs, such as steroids, can be used in some cases to reduce nerve inflammation but they have side effects and may spread the infection so that it affects the entire body system.

NATUROPATHY

CAUTION: *Read the information on page 167 before taking supplements.*

Take vitamin C (3000 mg per day), vitamin E (500 iu per day) and zinc (25 mg elemental per day) to build up your weak immune system and reduce your shingles. The amino acid L-lysine is excellent (1000 mg three times a day). Avoid arginine foods (see the entry for HERPES AND COLD SORES).

REFLEXOLOGY

Gently work points that correspond to the problem areas. Also all the points for the spine to encourage healthy nerve function and the pituitary for hormonal balance. If there is any infection, work the lymphatic system and spleen to boost the immune system and the adrenal glands to deal with any inflammation. Working the diaphragm point will assist with relaxation and stress reduction. Try this on both feet or hands for a total of 15 minutes twice a week — be careful not to overstimulate.

SINUSITIS

Sinusitis is an inflammation of the mucous membrane in the sinus cavities. If the passages from the sinuses to the nose become blocked, a vacuum can form in the cavity causing intense pressure. If infection occurs, pus and mucus can also build up. This is why there is often pain, tenderness and swelling in and around the nasal passages and face, HEADACHE, toothache, watery eyes, fever and chills as well as a congested and runny nose.

Sinusitis can accompany COLDS AND INFLUENZA or can occur from ALLERGIES or a sudden change in temperature; or it can be due to a structural defect in the nose. The condition may be acute or chronic. Chronic sufferers may have a permanent thickening of the sinus membranes, are more prone to colds and may develop further health complications.

Consult a doctor if:

- you have a fever, cough or headache that persists for more than two or three days
- the sinus pain persists for more than three days
- you have swelling along the sides of your nose and swollen eyelids
- you have blurred or double vision
- the discharge is green or yellowish with facial pain or headache.

WHAT YOU CAN DO

• As prevention and treatment, keep the sinuses moist and well drained by regularly inhaling steam over a bowl of hot water or by running a humidifier in your bedroom at night.

• To ease the flow of material from your nose, try gently flushing the nasal cavity with a warm saltwater solution. Dissolve ½ teaspoon salt in 1 cup warm water. Place in a shallow bowl and sniff up the water into one nostril, holding the other nostril closed. Repeat for the other nostril. For a child, a small bulb syringe could be used, with care. This can be done a couple of times an hour if desired.

• A warm, moist cloth placed on the cheekbones and nose can help relieve sinus pain. Heat from a hot water bottle (wrapped in a towel) or an electric pad may also bring relief.

• Drink plenty of water and fluids during the day to maintain hydration and keep mucus from clogging.

• Some foods are great sinus clearers — horseradish, wasabi, hot English mustard, cayenne pepper, garlic, pineapple, papaya.

• There are techniques that can help you breathe easier (see page 25).

• Use nose drops and sprays with caution as frequent use can injure the mucous membranes or create a cycle of swelling and shrinkage thereby triggering sinus troubles.

• Avoid irritants such as smoke and air pollution.

• Avoid animal milk products (milk, cheese and yogurt from cows, goats and sheep). These increase mucus production. Substitute with soya bean products such as soy milk and tofu.

• Avoid cold temperatures — if you are prone to sinusitis, wrap a scarf around your face when outside.

• Avoid alcohol as it dilates the blood vessels and closes cavities further. The histamines in wine can be a great aggravation.

• Some people's sinuses flare up in reaction to stress. See page 40 for advice on how to handle it.

• If you have a cold, blow your nose gently, one nostril at a time, or infectious mucus may be forced into the sinus cavities, leading to sinusitis.

• Some sinus trouble is actually a stuffed nose and tension headache — this will be eased if you lie down. Sinusitis becomes worse when you lie down as the sinuses can't drain.

• You should also have a health practitioner rule out dental and eye problems.

ACUPUNCTURE

Acupuncture is known to be an effective treatment in acute forms of sinusitis. See a qualified practitioner for advice and treatment.

AFFIRMATION

Problems with your sinuses may be caused by an emotional "irritant" as well as a physical one. If this applies to you, try repeating an affirmation like the following as many times a day as possible. "I accept myself and others easily and effortlessly".

AROMATHERAPY

CAUTION: *Read the information on pages 102 to 105 before using these essential oils.*

Essential oil steam inhalations are an effective way of clearing the nasal passages and relaxing the body to give it a chance to heal itself. Before you go to sleep, try adding 4 drops of eucalyptus to a bowl of steaming water. Inhale the steam deeply with a towel over your head. This mixture can clear your nose as well as reduce the pressure in your sinuses but make sure you use good quality eucalyptus essential oil.

BACH FLOWER REMEDIES

If your sinusitis is related to stress take rescue remedy and white chestnut.

CHINESE HERBS

Traditional Chinese Medicine is effective in supplementing and protecting the balance of your lung network. An imbalance will make you prone to sinusitis. See a Chinese herbalist for advice and a specific herbal prescription.

CHIROPRACTIC

Many people have had success reducing their sinusitis with the help of chiropractic adjustment to their neck, shoulders and head. This increases the function of the nervous system to these areas and improves circulation.

HEALING MEDITATION

Read the chapter on Healing Energies and learn the self-healing techniques. When you have the blue healing energy flowing concentrate it in the area of your face and feel the blue light clearing, calming and soothing your sinus area.

HERBALISM

Herbs that help relieve sinusitis include echinacea, horseradish and garlic to combat the infection, marshmallow and comfrey to soothe irritation and soreness, golden seal and eyebright for their astringent qualities and chamomile, peppermint, hyssop, ginger and cinnamon to loosen the mucus.

Try drinking 3 cups of herbal sinus tea that has a selection of these herbs in it. It will also help if you take echinacea, and garlic and horseradish tablets (these two herbs come in the one tablet) to strengthen your immune system against the infection. Take them according to the instructions on the bottle.

HOMOEOPATHY

Homoeopathic remedies have helped many people with the pain of sinusitis.

If your sinusitis makes you dizzy and your nose is constantly blocked, take one 6C preparation of *Sticta pulmonaria* every hour for four doses.

If your sinusitis is felt as an ache and tension across the bridge of your nose, take one 6C potency of *Kali bichromicum* every hour for four doses.

If your condition does not improve within a few days see a homoeopath for a remedy more specific to your holistic set of symptoms.

MASSAGE

Massage may be of benefit in clearing the sinus passages and relieving sinus headache — try massaging the face and neck area. You can follow the steps for facial massage detailed in the full-body massage on page 140.

MODERN MEDICINE

Over-the-counter tablets, drops and sprays that contain a decongestant can be effective in relieving pressure, but not the infection. Steam inhalations containing menthol are the general recommendation as well as antibiotics to clear infection. Antihistamines are also recommended if the sinusitis has an allergic component, but these can also dry out the mucous membrane and exacerbate the problem. In some severe cases, surgical drainage may be suggested.

NATUROPATHY

CAUTION: *Read the information on page 167 before taking supplements.*

Naturopaths would look to build up the immune system and clean out the liver. They would suggest eliminating dairy products from your diet when you have sinusitus because they produce mucus. Similarly, sugar should be avoided; it also decreases immune function. Food sensitivity tests would be carried out as other foods could be a problem.

Vitamins and minerals that may help reduce sinusitis include vitamin A (5000 iu per day), vitamin C (3000 mg per day), vitamin E (500 iu per day) and zinc (25 mg elemental per day).

OSTEOPATHY

Cranial osteopathy can be particularly effective in relieving sinusitis. For advice, see an osteopath who practises this kind of treatment.

REFLEXOLOGY

Your major focus should be to work all your toes/fingers as they correspond to your head region. You can also work points for the ileocecal valve to help control excess mucus, the adrenal glands to deal with inflammation and the lymphatic system if there is an infection. Work the chest/lungs to aid breathing and the small intestine and colon for elimination of waste. Try this on both feet or hands for a total of 20 minutes twice a week. Note, however, that it may get worse before it gets better.

SHIATSU

You may have particular problems with sinusitis if you eat a lot of mucus-producing foods, such as dairy products, or if your stomach and spleen are unable to cope with these rich foods. In this case a shiatsu practitioner can advise you on diet. Congestion in the large intestine and lung meridians can also contribute to sinusitis and a therapist would treat these channels. They will also balance the stomach and spleen to aid your general digestion and increase the flow of Ki energy around your body.

YOGA

Yoga breathing exercises can be effective in clearing the sinuses, but do them under the supervision of a yoga teacher who will advise you on how to avoid hyperventilation. They may also instruct you in yoga neti, cleansing the sinus with salt water.

SMOKING

Tobacco contains about 2000 dangerous toxic compounds other than tar, cyanide, carbon monoxide and highly-addictive nicotine. Among these chemicals are carcinogens (cancer-causing substances) and stimulants that place undue pressure on the circulatory system, toxins that must be flushed from the body, and substances that constrict blood vessels, inhibit the transfer of oxygen, cause the build up of fatty materials in your blood and irritate the respiratory system.

Smoking is associated with a vast range of conditions including 50 percent of all types of CANCER as well as ASTHMA, bad breath, birth problems, BRONCHITIS, emphysema, HEADACHE, HEART PROBLEMS, IMPOTENCE, IRRITABLE BOWEL SYNDROME, NOSEBLEED, stroke, teeth and gum problems, ULCERS and wrinkles. However, the good news is that after giving up smoking for a significant period, the risk of contracting such diseases as lung cancer decreases again.

Some smokers give up smoking through willpower and discipline. However, as most of us are creatures of habit and comfort, we often need help if we are to break our smoking dependency. But just because it can be hard, doesn't mean it can't be done. There are many foundations, courses and support groups that offer advice and support to people who would like to give up. Different smokers need different ways of quitting, and there are so many alternatives available you will find one to suit you. Highly addicted smokers may have no alternative but to go "cold turkey" whereas someone who smokes for the pleasurable effect may be able to taper off. Ask your health practitioner for a recommendation or contact your local community health centre.

WHAT YOU CAN DO

- Cigarettes that have less tar and nicotine may be a small improvement, but you may smoke more of them or inhale deeper which could be worse than the "saving". Take fewer draws on each cigarette and don't smoke a cigarette all the way down; chemicals concentrate in the remaining tobacco as it is smoked.
- Change to a less palatable brand of cigarettes.
- You need to become aware of when you smoke before you can control your actions.
- Learning how to relax and deal with stress is one of the most important steps you can take (see page 40). Not only do many smokers habitually turn to cigarettes for this release, the process of giving up smoking can be stressful in itself!
- Set a day to stop smoking altogether — it doesn't have to be New Years Day or your birthday but it shouldn't be a stressful time such as when you change jobs or around a big party.
- Take it one day at a time.
- When you first give up, keep yourself busy with enjoyable activity. Those that don't allow you to smoke such as going to the cinema or library are best. Socialising with non-smokers could make it easier.
- Keep your hands busy too. Try sketching, sewing, playing an instrument or playing with worry beads.
- Exercise. You can't smoke while you are active and it will ease tension and release the natural "feel good" chemical endorphins in your body.
- Concentrate on your breathing (see page 25).
- Avoid things that you associate with cigarettes such as alcohol and coffee.
- Instead of a cigarette after a meal, brush your teeth and use a mouthwash. Tobacco tastes terrible with these flavours in your mouth.
- Remember that sudden cravings usually pass within 10 minutes. Distract yourself, or chew gum, eat celery and carrot sticks, suck on a piece of fresh ginger, even chew a pen.
- Hypnotherapy is a popular technique that has met

with some success in breaking the habit (see page 208). At home, try AFFIRMATIONS AND VISUALISATIONS — visualise yourself as a non-smoker.

- Smoking can be a subtle form of self-abuse. COUNSELLING may help you discover and resolve any underlying issues
- Use the money you save on tobacco to buy yourself a treat.

ACUPUNCTURE

Acupuncture is renowned for its ability to help people with addictions of all kinds, including smoking.

AFFIRMATION

An affirmation like the following may assist you to give up smoking. Repeat it as many times a day as possible. "I live totally in the present, experiencing all my feelings as they arise. It is safe to be me and I celebrate my body by filling my lungs with pure air".

AROMATHERAPY

Regular aromatherapy massage can help relax you and relieve symptoms such as irritability and stress. Any of the relaxing oils such as lavender, chamomile, marjoram and vetivert can be used and sandalwood can help on an emotional level in letting go of the past.

BACH FLOWER REMEDIES

Bach flower remedies can assist with the emotional states that may be behind your desire to smoke. See page 106. Some you might like to try include rescue remedy for all symptoms, crab apple to cleanse the mind and body, walnut for breaking links, impatiens for irritability and white chestnut for recurring thought patterns and to help "switch off" mentally.

HERBALISM

A variety of herbal remedies are available from herbalists that will help if you want to quit.

HOMOEOPATHY

If your reasons for smoking match those below, take one of the appropriate homoeopathic remedies to help you give up the addiction. If there is no progress after a few days stop the remedy and see a homoeopath for a remedy that may be better suited to you.

If you smoke to block your feelings of indignation and anger, try taking one 6C potency of Staphisagria three times a day for two days.

If you smoke because of overindulgence or self abuse and you are experiencing withdrawal symptoms, try taking one 6C potency of *Nux vomica* three times a day for two days.

MASSAGE

Massage can help you relax and calm your nerves which will assist in the process of giving up. It will also feel like an indulgence so should counter any feeling of self-denial.

MODERN MEDICINE

Doctors can advise patients on the use of nicotine patches and nicotine gum. These deliver nicotine via the skin or saliva, thus avoiding smoke damage to the lungs. However, it does not avoid the problems of nicotine such as reduced circulation, skin aging, stomach ulcers and angina, and the risks during pregnancy are the same. Doctors may also recommend a suitable form of counselling.

NATUROPATHY

CAUTION: *Read the information on page 167 before taking supplements.*

Supplements can be helpful if you are giving up because smoking will have depleted your body of vitamins and minerals. Those that will be especially helpful to you include vitamin A (5000 iu per day), vitamin E (500 iu per day), high potency B complex (take as directed on the label), zinc (25 mg elemental per day), beta carotene (20 mg per day) and vitamin C (3000 mg per day).

REFLEXOLOGY

Work these points: the throat, the chest/lung area to assist in breathing, all the fingers or toes as they correspond to the sinus area, the diaphragm and solar plexus for relaxation and stress reduction, the thoracic spine for nerve function in the chest area, and the liver to detoxify the blood. Try this on both feet or hands for a total of 15 to 20 minutes twice a week or when you feel the urge to smoke.

SHIATSU

Shiatsu treatment can be useful in strengthening the lungs and helping the liver with detoxification.

YOGA

Yoga can be used to help you give up all kinds of addictions. It disciplines the mind and helps you gain confidence in your ability to go without the addictive substance. Yoga can become a "positive addiction" and by substituting a good habit for smoking you will build up self-esteem. Ask a yoga teacher to direct you in fairly active yogic exercises to get your blood flowing and relaxation techniques to calm your mind.

HERBAL, HOMOEOPATHIC AND BACH FLOWER REMEDY FOR GIVING UP SMOKING

Mix together the following combination: 40 per cent *Nicotiana tabacum* 6C (homoeopathic), 30 per cent *Nux vomica* 6C (homoeopathic), 10 per cent rock rose, 10 per cent walnut and 10 per cent crab apple. Take 4 to 6 drops of this mixture under your tongue as often as required to help you break the habit.

SNORING

Snoring may occur when the nasal passage is obstructed while you are asleep. In some cases, excess body fluid may cause the nasal passages to swell. Respiratory conditions such as ALLERGIES, BRONCHITIS, COLDS, SINUSITIS and other sinus problems have this effect. Anything else that causes fluid or mucus build-up, such as alcohol or dairy foods, will have an impact. See FLUID RETENTION.

If you are lying on your back, your tongue may fall back and block breathing. In elderly people, the outer sides of the nostrils may have softened, causing them to be drawn in with each breath.

WHAT YOU CAN DO

- Keep your weight down to normal. Even people who are only a little overweight often have swollen nasal passages due to excess fluid. Their body shape also means they tend to sleep on their backs for comfort.
- Avoid salt in food and drink such as mineral waters, especially before bed, as it causes fluid retention.
- Avoid dairy foods as they produce mucus in the body. Substitute with soya bean products.
- Avoid alcohol before sleeping.
- Medications such as sleeping pills and antihistamines relax the muscles in the head and neck and can make snoring worse.
- You can try elevating the head end of your bed — try a brick or two under the legs.
- Change your pillow, especially if you are using a large thick one, as a bend in your neck will cause some obstruction.
- Sleep on your side — it will reduce the vibrations on your palate.
- If you tend to sleep on your back, try tying a piece of fabric around your middle with a knot at the back. This should prevent you rolling on to your back for long as the knot will press into you, causing discomfort.
- Nose splints that keep the nasal passages open are available from pharmacists.

CHINESE HERBS

Chinese herbs can work to reduce snoring by reducing mucus and strengthening the supporting musculature. See a Chinese herbalist for details.

MODERN MEDICINE

If you still snore while sleeping on your side, consult a medical practitioner as you could have an obstruction in your respiratory system. Operations to reduce the size of the soft palate are currently being trialled to bring relief from snoring when the self-help measures don't assist.

NATUROPATHY

Naturopaths have had reasonable results with reducing snoring. They will adjust your diet to check if your snoring is caused by a build-up of mucus in your mouth and throat. They will also prescribe vitamins and minerals that help clear the mucous membrane.

REFLEXOLOGY

Work the points for the throat and, for relaxation, the diaphragm. Also work the toes or fingers as these correspond to the head. Try this on both feet or hands for 10 to 15 minutes two or three times a week.

SORE THROAT

A sore throat and pain on swallowing can be symptoms of a range of conditions including COLDS AND INFLUENZA, LARYNGITIS and TONSILLITIS.

The inflammation can be caused by a number of factors including viral and bacterial infection, irritation or strain to the voice, from shouting or overuse, for example.

Most sore throats will heal by themselves although various remedies can make you more comfortable. Some cases, such as strep throat, can be more serious.

Seek medical advice if your sore throat or laryngitis, even if mild:

- persists for more than four days
- is accompanied by a rash or high fever
- is accompanied by coughing, hoarseness and difficulty in breathing
- is accompanied by earache, joint pain or a lump in the neck
- causes extreme fatigue, nausea and loss of appetite
- recurs frequently.

WHAT YOU CAN DO

- Avoid irritants such as smoking, alcohol, dust and polluted environments.
- Be quiet. Rest your voice until your throat returns to normal. Try to be silent, and use a pad and pencil where possible.
- Gargle with saltwater every few hours. Dissolve 1/2 teaspoon salt in a glass of lukewarm water. This can bring relief from discomfort by clearing the throat. Note that no gargling (even with antiseptic gargles) will rid the throat of germs, nor will it help if the soreness is lower down the throat.
- Keep the throat from drying out by drinking plenty of fluids, but avoid cold, very hot or carbonated drinks as they could cause further irritation. Warm drinks are best as they increase circulation to the area which promotes healing. Avoid tea and coffee as the caffeine will dehydrate you further. Water is perfect as are fresh juices and vegetable broths. Sip lemon juice, ginger and honey in warm tea or water, or dissolve a tablespoon of bicarbonate of soda (baking powder) in the water. A pinch of cayenne pepper in a hot lemon drink is another trusted remedy.
- You can suck hard candies such as honey and eucalyptus drops to keep the throat moist. Sugar, however, encourages infection. Try pure licorice sweets from health food stores as they are anti-inflammatory.
- Try a cold-air humidifier to keep the air and the mucus around your vocal chords moist. Some cases may be eased by steam from a shower or Turkish bath.
- Steam inhalations can help too. Make a "tent" with a towel over your head and a bowl of very hot water. Breathe in the steam deeply for 5 to 10 minutes several times a day.
- If you tend to wake up with a sore throat, it could be that stomach acids are backing up into your throat at night. Avoid eating or drinking for 1 to 2 hours before going to bed. Try tilting your bed (bricks under the legs work well) so the head is about 10 cm higher than the foot. It could also mean that blocked air passages are causing you to breathe through your mouth, leaving your throat dry and sore.

• How you breathe can affect this condition. You should breathe through your nose as breathing through your mouth will dry your throat. See THE IMPORTANCE OF BREATH.

ACUPUNCTURE

A sore throat or bout of laryngitis can be relieved by acupuncture. An acupuncturist will give you specific advice and treatment.

AFFIRMATION

If you think there is an emotional aspect to your condition, affirmations may help (see page 48). Try repeating the following to yourself, as often as possible, if you feel it's appropriate: "I fully express myself, secure in the knowledge that it's okay to be me".

THE ALEXANDER TECHNIQUE AND FELDENKRAIS METHOD

Both Alexander and Feldenkrais practitioners have strategies for teaching you about the use of your neck and jaw during speech and how this relates to the organisation of your entire body. With this knowledge you may be able to prevent or reduce the tension in the area of your throat.

AROMATHERAPY

The vapour from essential oil steam inhalations helps clear the breathing passage and soothes inflammation in the throat. Add 2 drops each of benzoin, lavender and sandalwood to a bowl of steaming water. Breathe this in with a towel over your head for about 10 minutes then give yourself a break and breathe in some more. Do this every night before you go to bed until the condition clears.

Tea tree and eucalyptus can also help, either as inhalations or in oil burners. Tea tree oil lozenges are available commercially.

CHINESE HERBS

If you are prone to throat problems you may have an imbalance in your lung network. This can be put back into balance with herbs from a Chinese herbalist that supplement and protect the lungs.

CHIROPRACTIC

Chiropractic spinal adjustments increase nerve flow to organs of the throat and so increase your immunity and resistance to such conditions.

COUNSELLING

If you have a recurring problem with laryngitis, it may have an emotional aspect. It could be worthwhile seeking counselling to resolve this.

HERBALISM

Propolis lozenges and gargle are extremely effective as is drinking marshmallow tea, either on its own or with calendula. Simply gargling with warm sage tea can help as can wrapping a compress made in the tea around your neck. Better yet, gargle a sage, thyme and myrrh herbal infusion with a teaspoon of glycerine, three times a day, or one with golden seal or sanguinaria. Other herbs would be prescribed by a herbalist depending on the cause and other symptoms.

HOMOEOPATHY

Homoeopathics are effective in promoting recovery because the remedies prompt your body to fight the condition. If the problem is caused from overusing your voice and your throat hurts when you swallow, take one 6C potency of *Argentum nitricum* every hour for five doses. If it comes about after you have been in a cold wind and your cough is hoarse and your throat burns when you cough, take one 6C potency of *Aconitum napellus* every hour for five doses. If you feel no better in a few days, a homoeopath can give further advice and treatment.

MODERN MEDICINE

Antibiotics may be prescribed to reduce infection if there is a bacterial infection, but in many cases the cause is viral. Medicated anaesthetic lozenges and sprays are available over the counter and may bring relief from pain by numbing the area, but they only destroy surface germs and do not solve the problem. If you use a decongestant nasal spray, do so with caution as they can be addictive. Try a simple saline one instead.

A doctor will usually recommend an anti-inflammatory and analgesic such as aspirin, as well as steam inhalations.

NATUROPATHY

You can buy lozenges containing zinc or just dissolve tablets of zinc gluconate slowly in your mouth. Take 1/4 teaspoon (1000 mg) of non-acidic vitamin C powder hourly and 5000 iu vitamin A daily. Cell salts (iron phosphate and potassium chloride) and L-lysine are also recommended.

OSTEOPATHY

Osteopathic treatment can assist in boosting your body's immune defences so it can help to combat these conditions by treatment of mechanical stresses along with diet and lifestyle advice.

REFLEXOLOGY

Work the throat/neck as the main reflex for this problem. In addition, work all your toes or fingers—these correspond to your head and sinus areas—as well as the points for the lymphatic system, thymus and spleen (to boost the immune system), the adrenal glands (against inflammation) and the cervical spine (for nerve function in the throat area). Try this on both feet or hands for a total of 15 minutes three times a week.

SHIATSU

A shiatsu practitioner would work your lung and stomach meridians to reduce inflammation.

YOGA

Your yoga teacher can instruct you in yoga neti, cleansing your throat and sinus system with salt water.

STOMACH ACHE

Pain in your stomach, or in the general abdominal area, can involve many organs other than your stomach including your intestines, liver (see page 329), gall bladder (see page 287), kidneys (see page 326), pancreas and spleen. In the lower abdomen, it may be your bladder (see page 231) or reproductive organs that are involved. Stomach ache may also be a sign of spinal problems.

The pain can be the result of many different factors: ALLERGIES, CONSTIPATION, DIARRHOEA, FOOD POISONING, PERIOD PAIN, ULCERS, flu, food, stress or emotional upheaval.

Treatment will depend on the cause. As stomach problems are often at least partly diet-related, many treatments will only work if you eat a sensible diet. The self-help remedies for DIGESTIVE PROBLEMS, including aromatherapy, can be effective.

Seek medical advice if the pain:

- becomes a recurring problem
- lasts more than 24 hours
- occurs suddenly and is severe
- is severe enough to interfere with daily activities or sleep
- remains severe or gets worse over a few hours
- is persistent, even if not severe, in an elderly person or young child
- is preceded by injury to the abdomen or back
- is associated with vomiting (particularly if there is blood), fever, fainting, rectal bleeding or, if over time, there is weight loss
- if you are or may be pregnant, especially if there is dizziness or bleeding.

See also CANDIDIASIS, COLITIS, ENDOMETRIOSIS, FLATULENCE, HANGOVER, NAUSEA, PELVIC INFLAMMATORY DISEASE.

ACUPUNCTURE

Acupuncture is known to be effective in relieving stomach pains.

AFFIRMATION

There may be an emotional component to your upset stomach. If you relate to either of these affirmations repeat them to yourself as many times as possible.

"I am in perfect balance at all times. I only take into my body substances that are nourishing and harmonious." "I happily release my emotions and forgive myself and others."

BACH FLOWER REMEDIES

Stomach aches are often linked to worried minds. You could try white chestnut, rescue remedy or impatiens to relieve this.

CHIROPRACTIC

Chiropractic adjustment will improve the function of your nervous system which will make you less prone to stomach upsets.

THE FELDENKRAIS METHOD

If you have a problem with abdominal muscle spasms, Feldenkrais practitioners can teach you breathing and body awareness strategies to reduce these.

HEALING MEDITATION

Stomach problems can be assisted by healing energy. Consult a therapist or read the chapter on HEALING ENERGIES and channel energy to yourself. When the blue light is flowing strongly, concentrate it in your stomach area and feel it restore your internal balance.

HERBALISM

Herbal teas such as chamomile and meadowsweet are effective because of their soothing effects and the warmth they create in your body. Drink 1 cup three times a day when you have a stomach ache to ease discomfort. Drink peppermint tea if your stomach ache is accompanied by wind. Slippery elm powder is also effective for stomach aches when a spoonful is taken in half a glass of water.

To prevent a stomach ache related to indigestion, take gentian in a tincture — 30 drops before meals mixed in a glass of water. This will stimulate your correct digestive process.

HOMOEOPATHY

Homoeopaths will leave a mild stomach ache to right itself as it is the body's signal that you have overeaten or eaten the wrong thing. But if your stomach ache is a problem, you could try one of the following remedies if it fits the description of your condition or see a homoeopath for a complete diagnosis.

If your stomach ache occurs after eating unfamiliar food, take one 6C potency of *Nux vomica* every half an hour for five doses.

If your stomach ache is accompanied by wind and belching, take one 6C tablet or liquid form of *Carbo vegetabilis* every half hour for four doses.

If your stomach ache happens in the middle of the night and is a sharp pain in the pit of your stomach, take one 6C potency tablet or liquid form of *Arsenium album* every half hour for four doses.

MASSAGE

General stomach ache may respond to gentle lower back and abdominal massage (see pages 137, 143 147).

MODERN MEDICINE

Doctors will carry out a medical investigation to assess the cause of your stomach ache and suggest the appropriate treatment, perhaps a change of diet or prescription of antacids or analgesics. You should avoid using analgesics without a doctor's advice as they could make the problem worse. There are over-the-counter medications for mild aches: peppermint oil capsules for spasms or irritable colon, antacid emulsions and tablets for acidity, laxatives for constipation and drugs for indigestion pain.

REFLEXOLOGY

Work the point for the stomach as the main reflex plus the liver for digestion, metabolism and detoxification, and the diaphragm and solar plexus for relaxation and stress reduction. Try this on both feet or hands for a total of 15 minutes daily while the problem lasts. If you are prone to indigestion, work these points for 15 minutes before a meal.

SHIATSU

Dispersion of the Ki in your stomach meridian is effective in relieving pain from a stomach ache. See a shiatsu practitioner for treatment and advice on foods that hinder your stomach's natural function.

YOGA

The nausea relief exercise on page 200 will help with stomach ache as it stretches the stomach meridian.

THRUSH

Thrush (the common name for moniliasis) is an inflammation of the mucous membrane in either the mouth or vagina that is caused by the yeast-like fungus *Candida albicans.* See CANDIDIASIS for details and treatments.

In addition to the reasons outlined on page 245, the *Candida albicans* balance can be affected by irritations in the mouth or vagina which change the acidity of the region.

Oral thrush forms a white coating inside the mouth. It is common in newborn babies who acquire the fungus from mothers with thrush as they pass through the birth canal.

Vaginal thrush produces a thick, white, cheesy-textured discharge and the vaginal area can be very itchy and sore.

As *Candida albicans* is always in the body, it is not surprising that thrush can be a recurring problem. Some women are prone to thrush, and would benefit from incorporating the treatment advice outlined here into their everyday lives.

IMPORTANT: *Vaginal discharges should be investigated by a health practitioner as there are numerous types with a variety of causes such as PELVIC INFLAMMATORY DISEASE.*

WHAT YOU CAN DO

- Wear loose clothing and cotton underpants so the vagina is kept cool and dry. Avoid pantyhose and Lycra exercise wear and swimming costumes.

- Yeast spores can remain on underpants to reinfect despite washing, so give them an extra scrub, soak them in boiling water or bleach or iron them to destroy the fungus.

- Sexual activity can also cause cross-infection. Both partners should seek treatment even though a man may show no signs. You may find it more comfortable to abstain from sex during an outbreak. Using a condom during sex is recommended. Clean your diaphragm scrupulously if you use one. Avoid spreading bacteria from the anal area to the vaginal area through secondary contact via hands, the penis or sex toys.

- Avoid spermicides and chemical lubricants as they can trigger an outbreak.

- Semen is alkaline and the vagina usually slightly acidic which is another reason why sex can trigger thrush. If this is the case, try a mild naturally acidic solution (see below) in a douche or sitz bath after intercourse.

- Use sanitary pads instead of tampons to avoid irritating the vagina.

- Ensure you wipe from front to back after using the toilet so bacteria are not introduced from the anus to the vagina.

- Keep your genital area very clean but don't douche the vagina with chemicals, or wash with soap, or use feminine deodorants — the vagina naturally cleans itself and a foreign substance may aggravate or bring on an infection. For chronic thrush, however, regular douching with a naturally acidic solution may be recommended by your health practitioner.

- In a warm, shallow bath place ½ cup salt and ½ cup of apple cider vinegar and sit with the knees apart, allowing contact with the vagina.

- Eat acidophilus yogurt every day or take acidophilus tablets. The yogurt can be applied in and around the vagina, where the cold will also soothe the itch.

- Control the yeast level in your body by avoiding foods that contain yeasts, fungus and high levels of sugar (see page 245).

AFFIRMATION

As thrush may prevent you from fully enjoying sex this affirmation may help. Repeat it as many times as possible throughout the day: "I am a wonderful person who deserves all the joys that a sexual relationship can bring".

AROMATHERAPY

Vaginal thrush can be relieved by certain antiseptic

essential oils. These include myrrh, tea tree and lavender. Add 2 drops each of myrrh and tea tree to your bath, making sure the oils are well dispersed in the water. Before you sit fully in the bath swish the water towards your vagina to ensure contact. These oils will reduce infection and soothe the itching and soreness of the outer areas of the vagina.

BACH FLOWER REMEDIES

For the treatment and prevention of thrush, try crab apple to cleanse the mind and body, sweet chestnut for emotional despair and impatiens with cherry plum for emotional calm, patience and trust in oneself.

CHIROPRACTIC

Chiropractic adjustment on the pelvic area can increase the resistance of the immune system which will make your body less prone to thrush.

COUNSELLING

If your thrush is chronic and recurring, it may be an indication that you are feeling irritated by or uncomfortable with your sexual partner, or insecure about that relationship. Counselling may help resolve this issue.

HERBALISM

The astringent herbs such as oak bark, golden seal, thyme and witch hazel will help reduce the occurrence of thrush. Antifungal herbs include pau d'arco, echinacea and garlic, taken internally. Apply calendula ointment locally to your vagina to reduce the irritation and itchiness.

HOMOEOPATHY

Homoeopathic remedies such as *Borax veneta* are often used to help reduce thrush. They should be prescribed by a homoeopath who will fully assess your physical state and determine what other factors are influencing your condition.

MASSAGE

Lymphatic drainage or aromatherapy massage from a professional therapist can often be of assistance.

MODERN MEDICINE

Antifungal creams and tablets are prescribed for thrush and can clear away the infection and physical signs within a few days, however, they will not prevent recurrence. Both partners should be treated to prevent reinfection, and the course of treatment may take a month.

NATUROPATHY

In addition to the natural topical applications and douches recommended, a naturopath will treat the *Candida albicans* imbalance in your body through diet (see page 245).

REFLEXOLOGY

If you have vaginal thrush, work the point for your uterus. If it is oral thrush, work all the toes/fingers as these correspond to the head/throat area. You can also work the lymphatic system (especially the pelvis) to help fight the infection, the adrenal glands to help deal with inflammation, the spleen and thymus to assist the immune system, and the diaphragm for relaxation and stress reduction. Try this on both feet or hands for a total of 10 to 15 minutes two or three times a week.

SHIATSU

A shiatsu practitioner would work on "tonifying" the kidney, bladder, spleen and large intestine meridians and sedating the liver and gall bladder meridians to remove "damp heat" from the body.

THYROID PROBLEMS

The thyroid is the small gland located at the base of the front of the neck. It uses iodine to produce two hormones that control the rate of metabolism in your body and regulate growth.

People with underactive thyroids may show symptoms of FATIGUE, CONSTIPATION, weight gain, muscular aches, pins and needles, an excessive sensitivity to the cold, INFERTILITY and scanty or absent menstrual periods. This condition causes both mental and physical activity to slow down.

In addition, the skin dries out and thickens, the hair thins, the voice deepens and speech slows. The onset of symptoms can be gradual, making diagnosis difficult.

Causes for underactivity can include inflammation of the thyroid gland, autoimmune destruction of the gland, malfunction of the pituitary gland (which controls hormone production in the thyroid), excess treatment of an overactive thyroid or, in rare cases, a dietary deficiency. Pregnancy can cause a temporary underfunction. This condition is known as *hypothyroidism* or myxoedema.

Underactivity can also occur from a deficiency of the thyroid hormone at birth. Known as cretinism, it can lead to permanent problems with mental and physical development if not treated, although it is now usually detected within a few days of birth.

People with overactive thyroids may have problems with INSOMNIA, hyperactivity, tremors, palpitations, sweating, sensitivity to heat, DIARRHOEA, MENSTRUAL PROBLEMS and weight loss (despite a healthy appetite). The eyes may bulge and the thyroid gland itself may be enlarged.

Overactive thyroids are a result of excessive production of the thyroid hormone, causing physical and mental processes to speed up. This can place an extra burden on the heart. *Hyperthyroidism* or thyrotoxicosis, as it is known, may sometimes be brought on by emotional stress. It is five times more likely to affect women than men. In long-term severe cases, the symptoms can worsen with a "thyroid crisis" producing fever, delirium, vomiting and shock.

An enlarged thyroid is known as *goitre* and may be associated with either insufficient iodine in the diet, excess thyroid hormone or a tumour.

Thyroid dysfunction can vary in severity, from mild to extreme.

IMPORTANT: *Before beginning any treatment your thyroid condition should be diagnosed medically by a doctor. If your thyroid is overactive or underactive, a doctor should also continue to supervise your health.*

ACUPUNCTURE

In mild cases, acupuncture can help to regulate thyroid function.

AFFIRMATION

As your thyroid gland affects the whole body, some believe an imbalance may be connected with feelings of lack of control. If this applies to you, try repeating this affirmation to yourself as many times a day as possible: "I am in control of my life. It is safe for me to fully express myself."

CHINESE HERBS

Chinese herbal medicine is effective in healing overactive and underactive thyroids. See a Chinese herbalist for advice and specific herbal prescription.

HERBALISM

An overactive thyroid may be assisted with bugleweed, although it may increase the size of the thyroid. Bladderwrack is the specific herb that can help balance thyroid activity, whether overactive or underactive. A qualified herbalist will be able to advise you further.

HOMOEOPATHY

Homoeopaths recognise that thyroid problems can be complex and will prescribe remedies very carefully for the specifics of your condition, often with good results.

MODERN MEDICINE

Blood tests will confirm thyroid hormone levels, and are used to monitor any disorder. They can also indicate thyroid inflammation through the presence of antibodies.

Surgery is sometimes used by doctors to remove all or part of an overactive thyroid gland. Radiation treatment may be used to kill the overactive cells in the thyroid. However, medication is commonly prescribed to block the production of the hormone.

An underactive thyroid can be temporary and may not require medical treatment. In other cases, an oral form of thyroid hormone may be prescribed, and may need to be taken daily for the rest of the patient's life.

Goitre is also usually treated by thyroid hormone medication.

IMPORTANT: *Only in a few cases is a weight problem due to a thyroid problem. Thyroid hormone medication can be dangerous if used with the idea of reducing weight.*

NATUROPATHY

A naturopath is likely to treat an overactive thyroid with herbal or homoeopathic treatments. They can also give dietary advice. For example, iodine rich foods include seaweed (kelp), seafood and fish. For an underactive thyroid, take tyrosine (500 mg three times a day) and kelp tablets (1200 mg per day) that have been standardised with iodine.

REFLEXOLOGY

Work the thyroid as the main reflex for this condition. Also the pituitary for thyroid function, the heart for circulation, the adrenal glands for energy and the solar plexus for stress reduction. Try this on both feet or hands for a total of 10 minutes three times a week.

YOGA

As yoga is helpful in bringing your body systems into balance, consider regularly attending a yoga class if your thyroid is underactive. Yoga may be beneficial for an overactive thyroid. The salute to the sun (see page 190), for example, is an excellent toner of all glands.

Try the plough pose on page 202 as it will flush the head and neck with blood, nourishing the thyroid, helping it achieve a balance in secretions, whether it is underactive or overactive. You can also try the half-shoulder stand on page 197.

TONSILLITIS

Tonsillitis is an inflammation of the tonsils (an important part of your body's immune system) which causes the back of the throat to become red and sore. It is often caused by a bacterial or viral infection and can be a complication of various infectious diseases such as measles (see page 82), influenza (see page 253) and GLANDULAR FEVER.

You may have difficulty swallowing due to the enlarged size of your tonsils, as well as a dry cough, fever, chills, HEADACHE and other pains, and swollen neck glands. The tongue may develop a white coating of toxins. In cases of glandular fever, white spots appear on the tonsils.

Inflammation and swelling of the adenoids (tissue pads at the back of the nose) may also be involved. This can obstruct breathing.

Tonsillitis is most common in children but adults are also affected. After a sudden onset, the worst symptoms usually pass within two days and medical advice should be sought if the attack lasts longer than three days or if green or yellow phlegm is coughed up.

WHAT YOU CAN DO

- Rest in bed while the symptoms are at their worst.
- Drink plenty of fluids, especially if you have a fever. You may not feel like eating so try herbal teas or non-acidic juices such as apricot, mango, pear, beetroot or carrot juice (these are also good sources of vitamin A and iron). Carbonated and acidic drinks can be irritating.

ACUPUNCTURE

Acupuncture is useful in treating acute tonsillitis and also during recovery.

AFFIRMATION

Some believe that problems relating to your throat may be connected with stifled creativity or fears around self expression. If this applies to you, try an affirmation like one of the following and repeat it as many times as possible: "It is OK for me to speak my mind and I use my words wisely and gently." "My creativity flows easily and naturally. I fully express myself at all times."

AROMATHERAPY

CAUTION: *Read the information on pages 102 to 105 before using these essential oils*

The essential oils of peppermint and eucalyptus help

soothe the throat and combat any infection when absorbed through the skin from a bath.

For some relief from tonsillitis and to relax the body to aid the healing process, take a bath containing 2 drops of eucalyptus and 1 drop of peppermint, making sure the oil is fully dispersed in the water. Sit in it for as long as you can to get the full benefit of the oil.

BACH FLOWER REMEDY

Take rescue remedy if there is stress involved with the tonsillitis.

CHINESE HERBS

A Chinese herbalist can prescribe herbs and give advice on what to do when you are displaying symptoms. If taken over a long period Chinese herbs are effective in building up your immune system which will guard against infections like tonsillitis.

HERBALISM

Try herbal infusions containing the herbs calendula, echinacea or golden seal. For example, make a mixture of four parts of echinacea and one part poke root tinctures and take 30 drops in a glass of water three times a day.

You can also make up the following combination for a throat spray: 5 ml (1/6 fl oz) each glycerine and sanguinaria tincture, and 10 ml (1/3 fl oz) each of golden seal, echinacea and myrrh tinctures.

HOMOEOPATHY

Homoeopaths have had success in reducing the symptoms of tonsillitis using various homoeopathic remedies. The prescription depends very much on the symptoms you are displaying.

MODERN MEDICINE

Tonsillitis is usually treated with analgesics such as aspirin to relieve pain and inflammation in the throat. Antibiotics may be prescribed if there is bacterial infection involved, the symptoms are prolonged or there is fever.

If the tonsillitis is a recurring problem then surgery can be carried out to remove the tonsils. There is much debate as to whether infected tonsils should be removed and the option is not as readily suggested as it once was. Mere swelling, without complications, should be no basis for surgery. The tonsils are part of the lymphatic system which plays a large part in fighting and filtering potential infections. When they are removed one line of the body's defence system is destroyed. There is no indication that removal will make a child less susceptible to other respiratory conditions. If surgery is advised, seek a second opinion and guidance from other therapists so you can make an informed decision. The operation under general anaesthetic is very painful and carries risks of post-operative bleeding and aspiration.

NATUROPATHY

Once you have tonsillitis naturopaths recommend you drink plenty of water and eat lots of fresh fruit and vegetables, especially when juiced which is easier on your throat. Avoid dairy products because these are mucus-producing and can add to your problem, particularly if adenoids are involved — the traditional ice-cream treat can actually make things worse. Vitamin C powder (1/4 teaspoon or 1000 mg every hour when the condition is chronic) can also help.

REFLEXOLOGY

Work the points for the throat and head area as the main reflex. In addition, work the lymphatic glands to help deal with the infection, the adrenal glands for the inflammation, the spleen and thymus to boost the immune system, the cervical spine for nerve function to the throat, and the diaphragm for relaxation. Try this on both feet or hands for a total of 15 minutes twice a week.

SHIATSU

A shiatsu practitioner can help build up your immune system to guard against throat infections such as tonsillitis as well as improve the flow of Ki energy in your body.

Once you have tonsillitis a shiatsu practitioner can help by unblocking your lung meridian, through subtle pressure on your body, and increasing the flow of Ki energy along this meridian.

At home, you can try the shiatsu pressure point called Lung 6 for relief from the pain of tonsillitis. It is located on the front of your arm, one hand width and two thumb widths below your elbow crease. Hold it down for about 1 minute then rest for 1 minute and hold it again.

YOGA

If there is no fever, try the plough pose and the half-shoulder stand on pages 197 and 202 as they will flush the head and neck with blood, nourishing the area.

ULCERS

An ulcer is an open sore on a mucous membrane or on the skin. Ulcers can occur on many different parts of the body including the digestive system and the mouth.

Peptic ulcers result from damage to the intestinal lining, caused by the action of stomach acid and pepsin. This follows an imbalance between the amount of gastric juice produced and the protective elements of the lining (e.g. mucus). There may be a lack of mucus, excess acid production or weakness in the lining.

Stress or drugs such as alcohol, aspirin and tobacco are common factors in this imbalance, and heredity may play a role in predisposing someone to ulcers. In some cases, bacteria or a virus may be involved.

Peptic ulcers can affect the stomach (gastric ulcers) or, more commonly, part of the small intestine (duodenal ulcers). They are characterised by upper abdominal cramping or burning, often after meals, which is relieved by antacids and sometimes by vomiting or eating. There may be no pain but your stools may be dark and tarry. Some people do not display any symptoms.

You will need to seek medical advice if you suspect this condition. A doctor can determine if you have an ulcer by taking an X-ray or a gastroscopy. In some cases, gastric ulcers are associated with stomach cancer and this needs to be ruled out.

In many cases, the ulcer will heal on its own in about six weeks, once the underlying factors have been dealt with. There is a tendency, however, for them to recur. Any severe abdominal pain should receive immediate medical attention.

Mouth or aphthous ulcers (also known as canker sores) are inflamed sores inside your mouth that sting when touched by your tongue or by food. In severe cases, they can interfere with aspects of daily life such as eating and speaking. They can result from biting the side of your mouth, from stress or a virus, or they may be due to general poor health or a zinc or vitamin B deficiency. An imbalance in stomach acidity can impact on the acidity of the whole digestive system, irritating the mucous membranes in the mouth and contributing to mouth ulcers. Some people are prone to them when stressed, although persistent ulcers can indicate a serious disease.

Skin ulcers may develop from poor circulation. They can be associated with conditions such as SMOKING, VARICOSE VEINS, DIABETES and HEART PROBLEMS. Bedsores are one form of skin ulceration, caused by continual pressure cutting off circulation to the tissues. This is usually due to immobility, among the bedridden and elderly, for example.

WHAT YOU CAN DO FOR PEPTIC ULCERS

- Learn how to relax (see page 40).
- Eat a natural, healthy and balanced diet as it is now clear that a varied diet promotes healing as fast or faster than the once-advised bland diet.
- Avoid hot spicy foods, highly acid foods and junk food high in sugar. Monitor what aggravates your condition and steer clear of those items.
- Milk should also be avoided as despite its initial soothing effect it causes more stomach acid production.
- Avoid caffeine drinks, decaffeinated coffee and alcohol as they stimulate acid secretion.
- Eating smaller meals more often may reduce ulcer upsets because there is food for the acid to work on.

• Stop SMOKING as this will improve circulation and promote healing.

• Practise breathing techniques and exercise regularly to increase circulation and reduce stress.

• Avoid aspirin and anti-inflammatory drugs as these may erode the intestinal lining.

WHAT YOU CAN DO FOR SKIN ULCERS

• To prevent bedsores, ensure a bedridden person changes position. Areas of pressure should be massaged every two hours.

• To prevent skin ulcers, ensure you get regular exercise and wear support hose if you have varicose veins. Take care to avoid injury to fragile skin.

• Avoid regular use of topical steroid creams for skin conditions such as dermatitis. These weaken the skin.

• Be strict with hygiene when treating skin ulcers, changing dressings regularly. Compression bandages can increase circulation and aid healing.

WHAT YOU CAN DO FOR MOUTH ULCERS

• Over-the-counter preparations are available. There are liquids and gels containing menthol, camphor, eucalyptus, benzocaine and/or alcohol. Many people find these helpful, although for some they may cause further irritation.

• One home remedy is a mouthwash of 1 tablespoon hydrogen peroxide in a glass of water. If this is too harsh, just rinse with water several times a day.

• If applying a protective cream to a new sore, dab the ulcer dry with a cotton bud then use the other end to apply the cream.

• Try applying a wet tea bag to the ulcer. Ordinary black tea contains tannin, a pain-relieving astringent.

• Eating acidophilus yogurt daily can help fight problem-causing bacteria in your mouth to prevent and heal ulcers.

• Coffee, chocolate, acidic fruit (including pineapples, tomatoes, grapes and citrus), strawberries, spices, coconut and nuts (especially walnuts and pecans) should be avoided by people prone to mouth ulcers or during the ulceration.

• Replace shaggy old toothbrushes and choose ones with soft bristles.

ACUPUNCTURE

Acupuncturists have had success in healing gastric and duodenal ulcers. Ulcers on the surface of the body can be treated — laser acupuncture is often used. An acupuncturist sees ulcers in the mouth as associated with stomach heat and will advise accordingly.

AFFIRMATION

Some believe there is a connection between ulcers and the emotional state of "eating away" at yourself. If this applies to you try an affirmation like one of the following and repeat as many times a day as possible. "I have all the skills and resources I need to make a success of my life." "I release my inadequacies, acknowledge my strength and open myself up to all that life has to offer."

AROMATHERAPY

For mouth ulcers, make up a mouthwash of 2 drops of peppermint, geranium and thyme and 4 drops of lemon essential oils diluted in 1 tablespoon of brandy. Add 1 teaspoon of this mixture to a glass of warm water and swish around the mouth. Tea tree oil gargles are excellent as they kill the virus which causes some ulcers. *Do not swallow.*

Tea tree oil is also useful for sterilising and healing skin ulcers.

BACH FLOWER REMEDIES

Take rescue remedy and white chestnut for the stress associated with mouth and peptic ulcers, and aspen for anxiety.

CHINESE HERBS

Ulcers in both your mouth and digestive system can be relieved by Chinese herbs. See a Chinese herbalist for further advice and specific herbal prescription.

The patent medicine Yunnan Pai Yao can provide an effective over-the-counter first aid treatment for some ulcers.

CHIROPRACTIC

Your stomach is prone to becoming more acid and producing ulcers if your nervous system is not functioning properly. Chiropractic adjustment can improve the function of your nervous system.

COUNSELLING

As ulcers can be stress-related and commonly occur in people who are "overdoing it", counselling may help you reorganise your priorities and deal with stress more effectively.

HERBALISM

Mouth ulcers may be caused by poor digestive function causing malabsorption of essential nutrients. The herb gentian is useful in relieving the problem. Take 10 to 15 drops of gentian tincture in a glass of water twice a day to reduce the occurrence of mouth ulcers. Alternatively, before meals, gargle equal parts of thyme, sage and myrrh tincture with a teaspoon of glycerine to relieve the pain of your mouth ulcer. Golden seal is also an excellent herbal treatment.

Peptic ulcers can be relieved by the juice from about 1/6 of a cabbage and 1/2 a raw potato. Drink it once a day for three weeks. The herbs meadowsweet and chamomile can also be of assistance.

HOMOEOPATHY

Some homoeopathic remedies used to treat both stomach and mouth ulcers include *Borax veneta, Nux vomica, Arsenicum album* and *Mercurius solubilis.* The appropriate remedy for you depends on the particular symptoms you are displaying, among many other factors. See a homoeopath for a full assessment.

MODERN MEDICINE

Antacids are prescribed for most peptic ulcers, and may also relieve the pain of mouth ulcers by reducing acid levels in the mouth. Medications such as cimetidine and ranitidine that reduce the gastric secretions are also available. Surgery may be required in a few cases where there are complications.

For mouth ulcers local creams may be prescribed to relieve the pain and to provide a protective covering. A mouthwash containing an anaesthetic, used before meals, may be recommended if eating is difficult. For persistent sores, a steroid cream may be prescribed and/or an antibiotic to treat any oral bacteria that is preventing healing.

Medical attention may be required for ulcers on the legs caused by varicose veins as healing can be slow and difficult.

NATUROPATHY

CAUTION: *Read the information on page 167 before taking supplements.*

Naturopaths will usually treat mouth ulcers as a sign of a vitamin B deficiency — this can sometimes be caused by stress. You can try rubbing oil from a vitamin E capsule into the sores three times per day. Vitamin C mouthwash is also effective. Lozenges of zinc, vitamin C and L-lysine can help ulcers to heal.

If your mouth ulcer is related to excess stomach acidity, you can try drinking 4 cups of meadowsweet tea per day and take sodium phosphate as directed to balance the acidity in your mouth.

Peptic ulcers are also related to stress. Take sodium phosphate as directed to balance the acidity in your stomach.

REFLEXOLOGY

For peptic ulcers, gently work the point for the stomach as the main reflex as well as the adrenal glands for dealing with the inflammation, the thoracic spine for the nervous system and the lymphatic system for any infection.

If the ulcer is duodenal, work these same points as well as the pancreas — it neutralises digestive juices.

For mouth ulcers, have a friend work the reflex points on your big toes or thumbs.

In all cases, also work the points for the diaphragm and solar plexus for relaxation and stress reduction. Try this on both feet or hands for a total of 15 minutes twice a week.

SHIATSU

Boosting the Ki energy in your body can be used as a preventive measure to reduce the occurrence of mouth and peptic ulcers because you will be less stressed once the Ki is balanced. To achieve this a practitioner will mostly work on the digestive organs and the spleen.

YOGA

Peptic ulcers often occur in people as a result of low physical activity. Yoga is a gentle form of exercise that provides excellent blood flow to the stomach thus reducing your chances of forming an ulcer. If you have already developed an ulcer, yoga can help healing by restoring your body's balance and reducing inflammation. Consult a yoga teacher for specific exercises.

VARICOSE VEINS

Varicose veins are prominent, enlarged veins, often blue and "knotted", mostly found on the legs. They are caused by weak valves in the veins and/or a partial obstruction of blood flow. This occurs when an organ presses on nearby vessels, usually the rectum when the legs are involved.

CONSTIPATION (which also causes pressure due to straining) and pregnancy are frequent reasons behind this obstruction. LIVER PROBLEMS can also create pressure in the veins.

Varicose veins are more common in women, the elderly, overweight people and those who stand for a long time. Some people have a weakness in their veins or valves due to genetics or to poor nutritional intake when they were young, and should take preventive measures.

Varicose veins can be itchy and sore. There may also be tiredness, heaviness and aching in the legs and swelling in the ankles after standing. Varicose veins are not dangerous if near the surface of the skin. However, leg ulcers, blood clots, infected clots and bleeding can be complications and require medical attention.

Varicose veins can also be found in the scrotum and vulva as well as the rectum where they are known as HAEMORRHOIDS.

WHAT YOU CAN DO

To avoid varicose veins, alleviate the condition or stop it getting worse, you should:

- Avoid prolonged standing or sitting. Stretch your legs and get the blood flowing by taking regular short walks. Sit down regularly if you have been standing.
- To relieve tired aching legs, lie on the floor with your legs elevated, either up a wall or on a chair, preferably above your heart.
- Avoid sitting with your legs or ankles crossed.
- Exercise regularly to improve blood circulation. Thirty minutes each day of walking or swimming is highly recommended.
- Try alternating hot and cold leg baths to stimulate circulation.
- If you're overweight this will add pressure on your legs. Try to lose any excess weight.
- Eat a healthy, high-fibre diet to avoid constipation and keep your liver and heart in good order.
- Avoid tight clothes such as knee-high socks or stockings that interfere with circulation. Wear support stockings or socks (these support the vein walls) and comfortable shoes with support for your arch and heel.
- See also FOOT SORENESS.

MASSAGE AND APPLYING OINTMENT

Massaging above the affected area may give relief by improving blood and lymph flow to the region. Incorrect massage on varicose veins can make the condition worse.

When massaging ointment into your legs, remember to:

- only massage if you have no dark blue lumps
- always move your massage strokes upwards towards the heart, from ankle to thigh
- don't actually massage the veins themselves but work around them or only above them.
- use gentle, light strokes so that additional pressure is not placed on faulty valves
- use the palms of your hands to apply the ointment.

AFFIRMATION

As varicose veins can indicate problems with circulation and this may be linked to feelings of being burdened, the following affirmation may help. Repeat it as many times a day as possible: "I trust my ability to look after myself. I flow easily with life."

AROMATHERAPY

Aromatherapy can help encourage circulation and soothe irritation. Combine 3 drops of cypress, 3 drops of sandalwood and 1 drop of peppermint in 5 teaspoons of calendula base carrier oil and apply every morning. Geranium and lavender along with cypress is another possible combination. Remember that in all cases you should not use the same type of oil continually for a prolonged period.

THE FELDENKRAIS METHOD

The gentle exercises that are part of the Feldenkrais Method can help you learn new ways of weight bearing which put less strain on your varicose veins. These movement and posture techniques may prevent varicose veins if they run in your family or you have to spend a lot of time standing.

HERBALISM

There are many herbs that improve circulation and some of these are ginger, prickly ash and chilli. Try drinking three cups a day of ginger herbal tea and adding chilli and ginger to your meals.

Horsechestnut strengthens the capillaries. Yarrow and rue may be used internally and externally. Calendula, in the form of an ointment used for massage, relieves the itchiness and pain.

MODERN MEDICINE

In severe cases surgery is undertaken which "strips" (removes) the veins. This should not be done unnecessarily as it can impair circulation to the legs. Some small veins are treated, with limited success, with injections of a hardening material that cause the veins to wither and disappear. Recently, surgical techniques have been developed that repair valves in large leg veins to reverse the condition.

NATUROPATHY

CAUTION: *Read the information on page 167 before taking supplements.*

You can strengthen your veins with high doses of bioflavinoids (1000 mg three times a day). Vitamin E (500 iu per day) is also good for varicose veins because it will improve circulation. If dysfunction of the liver and constipation are involved, a naturopath will treat these conditions.

REFLEXOLOGY

Work these points: the large intestine for elimination, the heart and liver for circulation and the adrenal glands to deal with any inflammation. In addition, work the reflex that corresponds to the affected area e.g. if the problem is in your leg, work the points for the knee, leg, hip and lower spine areas. Try this on both feet or hands for a total of 15 minutes twice a week.

SHIATSU

In shiatsu terms varicose veins occur because of a weakness of Ki in the spleen, kidneys and heart. A shiatsu practitioner will work on these areas to strengthen your veins. Shiatsu is more effective as a preventive measure than a treatment in this case.

YOGA

The yoga posture known as the inverted corpse position (see page 199) is beneficial as it helps prevent further deterioration of the veins. It improves drainage and reduces stagnation of the blood in your legs. Before you start yoga be sure to see a doctor who will check if you have any clots in your deep veins.

WARTS

Warts are rough, pitted raised spots that can appear anywhere on the body. Warts in the soles of the feet are called plantar warts or veruccas; they grow inwards, causing painful pressure.

Different kinds of warts are caused by different strains of the papilloma virus. They are contagious, but rarely seem to be passed by contact such as shaking hands, as the virus usually enters through an opening in the skin. Scratching warts can cause them to spread.

Warts are usually not a problem unless they itch or get in the way. Some warts persist for years but most will go away of their own accord.

Warts around the genital area can be cause for concern as they can be transferred to the cervix, predisposing women to cervical cancer, although some versions of the virus seem to be more of a problem than others. Genital wart virus is highly contagious via sexual contact so use condoms.

IMPORTANT: *Warts do not lead to skin cancer but some flat brownish warts may not be warts at all but melanomas and should be checked by a doctor. If a wart changes shape or colour, or bleeds, consult your doctor. If you are unsure about identifying a wart, check with a doctor before any treatment.*

WHAT YOU CAN DO

- The wart virus breeds in moist areas so change shoes and socks regularly and wear footwear in places such as gym change rooms to avoid infection.
- Avoid touching warts, especially if you have a wound of any kind, and do not scratch. Use a cotton bud or tissue to apply all treatments.
- Go easy on treatments; try gentle ones first. Harsh chemicals can cause ulceration of surrounding skin.
- Try rubbing on vitamin A or E oil and covering with a bandage. Alternatively, vitamin C tablets ground and mixed with water can be applied and covered. Sometimes simply covering a wart tightly with a bandage for at least three weeks can work.
- Saliva is a popular folk remedy — apply as often as possible with a cotton bud.
- Warts seem to have a strong psychological link and hypnotherapy (see page 208) has been very successful in banishing warts. Suggestion therapy often works and can be tried at home: you can "wish" the warts away, for example. Try a visualisation (see page 48) that imagines the wart disappearing in some way and repeat it regularly. The secret is believing.

AFFIRMATION

Some people believe warts may be a symptom of feeling unattractive. If this affirmation feels right for you repeat it as many times as you can during the day: "I release my weaknesses and limitations and move into a new and positive state of being."

AROMATHERAPY

CAUTION: *Read the information on pages 102 to 105 before using these essential oils.*

Lemon is the most effective essential oil for treating warts because it strengthens the body's resistance to the virus. Mix 7 drops of lemon with 2 teaspoons of base carrier oil. Apply to the wart then cover with sticking plaster. Repeat daily until the wart drops off.

BACH FLOWER REMEDIES

Take crab apple remedy for its cleansing effect.

HERBALISM

Comfrey and thuja are the herbs that will fight a wart infection. Put a lump of comfrey or thuja ointment on your wart and cover it with a sticking plaster each night before you go to bed. Repeat nightly.

HOMOEOPATHY

There are many homoeopathic remedies used to treat holistically the person who has wart virus. They include *Antimonium crudum, Natrum muriaticum, Thuja occidentalis* and *Nitricum acidum.* See a homoeopath for the remedy that is best for you.

MODERN MEDICINE

Scarring can occur from wart removal and this possibility should be discussed with your doctor. Prescription or over-the-counter ointments containing salicyclic acid or a similar substance can be applied to warts on sticking plasters or corn pads, causing them to wither so they can be scraped off. If using at home, a thin layer of petroleum jelly should be applied to the surrounding healthy skin as protection. Freezing off warts, burning them off with electric current, laser treatment and minor surgery are other options.

FIRST AID

PAGE 385

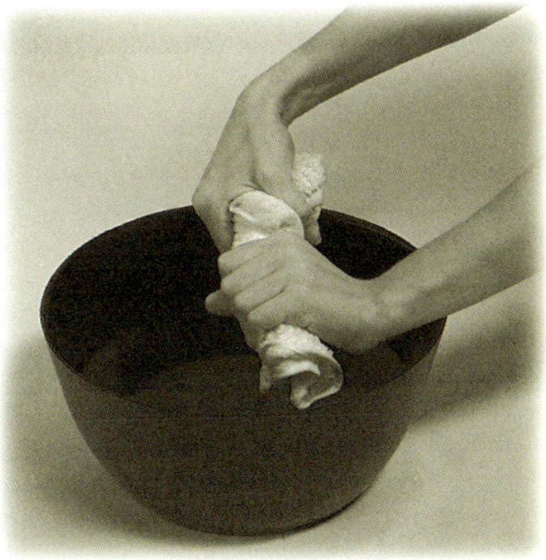

FIRST AID KIT

First aid materials should be stored inside a clearly marked, secure box, out of the reach of children. Items such as dressings and bandages should be kept in moisture-proof coverings. Any medication should be replaced regularly.

It is handy to have separate kits in the home, car and boat, and to have a smaller version of the kit for leisure activities such as hiking. Kits can be purchased ready-made from first aid associations or pharmacists.

- sterile non-adhesive dressings (assorted sizes)
- adhesive tape
- elastic bandages
- triangular bandage (sling)
- adhesive plasters (assorted sizes)
- gauze swabs
- sterile saline solution (for irrigation)
- antiseptic solution
- analgesics (e.g. paracetamol liquid, paracetamol tablets, soluble aspirin tablets)
- soothing skin lotion for itching, rashes, bites and stings (e.g. calamine lotion or a commercial preparation)
- measure for medicines
- sharp scissors with rounded tips
- sterile plastic gloves
- tweezers (forceps)
- thermometer
- splints (small and large)

FIRST AID PRIORITIES

- Remember when you are making first aid decisions that no matter what the injury, you have to keep the victim alive — breathing and heartbeat are your main priorities.
- Keep calm and work methodically.
- Do not move the person unless necessary.
- Do not leave the person alone.

ASSESSING INJURIES OR ILLNESS

The order of priorities is DRABC.

1. **Danger** — is the situation dangerous to you or the victim? Unless moving is essential, deal with ABC (Airways, Breathing, Circulation) first.
   See page 387 for moving an injured person.
2. **Response** — is the person conscious?
   See page 388 for more information, including positioning an unconscious person.
3. **Airways** — clear the airways of any obstruction.
   See page 388.
4. **Breathing** — check for 10 seconds by looking, listening and feeling.
   See page 388.
5. **Circulation** — check for 5 seconds at the carotid pulse in the neck.
   See page 389.

Then:

6. Is there blood, obvious wounds or broken bones?
   See page 390 for controlling bleeding, page 396 for treating fractures.
7. Is the person in shock?
   See page 391 for treating shock.

WHEN TO CALL THE DOCTOR

Seek immediate medical attention in cases of obvious injury and distress e.g. severe burns, head injuries, heavy bleeding, suspected fractures, possible poisoning, choking or suffocation. Also seek medical attention if there is a change to vital function, such as a rise or fall in pulse rate, even brief unconsciousness. See First Aid entries for what you can do in the meantime.

"Every-day" symptoms can be signals to seek medical attention when they are acute, prolonged, suddenly get worse or don't seem to have a cause. Such signs include:

- impairment of hearing or vision
- numbness
- dizziness
- confusion or amnesia
- spasms or convulsion.

Also, if there are two or more of the following symptoms:

- fever
- rash
- bad cough
- swollen glands
- stiff neck
- no appetite
- general feeling of sickness.

If you are concerned about any symptom, get professional advice. Do not ignore symptoms and do not think that you are wasting the doctor's/therapist's time. Advice on when to seek medical attention is also listed in the entries in the A–Z OF HEALTH CONDITIONS and NATURAL HEALTH FOR CHILDREN (e.g. EARACHE).

Bleeding: blood in urine, faeces or vomit; unexplained blood or other discharge from any body opening.
Breathing difficulties: shortness of breath even when resting or if accompanied by drowsiness; persistant wheezing over a few hours.
Diarrhoea: any in an infant; if it continues longer than 12 hours in children and 24 hours in adults; if accompanied by severe discomfort or vomiting; if there is blood in the faeces.
Headache: if it persists for 24 hours or recurs repeatedly over 3 days.
Pain: if it persists for 48 hours, especially without obvious cause; if it is severe enough to interfere with normal activity and/or sleep. Seek immediate medical attention if it is sudden and severe (especially in abdomen or chest) or involves pressure in the chest (particularly, if combined with shortness of breath).
Temperature: normal body temperature is 37°C; if temperature is above 40°C, seek immediate medical attention; if it is above 38°C, monitor for up to 24 hours; if it is below 38°C, seek medical attention if it is accompanied by other symptoms, particularly pain or swelling, or it persists for several days; any fever in an infant under 3 months.
Vomiting: if it is continual or severe; if an adult has vomited more than six times within a day; if a child has vomited more than three times within a day; any vomiting by an infant; if you suspect poisoning, seek immediate medical attention (see page 399).

MOVING AN INJURED PERSON

Only move injured people:
- to remove them from immediate danger (e.g. fire, electricity, traffic)
- to place them on their side if unconscious
- to place them on their back for resuscitation.

1. Place the person's arms by their sides.
2. Crouch behind their head and take hold of the clothing by the shoulders, if it it strong enough. Alternatively, take hold of the wrists.
3. Slide the person backwards. Drag, rather than lift. Keep the body as level as possible but do not let the head bump the ground.

If the person can walk with assistance, and does not have an arm or shoulder injury:

1. Stand beside them on the injured side.
2. Place your inside arm across their back and grip the clothes at hip-level on the uninjured side.
3. Drape the person's inside arm around your neck and over your outside shoulder, holding the hand to keep this position. In this way you can give support with your inside shoulder.
4. When walking, both you and the other person should step forward first with the inside foot.

UNCONSCIOUSNESS

Unconsciousness occurs when a person cannot respond to normal stimuli. Even if unconsciousness is only temporary, medical aid should be sought. Try to establish the cause of unconsciousness. Observe the person's appearance:

- red and flushed — could indicate diabetic coma, epilepsy, heat stroke, hypertension, skull fracture, stroke.
- pale — could indicate bleeding, convulsions, frostbite, heat exhaustion, insulin shock, poisoning, shock.
- blue — could indicate choking, drowning, electric shock, heart attack, gas poisoning.

The reflexes of an unconscious person may not be functioning normally which may lead to breathing difficulties. In all cases, the person must be placed in the stable side position (see below) to prevent choking or inhalation of vomit when they start to regain consciousness.

Steps to take

1. If the person is in immediate danger (from traffic, for example), move them. See page 387.
2. Assess unconsciousness by speaking very loudly to the person. Shake them gently if you do not suspect head, neck or back injuries.
2. Send for medical assistance but do not leave the person alone if at all possible.
3. Place the person in the stable side position (see below).
4. (a) **Airway** — clear their airway of any foreign material (see next column).
   (b) **Breathing** — check for 10 seconds by looking, listening and feeling. Resuscitate if necessary (see next column).
   (c) **Circulation** — check pulse for 5 seconds at the carotid muscle at the neck (see page 389). Begin CPR if necessary (see page 390).
5. Loosen tight clothing.
6. Do not try to give any drink or food — the person may choke.
7. Treat any injuries.
8. Monitor breathing and pulse until help arrives.

Stable side position

1. Place the person on the back. Kneel beside.
2. Place the person's far arm at right angles to the body.
3. Bend the near arm across the chest.
4. Bend the near knee so that the leg is at right angles to the body.

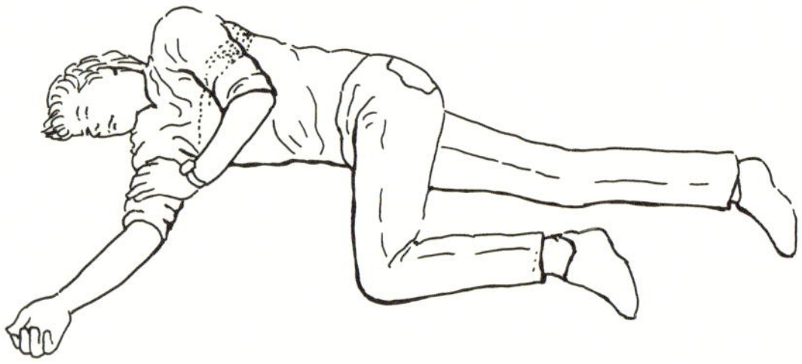

5. Maintain control over the head and, pushing on the knee as a lever, turn the person onto the side.
6. Bend the top arm across the bottom straight arm.
7. Open the mouth and clear the airway of any foreign material with your finger.
8. Check the head is tilted backwards with the face slightly downwards to keep the airway clear.

RESUSCITATION

The ABC of first aid involves A for airway, B for breathing and C for circulation:

A — AIRWAY

To ensure the airway is clear.

1. Place the casualty in the stable side position (see previous column).
2. Open the mouth and clear out any foreign material with your finger (including dentures if they are loose or broken).
3. Ensure the tongue is not blocking the airway. Place one of your hands on the forehead and the other hand under the lower jaw, and gently tilt the head back by lifting the jaw upwards and forwards.
4. Loosen any clothing around the neck.

B — BREATHING

While in the stable side position, check that the person is breathing. Watch or feel for chest movements, listen or feel for breath for 10 seconds. If there is no sign, turn onto the back and start expired air resuscitation (EAR) — which involves one of the following techniques.

EAR version 1: Mouth-to-mouth resuscitation

1. Pinch the person's nostrils to prevent air escaping.
2. Take a deep breath and seal your lips around the person's lips. Exhale firmly into the mouth.
3. If the chest does not rise, check head tilt and again look for obstructions of the airway.

   If the chest does rise, remove your lips and watch the chest fall. At the same time, place your ear close to the mouth, listening and feeling for the air leaving the lungs.

4. Repeat the procedure for 5 quick breaths (about 2 seconds for each cycle).
5. If there are no signs of breathing resuming, continue EAR at a rate of 1 breath every 4 seconds.
6. Check the pulse after 1 minute (see next column).

If there is one, continue applying mouth-to-mouth at this 4-second rate, monitoring the pulse every 2 minutes, until breathing begins independently. Then place the person in the stable side position (see page 388).

If there is no pulse, begin CPR (see page 390).

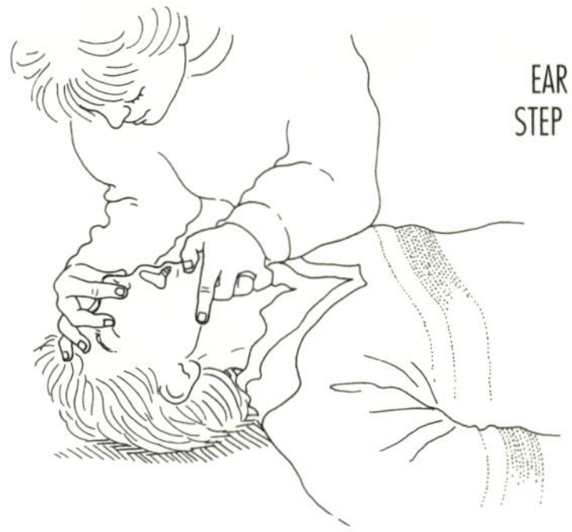

EAR STEP 1

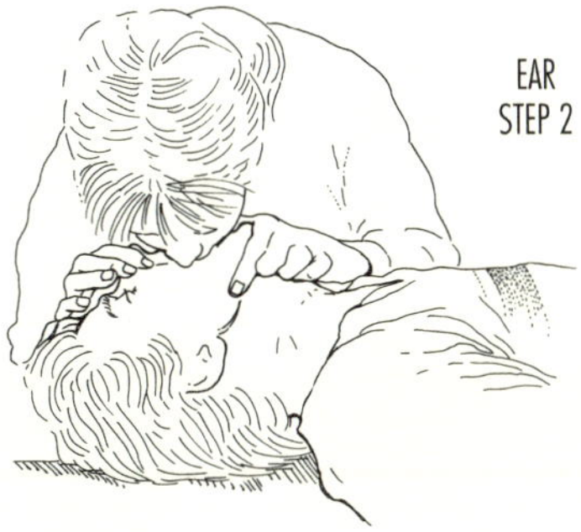

EAR STEP 2

EAR version 2: Mouth-to-nose resuscitation

This follows the same technique as mouth-to-mouth except your mouth is sealed over the person's nose and the mouth is held shut. Take care that even the bridge of the nose is completely covered but not to press the nostrils together.

This method is used when mouth-to-mouth is inappropriate e.g when the jaw is injured, the mouth is obstructed, the lips are coated with poison, or resuscitation is carried out in deep water.

For babies and small children

This follows the same technique as for an adult, except:

- do not tilt the head back
- it may be easier to seal your mouth over a child's mouth and nose
- breathe more gently than for an adult
- each breath cycle should take only 3 seconds (20 cycles in 1 minute).
- if you fail to clear a child's airways with your finger, the child may be held head-down and give several firm hits between the shoulder blades.

C — CIRCULATION

Heartbeat is indicated by pulse rate which is normally regular and strong, although it can increase dramatically during excitement or physical effort. The average resting rate is 60–80 beats per minute for adults (increasing up to 180 beats per minute during exercise or heightened emotional state), up to 100 beats per minute for children, and up to 140 beats per minute for babies. Injury or illness may cause changes to the pulse, making it weak and rapid, slow and pounding, or irregular.

Checking the pulse

- Monitor the pulse of a seriously injured or ill person every few minutes
- Check the neck pulse rather than the wrist pulse if possible as it is easier to detect in severe conditions.
- Use the three middle fingers of one hand to feel the pulse in the hollow of the neck just to one side of the Adam's apple. Do not press on the other side of the neck while you are doing this.
- Count the beats for 1 minute.
- Time the pulse with the second-hand on a watch if possible, or get someone else to count regularly ("One and then two and then three and then...").
- If checking the wrist pulse: feel the underside of the wrist about 2.5 cm (1 inch) from the base of the thumb and 1 cm (1/2 inch) from the side.
- If the pulse is absent, begin CPR (cardio-pulmonary resuscitation).

Cardio-pulmonary resuscitation (CPR)
This is a combination of expired air resuscitation (EAR) as described under Breathing and external cardiac compression (ECC). Use only when the heart has stopped beating and the person is likely to die if no assistance is given. CPR should be learned from a qualified instructor, and is best carried out by a team of two.

Steps to take
1. Check the pulse and if it is absent, begin CPR immediately.
2. Place the casualty on the back. Take up a kneeling position next to the chest.
3. Feel for the breastbone. Position one hand on the person's chest, two fingers' distance from the bottom of the breastbone. Have your fingers and thumb raised off the chest but hold the heel of the hand in place. Position your other hand over the top with the fingers interlocked — keep the bottom hand's thumb and fingers raised.

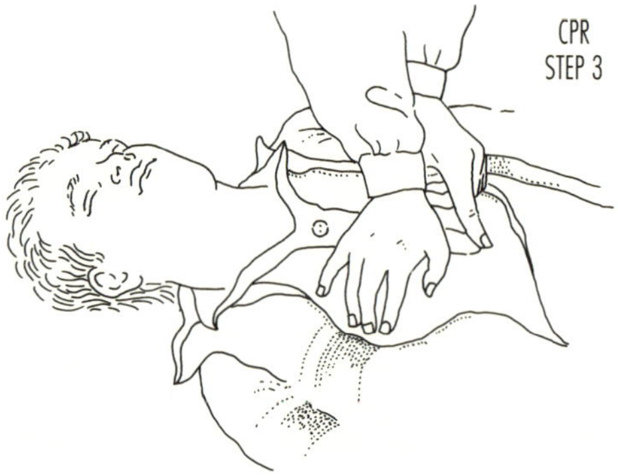
CPR
STEP 3

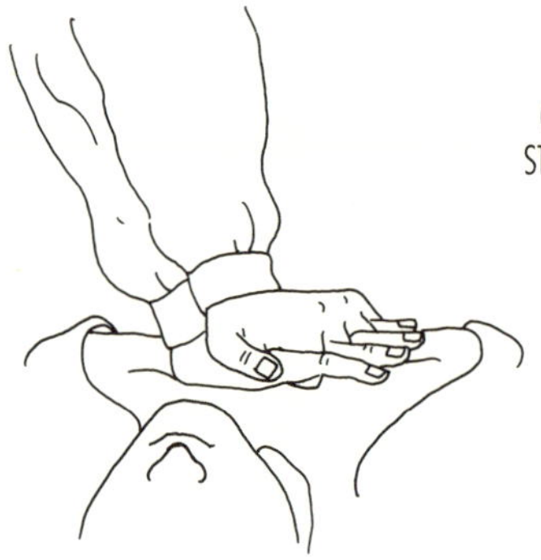
CPR
STEP 3

4. Press down about 5 cm then release pressure to let the chest rise — do not remove your hands. This is performed 15 times. Follow these compressions with 2 breaths. This is 1 cycle. Do 4 cycles each minute.
   If doing CPR in a pair: A cycle should be made up of 5 compressions followed by 1 breath, taking a total of 5 seconds (i.e. 1 compression per second with equal time for pressure and relaxation).
6. Check the pulse after 1 minute. If not present, continue CPR. If present but still not breathing, stop ECC but continue with EAR.
7. When pulse and breathing has resumed, place person in the stable side position (see page 388) and monitor closely.

For children
- Use only the heel of one hand and position it on the lower half of the breastbone.
- Press down only 2 to 4 cm.
- Use a cycle of 5 compressions followed by 1 breath. The younger the person the faster the rate — up to 100 compressions per minute.

For babies
- Support the baby along your arm with your hand cradling the head.
- Use only two fingers and position them on the lower half of the breastbone.
- Press down only a little more than 1 cm.
- Use a cycle of 5 compressions followed by 1 breath at a rate of 120 compressions per minute (i.e. 2 per second).

BLEEDING

Bleeding can look alarming but can be treated simply — normally healthy people can lose about one-fifth of their blood without serious effects. It is recommended where possible to wear rubber gloves.

1. Stay calm.
1. Check breathing and pulse. If necessary, start resuscitation (see page 388).
2. Do NOT use a tourniquet.

3. Lie the person flat, unless there are chest injuries, and elevate the bleeding area if possible.
4. If there are no embedded objects in the wound, apply direct pressure until the bleeding stops. Ideally use clean cloth but otherwise just your hand (do not waste time in an emergency situation searching for dressing or washing your hands). If it is a gaping wound, press the edges together.
5. If there is a foreign object in the wound, do not remove. Press around the wound.
6. Apply a pad of clean absorbent material and bind the wound to maintain pressure. If blood oozes through, do not remove dressing — apply more.
7. Seek medical attention for severe bleeding and continue to monitor for signs of shock (see below) and further bleeding. Do not give anything to eat or drink.

SHOCK

The medical condition known as shock refers to the insufficient circulation of blood to the brain and body.

Shock can be caused by:
- severe bleeding (sometimes internal)
- heart attack
- spinal injury
- poisoning
- fluid loss from diarrhoea, vomiting or major burns.

Shock is progressive. It may begin with pallor and lead to unconsciousness and even death. Signs include:

- paleness
- cold, clammy skin
- feeling faint or dizzy
- feeling anxious or agitated
- shallow breath
- rapid but weak pulse
- thirst, nausea
- feeling confused or drowsy
- unconsciousness.

1. Try to identify the cause and determine other first aid requirements and their priority (see page 386).
2. If conscious, lay the person on the back with the head flat and legs elevated above the level of the heart (except in case of leg fracture) to maintain blood flow to brain. If unconscious, lay the person in the stable side position (see page 388).
3. Loosen clothing but keep the person warm, not hot, with a blanket or coat.
4. Do not give anything to eat or drink.
5. Seek medical attention and continue to monitor pulse and breathing, remembering that shock is progressive.

CHOKING

Choking is usually caused by a foreign object such as a piece of food becoming lodged in the airway, obstructing breathing. There are manoeuvres in addition to those listed here but they are best learned under the supervision of a first aid trainer.

Signs include:
- violent fit of coughing
- face and neck become red then purple
- extreme attempts to breathe

1. It is crucial that you remove the object immediately. Coughing should be the first attempt at dislodging.
2. If coughing fails, try to remove it with your finger — but be careful not to push it down further.
3. If this fails, position the person so that the object can fall out: either bent forward over the back of the chair, or sitting in a chair and leaning forward, or turned to the side if lying down. Try two or three sharp slaps between the shoulder blades.
4. If you fail to dislodge the object, you will have to gently blow air into the lungs past the object using mouth-to-mouth resuscitation techniques (see page 388) until medical attention is received.

For babies and children
1. Sit down and place the child face-down across your knees with the head low. Slap two or three times between the shoulder blades with the heel of your hand.
2. Alternatively, hold the child in your arms with the head down and slap between the shoulder blades.

ABDOMINAL INJURIES

If there has been a deep cut to the abdomen and organs are protruding:

- Do not touch the organs or try to put them back (you may cause further injury).
- Gently cover exposed organs with a non-sticking material such as foil, plastic wrap, damp cloth.
- If using cloth, keep it warm and moist.
- Position the person on the back with quite a high support under the shoulders and another under the knees.

BITES AND STINGS

Bees, wasps, centipedes and scorpions

1. Do not pull or squeeze the bee or wasp sting. Remove it by scraping sideways with a fingernail, blunt knife or similar object.
2. Wipe area clean and apply ice wrapped in clean fabric to relieve pain. Reapply as needed but take care not to actually freeze the skin.
3. Monitor for allergic reaction (see Box). If severe, apply pressure immobilisation (see Box), seek urgent medical attention and monitor pulse and breathing.

Ticks

Ticks, which are active in spring and summer, can drop onto a person from surrounding bush and burrow into the skin. The tick's end remains visible. If you find one tick, search carefully for others. The venom can cause irritation and a lump. Occasionally, if left untreated, paralysis can occur from a bush tick. Seek urgent medical attention if any of the following signs are displayed:

- irritation and prickling sensations in the affected area
- double vision
- unsteadiness
- weakness of the face and eyelids which can progress to the breathing muscles and the upper limbs.

1. Do not pull or cut or squeeze to get the tick out.
2. Slide the two open blades of splinter tweezers around the sides of the tick and lever it outwards, making sure the mouth is not left behind in the skin. Or seek medical assistance for this procedure.
3. Wash area with soap and water and dry gently.

Snakes

Attend to the person rather than trying to find the snake as the type of venom can now be detected through tests. Treat all snake bites as serious and seek medical attention, even if you believe the snake to be non-poisonous. Symptoms can take up to 2 hours to develop.

1. Do not move the person or raise the limb as this will distribute the poison. Rest him comfortably and reassure him.
2. Do not wash the venom from the skin (it may help identification). Do not cut or cauterise the bite or try to suck out the venom.
3. Apply pressure immobilisation (see Box).
4. Seek urgent medical attention. Monitor pulse and breathing (see page 388).

Funnel-web spider

1. Treat as for snake bite. Urgent medical attention is crucial as the bite is life-threatening but an antivenom is available.

Red-back spider

1. Apply an ice-cube wrapped in damp fabric to relieve the pain. Reapply as needed but do not freeze the skin.
2. Do NOT apply pressure immobilisation.
3. Medical attention is necessary within 24 hours; antivenom is available. Monitor pulse and breathing (see page 388).

SIGNS OF AN ALLERGIC REACTION

- Pain, swelling and itchiness
- Puffy eyelids
- Wheezing and breathing difficulties

PRESSURE IMMOBILISATION

1. Apply pressure to the area with hands until a bandage can be applied.

2. Use a firm bandage, either commercial (e.g. crepe or one constructed specifically for pressure immobilisation) or improvised (e.g. fabric strips, pantyhose).

3. Start at the bite area and bandage limb down to extremeties (in the case of the limb, to the fingers or toes) then continue to bandage upwards (to the armpit or groin). Immobilise limb using a splint. See page 402 for details.

5. Seek medical attention, preferably without moving the patient.

Portuguese man-of-war (blue-bottle)

1. Do not attempt to remove tentacles with fingers or to rub the affected area.
2. Apply an ice cube wrapped in damp fabric to relieve the pain. Reapply as needed but do not freeze the skin. Alternatively, use cold compresses.
3. Do NOT apply pressure immobilisation.
4. Watch for allergic reaction. If so, apply pressure immobilisation and cold compresses to the throat.

Box jellyfish

1. Do not attempt to remove tentacles with fingers or to rub the affected area.
2. Flood the tentacles with vinegar which neutralises any active sting cells. Apply a pressure immobilisation bandage to the area (see BOX).
3. If no vinegar is available, apply the firm compression bandage above the sting. Gently remove any tentacles with tweezers (not fingers) then apply a firm compression bandage to the area.
4. Monitor pulse and breathing (see page 388) as this sting can be life-threatening.

Blue-ringed octopus and cone shell

1. Reassure the person.
2. Send for medical assistance urgently but do not leave person alone. Respiratory failure can occur rapidly.
3. Apply pressure immobilisation (see BOX).
4. Apply mouth-to-mouth or mouth-to-nose resuscitation (see page 388) as soon as breathing weakens and continue until medical assistance takes over.

Stonefish and bullrout

1. Bathe the area in hot (not scalding) water to relieve pain.
2. Remove any foreign body.
3. Do NOT apply pressure immobilisation (it will increase pain and tissue damage).
4. Seek urgent medical attention. Treat for shock (see page 391).

BURNS

In emergency cases, deal with the dangerous situation first and check the patient's condition — conscious, breathing, heartbeat (see page 386).

1. The most effective treatment of all is to immediately flush the entire area with cold water for at least 10 minutes (twice as long for chemical and corrosive burns) to stop the burning process. Do not apply butter or other fat, or any lotions or ointments.
2. Lightly wrap the burn with a sterile, non-stick dressing (e.g. a clean, moist piece of thick gauze). Do not use towels, cotton wool, adhesive dressing or blankets directly on the wound.
3. For severe burns, seek medical attention. Provide support for the injured body part (rest it on pillows, for example). Do not give alcohol but do give frequent sips of water and monitor for signs of shock (see page 391). Alleviate extreme pain by gently pouring cold water over the dressing. Do not overcool, particularly if the person is very young or burns are extensive — watch for shivering.
4. If the burn is minor, leave lightly bandaged for the first 24 hours to allow the healing process to begin.
5. Do not break blisters.

SUNBURN

• To prevent sunburn, use a high protection sunscreen or remain covered by clothing, a hat or shade. If you do become sunburnt, make sure you drink plenty of water to replace the fluid you have lost in the sun.

• To help protect your skin from the inside against sunburn, take regular doses of vitamins C and E and beta carotene according to the instructions on the bottle.

• To alleviate the stinging of sunburn, shower in cool or tepid water (not cold).

• Alternative follow-up treatment options include a compress of mild vinegar and water solution or a covering of yogurt.

FOLLOW-UP TREATMENT

After first aid procedures, consider the following treatment for minor burns:

- After 24 hours, gently wash and dry the area and apply an antimicrobial cream, a mild cream containing aloe vera, or else a little essential oil of lavender diluted in base carrier oil. Re-cover with a fresh gauze.
- As the burn heals, change dressing and ointment daily. Don't pop blisters — they are a natural protection.
- You can try Bach flower remedies. Rescue remedy is effective to reduce the shock from a burn and holly and willow are for the anger and bitterness which can accompany the trauma of being burnt.
- Aloe vera is an analgesic and healer. The pain of a burn, especially sunburn, can be significantly relieved by taking a leaf of an aloe plant, peeling it, and applying it to the burn 3 times a day for about 30 minutes at a time. Comfrey ointment can be used after the wound has closed. It will help reduce scarring.
- Some homoeopathic remedies which relieve burns include *Calendula officinalis* (otherwise known as calendula) and *Urtica urens*. Apply homoeopathic cream containing one of these to the burn immediately after it has occurred. Apply every hour for the first couple of days and then every morning and night until the burn heals.
- After your burn has started to heal apply vitamin E (use the oil from capsules for greater strength) to reduce scarring.

ELECTROCUTION

1. Do not touch the victim — you could also receive a shock.
2. If the current is high voltage (such as power lines), wait for experts to turn it off as the ground around the area could be conducting a strong current.
2. If low current is involved (as in a home or office), turn off the power or move the victim from the source with something made from dry wood like a broom handle or chair. Avoid anything wet and try to stand on a non-conducting surface like rubber.
3. Smother any burning clothing with a blanket or similar material.
4. Check breathing and start EAR if necessary (see page 388).
5. Check pulse after 5 breaths and start CPR if necessary (see page 390).
6. Once breathing has resumed, place the person in the stable side position (see page 388) and check for other injuries such as burns (see page 393).
7. Call an ambulance or get urgent medical attention. Although there may be only minor burns, electric shock can cause serious internal injuries.

EYE INJURIES

- Eye injuries are potentially serious and should receive expert medical attention.
- Do not rub or touch an injured eye.
- Do not open a closed eye as you could do further damage.
- Do not remove contact lenses unless the wearer can easily remove lenses themselves.
- Lie the person flat and cover both eyes.

CHEMICAL INJURIES

Chemical and heat burns should be washed immediately to prevent further damage.

Tilt the person's head to the affected side, hold the eyelids apart with thumb and forefinger, and rinse the eye with a gentle stream of lukewarm water for at least 20 minutes. Make sure the water does not flow into the other eye. When rinsed clean, cover eye with a clean cloth and seek medical attention.

Do not wash a flash burn.

FOREIGN BODIES

Simply splashing open eyes with water can be enough to rinse away loose surface irritants. Otherwise, tilt the head to the affected side and rinse the eye with a gentle stream of lukewarm water, blinking at the same time.

If this does not work, the object may be removed by touching it with a moistened piece of clean cloth. The eye should look down if the object is under the upper lid, or up if the object is under the lower lid.

Do not touch any part of the eye other than the white and the eyelids.

If an object is stuck or embedded, do not try to remove. Cover both eyes with a clean cloth and seek medical attention.

BLACK EYE

Check the eyeball for any damage. If there is, or if the person cannot see properly, cover the eye with a clean cloth and seek medical attention.

If the eyeball is not damaged, treat with a cold compress intermittently — apply to the eye area for 20 minute intervals, removing for 2 hours in between.

FAINTING

Fainting is caused by a temporary drop in the blood supply to the brain and is usually triggered by heat, lack of air, over-exertion or extreme emotion, although it can be a sign of illness or injury.

Warning signs before a faint:
- dizziness, weakness, hot and cold flushes
- pale, clammy skin
- sweating
- frequent yawning
- blurred vision.

If you feel these sensations, lie down until the signs have passed then rise slowly.

If a person has fainted but is breathing normally:
1. Lie the person flat with legs raised higher than the heart to increase blood supply to the brain.
2. Loosen any tight clothing and make sure he can get plenty of air.
3. Check that the person has not injured himself as he fainted.
4. Recovery should happen spontaneously within a few minutes but if it does not, place the person in the stable side position (see page 388) and seek immediate medical attention.

FITS AND CONVULSIONS

A fit or convulsion is a disturbance in the functioning of the brain. There may be a number of causes, including head injury or poison, although a common cause is epilepsy.

EPILEPTIC FIT

In an epileptic fit, a sufferer will usually lose consciousness and collapse, lying rigid for a few seconds with the back arched and the jaw clamped shut. They may hold their breath, causing the face to turn blue. As breathing resumes, there may be jerking muscular movements and frothing at the mouth. The casualty may bite their tongue or lose control of bladder or bowel. After consciousness has been regained, they may be confused and unable to remember the event for about 15 to 20 minutes, and will continue to feel exhausted afterwards.

- Protect the casualty from injury but do not restrict movements.
- Remove any surrounding objects that may be dangerous.
- Do not pry mouth open or force objects into it.
- Protect the head by placing something flat and soft (like a folded sweater) underneath.

- Loosen the collar if possible to allow easier breathing.
- The casualty will breathe normally again at the end of the seizure, but may fall asleep. Place them in the stable side position (see page 388) and monitor breathing and pulse.
- Look for any card or tag on the person that may give instructions as to what action to take when a siezure has occurred. If the person is a known epileptic, ask if they wish to consult a doctor. Otherwise, seek medical attention.

FEBRILE CONVULSIONS

This kind of convulsion is experienced by some children under the age of about four and is associated with high temperatures caused by infection. The signs of febrile convulsion include a rigid body with twitching, rolling eyes, an arched head and back, a congested face and neck, and bluish face and lips.

1. Ensure the airway is clear and turn the child on the side if necessary.
2. Remove all clothing.
3. Bathe or sponge the child with tepid water.
4. Fan the child.
5. When the temperature has been lowered, cover the child lightly.
6. Seek medical attention.

FRACTURE

A fracture is just another term for a broken bone. There are three main kinds:

- greenstick fractures — in young people the flexible bones may bend without breaking completely.
- closed fractures — the skin around the fracture remains unbroken but the bone can cause serious damage to tissue.
- open fractures — the bone protrudes through the skin or wound, risking serious blood loss and infection.

Signs of a fracture include:
- the snapping sound of a bone breaking
- the dry grating noise of broken bone rubbing together
- pain which is made worse by movement of the part
- unnatural appearance or movement of the part, or the inability to move it
- tenderness under gentle pressure
- swelling.

1. Do not move a person with a suspected back or neck fracture unless he is in immediate danger. Other fractures should be moved as little as possible and treated very gently.
2. Do not try to manipulate the bone or joint yourself as you could cause further damage.
3. Make the person as comfortable as possible; give the fractured limb as much support as possible.
4. Carefully remove clothing from any open wound around the break, and apply a ringpad bandage (a bandage wrapped around the area to form padding).
5. Immobilise the fracture using bandages, slings and splints (see pages 401 to 402).
6. Do not give anything to eat or drink (the setting of the fracture may require an anaesthetic). Seek medical attention.

FROSTBITE

Frostbite results in the freezing of body tissue, usually in the toes, fingers or other extremeties. Deep frostbite may affect the blood supply so seriously that amputation may be necessary.

Signs include:
- skin appears waxy and turns suddenly white
- skin is firm to touch
- area feels numb or tingling until warmed, then there is pain
- possible blistering.

1. Keep the casualty warm and dry. Move them to a warm dry place if possible.
2. Remove anything constricting the affected area.
3. Rewarm the area by body heat — cover with a hand, for example, or hold fingers under an armpit.
4. Do not rub or massage the area. Do not apply direct heat (such as hot water bottles), snow or cold water. Do not give alcohol.
5. Cover any blisters with dry sterile dressings.
6. Seek medical attention.

FOR DEEP FROSTBITE

In addition to the normal signs of frostbite, the area is white, hard to the touch, and painless.

1. Do NOT attempt to thaw.
2. Keep the casualty warm and dry.
3. Protect the injured area from further injury, particularly as the person will not be able to feel if more damage is being done.
4. Seek urgent medical attention.

HEAD INJURIES

Never disregard a head injury, no matter how insignificant it may first appear. Fatal injuries may not be apparent immediately, and unconsciousness and concussion may not occur for hours. Medical attention must be sought after even the briefest period of unconsciousness.

In cases of head injury:

1. Place the person in the stable side postion (see page 388) even if not unconscious. Support the head and neck. Be gentle, as there may be neck and back injuries.
2. Clear the airway (see page 388). In some cases of injury, you may need to keep the airway open with your fingers.
3. Monitor breathing and pulse.
4. Control any external bleeding (see page 390) but do not exert pressure on a suspected skull fracture. For scalp injuries, cover with a bulky, clean dressing and bandage lightly.
5. Keep the head as steady as possible.

CONCUSSION

Concussion is an altered mental state caused by a blow to the head or a severe shake of the body. The severity may vary from slight giddiness to complete loss of consciousness and memory loss. Symptoms may include: some loss of consciousness, confusion, slurred speech, difficulty with vision, shallow breathing, unsteadiness, nausea or vomiting, and pale, cold and clammy skin.

1. The person should lie down and be kept warm and comfortable.
2. Cold compresses to the forehead or site of injury may help.
3. Do not give anything to eat or drink.
4. If the person becomes unconscious, place in the stable side position (see page 388), monitor breathing and pulse, and seek immediate medical attention.

WARNING SIGNS OF SERIOUS INJURY

If any of these symptoms occur, seek medical attention immediately:

- worsened headache
- continued vomiting
- weakness down one side
- restlessness
- twitching of the limbs or convulsions
- drowsiness or stupor
- abnormal rcsponses and incoherent speech
- deliriousness
- noisy breathing
- collapse, fits or blackouts
- bruising around the eyes
- dilated pupils
- blurred vision
- clear or blood-stained fluid draining from the nose or ears.

HEART ATTACK

A heart attack occurs when the supply of blood to the heart is reduced by narrowing or hardening of the arteries, or because a clot has formed. The symptoms include:

- sudden chest pain which may be an ache or pressure, usually spreading to the arms, neck or jaw
- breathlessness
- weak or irregular pulse
- nausea or vomiting
- pale, cold, clammy skin
- anxiety
- shock (see page 391)

- unconscious collapse followed by the heart stopping (cardiac arrest).

1. Start the ABC of first aid (see page 388). If necessary, start resuscitation.
2. If the person is conscious, help them into a comfortable position — try a half-sitting posture with the head and shoulders supported by pillows and a pillow under the knees. Loosen clothing around the neck, chest and waist. Ensure there is plenty of air.
   If the person is unconscious but breathing, place them in the stable side postion (see page 388).
3. Seek medical attention urgently.
4. Comfort and reassure the person.

Heart failure sometimes occurs after a heart attack, or due to disease or old age, when the heart is less able to pump blood around the body leading to congestion of the lungs and other organs. Symptoms may include:

- bluish lips and extremities
- congested veins in the neck and swelling in the neck, legs and ankles
- severe shortage of breath
- noisy breathing
- weak but rapid pulse
- frothy, blood-stained mucus.

Treatment is similar to that for heart attack.

HEAT ILLNESS

HEAT EXHAUSTION

This is caused by dehydration or excessive loss of body fluids through perspiration. Symptoms include:

- exhaustion and faintness
- muscular weakness and lack of co-ordination
- muscle and stomach cramps
- headache
- nausea
- sweating
- pale, clammy skin
- rapid pulse
- irritability and confusion.

1. Rest the person in a cool airy place.
2. Check temperature and pulse.
3. Undress the person and sponge down with tepid water.
4. Give frequent small drinks, preferably water.
5. If condition does not improve, seek medical attention.

HEAT STROKE

Heat stroke is a complete breakdown of the body's heat-control mechanism and is more serious than (and often follows) heat exhaustion. Symptoms include:

- body temperature of 40°C or more
- hot, flushed dry skin
- strong and rapid pulse
- rapid breathing
- rapid onset of nausea
- headache
- restlessness
- confusion
- dilated pupils
- loss of consciousness.

1. Rest the person in a cool airy place.
2. If unconscious, place in the stable side position (see page 388).
3. Undress the person and sponge with cold water. Apply ice packs to the neck, groin and armpits.
4. Wrap in sheet or towels soaked in tepid water and fan regularly.
5. Seek medical attention.
6. Check temperature every 5 minutes. When temperature drops to 38°C, remove sheet but continue fanning. If temperature rises again, resume cooling procedures.
7. When person regains consciousness, give frequent drinks as tolerated.

HYPOTHERMIA

Prolonged over-exposure to cold can cause the body's internal (as well as surface) temperature to drop.

Symptoms can include:

- slow, shallow breathing
- weak pulse
- pale skin that feels cold and waxy
- shivering and numbness in some cases, although others may not actually feel cold
- confusion, lack of co-ordination, drowsiness, even loss of consciousness.

1. If unconscious, place in the stable side position (see page 388).
2. Slow gentle heating is required. Place person in warm, sheltered environment, if possible. Remove any wet clothing. Wrap in blankets or extra clothing, or place in a sleeping bag with another person (naked or in underwear) to share body heat.
3. Do not massage or warm via direct heat (such as a fire or heater).
4. If conscious, give sweet warm drinks. Do not give alcohol.
5. Check for frostbite. Seek medical attention.

OVERDOSE

The symptoms of overdose vary depending on the drug involved but can include:

- faintness
- slurred speech
- slow shallow breathing
- rapid but weak pulse
- twitching muscles and convulsions
- blue tinge to skin
- unconsciousness.

1. Check breathing and pulse. If necessary, start resuscitation (see page 388).
2. If person is breathing but unconscious, place in the stable side position and monitor (see page 388).
3. If person is conscious, treat for poisoning (see next column). Do not induce vomiting unless advised. Contact a poisons information centre or other emergency medical advice.
4. Seek immediate medical attention, even if person seems to have recovered.
5. Try to keep person awake but do not give coffee or help them walk about, unless stomach contents have been emptied.
6. Keep anything that will help identify the drug (e.g. samples of vomit, tablets, containers).

POISONING

In addition to the symptoms of overdose, signs of poisoning can include:

- ringing in the ears
- abdominal pain
- bite or injection marks
- burns around mouth or tongue
- change of skin colour
- odours of poison on breath.

1. If the person is unconscious, place in the stable side position (see page 388).
2. Monitor breathing and pulse. Wipe any remnant of the substance away from mouth, face or skin. If necessary, start resuscitation (see page 388) — using mouth-to-nose resuscitation if poison remains around the mouth.
3. Give nothing by mouth.
4. Seek medical attention urgently and contact a poisons information centre.
5. If the poison is a medicinal or similar substance, keep a sample of the vomit for medical examination.

If the poison has been inhaled

- Turn off the source (e.g. if it is gas) or remove the person to fresh air. Take care that you are not at risk — hold a deep breath, wear a wet cloth over your mouth and nose, or call the fire department.
- Loosen clothing and seek medical attention.
- Follow the ABC of first aid (see page 388).

If the poison has been absorbed through the skin

- Remove clothes and shower or wash thoroughly.
- Monitor the person's condition and seek medical attention.
- Wash the contaminated clothing separately from other clothes.

SEVERED BODY PARTS

Your first priority is to save the person, then to preserve the severed part of the body (limb, finger etc) for possible surgical re-attachment.

1. Do not attempt to restore the severed part yourself.
2. Put on gloves if possible.
3. Lay the person down, elevating the bleeding area.
4. Apply direct pressure until the bleeding stops. Ideally use clean cloth but otherwise just your hand (do not waste time searching for dressing or washing your hands).
5. Apply a pad of clean absorbent material and bind the wound to maintain pressure. If blood oozes through, do not remove dressing — just apply more.
6. Seek medical attention while treating for shock (see page 391).
7. Wrap severed body part in clean material. Place in plastic bag. Place bag in cold water to which ice has been added and send with person to hospital.

SPRAINS, STRAINS AND DISLOCATIONS

A strain occurs when a muscle or tendon is overstretched. A sprain occurs when ligaments connected to a joint are wrenched or torn. Dislocation occurs when the ligaments are stretched so far that the bones of a joint are forced out of contact with each other.

Sprains and dislocations display many of the same symptoms as fractures (see page 396) so if there is any doubt, medical attention should be sought.

STRAINS AND SPRAINS

1. Make the person comfortable. Remove or loosen clothing around the injury. Handle the injured muscle gently and support it carefully.
2. If there is any suspicion that a fracture may be involved, treat as a fracture (see page 396).
3. If a fracture is not involved, gently apply an ice pack or cold compress to the injured area for a maximum of 20 minutes, then remove for 2 hours. Wrap ice in damp cloth before applying to skin.
4. Bandage firmly but not too tightly as muscles may swell (see bandaging, page 401).
5. Elevate the injured part using a sling (see page 402) or pillows to reduce pressure and swelling.

DISLOCATIONS

1. Never try to push a dislocated bone back into place.
2. Rest the joint in the most comfortable position and treat as for fractures (see page 396).
3. Using a splint and soft padding, splint the bone in the position in which it was found (see page 402).
4. Seek medical attention.

SUFFOCATION

A person's supply of oxygen may be cut off due to blockage of the mouth and nose, chest injury, collapse of the lungs, liquid in the lungs (drowning), smoke inhalation or toxic fumes.

Signs include:

- swollen veins in the head and neck
- blue around the lips and nails
- difficult, noisy breathing becoming spasms and then stopping
- rapid pulse becoming weak and then stopping.

1. Remove any obstruction. If the cause is smoke or fumes, transfer the person to a safe place (keep low and cover your mouth and nose with cloth). If there is smoke, do not open windows or doors as this can increase the fire-risk.
2. Check breathing and pulse. If necessary, start resuscitation (see page 388).
3. If person is breathing but still unconscious, place in the stable side position and treat for unconsciousness (see page 388).
4. Seek medical attention and continue to monitor breathing and pulse.

Skills

TAKING A TEMPERATURE

Although it can vary with activity and time of day, average body temperature is 37°C. Changes due to injury or illness may include:

- low temperature (after shock, page 391; bleeding, page 390; or hypothermia, page 389)
- high temperature (indicating severe infection).

ADVICE ON TAKING TEMPERATURE

- Use a mercury thermometer for an accurate reading.
- Wash and dry the thermometer then shake it (holding the rounded glass end) until the reading is lower than 37°C.
- For adults and older children, place the thermometer under the tongue with the lips closed gently around it. Do not use this method within 20 minutes after consuming hot or cold substances.
- Leave the thermometer in place for 3 minutes before reading.
- Wash the thermometer with soap and warm water (not hot water as it may break the glass). Rinse and store in its case.
- For those who may bite the thermometer but for whom rectal readings are not possible, place the thermometer high up under the arm and hold the arm gently but firmly by the side of the body. The same method can be used in the groin crease. Wait 10 minutes before reading. These methods are less accurate than the oral method.

BANDAGING

DRESSINGS

Dressings are placed over wounds before bandaging to absorb discharges, and prevent infection and further damage.

- Use clean non-stick material. If commercial dressings are unavailable, you can use handkerchiefs or towels. Do not place material that sheds fibres (e.g. cotton wool) in direct contact with a wound.
- Wash hands before touching either wound or dressing, and wear gloves if at all possible. Avoid breathing or coughing on the dressing.
- Pads of clean material can be used on top of the dressing to increase pressure and absorption.

BANDAGES

Bandages are used to:

- keep dressings and splints in place
- prevent and reduce swelling
- control bleeding through pressure
- support or immobilise an injury.

Elasticated bandages are recommended for injured joints and crepe bandages serve well as compression bandages. In the absence of commercial bandages, improvise with clean fabric (such as sheets) or even belts and pantyhose.

What you should do

1. Position yourself opposite the person and make sure the injured part is supported.
2. Hold the bandage (ideally in a roll) in one hand and, with your other hand, place the end of the bandage at a place just below the injury.
3. Unroll the bandage a few centimetres at a time, bandaging outwards from the person's body. Overlap each turn slightly and keep an even pressure.
4. Finish just above the injury and fasten the bandage securely. To tie off, cut the end into two strips and make a reef knot. Otherwise, fold in the end of the bandage and secure with a safety pin or adhesive tape.
5. Bandages should be firm but not too tight — the surrounding areas or extremities should not become numb or turn blue-white.

SLINGS

Arm sling for an injured forearm

1. The injured person should support the arm, raising the wrist and hand higher than the elbow.
2. Use a bandage that is in the shape of a large triangle. Place it between the chest and the forearm so that the top of the triangle (A) is stretched well beyond the elbow, the uppermost point (B) hangs over the shoulder and the bottom point (C) hangs towards the ground.

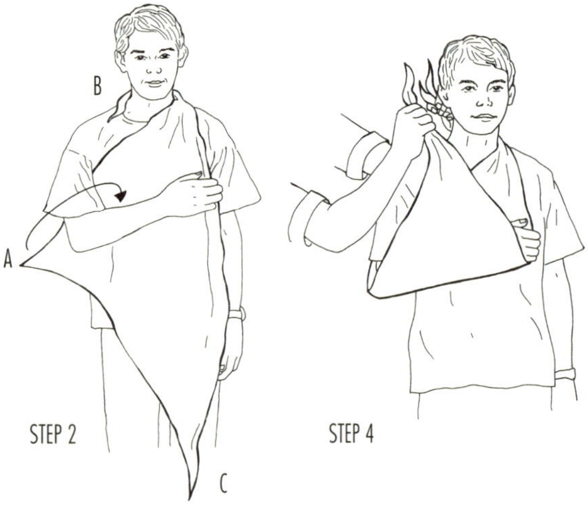

3. Bring point A over the elbow and tuck between the arm and the sling.
4. Bring point C over the forearm and bring point B behind the neck so that the two points meet in the hollow of the neck just above the collar bone on the injured side. Tie the ends with a reef knot.
5. Monitor the colour of the fingernails. If they turn white or blue, loosen the bandage or change the position of the arm.

Elevation sling for an injured hand, forearm or shoulder

1. The injured person should rest the hand of the injured side on the opposite shoulder with the upper arm by the side of the body.
2. Cover the forearm and hand with a bandage in the shape of a large triangle. The top point of the triangle (A) should be towards the bent elbow. The upper point (B) hangs over the shoulder and the lower point (C) hangs towards the ground.
3. Place one of your hands on the person's shoulder to hold both the person's hand and point B. Keep your hand here.
4. With your other hand, tuck point A firmly under the upper arm.
5. Now, bring point C up under the upper arm and then around the person's back to meet up with point B on the uninjured side.
6. Tie point B and point C together in a reef knot.
7. Monitor the colour of the fingernails. If they turn white or blue, loosen the bandage or change the position of the arm.

If you do not have a piece of material you can use for a sling, you can turn up and pin the person's shirt or, if the sleeves are long, pin the sleeve to the front of the shirt on the opposite side. If even this is not possible, tuck the wrist inside the buttoned shirt-front.

SPLINTS

Splints are used to support or immobilise limbs, especially in case of Fracture. You can use any rigid item such as a piece of wood or cardboard, a rolled up newspaper or blanket — as long as it is long enough to reach above and below the fracture. The body itself can also be used, e.g. the other leg (in the case of an injured leg) or the trunk of the body (in the case of an injured arm).

1. Move the limb as little as you can (avoid removing clothing if possible).
2. Pad the area with clean folded fabric, especially between the splint and natural hollows, and on the bony points.
3. Bandage the splint firmly to the limb at the top and bottom and points in between but NOT over the wound area.
4. Monitor the bandages to check they are firm enough to immobilise effectively but are not causing pain or cutting off circulation (check the fingernails have not turned blue-white).

LIST OF HERBS

The botanical name for these herbs appears in parenthesis after the common name.

agrimony (*Agrimonia eupatoria*)
aloe vera (*Aloe barbadenis*)
astragalus (*Astragalus membranaceous* — also known as Huang Qi)
balm (*Melissa officinalis*)
barberry (*Berberis vulgaris*)
bearberry (*Arctostaphylos uva ursi* — also known as uva ursi)
bittersweet (*Solanum nigrum*)
black cohosh (*Cimicifuga racemosa*)
black horehound (*Ballota nigra*)
bladderwrack (*Fucus vesiculosus* — also known as kelp or seaweed)
bloodroot (*Sanguinaria canadensis*)
blue cohosh (*Caulophyllum thalictriodes*)
blue flag (*Iris versicolor*)
boneset (*Eupatorium perfoliatum*)
borage (*Borago officinalis*)
buchu (*Agathosma betulina*)
burdock (*Arctium lappa*)
calendula (*Calendula officinalis* — also known as marigold)
cascara sagrada (*Rhamnus purshiana*)
celandine (*Chelidonium majus*)
celery (*Apium graveolens*)
chamomile, German (*Matricaria chamomilla*)
chamomile, Roman (*Anthemis nobilis*)
chaste tree (*Vitex agnus castus*)
chickweed (*Stellaria media*)
chilli (*Capsicum annum*)
cinnamon (*Cinnamonum zeylandica*)
cleavers (*Galium aparine*)
coltsfoot (*Tussilago farfara*)
comfrey (*Symphytum officinale*)
corn silk (*Zea mays*)
cramp bark (*Viburnum opulus*)
cranesbill (*Geranium maculatum*)
damiana (*Turnera aphrodisiaca*)
dandelion (*Taraxacum officinale*)
devil's claw (*Harpagophytum procumbens*)
dill (*Anethum graveolens*)
dong quai (*Angelica sinensis*)
echinacea (*Echinacea angustifolia*)
elder (*Sambucus nigra*)
elecampane (*Inula helenium*)
epilobium (*Epilobium parviflorum*)
euphorbia (*Euphorbia hirta*)
evening primrose (*Oenothera biennis*)
eyebright (*Euphrasia officinalis*)
false unicorn root (*Chamaelirium luteum*)
fennel (*Foeniculum vulgare*)
feverfew (*Tanacetum parthenium*)
fringetree (*Chionanthus virginicus*)
fenugreek (*Trigonella foenum-graecum*)
garlic (*Allium sativum*)
gentian root (*Gentiana lutea*)
ginger (*Zingiber officinale*)
ginseng (*Panax ginseng*)
golden rod (*Solidago virgauria*)
golden seal (*Hydrastis canadensis*)
gravel root (*Eupatorium purpureum*)
greater celandine (*Chelidonium majus*)
grindelia (*Grindelia camporum*)
guaiacum (*Guaiacum officinale*)
gymnema (*Gymnema sylvestre*)
hawthorn berries (*Crataegus oxyacanthoides*)
hops (*Humulus lupulus*)
horsechestnut (*Aesculus hippocastanum*)
horseradish (*Armoracia rusticana*)
horsetail (*Equisetum arvense*)
hydrangea (*Hydrangea aborescens*)
hyssop (*Hyssopus officinalis*)
jamaican dogwood (*Piscidia erythrina*)
lemon balm (*Melissa officinalis*)
lime blossom (*Tilia europea* — also known as Linden blossom)
liquorice (*Glycyrrhiza glabra*)
lobelia (*Lobelia inflata*)
marshmallow (*Althaea officinalis*)
meadowsweet (*Filipendula ulmaria*)
motherwort (*Leonurus cardiaca*)
mullein (*Verbascum thapsus*)
myrrh (*Commiphora molmol*)
nettle (*Urtica dioica*)
oak bark (*Quercus robur*)
oats (*Avena sativa*)
passion flower (*Passiflora incarnata*)
pau d'arco (*Tabecuia impetiginosa*)
peppermint (*Mentha piperita*)
plantain (*Plantago major*)
pleurisy root (*Asclepias tuberosa*)
poke root (*Phytolacca decandra*)
prickly ash (*Zanthoxlyn americanum*)
psyllium husks (*Plantago psyllium*)
red clover (*Trifolium pratense*)

red raspberry (*Rubus idaeus*)
rhubarb root (*Rheum palmatum*)
rosemary (*Rosmarinus officinalis*)
rue (*Ruta graveolens*)
sage (*Salvia officinalis*)
saw palmetto berries (*Serenoa serrulata*)
senna pods (*Cassas senna*)
silymarin (*Silybum marianum*)
skullcap (*Scutellaria laterifolia*)
slippery elm bark (*Ulmus fulva*)
squaw vine (*Mitchella repens*)
sweet sumach (*Rhus aromatica*)
St John's wort (*Hypericum perforatum —* also known as hypericum)
St Mary's thistle (*Silybum marianum*)
thuja (*Thuja occidentalis*)
thyme (*Thymus vulgaris*)
true unicorn root (*Aletris farinosa*)
valerian (*Valeriana officinalis*)
vervain (*Verbena officialis — also known as lemon verbena*)
vitex (*Agnus castus*)
wild carrot (*Daucus carrota*)
wild cherry bark (*Prunus serotina*)
wild yam (*Dioscorea villosa*)
witch hazel (*Hamamelia virginiana*)
wormwood (*Artemisia absinthium*)
wood betony (*Betonica officinalis*)
yarrow (*Achillea millefolium*)
yellow dock (*Rumex crispus*)

LIST OF HOMOEOPATHIC REMEDIES

The commonly used name for these homoeopathic remedies appears in parenthesis after the botanical name.

Aconitum napellus (Aconite)
Aesculus hippocastanum (Aesculus)
Agaricus muscarius (Agaricus)
Allium cepa (Allium)
Aloe socotrina (Aloe)
Antimonium crudum (Antimodium)
Apis mellifica (Apis)
Argentum nitricum (Arg-nit.)
Arnica montana (Arnica)
Arsenicum album (Arsenicum)
Atropa belladonna (Belladonna)
Baryta carbonica (Baryta carb.)
Berberis vulgaris (Berberis)
Borax veneta (Borax)
Bryonia alba (Bryonia)
Calcarea carbonica (Calc-carb.)
Calcarea fluorata (Calc-f.)
Cantharis vesicatoria (Cantharis)
Carbo vegetabilis (Carbo-veg.)
Carduus marianus (Carduus)
Causticum (Causticum)
Chamomilla vulgaris (Chamomilla)
Chelidonium majus (Chelidonium)
Cina (Cina)
Coffea cruda (Coffea)
Colchicum autumnale (Colchicum)
Colocynthis (Coloc.)
Cuprum metallicum (Cuprum)
Datura stramonium (Stramonium)
Eupatorium perfoliatum (Eupatorium)
Euphrasia officinalis (Euphrasia)
Ferrum metallicum (Ferrum)
Ferrum phosphoricum (Ferrum-phos.)
Folliculinum (Folliculinum)
Gelsemium sempervirens (Gelsemium)
Graphites (Graphites)
Hamamelis virginica (Hamamelis)
Hypericum perforatum (Hypericum)
Kali bichromicum (Kali-bi.)
Lacticum acidum (Lacticum)
Lycopodium clavatum (Lycopodium)
Mercurius corrosivus (Merc-corr.)
Natrum muriaticum (Nat-mur.)
Nicotiana tabacum (Tabacum)
Nitricum acidum (Nitric-ac.)
Nux vomica (Nux)
Petroleum (Petroleum)
Phosphoricum acidum (Phos-ac)
Phosphorus (Phos.)
Podophyllum peltatum (Podophyllum)
Pulsatilla nigricans (Pulsatilla)
Rheum officinale (Rheum)
Rhus toxicondendrona (Rhus-tox)
Ruta graveolens (Ruta)
Sabina (Sabina)
Sarsaparilla (Sarasparilla)
Sepia officinalis (Sepia)
Silicea (Silicea)
Staphisagria (Staph.)
Sticta pulmonaria (Sticta)
Thuja occidentalis (Thuja)
Urtica urens (Urtica)
Veratrum album (Veratrum)

NUTRIENTS GLOSSARY

acidophilus: lactobacillus acidophilus — its full name — is a strain of "friendly" bacteria which is very beneficial to the digestive system. Long-term use of antibiotics or the contraceptive pill, or bouts of diarrhoea can destroy acidophilus. In these cases powder or tablet supplements are recommended to promote regrowth; they should be taken 30 minutes before food. Acidophilus can be included in the diet in "live culture" yogurts.

amino acids: the building blocks for protein. There are 20 amino acids necessary for human metabolism. Some can be produced by the body, while others are only found in food. The latter are known as essential amino acids. Food which contains all the essential amino acids are called complete proteins and include meat, milk, cheese and eggs. Incomplete proteins such as grains, pulses and vegetables contain only some of the amino acids and need to be eaten in proper combinations (see page 9).

beta carotene: a yellow pigment found in plant and animal tissue, especially red/yellow/orange vegetables such as carrots, corn and squash. It is stored and converted to vitamin A in the liver. A powerful antioxidant, it is recommended for protection against heart disease and cancer.

bifidus: a friendly bacteria (bifidobacterium bifidus) that is often incorporated with acidophilus into a supplement.

bioflavinoids: nutrients which aid the proper use of vitamin C. Recommended for blood capillary health (e.g. prevention of blood clots, stroke, coronary thrombosis).

bromelain: an enzyme found in pineapple that speeds up the conversion of proteins to amino acids. Recommended in some cases of heart disease.

calcium fluoride: this celloid affects the elasticity of tissues and is recommended for VARICOSE VEINS, HAEMORRHOIDS, CHAPPED SKIN, muscle strain and ache, torn ligaments and to help blood circulation.

celloids: also known as cell salts or tissue salts, these mineral salts occur naturally in human cells. There are 12 different cell salts, all with varying functions. An imbalance in any of the cell salts can lead to illness, so supplements have been developed to counterbalance deficiencies.

cod liver oil: an oil from the fresh liver of the codfish which is very high in vitamins A and D. It can be used to supplement these vitamins.

coenzyme Q10: also known as ubicaronine, this naturally occurring enzyme is involved in the production of energy. It is found in every cell in the body but is especially prevalent in the heart and liver. Low levels of coenzyme Q10 inhibits the conversion of food into energy. Recommended for FATIGUE, low energy levels, HEART PROBLEMS, weight control (see page 345), gum disease (see page 289) and boosting the immune system.

evening primrose oil: oil from the seed of the evening primrose plant which is converted by the body into a hormone-like substance (prostaglandin). Recommended for the regulation of the menstrual system and to alleviate PRE-MENSTRUAL TENSION and reduce breast tenderness. It helps maintain healthy arteries and is used to treat ARTHRITIS, ECZEMA and high cholesterol levels (see page 234). It also has general anti-inflammatory properties.

fish oil: fish oils, especially those from deep sea fish, contain the omega-3 fatty acids which regulate blood clotting, control cholesterol levels and reduce arterial clotting. The oils have been associated with low levels of heart disease.

lecithin: naturally occurring in every cell in the body, especially the brain, kidneys and endocrine glands. This substance has many functions, particularly ones associated with the nervous system. Lecithin supplement is sourced from the soya bean and is recommended for memory problems, neurological disorders, drug and alcohol rehabilitation and high cholesterol levels (see page 234). It is often used as an emulsifier in beauty products and as a treatment for some skin problems.

linseed oil: oil from the seeds of the linseed plant. Used to soften the skin and mucous membranes, as a mild laxative, to soothe dry coughs and the chest pain of BRONCHITIS, and to draw boils.

liquid chlorophyll: this is concentrated chlorophyll in liquid form. It is sourced from plants (usually alfalfa) and is used as a general nutritional supplement. It "imitates" human blood, containing all the essential minerals.

lysine: an essential amino acid, produced in the body and necessary for the growth and repair of tissues. Recommended for treatment of HERPES and to help fight any infection.

magnesium phosphate: this celloid is found in bones, teeth, muscle cells, nerve cells and the brain. Recommended in the treatment of twitching and CRAMPS (including menstrual), toothache, hiccups, colic and palpitations.

phenylalanine: an amino acid which is involved in brain function. It extends the lifespan of naturally occurring painkillers known as endorphins. It is used in supplement form as a natural painkiller. It cannot be synthesised by the body but is found in cheese, nuts, bananas, avocados, sesame seeds and other foods.

potassium acetate: a potassium supplement that is taken in powder or crystal form.

potassium chloride: a celloid that is useful for relieving congestion. Recommended for sore throat, TONSILLITIS, ear infection, swollen glands and the congestion of COLDS and SINUSITIS.

potassium phosphate: this celloid raises energy and is used for DEPRESSION and lack of motivation.

potassium sulphate: this oxygenating celloid is used for dry, flaky skin, inflammation, fungal infections, DANDRUFF, and respiratory and circulatory problems.

propolis: a resin substance from trees that has anti-viral properties.

psyllium: seeds that are used as a laxative and to treat wounds and skin infections.

silica: also known as silic oxide, this celloid aids cleansing and elimination. Recommended for FLUID RETENTION, abscesses, boils, brittle bones, poor hair and nail condition, excess perspiration, skin problems and CONSTIPATION.

sodium phosphate: this celloid maintains the alkalinity of the blood and is recommended in conditions where there is over-acidity, such as ARTHRITIS and DIGESTIVE PROBLEMS. Also used for worms, NAUSEA and CONSTIPATION.

tyrosine: an amino acid involved in neurological activity. Used as a natural alternative to anti-depressants, it can also be of benefit in the treatment of ALLERGIES, high blood pressure (see page 234), INSOMNIA and memory problems.

GLOSSARY

acute: an acute health condition is one that appears to begin suddenly, and the symptoms are severe. The problem is usually short-term unless it becomes chronic.

allergen: any substance that might cause an allergic reaction.

analgesic: a remedy that relieves pain (but does not treat its cause). The term is most commonly applied to a group of drugs that can range in strength from aspirin to morphine, for example. Other substances can have analgesic properties, e.g. the herbs chamomile, clove, juniper and sage.

anti-inflammatory: substances that reduce inflammation in body tissues. Anti-inflammatory medication is available. Other remedies, e.g. peppermint essential oil can also have an anti-inflammatory effect. See also NSAIDS and steroids (page 163).

antibacterial: stopping the growth of, or destroying, some bacteria. This can apply to drugs or to natural substances such as lavender essential oil.

antifungal: stopping the growth of, or destroying, some fungus. This can apply to drugs or to natural substances such as tea tree essential oil.

antigen: a substance that causes the immune system to produce antibodies when it enters the body.

antioxidants: any substance which prevents or inhibits oxidation by neutralising free radicals.

Examples include vitamins A, C, and E, beta-carotene, selenium, copper, zinc and herbs such as garlic, ginger, echinacea and rosemary.

antiseptic: a substance that stops the growth of, or destroys, bacteria and some other micro-organisms. It is used to disinfect skin and other surfaces. There are natural antiseptic products including pine and eucalyptus essential oils.

antispasmodic: a substance that prevents or eases spasms in muscles such as the gut.

antiviral: stopping the growth of, or destroying, some viruses.

astringent: a substance that contracts the tissues or canals of the body, e.g. witch hazel has an astringent action on the skin.

bronchodilator: a drug that causes the bronchial muscle to relax and the air passages of the bronchi to expand. See ASTHMA.

carminative: a substance that relieves flatulence by causing gas to be expelled from the body.

chronic: a chronic health condition is one that continues over a long period of time (in contrast to an acute conditon). The term does not refer to the severity of the problem.

contraindicated: when it is advised NOT to use a particular remedy to treat a symptom or condition

diuretic: a substance that increases the amount of urine produced by the kidneys.

douche: a jet or shower of water is applied to a body part. Vaginal douches are quite common and suitable containers are available commercially; they should not be used during pregnancy and may not be advised during menstruation or when infection is present.

expectorant: a substance that helps remove mucus and phlegm from the lungs and throat through coughing. Anti-expectorants work to supress coughing.

nervine: soothing to the nerves

oral: associated with the mouth. If a substance is taken orally, it is swallowed.

oxidation: a very important energy-giving process in the body. Too much oxidation, however, can lead to the degeneration of cells. Oxidation is caused by the production of "free radicals" — extremely unstable molecules which steal electrons from healthy cells in order to balance themselves. Free radicals can be encouraged by chemicals, X-rays, preservatives, alcohol, fever, fasting and even excessive exercise.

pathological condition: this is a health problem that is caused by a disease. Examples would include tuberculosis, typhoid and malaria. Medical advice should be sought for pathological conditions, although other therapies can assist recovery.

photosensitivity: sensitive to light. The use of some substances can trigger reactions when the skin is exposed to sunlight.

prostaglandins: a variety of hormone-like substances produced by the body. They act as regulators and have a powerful effect on the muscles in the reproductive, digestive and urinary systems. Synthetic prostaglandins and antiprostaglandins have been developed.

salicylates: a group of plant chemicals found naturally in some food, including many herbs, spices and condiments, snack foods, jams, honey, yeast extract, coffee, tea, wine, beer and a large variety of fruit and vegetables such as tomato, mushroom, spinach, cauliflower, broccoli, oranges, pineapple, avocado, grapes and plums. Some people are sensitive to salicylates — consult a doctor or naturopath for details.

topical: applied to a particular part of the body. A substance may be applied topically as an ointment to a rash rather than taken orally (i.e. swallowed).

ultrasound: a tool for diagnosis and investigation. High frequency sound waves are used to provide a "picture" of deep body tissues. They are quite different to — and much safer than — X-rays.

X-rays: a tool for diagnosis and investigation that gets through deep tissue to provide a clear "picture" of bones. X-rays are a form of radiation and thus must be used with caution.

INDEX

CONSULTANTS AND CONTRIBUTORS

TONI EATTS has over 20 years experience as a journalist in newspapers, magazines, television, and radio. Her work has covered many areas of health and personal growth, including investigative articles, feature stories and books. She produced a top-rating radio program on holistic health and personal growth for five years, has worked as deputy editor of *New Woman* magazine, and is currently editor of *Better Homes and Gardens.*
Originating Author

DR GISELLE COOKE has worked as an holistic general practitioner for 16 years and, for nine years, has been the director of a large holistic health centre, incorporating all the treatment modalities in this book. She lectured naturopathic students on medical diagnosis for seven years and has spoken on natural therapies to medical practitioners and the general public at conferences and seminars in Australia, New Zealand and Asia. She is also well-known for her work in the media.
Medical and General Consultant

KAREN BAILEY is a homoeopath, remedial massage therapist and reflexologist with over 7 years experience. She is author of *The Gentle Art of Yoga* (Lansdowne).
General Consultant

PETER BERRYMAN has practised as a homoeopath and taught in the area for over 12 years. He currently lectures at Sydney's Naturecare College and Australasian College, where he is also supervisor of the student homoeopathic clinic.
Homoeopathy Consultant

KERRIN BOOTH is a naturopath with over six years experience. She currently practises in the Sydney area and specialises in women's health, preconceptual care and health care during pregnancy.
Herbalism and Naturopathy Consultant

JEREMY CHANCE is a practitioner of the Alexander Technique with over 17 years experience. He is editor and publisher of *Direction: A Journal on the Alexander Technique.*
Alexander Technique Consultant

ROSALBA COURTNEY-BELFORD is an osteopath and Buteyko practitioner with over 20 years of experience who also lectured at Naturecare College, Sydney, and the NSW School of Osteopathy and Naturopathy.
Buteyko Method Consultant

JOHN F. DE VOY is qualified both as a chiropractor and osteopath. With 15 years clinical experience, he lectures widely on spinal and preventitive health care to many corporate bodies, sporting bodies and schools.
Chiropractic Consultant

JULIE M. FENDALL has spent over 15 years in private practice as an osteopath and held teaching positions in Australia, New Zealand and the United Kingdom.
Osteopathy Consultant

DOROTHY GOLDBERT has over seven years experience as a naturopath and herbalist.
Herbalism Consultant

EVE GRZYBOWSKI, author of *Teach Yourself Yoga*, has been a yoga practitioner since 1971. She teaches yoga students and trains yoga

teachers at the Sydney Yoga Centre, which she founded in 1985.
Yoga Consultant

AURORA HAMMOND has 22 years of professional experience and a Bachelor of Social Studies and an Masters in Psychology. She is director and principal lecturer of the College of Holistic Counselling, Sydney and the author of *Good Grief: The Healing Heart.*
Counselling Consultant

CONNIE HOWELL has a Diploma of Aromatherapy and a Certificate of Bach Flowers among her qualifications in holistic healing.
Aromatherapy and Bach Flower Remedies Consultant

ALLAN HUDSON has been involved with Naturecare College, Sydney, since its inception over 25 years ago, specialising in massage. He is the clinic manager and also supervisor of the student clinic and heads the faculty of tactile therapies.
Massage Consultant

MARGARET KAYE has been an Awareness through Movement teacher since 1989 and Feldenkrais practitioner since 1991.
Feldenkrais Method Consultant

MARGARET MAYO is a physiotherapist with over 30 years experience. She has been a practitioner of the Feldenkrais Method for more than seven years.
Feldenkrais Method Consultant

GRAEME MURRAY has been a qualified practitioner in remedial massage and reflexology for over nine years. He teaches at the Australasian College of Natural Therapies and is education co-ordinator for the Reflexology Association (NSW.).
Reflexology Consultant

FRANCESCA NAISH is an author of health books and an accredited herbalist, naturopath and hypnotherapist who has been in practice for over 21 years.
Consultant for Natural Approaches to Clear Sight

ROSS T. NEWBERY is the founder and principal of the Sydney Shiatsu College and Clinic and author of the *Somatic Shiatsu Therapists Manual.* He has over 16 years experience in shiatsu and oriental therapies.
Shiatsu Consultant

ASSOC. PROFESSOR CAROLE ROGERS is head of the College of Traditional Chinese Medicine at the University of Technology, Sydney and has professional qualifications from Hong Kong, Australia and the United States. She has over 20 years of teaching experience and is the author of two text books on acupuncture and traditional Chinese medicine.
Acupuncture and Traditional Chinese Medicine Consultant

PETER TOWNSEND has studied Chinese herbs since the late 1970s, both in Australia and Japan. He is in private practice in Sydney.
Chinese Herbs Consultant

ST JOHN'S AMBULANCE AUSTRALIA (NSW)
First Aid Consultant

CONTRIBUTING WRITERS, RESEARCHERS AND EDITORS

CYNTHIA BLANCHE
KATIE DAVIS
MARGARET GORE
KIRSTEN TILGALS

PROJECT CO-ORDINATOR/EDITOR: Kirsten Tilgals
DESIGNER: Liz Seymour

ACKNOWLEDGMENTS AND PICTURE CREDITS
Illustrations: Janet Jones, Sue Ninham
Photography: Andre Martin
Photographic libraries: Austral Photo Library (p 56); Image Bank (p 186—D Klump);
International Photographic Library (pp 49, 77);
The Photo Library (pp 8, 33, 57, 94, 108, 121, 158, 159, 160, 161, 162, 163, 171)

Special thanks to Katie Davis for her research and writing contributions,
and to herbalist Robyn Kirby for so generously sharing her expertise.

Thanks also to models Niki Barnes, Jenny Coren, Angelika Hilden, Benito Martin, Pablo Martin, Amalia Matheson, Lucille Nixon Pearson, Gillian Souter, Nicholas Szentkuti, Michael Tilgals, and to Belinda Cudmore, Mary-Anne Danaher, Glenda Downing and Megan Smith, for design, photographic and editorial assistance.

Published by Lansdowne Publishing Pty Ltd
Level 1, 18 Argyle Street, Sydney NSW 2000, Australia

First published 1998

Created and produced by Lansdowne Publishing Pty Ltd

Set in 10/12pt Life Roman, 8/12pt Gill Sans, 11/13pt Bembo,
9/10pt Futura Condensed, on Quark Xpress
Printed in Singapore by Tien Wah Press (Pte) Ltd

Cataloguing-in-Publication data
is available at the National Library of Australia

ISBN 1 86302 412 3

This book is intended to give general information only and is not a substitute for professional and medical advice. Consult your health provider before adopting any of the treatments contained in this book.
All liability to any person arising directly or indirectly from the use of, or for any errors or omissions in, the information in this book is expressly disclaimed.
The adoption and application of the information in this book is at the reader's discretion and is his or her sole responsibility.